CW00857852

BSAVA
Small Animal
Clinical Pathology
(formerly Manual of Laboratory Techniques)

General Editor

Malcolm G. Davidson
BVM&S CertVOphthal MRCVS
19 Hillhouse Road, Edinburgh
Midlothian EH4 3QP, UK

Scientific Editors

Roderick W. Else
BVSc PhD MRCVS MRCPath
Department of Veterinary Pathology
Royal (Dick) School of Veterinary Studies
Veterinary Field Station, Easter Bush
Midlothian EH25 9RG, UK

and

John H. Lumsden
DVM MSc DipAVCP
Department of Pathology
Ontario Veterinary College
University of Guelph
Guelph, Ontario, CANADA N1G 2W1

Published by:

British Small Animal Veterinary Association
Kingsley House, Church Lane
Shurdington, Cheltenham
GL51 5TQ, United Kingdom

A Company Limited by Guarantee in England.
Registered Company No. 2837793.
Registered as a Charity.

A catalogue record for this book is available from the British Library

ISBN 0 905214 41 2

The publishers and contributors cannot take responsibility for
information provided on dosages and methods of application of drugs
mentioned in this publication. Details of this kind must be verified by
individual users from the appropriate literature.

Typeset by: Fusion Design, Fordingbridge, Hampshire, UK

Printed by: Lookers, Upton, Poole, Dorset, UK

Other Manuals

Other titles in the BSAVA Manuals series:

Manual of Anaesthesia for Small Animal Practice
Manual of Canine and Feline Gastroenterology
Manual of Canine and Feline Nephrology and Urology
Manual of Companion Animal Nutrition and Feeding
Manual of Canine Behaviour
Manual of Exotic Pets
Manual of Feline Behaviour
Manual of Ornamental Fish
Manual of Psittacine Birds
Manual of Raptors, Pigeons and Waterfowl
Manual of Reptiles
Manual of Small Animal Arthrology
Manual of Small Animal Cardiorespiratory Medicine and Surgery
Manual of Small Animal Dentistry, 2nd edition
Manual of Small Animal Dermatology
Manual of Small Animal Diagnostic Imaging
Manual of Small Animal Endocrinology, 2nd edition
Manual of Small Animal Neurology, 2nd edition
Manual of Small Animal Fracture Repair and Management
Manual of Small Animal Oncology
Manual of Small Animal Ophthalmology
Manual of Small Animal Reproduction and Neonatology

Contents

Contributors

Christopher J. Belford DipWildlMgt DVSc FACVS MRCVS
Cytopath, PO Box 24, Ledbury, Herts, HR8 2BR, UK

Nicholas Carmichael BScVetSci BVM&S MRCVS
Grange Laboratories, Grange House, Sandbeck Way, Wetherby, West Yorkshire LS22 4DN, UK

Christopher J. Clarke BVetMed MSc PhD MRCPath MRCVS
Department of Veterinary Pathology, Royal (Dick) School of Veterinary Studies, University of Edinburgh,
Veterinary Field Station, Easter Bush, Near Roslin, Midlothian EH25 9RG, UK

Malcolm A. Cobb MA VetMB DVC PhD MRCVS
Leo Animal Health, Longwick Road, Princes Risborough, Bucks HP27 9RR, UK

Mike Davies BVetMed CertVR CertSAO FRCVS
Provet, Kingfishers, Kings Court Road, Gillingham, Dorset SP8 4LD, UK

Michael J. Day BSc BVMS PhD MASM FRCVS
University of Bristol Department of Veterinary Medicine, Langford House, Langford, Bristol BS18 7DU, UK

Joan Duncan BVMS MRCVS
Grange Laboratories, Grange House, Sandbeck Way, Wetherby, West Yorkshire LS22 4DN, UK

John K. Dunn MA BVM&S MVetSc MRCVS
Department of Clinical Veterinary Medicine, University of Cambridge, Madingley Road,
Cambridge CB3 0ES, UK

Rod W. Else BVSc PhD MRCVS MRCPath
Department of Veterinary Pathology, Royal (Dick) School of Veterinary Studies, University of Edinburgh,
Veterinary Field Station, Easter Bush, Near Roslin, Midlothian EH25 9RG, UK

Robert A. Foster BVSc PhD MACVSc DipACVP
Ontario Veterinary College, University of Guelph, Guelph, Ontario N1G 2W1, Canada

Edward J. Hall MA VetMB PhD MRCVS
University of Bristol Department of Veterinary Medicine, Langford House, Langford, Bristol BS18 7DU, UK

Michael E. Herrtage MA BVSc DVR DVD DSAM MRCVS
Department of Clinical Veterinary Medicine, University of Cambridge, Madingley Road,
Cambridge CB3 0ES, UK

John H. Lumsden DVM MSc DipAVCP
Department of Pathology, Ontario Veterinary College, University of Guelph, Guelph,
Ontario N1G 2W1, Canada

Kenneth Mason BVSc MSc FACVS MRCVS
Albert Animal Hospital, 3331 Pacific Highway, Springwood, Queensland 4127, Australia

Irene A. P. McCandlish BVMS PhD MRCVS
Grange Laboratories, Grange House, Sandbeck Way, Wetherby, West Yorkshire LS22 4DN, UK

Carmel T. Mooney MVB MPhil PhD MRCVS
Department of Small Animal Clinical Sciences, University College Dublin, Ballsbridge,
Dublin 4, Republic of Ireland

James W. Simpson SDA BVM&S MPhil MRCVS
Department of Clinical Studies, Royal (Dick) School of Veterinary Studies, University of Edinburgh,
Summerhall, Edinburgh EH9 1QH, UK

David J. Taylor MA VetMB PhD
Department of Veterinary Pathology, University of Glasgow Veterinary School, Bearsden Road, Bearsden,
Glasgow G61 1QH

Elizabeth Villiers BVSc CertVR CertSAM MRCVS
Chesterford Cytology Service, Hills Cottage, Carmen Street, Great Chesterford, Saffron Waldon,
Essex CB10 1NR, UK

Brian Wilcock DVM PhD
Ontario Veterinary College, University of Guelph, Guelph, Ontario N1G 2W1, Canada

Julie A. Yager BVSc PhD
Ontario Veterinary College, University of Guelph, Guelph, Ontario N1G 2W1, Canada

Foreword

The standard of care demanded of the veterinary surgeon in practice today, by clients who have a much greater understanding of what can be achieved for their companion animals, has led to an ever increasing reliance on clinical pathology. The *Manual of Small Animal Clinical Pathology* replaces A Manual of Laboratory Techniques and reflects the considerable advances in the field which have occurred in the last nine years.

The first section gives clear and precise guidance on sample collection and handling which will allow accurate results to be obtained to support one's clinical examination. The various fields which comprise the science of Clinical Pathology are reviewed and the logical interpretation of the results obtained is considered. The Health and Safety considerations of laboratory practice are also highlighted.

The second section goes on to consider in detail how laboratory investigation can aid in the diagnosis of clinical problems of different organ systems. The Manual's approach should allow the clinician to use his or her skill to select the assays required, to interpret the results obtained and apply them to each individual case. The full-colour format and the use of plentiful charts and tables, highlighting key points from the text, guide the user rapidly to the relevant information.

The Editors have brought together expert authors from the UK and abroad to produce a comprehensive guide to the subject in its present state of development and to consider which techniques might gain importance in the near future. The logical and user-friendly approach adopted in this Manual is the hallmark of the BSAVA Manual Series and I am sure that the busy practising veterinary surgeon, as well as veterinary students, veterinary nurses and laboratory staff, will find this book an invaluable addition to their reference materials.

H. Simon Orr BVSc DVR MRCVS
BSAVA Senior Vice-President 1997-98

Preface

Modern small animal practice makes heavy demands on the diagnostic skills of the veterinary surgeon but whilst there is an increase in the availability of sophisticated procedures such as flexible endoscopy and ultrasonic and other imaging devices, haematological, microbiological, biochemical, parasitological and tissue pathology examinations remain the cornerstones of the discipline of clinical pathology.

In North America the concept of total body diagnostic 'work up' procedures is well established although in Europe veterinarians have been more selective in the use of assays. Recently, however, escalating demand, the advent of cost-effective test kits and analytical equipment and the ability to perform a wide range of screening tests has resulted in a major increase in interest in clinical pathology.

This manual presents the veterinary surgeon in practice with a review of clinical pathology procedures and assays that are currently available, together with information on techniques that may be available in the near future. It is not intended to be a 'recipe book' of every diagnostic test but rather to indicate the logical basis for selecting appropriate assays. The manual is divided into two parts, the first giving a general outline of collection and interpretation of laboratory test samples and biochemical, haematological and microbiological procedures. The second part is divided into fifteen chapters, each dedicated to a separate body system. It is hoped that this approach, as opposed to a 'problem–oriented' approach, will find favour with the users of this manual.

We have invited contributors from authors in North America and the UK. Inevitably with a multi-author book there are differences in style and emphasis between chapters as well as some overlap between the chapters. It is hoped this will be seen as a strength rather than a weakness as it allows each author's individual approach to be appreciated and prevents this manual from being simply a long list of facts and figures.

We are indebted to our contributing authors for all their hard work and it is our hope that readers of this manual will find it useful and stimulating. In a rapidly expanding subject like clinical pathology it is inevitable that there will be omissions and possibly contentious contributions in this manual. We trust that colleagues will inform us of any changes that they consider relevant for any future edition.

Malcolm G. Davidson
Rod W. Else
John H. Lumsden

February 1998

PART ONE

Principles and Techniques in Clinical Pathology

CHAPTER ONE

Collection and Handling of Samples for Diagnosis

Roderick W. Else and Brian G. Kelly

INTRODUCTION

There can be very few veterinary surgeons today in general or specialist veterinary practice who do not use diagnostic assays or tests, performed as laboratory or 'side room' examinations, as an aid to making accurate clinical diagnoses and assisting in assessing prognosis. Clinical pathology assays are particularly powerful adjuncts to clinical diagnosis in the canine and feline patient. It is important to remember, however, that laboratory tests are *additional* aids to diagnosis and should never supplant the important fundamental skills of clinical examination and diagnosis, supported by clinical history and clinical signs.

The application of laboratory assays in canine and feline diagnostic work provides interesting comparisons with the larger companion species the horse and with the farm species. Unlike farm animals, dogs and cats are usually presented as individual patients rather than groups of animals. They, therefore, cannot act as their own controls or provide a local baseline for parameters that may be measured in, say, blood or urine. This difference generated some angst in previous decades in consideration of the reliability of values of measurements and generated considerable activity of validation of results and debate regarding 'normal' values and ranges of normality against which any one individual patient could be assessed. Much of this controversy has been resolved by the adoption of the concept of reference values or ranges for a species as measured by a particular laboratory.

This point is discussed more fully in Chapter 2 but veterinary surgeons who regularly employ laboratory assays as part of their diagnostic armoury are aware of the importance of interpreting an individual animal's laboratory results in the knowledge of the reference values and ranges used by the laboratory that carried out the assay(s) rather than comparing them with figures from a textbook or another laboratory's set of figures.

An important additional point here is the establishment of a good working relationship between the clinician and the laboratory staff. Dialogue and communication between the two builds confidence. Most successes come from a situation where the clinician has 'shopped around', found a suitable laboratory and uses that facility (or several facilities depending on what the laboratory can offer) on a regular basis rather than using a series of different laboratories at random.

The above comments assume that the clinician is using a commercial laboratory rather than doing assays in-house. There are pros and cons for using either commercial or in-house arrangements and these considerations will be discussed at the end of this chapter, together with a consideration of the health and safety aspects of laboratory work.

This chapter gives an introductory overview of the types of samples that may be taken from dogs and cats as aids to diagnosis, discusses how to handle and present samples so as to obtain the best results, and reviews tissue biopsy procedures. Many of the assays and techniques will be covered in greater detail, together with the appropriateness of their applications, in later chapters.

SAMPLE COLLECTION

The type of sample collected from a patient is governed by whether there is a firm clinical diagnosis that requires absolute confirmation, a more tentative diagnosis or whether the case is undiagnosed and the clinician wishes to use one or more assays to assist in making the diagnosis. In the latter case, several different types of sample may be collected but many clinicians will be aware of the financial considerations inevitably involved in deciding how many laboratory tests are needed. In the UK particularly, where complete 'profiling' of a patient is not generally the normal procedure, the choice of tests requested is an important aspect of successful practice. In short, many UK animal owners are prepared to pay for relevant tests rather than a set of complete screening procedures.

The types of samples that are submitted for laboratory assessments are shown in Table 1.1. As will be seen in the following account, some samples can be used for more than one type of examination, e.g. blood or serum can be used to measure haematological parameters and also for some biochemical assays. It is important, however, that the clinician should check carefully before submitting the sample whether a single type of sample (e.g. whole venous blood with ethylene diamine tetra-acetic acid (EDTA) anticoagulant) is suitable for use in all the required assays and, furthermore, that the amount of sample submitted is adequate. Wherever a clinician is uncertain, even after consulting a laboratory manual, as to the suitability or state of a sample intended for assay purposes, he/she should consult the laboratory verbally. This, of course, is easier where the practitioner and laboratory staff have cultivated the good relationship referred to above.

The general range of examinations and methods in veterinary clinical pathology is summarized in Table 1.2. In the UK microbiological assays carried out in dogs and cats are usually bacterial or virological in emphasis, with slightly greater numbers of bacteriological screens. This is probably because the strategies of prophylactic vaccination against the common viral diseases of dogs and cats in the UK have been conspicuously successful and diseases such as canine distemper, hepatitis and feline panleucopenia are not the major problems they were three decades or so ago. Outbreaks of the common viral diseases do still occur in susceptible populations but the detection of viral infections in affected animals is now easier (using serum assays such as antibody tests) and a lot cheaper and more efficient than was previously the case.

Bacteriological assays

Examinations are often carried out on faeces, urine, skin (swabs, scrapings or solid tissue samples), genital swabs or curettage samples. Samples may be presented as swabs, fluids or solid tissues (e.g. from skin punches, fragments of superficial abscesses).

Fluid and solid samples should be collected as aseptically as possible into suitable sterile containers;

Type of sample	Origin/State of sample
Skin scrapings	Superficial or deep parasitic, fungal, or bacterial inspection
Faeces (or large bowel contents)	Natural voidance or collected
Smears on glass slides (usually air-dried)	Impressions of surface lesions Abscesses or surface secretions Fine-needle aspirates
Fluids	Urine Cavity aspirates Synovial Respiratory (nasal or respiratory tract lavages)
Blood/serum	Intravenous withdrawal Clotted or unclotted Altered blood from serous (body) cavities

Table 1.1: Types of sample submitted for assays.

Examination	Type of sample	Nature of assay or examination
Haematology	Peripheral blood with anticoagulant (EDTA, heparin, citrate)	Cell counts (manual or automated) Haemaglobin assays Platelet counts
Serology	Peripheral clotted blood → serum/plasma	Antibody assay (viral or bacterial) Plasma protein levels Immunology (ELISA, precipitation tests, immunoelectrophoresis, immunohistology)
Biochemical	Serum/plasma or whole blood Urine	Wet and dry chemistry Stick tests ELISA Radioimmunoassay
Microbiological: Bacteriological	Faeces; urine; genital; skin; mucosae; lesions (swabs, fluids, tissue)	Smear examination Culture on agar ± selective media Antibiotic sensitivity
Mycological	Skin; aural; genital; ?urine (swabs, tissue)	Smear examination Culture
Virological (and Rickettsiae)	Faeces; secretions; vesicles; CSF	Antibody assay ELISA Polymerase chain reaction (PCR)
Parasitological (external and internal)	Faeces; tracheal lavage; skin	Faecal oocyte counts Currettage smears
Tissue pathology and cytology	Biopsy; cytology; necropsy (tissue, fluids, aspirates)	Histopathology sections Cytopathology smears Cryosections Electron microscopy

Table 1.2: *The general range of examinations used in veterinary clinical pathology.*

swabs should also be sealed immediately within containers to prevent contamination (Figure 1.1). It is important not to let small samples or swabs dry out. If swabs are to be posted to a laboratory or there is a risk of the material drying, transport medium (Figure1.1) may be used. Sample containers must always be labelled and it is important to remember to keep multiple samples separate; 'pooled' samples lead to confusion and misleading results which can hinder therapy and prognosis.

Bacteriological assay (see Chapter 5) involves well established, reliable techniques of smear production and staining plus examination by microscopy, followed where appropriate by culture on blood agar

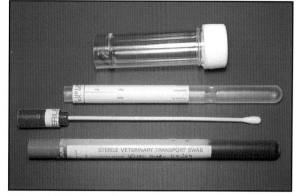

Figure 1.1: *Swabs and containers for bacteriological samples. The black material is transport medium.*

plates to identify or verify the pathogen(s). Special selective culture media can be used to identify unusual pathogens and to separate significant from non-significant bacteria (Figure 1.2).

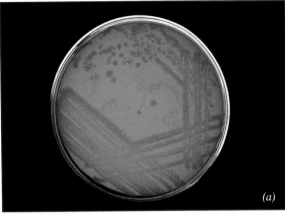
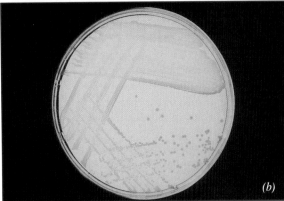

Figure 1.2: *Bacterial culture plates. (a) Routine blood agar plate with multiple colonies. (b) Plate with desoxycholate agar (DCA) selective for* Salmonella *spp.*

An important feature of bacteriological assays is the examination for antibiotic sensitivity (Figure 1.3). It is therefore important for the clinician to supply full details of any antibiotic therapy the patient may have already received. Antibiotic sensitivity testing can prove expensive if the clinician fails to supply information about antibiotics previously used to treat a case or demands that a wide spectrum of antibiotics is assessed for efficacy.

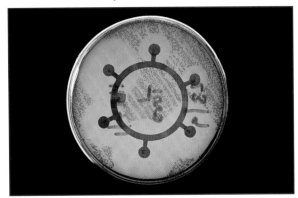

Figure 1.3: *Antibiotic sensitivity culture plate. Note the areas of non-growth around effective antibiotic discs.*

Where culture of blood samples is anticipated (e.g. in suspected bacterial endocarditis), rapid results can now be obtained using special culture apparatus (Figure 1.4) rather than serial cultures generated in nutrient broth.

Rapid identification of enterobacterial pathogens, especially *Salmonella* spp. and coliforms, can be achieved using identification kits that combine carbohydrate fermentation and biochemical reactions (Figure 1.5).

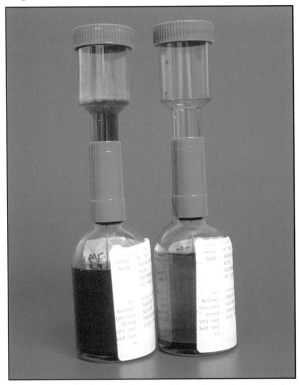

Figure 1.4: *Blood culture bottles. Where bacterial growth has occurred the fluid has been displaced into the upper chamber; an empty upper chamber indicates a negative sample.*

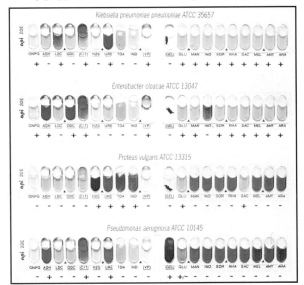

Figure 1.5: *Examples of identification of the presence of bacteria by the API 20E identification system.*
Courtesy of bio Merieux.

Mycological assays

Assays for the presence of fungal agents are often carried out on fresh skin samples (scrapings, swabs or tissue biopsy samples) and genital samples, usually from females (vaginal swabs or aspirates). In addition, urine samples may be concentrated and assayed for the presence of fungal agents or yeasts.

The usual method employs microscopic examination of smears using vital stains accompanied by culture on special media (Figure 1.6).

Fungal agents such as *Aspergillus*, *Trichophyton* and *Microsporum* are relatively easy to culture and identify by their hyphal growth or conidial features but the smaller fungi, such as *Malassezia* found on the surface of canine skin, may be difficult to identify. *Malassezia* infection (Figure 1.7) may sometimes be

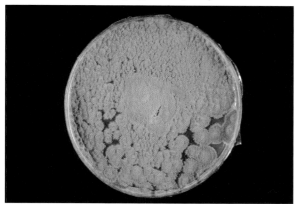

Figure 1.6: A culture of Aspergillus flavus *on Sabouraud's medium.*

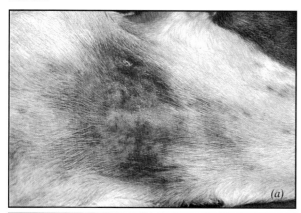

(a)

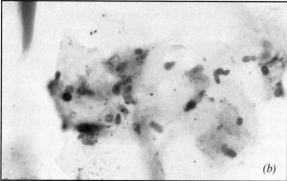

(b)

Figure 1.7: (a) Malassezia *dermatitis in a dog. (b) The* Malassezia *organism can be seen in a smear from a skin scraping.*
Courtesy of T. Nuttall.

more easily identified in skin biopsies (see below and Chapter 15) using special silver staining techniques (Grocott's method). The complex yeast-like fungal infections, such as *Cryptococcus neoformans*, do not present as problems in the UK, though they are important in areas of North America.

Virological assays

The gold standard for diagnosis of a viral infection is the isolation and identification of virus from an animal. Today, however, most evidence of viral infection is gleaned from examining secretions or tissues for evidence of the presence of either viral antigen or antibodies to a virus. The technique of isolation and growth of virus on cell culture monolayers is expensive and time-consuming and the range of viruses so great that few laboratories other than research institutes have the facilities to offer such a service.

Viruses or their antigens can be isolated from a variety of organ samples or body secretions (Table 1.3). Secretions such as nasopharyngeal aspirates or bronchoalveolar lavage samples are ideal sources of virus and are relatively easily obtained. Swabs provide a less efficient mode of sample collection from the respiratory or intestinal tract. Fluids or swabs should be placed in sterile leak-proof containers; if the specimen is likely to be in transit for some hours or is a tissue sample, the use of a sterile transport medium (Quinn *et al.*, 1994) should be considered.

Cell aspirates can be smeared on to glass microscope slides and fixed in acetone for fluorescent antibody or immunocytological antibody assay. Acetone-fixed smears should not be allowed to dry out and this clearly provides a transportation problem. Cryostat sections of viral-infected tissue provide good material for assay by fluorescent antibody or immunocytochemical techniques but the problems of handling, transport and processing of frozen tissue require immediate laboratory access not feasible in most practice situations.

A common technique employed is to use a serological or immunological assay to identify antibodies to a specific virus. The use of paired serum samples with a 4-fold rise in antibody titre over a period of 3–4 weeks usually indicates recent and active infection. This is known as the acute and convalescent samples procedure.

Many of the immunological assays now available can be used to give a rapid indication of the presence of viral antibody or antigen in a serum sample from a patient. Most laboratories are able to perform such tests as direct or indirect enzyme-linked immunosorbent assay (ELISA), fluorescent antibody or immunoperoxidase antibody assays, as well as the more traditional antibody precipitation tests such as agar gel immunodiffusion (AGIT), haemagglutination or complement fixation tests (see Chapter 6). Many laboratories are also able to carry out newer and more sensitive

Organ system	Type of sample
Generalized or multiorgan	Nasal secretion; faeces; blood (or white cells)
Gastrointestinal	Faeces
Respiratory: Upper	Nasal secretion; nasopharyngeal aspirate/lavage
Lower	Tracheal or bronchoalveolar endoscopic aspirate/ lavage
Genital Skin Ocular Central nervous system	Swab/lavage Scraping; vesicle contents (swab); biopsy Conjunctival swab Cerebrospinal fluid; nasal secretion; faeces

Table 1.3: Types of samples for virological examination.

tests, such as the polymerase chain reaction (PCR) and 'in situ' hybridization, for detecting very small quantities of viral nucleic acid. The types of assay available are shown in Figure 1.8 and their advantages and disadvantages in Table 1.4. Chapter 5 deals with these topics more specifically.

Canine and feline viral infections can now be diagnosed in practice laboratory situations using commercial kits. The majority of these tests employ ELISA methods to detect either antigen or antibody. The format was originally a solid microtitre plate (Figure 1.9) but some ELISA tests use membranes, 'sticks' or more specifically designed matrices (Figure 1.10). Other forms of kit available for detecting viral antigen or antibody are those using latex agglutination, complement fixation, haemagglutination and agar gel immunodiffusion (Figure 1.11). Immunofluorescence and immunoperoxidase tests are specific and sensitive but are currently only feasible in larger commercial laboratories rather than in veterinary practices.

Method	Advantages	Disadvantages
Virus isolation	Sensitive Further study of virus	Difficult? Slow Expense May not detect non-viable virus
Direct observation (electron microscopy)	Rapid Detects non-viable virus or virus that cannot be isolated	Expensive Insensitive (small tissue sampling)
Serological antigen identification (ELISA)	Rapid Sensitive Kits available	Difficult interpretation? Not all viruses detectable?
Nucleic acid probes (PCR)	Rapid Very sensitive	Special equipment Contamination by foreign DNA?
Light microscopy (histopathology)	Rapid Cheap	Not suitable for many viruses
Antibody seroconversion (acute/convalescent)	Group disease situations	Retrospective Slow

Table 1.4: Advantages and disadvantages of viral assays.

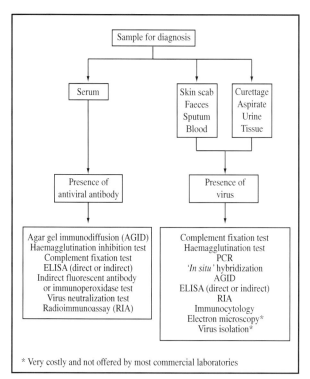

Figure 1.8: *Assays used for viral detection.*

Within the figure:

Sample for diagnosis

Serum

Skin scab
Faeces
Sputum
Blood

Curettage
Aspirate
Urine
Tissue

Presence of
antiviral antibody

Presence of
virus

Agar gel immunodiffusion (AGID)
Haemagglutination inhibition test
Complement fixation test
ELISA (direct or indirect)
Indirect fluorescent antibody
or immunoperoxidase test
Virus neutralization test
Radioimmunoassay (RIA)

Complement fixation test
Haemagglutination test
PCR
'*In situ*' hybridization
AGID
ELISA (direct or indirect)
RIA
Immunocytology
Electron microscopy*
Virus isolation*

* Very costly and not offered by most commercial laboratories

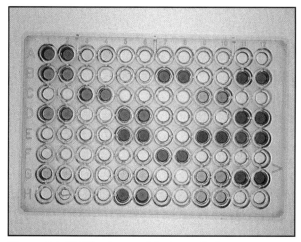

Figure 1.9: *ELISA using a solid microwell plate.*

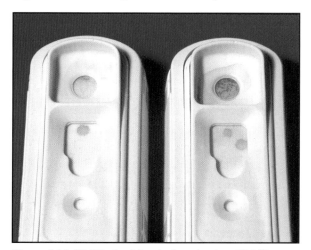

Figure 1.10: *ELISAs for feline leukaemia virus (FeLV) antigen and anti-feline immunodeficiency virus antibody. A positive test for FeLV antigen is shown on the right.*

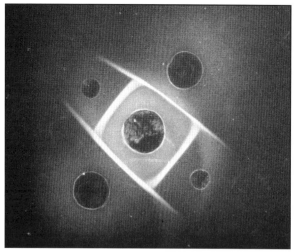

Figure 1.11: *A typical agar gel immunodiffusion test showing white lines of precipitation where an antigen–antibody reaction occurs.*

Assays for other infectious agents

Rickettsial agents such as *Chlamydia* spp. have been implicated in ocular and respiratory diseases in cats and dogs. Sampling for this type of infection can be done by taking swabs or lavages from ocular and respiratory tracts and submitting them for immuno-fluorescent or immunoperoxidase antibody assays, ELISA or PCR tests. Commercially available ELISA kits are probably the method of choice.

Haematological and serological assays

Haematological parameters and their significance in relation to specific diseases are discussed in detail in Chapter 3. Checking blood and serum parameters is an important and convenient method of assessing or confirming aspects of health in dogs and cats simply because the blood required for analysis is so readily accessible and the procedure repeatable with minimal discomfort to the patient. Manual counting and light microscope examination remain the principal means of determining red cell parameters (total count, reticulocyte count, packed cell count, red cell morphology), white cell parameters (total and differential counts, white cell morphology), and platelet counts. Commercial laboratories may have automated counting devices but reliance is still placed on manual methods. Other routinely performed assays measure haemoglobin values (mean cell haemoglobin - MCH, mean cell haemoglobin concentration - MCHC, mean cell volume - MCV), coagulation and plasma proteins (principally fibrinogen). Simple blood cell counts should be within the ability of most practitioners and veterinary nurses. The apparatus is simple but a good microscope and fresh stains for differential white cell counts are mandatory. Increasingly, busy veterinary practices are using automated haematology analysers and there are several designed for veterinary use. Many people, however, use commercial facilities because of time considerations.

Collection of blood is easily accomplished with simple apparatus (Figure 1.12). In dogs and cats small quantities (up to 10 ml) are usually collected from venous sites, such as the brachycephalic or jugular vein, using sterile hypodermic needles (20–25 gauge, 25–35 mm) and syringes. Some clinicians prefer the use of vacuum syringes and these have the advantage that the collection vessel is connected directly to the sampling needle, thereby obviating any transfer step in the collection procedure. The disadvantage of vacuum syringes is that in old or debilitated animals with poor circulation or narrow veins the suction effect is sufficient to collapse the blood vessel, thereby making collection more difficult. Only 'free-flow' blood should be collected; blood that is withdrawn with difficulty tends to be partially clotted and there is often damage to the cell morphology. Blood can be placed in traditional sterile containers. The use of 'gel bottles' (Figure 1.13) is popular now; the cellular component is separated from the plasma by the gel, rendering the plasma cleaner and easier to decant on receipt at the laboratory.

Depending on the assays required, blood is collected into containers with or without anticoagulant. Most laboratories prefer the use of ethylene diamine tetra-acetic acid (EDTA) as an anticoagulant, although

heparin is still acceptable and citrate-coated tubes are preferred for platelet counts. Where the clinician is unsure as to the type of blood sample (i.e. whole blood, plasma or serum) or which anticoagulant to use, the laboratory should be consulted prior to collecting the sample.

Bone marrow sampling falls somewhere between haematological sampling and biopsy (see Chapter 3). The technique involves using stout cannulated needles or trephines to penetrate the ischial bone of the pelvis or the femur via the trochanteric fossa in order to aspirate the bone marrow (Figure 1.14). Ideally the smeared sample should contain fatty marrow and bony spicules from cancellous bone but many samples are predominantly marrow blood samples. The technique is not as simply performed as some authorities would lead one to believe and it requires practice. Once the marrow has been acquired it should be smeared or crushed on microscope slides, rapidly air-dried and sent to the laboratory for staining (modified Romanowsky) and interpretation. Interpretation requires expertise.

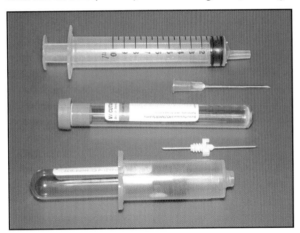

Figure 1.12: Apparatus for obtaining blood samples.

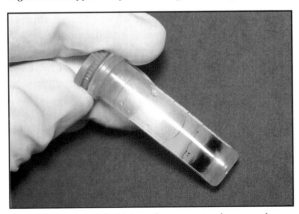

Figure 1.13: A 'gel bottle' used to separate plasma and blood cells. The pale orange top layer is the plasma and there is a dark red basal collection of blood cells, with the gel 'sandwiched' between.

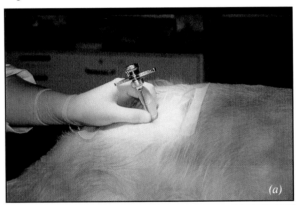

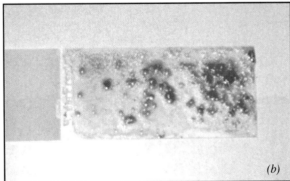

Figure 1.14: (a) Bone marrow aspiration technique in a dog. (b) Bone marrow aspirate on a microscope slide.

Biochemical assays

These analyses range from blood biochemistry, through urine analysis, to endocrinological and electrolyte assays. Many of the assays performed routinely nowadays are carried out on serum, plasma or urine; these assays are dealt with more fully in the respective chapters in this manual.

Many serum analyses are carried out as ELISA tests. In the case of endocrinological assays, radioimmunoassay (RIA) of plasma is important. The technique of RIA requires special conditions because of the isotopes involved and is only carried out in properly appointed laboratories.

The advent of 'wet and dry' chemistry kits and 'stick' tests has meant that many practitioners can perform several biochemical assays for a patient at economic rates with a high degree of accuracy. Dry reagent strips and dry chemistry analyser instruments are proving useful in some larger veterinary practices. Where there is doubt about a test kit result or the practitioner requires confirmation, samples can be referred to a commercial laboratory for more rigorous examination.

Parasitological assays

Tests for external parasites are reviewed in Chapter 15, together with methods of identification. Internal parasites such as helminths, coccidia and *Giardia* are usually identified by oocyst or egg counts in faeces (see Chapter 8), and lungworm detection is discussed in Chapter 10 of this Manual.

TISSUE AND CYTOLOGICAL EXAMINATIONS

Tissues for examination fall into two main categories:

- **Necropsy samples** - taken from postmortem examinations, usually to confirm an abnormality or to establish the nature and significance of an abnormal-looking tissue or organ
- **Biopsy samples** - taken from live patients to establish the nature of abnormal tissue that can be seen macroscopically, detected clinically or by using imaging techniques (radiography, tomography or ultrasonography). Tissue examination may also help in establishing the nature of a disease, i.e. differentiating neoplasia from inflammation or degenerative changes.

Although both types of sample may be subject to a degree of macroscopic assessment, the main objective is to determine any microscopic architectural changes by histological examination. This usually involves preparation and fixation of tissue prior to submission for preparation as paraffin wax-embedded tissue blocks which are cut and stained for histological examination. The latter procedures are specialist laboratory techniques, the description of which is outwith the scope of the present article. The handling and fixation of tissue are, however, important initial stages in which the sampling clinician plays a critical role and can make all the difference between success, mediocrity or even failure in results and diagnosis. The techniques of sampling and preparing necropsy and biopsy tissues for routine histopathological examinations are essen-

tially similar and are described below.

In contrast, cytological sampling and examination involves the acquisition and preparation of individual or small groups of cells. These cells are obtained *in vivo* from patients by a variety of routes (Table 1.5). These include: natural shedding or exfoliation (e.g. desquamation from skin or mucosae such as buccal, vaginal, anal); natural voidance in urine, sputum or other secretions (e.g. ocular, nasal, aural); or aspiration using needles of various bore, cannulae or catheters (e.g. from body cavities, solid organs).

The cell samples are aspirated immediately after collection on to glass microscope slides, smeared and rapidly air-dried or fixed in 95% alcohol, prior to staining and microscopic examination. Where the samples are predominantly fluid they are usually centrifuged gently to concentrate the cells or prepared by use of a cytocentrifuge. These techniques and the types of samples that may be examined are discussed at length in Chapter 7.

Types of biopsy

There are several types of biopsy, summarized in Table 1.6. The following is a general account of biopsy sampling; for specific organ sampling techniques the reader should consult individual chapters.

Excisional and incisional biopsies

The advantage of the excisional biopsy is that the whole lesion can be removed in one operation if correctly performed. In contrast, incisional biopsy deliberately removes only a piece (representative hopefully) of the lesion. This is usually sufficient tissue for diagnostic purposes or for 'planning' purposes, i.e. the whole lesion may be near a vital tissue or organ and removal may threaten that organ's integrity, or the lesion is infiltrating, or its nature (neoplastic, malignant or benign) requires to be established before proceeding further.

Full excision may not be possible because of site, size of lesion, other complicating disease (cardiac or metabolic), or where the patient is aged or debilitated and constitutes an anaesthetic risk since most excisional biopsies are performed under general anaesthetic.

No special instruments are required for excisional or incisional biopsies; standard surgical instruments are sufficient, i.e. scalpel, rat-toothed forceps, scissors, artery forceps and suture instruments.

Care should be exercised when contemplating excision biopsy if there is any doubt about the patient's blood clotting efficiency, particularly if a large lesion is likely to be removed. This also applies to incisional sampling. Clotting time or platelet count should be assessed accordingly.

Where an incision biopsy is taken for histopathological assessment prior to planning more radical surgery, it is recommended that the incised tissue includes a margin with normal tissue if possible. This assists the

Organ or site	Types of biopsy	Comment
Skin	Excision Incision	Site and size considerations Solitary, multiple or generalized lesions Needles not helpful usually Keyes punch
Peripheral lymph nodes	Exfoliation (impressions) Incision (needle) Excision (± impression)	Useful where ulcerated or neoplastic Needles useful
Reproductive system: 　　Male:　Testes 　　　　　Prostate 　　Female: Vagina 　　　　　Mammae	 Excision Incision (fine needle) Exfoliation Incision (needle) Exfoliation Excision/incision Excision; incision Excision Incision Exfoliation (secretions)	 Customary to perform bilateral orchidectomy Difficult to interpret fine needle Prostatic massage per rectum Needle techniques difficult; avoid per rectum Site and size considerations Include lymph node where appropriate Problems of healing Needles useful if patient aged or debilitated Helpful in mastitis or neoplasia
Urinary system: 　　Kidney 　　Bladder 　　Liver	 Incision Excision Exfoliation Incision Incision	 Usually Vim–Silverman-type needle — can haemorrhage If whole organ obviously abnormal Centrifuge or sediment whole sample — rapid deterioration Size and site considerations Wedge resection requires laparotomy Wide-bore needle useful (Menghini) Difficult to interpret fine needle

Table 1.5: Organ systems and their appropriate biopsy procedures. (Continued.)

pathologist in making a diagnosis and assessing the degree of circumscription of the lesion; this is particularly important in assessing neoplasms.

Punch and needle biopsies
Biopsy punches are not commonly used in veterinary practice, with the exception of the Keyes punch which is extensively used for obtaining circular cores of epidermis and dermis of 5 mm diameter or less. These punch instruments are suitable for multiple sampling of canine and feline skin or where the lesion is small, focal, and can be encompassed by the biopsy punch. By choice most veterinary pathologists prefer larger elliptical biopsies of skin which usually ensure adequate margins of excision around the lesion. The disadvantage of these ellipses, however, is that they require more sutures compared with using punches. Elliptical biopsies can be performed under sedation

Organ or site	Types of biopsy	Comment
Alimentary tract:		
Oral cavity	Exfoliation (impressions) Excision; incision	Useful if surface abrasion Site and size considerations
Upper tract: Oesophagus	Exfoliation Excision	Endoscopy and fibre optics with brush sampling or snaring lesions
Stomach	Excision; incision	Size considerations — endoscopy with snaring or forcep removal if small Usually requires laparotomy

Mid-tract:
      Small
      intestine
	Excision
	Rarely incision
		Cannot use endoscopy — requires
		laparotomy or biopsy capsule
		May reach into distal ileum?

Lower tract:
      Colon,
      Rectum
	Excision
	Rarely incision
		Size considerations - endoscopy
		with snaring or forceps removal
		if small

Anus	Excision; incision Exfoliation (impressions)	Site and size considerations Useful if accessible or with curettage of lesion
Respiratory tract:		
Nasal passages	Exfoliation Excision; incision	Nasal secretions or isotonic irrigation Size and degree of invasion
Airways	Exfoliation Excision; incision	Sputum or irrigation via bronchoscope Snaring or forceps sampling via bronchoscope
Lungs	Excision Incision	Lobectomy via thoracotomy Needles (wide-bore or fine) via open or percutaneous technique Resection via thoracotomy

Table 1.5 (continued).

and local anaesthetic, as is normally the procedure with punch sampling, and local anaesthetic agents do not, in the experience of the author, affect the histological quality of the biopsy.

Needles for biopsy purposes fall into two broad categories: wide bore and fine bore (Table 1.7), and range in length from 12 mm to 15 cm.

Fine needles are standard hypodermic needles and are used with 10–20 ml syringes to aspirate fluids, exudates or cell aspirates from cavities, organs or lesions (see Table 1.5 and Chapter 7). The great advantages (Figure 1.15) of the use of these needles are speed of sampling and cost-effectiveness (time and equipment), and ease of preparation by air-dried smearing (Figure 1.16). Assessment of fine-needle aspirates other than deciding if the sample is 'inflammatory or otherwise' is, however, a task for the trained pathologist (see Chapter 7).

Type of biopsy	Brief description and characteristics
Excisional	Complete removal surgically Often requires general anaesthesia Site and size considerations are important
Incisional	Removal of a portion of representative sample of lesion only Healing problems if neoplastic? Allows planning of further therapeutic approaches
Punch	Removal of a core of tissue Usually confined to skin
Needle	Removal of small cylindrical core of tissue or only cells Accuracy important; imaging-assisted helpful Minimally invasive
Endoscopic	Removal of small mucosal samples by avulsion, snaring or forceps excision from alimentary, respiratory systems and body orifices Small tissuc samples Minimally invasive Sedation or general anaesthesia depending on site sampled
Exfoliative	Collection of desquamated (natural or curretted) cells from external or internal surfaces Usually a cytological assessment Simple and easy, depending on site Minimally invasive, depending on site

Table 1.6: *Types of biopsy.*

Designation	Name	Gauge	Sample
Wide bore	Modified Vim–Silverman	14	Tissue core (kidney)
	'Tru-cut'	14	Tissue core (all tissues and organs)
	Osgood	15/16	Bone marrow (marrow plug + marrow blood)
	Jamshidi	15	Bone trephine (bone + marrow)
	Menghini	15	Tissue core (liver)
Fine bore	Hypodermic	21–25	Cells (aspiration of any organ)

Table 1.7: *Types of biopsy needle.*

Advantages	Disadvantages
Minimally invasive but depends on site	Size of sample small; may be fragmented
Rapid — fine-needle cytology within 1 hour	May not be representative of whole lesion
Repeatable — dependent on size, site and nature of lesion	May miss focal lesion unless imaging-assisted
Anaesthesia — sedation with local anaesthetic rather than general	May get 'false negatives'
Good for debilitated or geriatric patients	Interpretation requires expertise (especially fine needle)
Cost-effective because no expensive sampling equipment	Post-biopsy haemorrhage? 'Seeding' of cells from malignant neoplasms (rare)

Figure 1.15: *Advantages and disadvantages of needle techniques.*

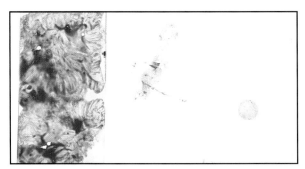

Figure 1.16: Aspirate smears. The purple-stained smear (left) is too dense to read easily; the central pale blue preparation (stained with Alcian blue) is about right; the sample on the right was fluid enough to be prepared by cytocentrifuge. Note the confined area rendering it easier to examine microscopically.

Wide-bore needles are specialized for different purposes and are designed to remove a small core of tissue for histopathological or other examination.

The Franklin-modified Vim–Silverman needle (Figure 1.17a) was designed for renal biopsy work, whilst the Menghini needle (Fig. 1.17b) has a specially modified convex cutting tip, designed to remove a core of liver tissue with minimal haemorrhage. The Osgood and Rosenthal needles are short (2.5 cm), 14–16 gauge bore with stylets, designed for bone marrow sampling from the pelvis. The Jamshidi trephine (14 gauge, 10 cm long) has become popular for sampling bone marrow (Figure 1.18).

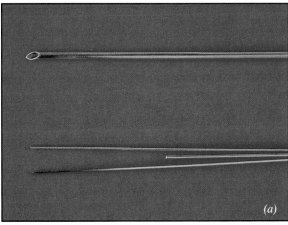

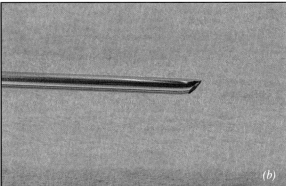

Figure 1.17: Biopsy needles. (a) Franklin-modified Vim–Silverman needle for renal biopsy. (b) The Menghini needle has a special tip to minimize hepatocellular damage.

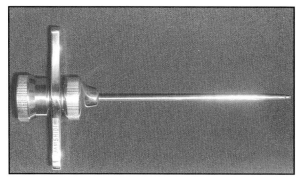

Figure 1.18: The Jamshidi trephine for bone marrow biopsy.

The most popular wide-bore needle, however, is probably the 'Tru-cut' (Travenol Laboratories, Inc., USA) since it has proved to be extremely adaptable for sampling many different types of tissue and lesions. The apparatus comprises an inner obturator specimen rod with a cutting point and a specimen trough located behind the point, enclosed in an outer protective 14 gauge cannula which also has a cutting leading edge (Figure 1.19). The needle is used to trap and excise a tissue plug in the trough (Figure 1.19). One of two basic techniques can be used (Fig. 1.20). More recently a mechanized version of the apparatus, known as the bioptome, has been introduced with which it is easier to obtain good samples. The plug sample can be used for histopathological assessment or divided and submitted for a number of other assays (Figure 1.21).

Whenever sampling using a wide-bore needle is contemplated, the clinician is well advised to check the blood clotting status of the patient.

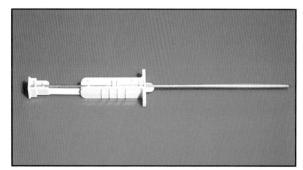

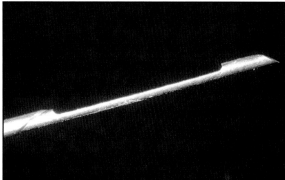

Figure 1.19: The 'Tru-cut' needle apparatus. The obturator cutting point and specimen trough are shown in the lower picture.

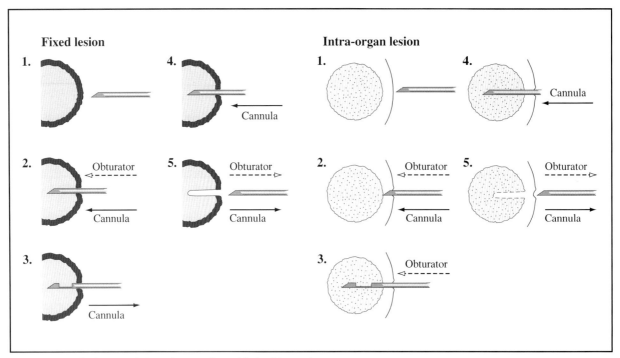

Figure 1.20: The basic technique for sampling with the 'Tru-cut' apparatus.

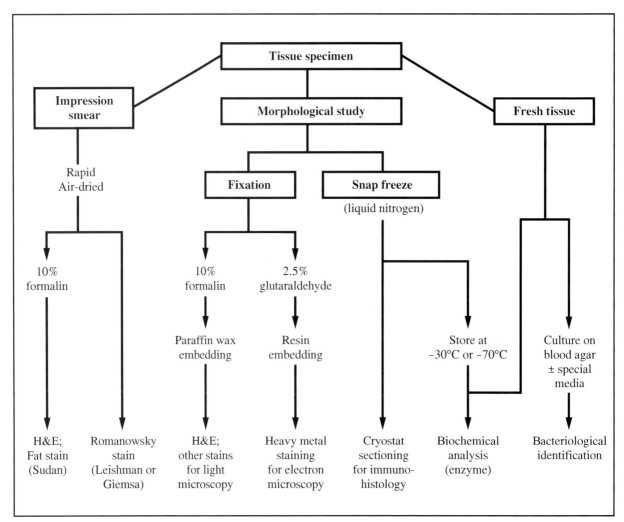

Figure 1.21: The assays possible for wide-bore needle samples.

Endoscopic biopsies

Rigid tube or, increasingly, flexible fibreoptic endoscopes are used to examine, evaluate and sample body orifices, hollow organs and tracts, and cavities. In the last 5 years there has been great development of the flexible fibreoptic endoscope in veterinary work, particularly in the investigation of the alimentary and respiratory tracts. Anatomical sites such as the oesophagus, stomach, upper small intestine, colon and rectum can be examined and sampled with minimal surgical invasion (see Table 1.5).

Additionally, the colon and rectum can usually be examined under sedation rather than with full anaesthesia. The small intestine has to be sampled by excision at laparotomy or by use of special peroral capsule sampling devices.

Biopsy by endoscopic apparatus involves sampling mucosal surfaces or lesions either by snaring focal lesions or by suction–avulsion using fine biting forceps on the tip of the endoscope. The biopsy samples are small (Figure 1.22) and the pathologist needs to have some experience in examining such samples since they are markedly different from the usual biopsy material received for histopathological examination.

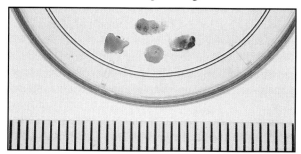

Figure 1.22: Typical endoscopic biopsy samples. Note the small size (scale shows mm).

Endoscopic biopsy is an important adjunct to investigation of alimentary problems in the dog and, to a lesser extent, the cat. The reader is referred to the *BSAVA Manual of Canine and Feline Gastroenterology* (Thomas *et al.*, 1996) for fuller expositions on the applications and methodology of endoscopy.

The respiratory tract can be examined using the same type of instrumentation, and endoscopic biopsy or bronchoalveolar lavage are commonly employed in investigation of respiratory conditions of the dog and cat (see Chapter 10).

Exfoliative samples

These samples consist of small tissue fragments or more often cells, desquamated from skin, body orifices (mouth, ears, genitalia, anus) or mucosae (lips, eyes), or naturally voided in fluids from organ systems such as the bladder, prostate, or respiratory system via the nose (see Table 1.5). An additional source of exfoliated cells may be from manually expressed fluids, such as those produced by prostatic massage or lavage using isotonic saline or cell culture fluids. Other samples

may be collected by scraping an accessible lesion (e.g. skin or anal tumour) with a spatula or curettage device, or swabbing the lesion and transferring collected cells to a microscope slide by rolling the swab over the slide's surface. In addition, and probably the easiest technique where the lesion is clearly accessible, it is possible to make an impression smear by touching a microscope slide directly but gently on to the lesion's surface and rapidly air-drying the smear. Moist, exudative or haemorrhagic lesions should be gently blotted dry with a non-fluffy paper towel prior to the impression process, and dry surfaces can be lightly scarified prior to sampling to ensure an adequate and representative cell yield.

Impression smears are easy to prepare and can yield considerable information cheaply in a short time. Most practising veterinarians can, with practice at the technique, produce good smears suitable for diagnostic purposes.

Smears should be rapidly air-dried and then sent to a pathologist for staining and interpretation. Some practitioners may have the time and inclination to stain and read their own smears. Simple one-step stains such as Leishman or modified Romanowsky stains (e.g. Diff-Quik®) can be used in the surgery but they do require practice in use. If clinicians examine their own smears, they should be able to distinguish between inflammatory and non-inflammatory states (e.g. Figure 1.23) but diagnosis beyond this is best left to the full-time cytopathologist.

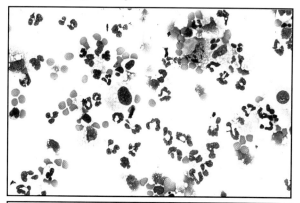

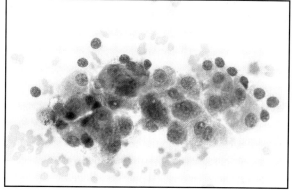

Figure 1.23: (a) Typical cytology from an inflammatory lesion with polymorphonuclear neutrophils predominating. (b) Cytological preparation from a non-inflammatory lesion; in this case a hepatoid adenoma adjacent to the anus.

The majority of exfoliative samples are essentially cellular in nature and are therefore treated as cytological samples (see Chapter 7). Where small tissue fragments are part of an exfoliation sample, these are best managed as tissue samples for histopathological examination, albeit they are of small size.

TISSUE AND BIOPSY MANAGEMENT

The correct management of fluid and tissue samples after biopsy or collection is an important stage that is often not given sufficient attention. Initial post-sampling handling, fixation and transportation of the sample can influence the success of diagnosis; improperly fixed or badly handled tissue samples, especially if small (e.g. endoscopic biopsies), can make meaningful diagnosis impossible. This wastes time and is economically unsound.

Fluid samples

The key to success here is rapid submission, ideally within the same working day. Where samples can be submitted to a laboratory for examination on the same day as they are obtained, a representative volume, no more than 20 ml, should be submitted in a sterile leak-proof container. Plastic containers are commonly used but care should be exercised as they are easily knocked over unless placed in a rack. If the fluid has a tendency to clot, EDTA or a similar anticoagulant should be employed.

Where it is not possible to submit fresh unfixed fluid, then smear preparations should be made on glass microscope slides. Where the fluid is densely cellular, a small drop of suspension may be smeared using the conventional haematological technique (see Chapter 7). Where cell density is low, if possible the cell content should be concentrated by centrifugation at 1500 rpm for 3–5 minutes or, failing the availability of a centrifuge, sedimentation of the sample under gravity for about 30 minutes. Samples of cerebrospinal fluid require special handling (Jannison and Lumsden, 1988) and need to be prepared for examination within one hour of sampling for best morphological results (see Chapter 13). Lavage specimens from the respiratory tract are discussed in Chapter 10 but they can basically be prepared as smears as described above (Rebar and De Nicola, 1988).

Smears should be rapidly air-dried by waving the smears vigorously or using a small hand hair-drier on *low* heat. The smears can then be sent to the laboratory in a suitable container. Fixation and transportation in 95% alcohol is not recommended since veterinary cytopathologists rarely use Papanicolaou's stain (unlike the case for human samples). Aerosol fixative and coating sprays are not recommended for veterinary work.

Tissue samples

Tissue samples range in size from endoscopic biopsies and exfoliated fragments a few millimetres in diameter, to large neoplastic masses of 15–20 cm diameter or more. In either case, what happens to the sample after removal from the patient is important; it is easy to lose or squash small pieces of tissue, or to allow them to desiccate. Small tissue samples should be placed in a Petri dish on a bed of non-fluffy foam matting or a similar base, moistened with sterile isotonic saline or tissue culture medium, pending fixation. Alternatively, if assistance is available, the sample should be placed in fixative within 5–20 minutes of removal.

Large samples can be placed on a clean, preferably sterile dish or tray (e.g. Petri dish or stainless steel instrument tray) pending selection of areas for fixation for histopathological or other examinations (e.g. bacteriological, biochemical). Large specimens always pose a problem for submitting clinicians since the traditional dogma of fixation of tissue samples in formalin fluid in terms of one 'volume' of tissue to 10 'volumes' of formalin, laid down by pathologists, is often nullified by the sheer size and complexity of such samples. In the case of well defined or encapsulated masses such as skin surface neoplasms of, say, 3–4 cm diameter, then fixation in a 1:10 ratio of formalin is still feasible but there remains the problem of adequate penetration of the sample by fixative. Without proper penetration the tissue sample undergoes autolysis and thereafter histopathological interpretation is difficult or impossible.

The solution to the problem is a logical one which can provide additional useful diagnostic information. In the case of smaller masses or well defined lesions, bisection alone is usually sufficient and the lesion can be fixed as two halves (preferably sectioned longitudinally). If the lesion is to be bisected then it should be done completely and uniformly. All too often the pathologist is presented with a distorted specimen (Figure 1.24) which is difficult to orientate and take blocks from because the fresh sample was improperly transected by a well-meaning clinician. Larger or irregular lesions may have to be subjected to more than one gross section, or sectioning in more than one plane. In these cases it is important that the submitting clinician informs the pathologist exactly what has been done and which bits of the lesion, if not the whole, have been sent. This can be done by a written description but probably the easiest and best way is to send an annotated diagram(s) (Figure 1.25) with a complete clinical history and signalment. Where several tissue blocks from the same specimen at different levels or sites in the sample are sent, it is better to submit them in separate labelled containers, again referencing them with a diagram. Multiple different tissue samples from the same animal (e.g. skin wart, epulis from the mouth, anal tumour) must *never* be placed in the same con-

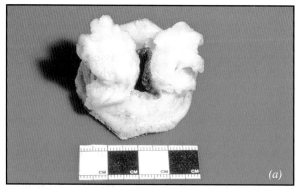

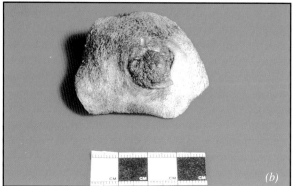

Figure 1.24: An excised mammary tumour that had been incompletely bisected prior to fixation. (a) The specimen as received, showing inversion and distortion; (b) the specimen after correction of the inversion.

tainer. The submission of multiple unlabelled samples from different sites in the same container causes great agitation to pathologists.

Very thin slices of tissue (e.g. liver), taken with the mistaken notion that their thinness will ensure correct fixation, will often distort in fixatives. Similarly, opened sections of gut and larger elliptical skin biopsy specimens often distort on immersion in fixative. Distortion can be minimized, if not entirely prevented, by pinning the edge of the opened bowel or ellipse onto a piece of thick card or air-drying the tissue on to card for a few minutes prior to immersion.

Fixation

Fixation is the process whereby the natural autolytic changes in tissues, often enhanced by infective agents, inflammation and physical mishandling post-sampling, are prevented or minimized. The aim is to use an agent to fix and preserve the cellular architecture for histopathological interpretation and assessment.

If additional assays are contemplated then parallel unfixed lesions should be collected or samples taken from the same lesion prior to the procedure, since histopathology fixatives render tissue samples unusable for microbiological, biochemical and many immunological assays. The common way around this

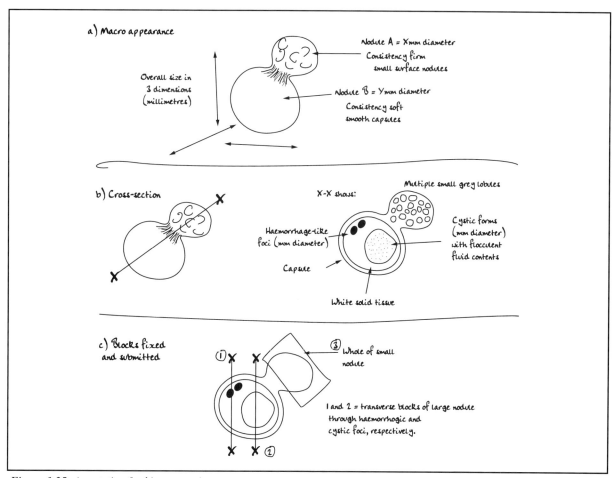

Figure 1.25: Annotation for biopsy specimens.

is to bisect a lesion and, assuming both halves are representative, use one half or representative portions for assays requiring unfixed tissue, and fix the remaining half. Impression smears should be made before tissue is fixed; fixation of smears should be done after rapid air-drying, usually with 95% alcohol. Where a modified Romanowsky stain is to be used, the fixation stage is incorporated in the application of the stain.

The best all-round fixative for most diagnostic purposes is still formalin solution. It is relatively cheap, easy to use and, if handled sensibly, is non-toxic and non-irritant to users. A major benefit is that formalin is a good preservative as well as a fixative, thereby allowing tissues fixed in formalin to be stored for months if necessary. The solution preferred by most pathologists is a 10% buffered solution which can be made up as follows:

40% commercial formalin concentrate	100 ml
Acid sodium phosphate monohydrate	4 g
Anhydrous disodium phosphate	6.5 g
Made up with water to 1 litre	

Other fixatives are sometimes used for specific purposes. Picric acid-containing solutions (e.g. Bouin's fixative) are often used for rapid fixation of, for example, skin samples. These fixatives do penetrate tissues rapidly but only to a limited extent. The disadvantages are that if tissues are left in the fixatives for more than 24 hours they become brittle and difficult to section for histology, plus the fact that the picric acid imparts a vivid yellow line to the tissue which can interfere with stains.

Alcohol (as opposed to aldehyde) fixatives are no longer recommended except for cytology (see Chapter 7).

Where ultrastructural examination is contemplated, tissues should ideally be fixed in freshly made 3–4% glutaraldehyde. Very small cubes (2–4 mm) of tissue are mandatory and fixation must be effected within a few minutes (up to 15 minutes) to make sure of the preservation of subcellular fine structure.

Glutaraldehyde (like other reagents used for ultrastructural preparation) is extremely irritant to mucosae and should be used with great care, preferably in a fume cupboard. Tissues that have been fixed in formalin very soon after removal can be thinly sliced and 'post-fixed' in glutaraldehyde for electron microscopy but this is less than satisfactory.

Tissue samples may also be 'fixed' by rapid (or 'snap') freezing, using liquid carbon dioxide sprays or liquid nitrogen and 'dry ice', and the tissues used for cryostat sections or histochemical/immunocytochemical examination. This method gives rapid results but requires specialized laboratory equipment and interpretation by an expert. Frozen sections are therefore only a serious option for clinicians in veterinary schools and research institutes, or where a suitably equipped laboratory is very close at hand. Some assays, e.g. antibody assessment of skin disease by immunohistology (see Chapter 6), do require frozen sections, although increasingly these assays can be performed on routinely fixed tissue.

Transportation and presentation

The majority of specimens, whether tissues for histopathology or samples for microbiological or biochemical analysis, are sent to the laboratory by postal services or public transport. Those fortunate clinicians who are geographically close to a diagnostic laboratory or work in an institute where the laboratory is an integral part of the organization can submit fresh unfixed (but hopefully not dehydrated or autolytic) tissues and other samples, and have the added benefit of being able to communicate directly with their pathologist colleagues. Where a delay in direct submission of 2–3 hours to a local laboratory may occur, fresh tissue may be held on ice prior to presentation. Some authorities have advocated the use of synthetic transport media (e.g. Michel's transport medium). Generally, however, it is inadvisable to prejudice good tissue preservation by delaying fixation in buffered formalin. Where microbiological assay from the same tissue is required then tissue subdivision as indicated above is the only option, with submission of unfixed material or swabs as soon as possible thereafter. A degree of common sense is needed in such cases to obtain the best results.

Containers

Samples should be submitted in suitable leak-proof and breakage-resistant containers (Table 1.8). There are many such containers in a range of sizes available commercially and many diagnostic laboratories provide their own containers and wrappings with suitable labels.

It is important to remember that fresh unfixed tissue samples swell and harden on fixation in formalin and therefore narrow-necked bottles and jars should not be used (Figure 1.26). Glass containers are not to be encouraged; metal or plastic tablet cannisters are often good cheap alternatives. Whatever type of container is used, it should be of sufficient volume to hold the specimen without distortion. Fresh unfixed tissue can be, and regrettably often is, crammed into a container that is too small and of the wrong shape. Once fixed, the result is a less than useful sample (Figure 1.27) that cannot be oriented by the receiving pathologist.

Suitable leak-proof, non-breakable containers should be placed in plastic bags and wrapped in padded material (e.g. plastic 'bubble wrap') prior to transportation. Padded bags approved by the postal services can be used. Packages should be clearly labelled as containing clinical or pathological specimens. Large specimens may present problems and may have to be sent by rail or courier services, and again, adequate

Characteristic	Comment
Resistance to breakage	Avoid glass Plastic or metal tablet containers ideal
Leak-proof lid	Screw-on or snap-top Seal with waterproof tape?
Wide neck i.e. uniform diameter with rest of container	Ease of specimen removal after fixation
Size of container	Must be adequate for specimen plus adequate fixative Fixed tissue swells and hardens
Packaging	Plastic bag to contain leakage Padding or wrapping to protect data sheet in separate plastic bag
Identification and documentation	Clear labelling Address of laboratory plus sender's address Check postal service regulations

Table 1.8: *Containers for transportation of biopsies.*

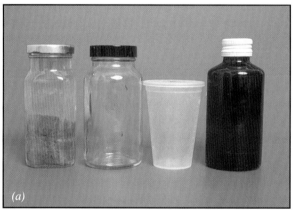

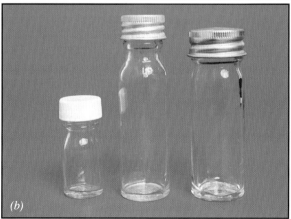

Figure 1.26: *Containers which are <u>not</u> suitable for transportation of biopsy samples. (a) The glass containers have narrow necks, and one is dark; the plastic container is unstable. Note the large piece of liver in the narrow-necked jar on the left. (b) These containers would only be suitable for very small tissues, fragments or skin punch biopsy specimens.*

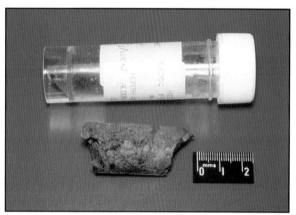

Figure 1.27: *Gross distortion of a tissue sample as a result of being crammed into an undersized container. The specimen was also incompletely fixed.*

leak-proof packaging and clear labelling are mandatory. Accurate destination addressing and labelling as to the originator of any package is very important; the author's experience is that this task is often best assigned to a reliable veterinary nurse or secretary. Postal agencies in different parts of the world may vary in their attitude and regulations about postal transport of samples, so it is advisable to check on these prior to posting specimens or samples.

Documentation

Equally important for successful diagnosis from a sample is the provision of accurate and full documentation. Ideally, this should be done on a standard form issued by the receiving laboratory but failing that a typed or legibly handwritten letter should accompany the specimen(s), preferably in a separate plastic bag to prevent damage if there is leakage of fixative or other fluid in transit.

Full clinical details for the animal, including the owner's name, patient's signalment (breed, age, sex), history and clinical findings and any treatment (especially antibiotics if bacteriology is required) should be given. Especially important are details of the lesion(s) submitted, i.e. size, site, consistency and appearance. A diagram is often helpful, particularly with skin neoplasms or biopsies where multiple samples are taken or where only parts of a large lesion are submitted. If previous samples have been submitted from the same patient, then the reference numbers or (if a different laboratory is involved) an indication of the previous diagnoses, should be quoted.

It is important to remember when giving case details to accompany a sample that information which may appear trivial to the clinician can provide the pathologist with important clues in making a diagnosis.

PRACTICE LABORATORIES *VERSUS* COMMERCIAL LABORATORIES

In large veterinary practices in the UK, particularly those dealing with farm animals and horses as well as the small companion animals, there is the possibility of setting up an in-house or practice laboratory rather than using a commercial, government or university veterinary school diagnostic laboratory. In this case the numbers of staff and financial turnover may justify such considerations. In smaller practices the practice laboratory may come about through the interest of one of the veterinary surgeons involved or as the result of a particular specialist interest, e.g. gastroenterology. In North America there has traditionally been more in-house assaying of patients because of the total animal 'work-up' approach to diagnosis and because of the relatively different expectations of many small animal owners.

The advent of wet and dry chemistry assays, serological tests and more user-friendly assay kits in the UK has resulted in more veterinary practices embarking on more of their own testing. At the same time a general raised awareness amongst the pet-owning general public has driven up the demand for diagnostic testing to complement clinical diagnosis as well as the more established aids to diagnosis such as radiography.

Much of the considerations involved in setting up a practice laboratory will depend on the financial balance involved together with time, workload and manpower, as well as decisions about the range of assays that the in-house facility can handle. Assays or investigations that are technologically demanding or expensive are really non-viable. Simple haematological and biochemical assays, particularly using commercial kits now available, can be undertaken in a cost- and time-effective

way, but histopathology and complex microbiological investigations should probably remain the province of the specialist and dedicated laboratory.

Setting up an in-house laboratory requires: suitable premises; staff ('omnipotential', full-time or part-time, veterinary or technical?); suitable equipment, such as a microscope, centrifuge, refractometer, photometer and laboratory glass and plasticware; and suitable commercially manufactured assay kits or expensive instruments such as cell counters or analysers. Running costs have to allow for reagents and disposable laboratoryware. Hard decisions are required as to which assay kits are likely to be cost-effective, i.e. can the capital outlay be justified by the likely number of patients likely to be sampled? Many practices in the UK increasingly use analytical instrumentation for assays and according to most users this provides a quick and cost-effective first-time assay system for many of the routine serum and urine biochemistry examinations that are required.

Added to the above considerations, there is now the additional requirement in the UK to observe the regulations of the Health and Safety at Work Act 1974 and to carry out risk assessment under the Control of Substances Hazardous to Health (COSHH) regulations. There are similar and more stringent legislative requirements governing diagnostic and private laboratories in North America. These regulations are serious considerations for both commercial and private practice laboratories.

In deciding on the advantages and disadvantages of using a commercial laboratory as opposed to an in-house facility, consideration has to be given to financial cost per case (or sample), convenience of use of an outside laboratory, speed of reporting, accuracy and reliability of laboratory results, and level of feedback, i.e. does the laboratory provide support other than a straight analysis of material. In the latter case many practitioners would be more inclined to use a laboratory where they can obtain expert advice to either explain or enlarge on laboratory results. The clinician has to weigh the benefits of gaining expertise, accuracy and rapidity against the relative cost of using a commercial laboratory. Most veterinary diagnostic laboratories nowadays provide a fully comprehensive and extensive range of assays for the practitioner and additionally will offer supporting advice. What does seem to be important is that because of the species variations involved and the increasing complexity of diagnostic problems, the practitioner uses a *veterinary* laboratory and one that is prepared to give advice and helpful back-up when required.

LABORATORY HEALTH AND SAFETY

As a society we are rightly becoming more aware of the everyday health and safety dangers we encounter and, consequently, legislation in this area has been tightened to reflect this awareness and concern. The nature of some of the material handled means that the laboratory environment poses a risk to persons working there. Laboratories and laboratory managers therefore have a duty of care to ensure that their employees and others who come in contact with the laboratory are protected from the potential hazards within that environment.

The Health and Safety at Work Act 1974 is a basic piece of legislation designed to protect all workers. Although this type of legislation and some of the points outlined below may seem more applicable to commercial diagnostic laboratories, or teaching and research institutes, the Act applies equally in the UK to private veterinary practice laboratories or those parts of a practice that may be used for diagnostic laboratory procedures. In thinking about health and safety in the laboratory, it is useful to consider the formation of a Health and Safety Policy Statement which will reflect, as reasonably as is practicable, the intention to achieve the safest possible environment for staff and others. This policy statement should include the following intentions:

- To provide and maintain plant and equipment that are safe and without risk to health
- To make arrangements for ensuring safety and absence of risk to health in the connection with the use, handling, storage and disposal of substances
- To provide and maintain an environment that is safe and without risk to health
- To provide such protective clothing and equipment as is necessary for safe working
- To monitor the effectiveness of measures put in place.

It is worth stressing that whilst it is the duty of laboratory managers to provide a safe working environment, it is the responsibility of individual workers to exercise care to ensure that they and others are not endangered by their acts and omissions. Once an agreed policy statement has been formulated there are measures that must be put in place to achieve the objectives of the policy.

General precautions

Fire safety
Regular fire prevention routines, e.g. the nightly unplugging of electrical equipment, checking gas taps, closing doors, storing reagents away properly, are the most effective means of preventing fire. There should be a well rehearsed 'in the event of a fire' routine in the laboratory, plus an easy means of escape from the premises.

First aid
It is desirable to have several members of staff trained in basic first aid and to have correctly stocked first aid kits available at various sites throughout the laboratory complex. The exact numbers of trained personnel and kits will be dependent on the total number of staff to be served.

Systems of work
Instructions should be laid down for the safe handling of equipment and substances, both chemical and biological, in the laboratory. No apparatus should be used or dangerous material handled until the user fully understands the hazard and the precautions to be taken.

Appropriate hand and eye protection must be used to protect from splashing. A major cause of accidents is poor housekeeping; as a general rule 'a tidy workplace is a safe one'. Apparatus and materials not required immediately should be returned to storage and waste materials should be disposed of promptly and safely. Spillages should be cleared up immediately. Appropriate signs should be used on all hazardous materials. Manual handling of loads should be carried out by first assessing the degree of difficult by doing a test lift and then seeking the correct level of help required.

Chemicals
The Control of Substances Hazardous to Health (COSHH) regulations were formulated to eliminate the risk to health through the contract with hazardous substances. The regulations require an assessment of the risk in the use of any substance. This assessment is comprised of: recognition; evaluation; consideration of precautions; and record keeping of the assessment for consultation. This is best achieved through the production of a standardized Risk Assessment Form (see Figures 1.28 and 1.29) for each reagent, group of

---

1. Identify and name activity
2. Identify and list all hazardous substances used in activity[*]
3. Identify by which route substances are hazardous[†]
4. Identify protection required[**]
5. Identify means of disposal
6 Complete a risk assessment form for each activity

[*] As determined by Approved list for the Classification, Packaging and Labelling of Dangerous Substances Regulations, 1984 and onwards. See warning labels on bottles etc. Substances with minimum exposure limits (MEL) and occupational exposure standard (OES) should also be included.

[†] e.g. Inhalation, ingestion, skin absorption, direct contact or injection (via 'sharps')

[**] e.g. Eye protection, face protection, hand protection, respiratory protection, microbiological safety cabinet.

Figure 1.28: Control of Substances Hazardous to Health risk assessment exercise. Risk assessment can be done on a form of your own design but must include all the elements listed.

PART A

Activity: Immunocytochemical Staining

Location: Room 49, Department of Veterinary Pathology, University of ???

PART B

Hazardous substances classification:

Very Toxic ☑   Toxic ☑   Harmful ☑   Corrosive ☑   Irritant ☑

Substances with MEL or OES ☐   Dust ☐   Carcinogenic (or suspected carcinogen) ☑

Micro-organism _____

PART C

Route by which substances are hazardous:

Inhalation ☑   Ingestion ☑   Skin absorption ☑   Direct contact (skin or eyes) ☐

Injection (via sharps) ☐

PART D

Effect of exposure:

Single acute: Serious ☐   Not serious ☐   Not known ☑

Repeated low: Serious ☑   Not serious ☐   Not known ☐

PART E

Protection required:

Eye protection ☑   Face protection ☐   Hand protection ☑

Respiratory protection ☑   Other, e.g. clothing _____

PART F

Is specific training required?   YES ☑   NO ☐

Level of supervision   Close ☐   Intermittent (after approval of scheme of work) ☐

Minimal (after approval of scheme of work) ☑

PART G

Waste disposal:

In-house via local authority after rendering safe ☑   To incinerator ☐

To specialist contractor ☐

PART H

List of hazardous substances:

Sodium azide	VERY TOXIC by ingestion and inhalation
FITC	Irritant
H202	Irritant, corrosive - burns skin/eyes
DAB	Irritant, possible carcinogen - ingestion, skin/eye contact.
Xylene	Harmful, possible carcinogen - inhalation, skin/eye contact. Vapour narcotic at high concentrations
Methanol	TOXIC by injection, inhalation, eyes. Can cause longterm CNS changes
DPX	Harmful
Tris Buffer	Irritant

Figure 1.29: Example of a risk assessment form.

reagents or procedure. Once an assessment has been made, this must be made available when work is to take place using the corresponding reagent(s). The assessments should be reviewed from time to time. No person should undertake a piece of work until he or she has read and understood the risk involved.

Whilst COSHH Risk Assessment should form the basis for the safe handling of chemicals and reagents, some general precautions will also be of use:

- Training and supervision of staff should be ongoing and increased when substances are being used for the first time
- Chemicals should be stored in appropriate areas and conditions, e.g. toxic and poisonous agents should be kept in secure storage, flammable/explosive chemicals should not be stored in a refrigerator unless it is sparkproof
- Waste chemicals should be disposed of in accordance with the Environmental Protection Act and may involve the use of a specialized chemical waste disposal company
- Hygiene: No eating or drinking should take place in the laboratory. No mouth pipetting should take place. Hands should be washed frequently and always before leaving the laboratory. Laboratory coats should be worn when working in the laboratory and should not be worn outside the laboratory.

Biological hazards

The COSHH regulations also cover biological substances and the risk associated with their use must be assessed in the same way as for chemicals. In addition, work involving dangerous pathogens is subject to the Dangerous Pathogens Regulations 1981. This document should be read in conjunction with another set of regulations, The Categorisation of Pathogens according to their Hazard and Category of Containment. It is worth remembering that the dividing line between pathogenic and non-pathogenic is often uncertain and that indeed the potential hazards associated with many biological materials are unknown. Benign organisms can cause sensitivity or an allergic response. The principles of good housekeeping and laboratory hygiene equally apply to biological safety as they do to chemical hazards. Specifically in considering biological safety, the safe disposal of waste

material must be given careful consideration and route of disposal established. Depending on the nature of the material involved, this will mean the use of chemical disinfectants, autoclaving or incineration. The Safe Disposal of Clinical Waste Guidelines issued by the Health and Safety Executive are designed to cover such material. Essential to all this is that clinical waste must be rendered safe *before* entering the domestic waste outflow.

REFERENCES AND FURTHER READING

Else RW (1986) Biopsy - principles and specimen management. *In Practice* **8**, 112-116

Else RW (1989) Biopsy - special techniques and tissues. *In Practice* **11**, 27-34

Jannison EM and Lumsden JH (1988) Cerebrospinal fluid analysis in the dog: methodology and interpretation. *Seminars in Veterinary Medicine and Surgery* **3**, 122-132

Kerwin SC (1995) Hepatic aspiration and biopsy techniques. *Veterinary Clinics of North America: Small Animal Practice* **25**, 275-291

Knoll JS and Rowell SL (1996) Clinical haematology - incline and analysis, quality control, reference values and system selection. *Veterinary Clinics of North America: Small Animal Practice* **26**, 981-1002

Murtaugh RJ (1993) Biopsy techniques. *Seminars in Veterinary Medicine and Surgery* **8**

O'Brien PT and Lumsden JH (1988) The cytological examination of body cavity fluids. *Seminars in Veterinary Medicine and Surgery* **3**, 140-156

Quinn PJ, Carter ME, Markey BK and Carter GR (1994) *Clinical Veterinary Microbiology*. Wolfe, London

Rebar AH and De Nicola DB (1988) The cytological examination of the respiratory tract. *Seminars in Veterinary Medicine and Surgery* **3**, 109-121

Thomas D, Simpson JW and Hall EJ (1996) *Manual of Canine and Feline Gastroenterology*. BSAVA, Cheltenham

Valli VEO (1988) Techniques in veterinary cytopathology. *Seminars in Veterinary Medicine and Surgery* **3**, 85-93

Vap, LM and Mitzwer B (1996) An update on chemistry analyzers. *Veterinary Clinics of North America: Small Animal Practice* **26**, 1129-1154

White RAS (1991) Biopsy techniques. In *Manual of Small Animal Oncology*, ed. RAS White, pp.87-97. BSAVA, Cheltenham

Further reading on laboratory health and safety: all the following statutory documents are available through HMSO in the UK.

Health and Safety at Work Act 1974

Control of Substances Hazardous to Health

Electricity at Work Act 1989

Dangerous Pathogens Regulations 1981

Categorisation of Pathogens according to their Hazard and Category of Containment, 4th edition, 1995

Controlled Waste Regulations 1992

Special Waste Regulations 1996

Safe Disposal of Clinical Waste 1992

Environmental Protection Act 1990

CHAPTER TWO

Laboratory Data Interpretation

John H. Lumsden

INTRODUCTION

Laboratory tests are used to assist diagnosis of disease. They are used also to screen for health or possible disease, to guide prognosis and to monitor response to therapy. These different clinical settings in which tests are used, and the questions asked, markedly influence the diagnostic utility and thus the interpretation of laboratory tests.

The traditional approach to interpreting laboratory data is to compare patient test results with 'normal values' for the species. The patient's results are considered abnormal and thus supportive of disease when outside the 'normal values' quoted by the laboratory. There are many reasons why this approach can lead to misinterpretation, especially if the degree of change is not considered. Is the patient similar, i.e. similar subset, to the 'normal' animals? Was a similar analytical method used? Was the sample size of normal animals large enough to establish reasonable confidence in the lower and upper limits quoted?

If the clinician is using the test results to help formulate a list of differential diagnosis, small increases in patient values may weigh heavily in interpretation. Alternatively, if a differential diagnosis was made initially on the basis of the clinical information, then small changes in laboratory values are less likely to be over-interpreted.

Many factors contribute to variation, or error, in laboratory results. Clinicians should understand how their actions may contribute to this laboratory error, how to investigate possible sources of error, and how this knowledge may affect their interpretation of laboratory data.

When monitoring a patient for response to therapy, differences in sequential values due to test imprecision, i.e. the analytical variation of the method used, should be allowed for before assuming a change in the patient. This information is generated daily within good laboratories and is available upon request. Simple guidelines can assist differentiation of analytical imprecision from real patient change.

The clinical utility of a laboratory test can be described by *diagnostic* characteristics. These include diagnostic sensitivity [Sn], specificity [Sp] and predictive values of positive [PVP] and negative tests [PVN].

Although the diagnostic process is complex, knowledge of basic analytical and diagnostic characteristics of tests simplifies the interpretation of laboratory data.

ANALYTICAL CHARACTERISTICS OF LABORATORY DATA

Laboratory error
Laboratory error is a broad term used to encompass all potential errors associated with laboratory testing. It is assumed that a degree of laboratory error (analytical imprecision) contributes to every test result. Laboratory error can be divided into pre-analytical, analytical and post-analytical error (Lumsden, 1989). The clinician is a major contributor to pre- and post-analytical error and can have direct influence on analytical error.

Although pre- and post-analytical errors are difficult to monitor, analytical error is assessed routinely using repeated testing of serum-based samples containing predetermined or unknown concentrations or activity (*known* and *unknown* controls). Daily plotting and examination of values obtained for the known controls provides both immediate and retrospective information regarding the likely reliability of results. The known control observations are assumed to represent the accuracy and precision expected for patient results. The unknown controls provide additional unbiased assessment of analytical reliability.

Differentiation of real changes in sequential patient observations requires knowing the analytical variation expected for the method. Is the patient's platelet or leucocyte count increasing or decreasing, or could the changes be due to inherent variation in the method? What information is required by the clinician to separate these sources of change and where is this information obtained?

Pre-analytical error

Pre-analytical errors occur during sample collection, separation and storage. Identification errors, incorrect anticoagulants, incorrect sampling times including inappropriate postprandial sampling, iatrogenic haemolysis during blood collection or serum separation, and leaching of cell components are frequently encountered contributors to pre-analytical and analytical error. The concentration of inorganic phosphorus is similar in erythrocytes and serum but when erythrocytes lyse or are left in serum overnight, organic phosphorus can be released and converted to inorganic phosphorus, resulting in analytical error. Samples obtained in the postprandial period have increased lipids, glucose and urea when compared to reference limits determined from fasting individuals. Lipaemia, bilirubinaemia and haemoglobinaemia create negative and positive interference for several routine clinical chemistry tests (Glick *et al.*, 1991; Jacobs *et al.*, 1992). The effect varies with the species and the analytical methods. The effects of major interferences such as haemolysis, icterus and lipaemia have been determined by kit manufacturers for human serum. This information, which may or may not be similar for animal species, is available from laboratory personnel.

Analytical error

Errors may be due to the operator (analyst), reagent, instrument or method (analytical). The training and experience of analysts are of primary concern, especially for in-clinic laboratories. The errors may be constant or random. Laboratory protocols, especially for in-clinic use, must be written in the detail appropriate for the training and experience of the analysts and made readily available in a laboratory manual of operating procedures. In laboratories these may be termed standard operating procedures (SOPs).

Analytical errors may occur due to: improper instrument calibration; errors in pipetting; use of outdated, contaminated or improperly stored reagents, standards and controls; inadequate time for reagents to reach room temperature after removal from

refrigerator or freezer prior to use; and errors in reaction time or temperature if not automatically controlled within the instrument. Current modular wet chemistry and dry reagent chemistry instruments manufactured for use in the clinic or at the point of care (POC) control time, temperature, wavelength and frequency of readings through microprocessors and barcoding on each module or reagent strip.

Analytical errors are detected through routine use of known and, for unbiased estimation, unknown serum-based controls. Manufacturers of instruments and reagents for use in the clinic often do not emphasize the importance of routine testing of 'known controls'. Routine use of 'known controls' is required to establish and to maintain confidence in test results. The clinician interpreting sequential patient values should be aware of the true in-clinic analytical precision of the tests used.

Interference

Many drugs interfere with analytical procedures. The effect may be direct or may be indirect, by initiating a physiological or pharmacological change within the patient (Young, 1990; Glick *et al.*, 1991). In the dog a common example is the induction of several liver-related enzymes following the administration of corticosteroid, anti-epileptic or anti-inflammatory drugs. The degree of influence of therapeutic agents on clinical chemistry and haematological values is often unpredictable. The most reliable laboratory values for diagnosis of disease are determined from blood samples obtained prior to initiating therapy. Unexpected test results should be reviewed for possible effects of medication.

Quality control

Quality control (QC) and quality assessment (QA) are procedures used to monitor, and minimize, laboratory analytical errors. Quality control procedures are described in Chapter 1. The principles of use are reviewed briefly here because of the implications for interpretation of laboratory data. Serum samples with *known* analyte concentration or activity are tested as for patient samples. In diagnostic laboratories three levels of each analyte are usually used, i.e. abnormally low, normal, and abnormally high. The resulting values are plotted on graphs containing the analyte mean, standard deviation and acceptable range as predetermined by the manufacturer of the known control sera for the specific methods used in that laboratory. Values will differ by method. If the known 'control' values are within expected limits, patient values are assumed to be acceptable. *Unknown* controls are used in addition in larger laboratories as an independent unbiased assessment of laboratory performance.

On a daily basis, the accuracy, or bias, and the precision of each method are assessed from the graph of the plotted observed known control values.

This provides immediate feedback to the chief technician, or clinician, allowing a decision to be made regarding the acceptability of patient values. The basic principle is that the values obtained within the laboratory should be within one standard deviation (SD) of the predetermined mean value 68% of the time and within 2 SD of the mean value 95% of the time. At regular intervals, e.g. each month, the mean, SD and coefficient of variation (CV) for each method at each concentration are calculated for comparison with the predetermined values. Examination of the charts and retrospective calculations of mean and SD provides a good estimation of within-laboratory accuracy and precision for each method.

Accuracy, the closeness of the observed value to the true value, is estimated by comparing the mean value obtained, after *repeated* measurements, with the manufacturer's expected value. *Precision*, the reproducibility of the test when measurements are repeated on aliquots of the same known control sera, may be expressed in percentage form as the coefficient of variation, calculated as follows:

$$CV = \frac{SD}{Mean} \times 100 \; (\%)$$

This formula allows the clinician readily to convert between absolute values (SD) and the percentage (CV) estimation of precision if either is known.

Laboratory personnel can provide information on precision for the concentrations used for the known controls. Calculations should include 20–30 replicates for estimating likely performance for patient samples. When the method's CV is calculated using 90 or more replicates, as may be determined during one month in a high-volume laboratory, the estimated CV will be smaller than expected for patient samples because the variation in known controls does not allow for other sources of error such as random interference (Kringle, 1994).

Besides within-day and between-day method variation, the clinician must consider within-day and between-day individual variation, as well as variation between individuals. Information may be obtained from the laboratory, or more often from the literature, for expected within-day and between-day variation for healthy individuals.

This information can have direct influence on clinical interpretation. Differences in *sequential* values for a sample must be greater than the expected within-day and between-day individual and analytical variation before the clinician can assume there is a real change in the patient. One rule of thumb suggests there must be a difference in sequential patient values of at least 3 SD observed for known controls before assuming there is real change in the patient's value. Thus, the method's *analytical variation* would predict a difference of less than ± 1 SD inherent in the method 68% of the time

and less than ± 2 SD 95% of the time. This also means that sequential patient values may differ by more than 2 SD and less than 3 SD, inherent in the method, about 5% of the time due entirely to analytical variation. As an example, if a patient has a cortisol concentration of 100 nmol/l and the CV of the method is 10%, sequential values as low as 70 nmol/l and as high as 130 nmol/l should be considered to be potentially due to analytical variation. This degree of analytical variation must be considered when interpreting dexamethasone suppression tests for suspect adrenocortical hyperfunction.

In very general terms, and depending very much on the instrumentation and method, the expected CV for many chemistry methods is about 5%. For some assays including electrolytes the CV may be lower, while for protein, urea, enzymes and especially hormones, the CV may be higher. Manual methods usually have a higher CV than automated and dry reagent assays. The CV for all methods, as determined using known controls, should be readily available from the laboratory and provided to the clinician upon request.

There is no external regulation of private or commercial veterinary diagnostic laboratories at present. Good commercial laboratories usually incorporate quality assessment procedures similar to those used in regulated research and human diagnostic laboratories. The clinician must ask for and obtain the necessary information to initiate and maintain confidence in laboratory test results. The routine use of control samples appears to be the exception rather than the rule for in-clinic laboratory testing.

As an initial source of information regarding the expected CV of a method, manufacturers provide tables for each lot of control sera that list, by method, the predetermined mean, SD and acceptable limits for each analyte. From the information contained in these tables, the analyte CV at specific concentrations can be calculated and used by clinicians until validated within the laboratory.

Post-analytical error

Post-analytical errors occur during reporting and interpretation of test results. Transcription errors may be due to transposition of numbers or intermixing of patient results. The clinician should question all suspicious reported values. The initial examination should begin in the laboratory log book or computer entry in order to rule out a reporting error. Unexplained or unanticipated test results should initiate a request to repeat the analysis using an aliquot of the *original* patient sample. If a discrepancy with clinical information persists, a separate blood sample should be obtained and analysed.

Errors of interpretation are considered to be post-analytical but may originate from pre-analytical errors contributing to sample haemolysis or lipaemia and resulting in analytical interference.

Post-analytical errors may occur when patient values are compared to inappropriate reference limits. For example, an incorrect interpretation of anaemia will occur if erythrocyte values for juvenile animals are compared to adult reference limits. Reference values may be quoted that have not been determined or have been determined inadequately for the particular method used in the laboratory.

Reference values

Reference values must be used to guide interpretation of patient test results when alternative test diagnostic characteristics have not been determined, e.g. predictive values of positive or negative tests using described decision limits, as discussed below. Also, reference values are used for initial assessment of patient test results if clinical differential diagnoses have not been established prior to data interpretation.

The term 'normal' is not recommended because of the ambiguity in meaning. Common definitions of 'normal' include: 'gaussian', in the statistical sense as when data form an evenly distributed bell curve; 'common' in the epidemiological sense; and 'non-pathological' in the clinical sense. A not uncommon supposition is that if a test is not 'normal' then it must be 'abnormal' and thus associated with disease. Such use places considerable reliance upon the lower and upper reference limits provided by the laboratory.

'Reference limits' are proposed as the preferred way to describe the *upper and lower limit for 95% of similar individuals* (Solberg, 1994). Alternative terms are *reference range* or *reference intervals*. The individual animals selected using defined criteria for establishing reference values are called *reference individuals*. The values obtained by observation or measurement of a particular type of quantity (analyte) for the reference individual are called *reference observations* or *reference values*. The value of a measurement or observation used to make a medical decision is called an *observed value*. The observed value is compared with the reference limits. As discussed later, the observed value may be compared with decision points other than the central 95% reference limits.

Sources of reference values are usually from healthy individuals and are used to derive population-based reference limits. Carefully considered guidelines have been established for the development and presentation of reference values (Solberg, 1994). Laboratory reference values should include a description of the source and state of health of the reference individuals, the fasting state of monogastric individuals, the sample size (*n*), sample collection and handling procedures, and the specific laboratory analytical methods. The procedures used for determining the lower and upper reference limits should be described, including identification and handling of outliers, data distribution, i.e. whether the observations were gaussian/non-gaussian before and/or after transformations, and

whether parametric or non-parametric methods were used for calculation of reference limits. Was the effect of sample size and probability incorporated into estimation of the central 95% reference interval? Were confidence limits determined for the reference limits? A DOS-based software program is available which will analyse reference observations and, if data distribution and sample size are adequate, will determine lower and upper reference limits as well as calculate the margin of error for each limit (Solberg, 1994).

As a minimum, the clinician should know if the described limits are expected to include 95% of similar healthy individuals. It is always surprising when one finds out that the range reported by a laboratory, or researcher, was calculated to include 90%, or less, of the reference observations and thus the population. Were the values developed in-house from original studies, from comparison of old and new methods, from 'experience', or were they extrapolated from the literature? This information should be known to everyone interpreting data from a laboratory. The age range may be important. Many young dogs are diagnosed as having anaemia when red cell values are compared with reference limits (normals) for mature dogs. In summary, the clinician must know the origin and the relative appropriateness of the reference limits from a laboratory in order to interpret observed patient values.

It is universally stated that each laboratory should determine reference limits for each species. A major reason for this is the effect of methodology, e.g. substrate and incubation temperature greatly alter enzyme activity; methods used for differentiating leucocyte types vary greatly between automated haematology instruments.

Unfortunately it is impractical for veterinary diagnostic laboratories to develop reference limits for all subsets of interest, e.g. species, breed, age, sex, pregnancy, lactation, nutrition. The statistically required number of healthy reference individuals may not be available; the cost of sampling and analyses may be prohibitive. Also, the frequent changes in instrumentation and reagents require repeat evaluation. As a minimum, the central 95% reference limits should be developed for one subset for each species of clinical interest. The clinician should be provided with: a description of the source and number of reference individuals; the statistical approach used to estimate the central 95% reference limits; and, where sample size is adequate, the margin of error for both the lower and the upper reference limit.

On a practical basis, unless more than 40 reference individuals are sampled, the lowest and highest *observed* values appear to be the best estimate of the central 95% reference limits, provided there are no obvious outliers. With large samples, *n* = 120–140, the probability can be calculated, i.e. with 0.9 probability, that 95% of the population lies between the lower and upper reference limits. Larger samples are required when the data are non-gaussian to obtain the same degree of confidence that the limits will include 95% of the population, e.g. $n = 120$ *vs* $n = 60$. The observed values for many analytes from healthy individuals are non-gaussian, i.e. skewed, and must be transformed to gaussian distribution or, if not, the central 95% range must be estimated using non-parametric methods. Parametric analysis permits calculation of the central 95% reference limits as the mean ± 1.96 SD. The multiples of SD must be increased as sample size decreases, e.g. for $n = 20$, use mean ± 2.56 SD to ensure a 0.9 probability that the lower and upper limits will include 95% of similar individuals (for gaussian data distributions).

Manufacturers of analytical systems often provide reference limits for the species but seldom include information describing the source of reference individuals, the state of health, age, management, sample size or the statistical procedures used.

When a new methodology is introduced into a laboratory, temporary reference limits for the new method may have to be estimated. Samples from healthy and sick individuals should be tested using the old and new method over a broad range of values. The observations are plotted on a graph and compared mathematically or visually to estimate reference limits for the new method for use until correctly validated reference values are determined.

There is another aspect that clinicians must consider when interpreting laboratory data. When reference limits are calculated to include 95% of healthy individuals, 5% of similar individuals are excluded. Thus, an individual with characteristics similar to the reference individuals, but without disease, may have an observed value up to 1 SD outside the reference limits 5 in 100 times. When using multiple tests, such as clinical chemistry profiles, there is an increasing probability that one or more observed value from a healthy individual will be outside the reference limits. In a 20-test profile from a healthy individual, there is a 64% probability ($p = 0.64$) that one or more observed value may be one SD outside the reference limits (calculated as $(0.95)^n$ for independent variables, where n is the sample size).

The greater the understanding of the source and confidence in reference limits, the greater the probability of correct interpretation of observed patient values.

What are the alternatives to comparing observed patient values with reference limits? There are two major alternatives. One is to report all patient observations as a percentile relative to previous observations (Little, 1997). Electronic databases allow comparison to be made with similar species and possibly specific subsets including breed, age and sex. When a new method is introduced data must be accumulated before percentiles can be calculated.

The clinician must be aware of the demographics of the database in order to apply decision limits. Laboratories differ with geographical area and whether they are serving primary, secondary or even tertiary care patients. Clinicians will require training to use this alternative to reference values.

The other major alternative approach is to develop and use diagnostic characteristics of laboratory tests, as increasingly described in clinical reports. Some are simple, such as diagnostic sensitivity and specificity. Others are more complex, such as the predictive value of positive and negative tests, or likelihood ratios, at specific cut-off points or decision limits.

For example, if the clinician has predetermined the likelihood of a specific disease being present, and the diagnostic value of a laboratory test has been predetermined for that disease at specific cut-off points or decision limits, then the post-test probability of disease can be determined.

DIAGNOSTIC CHARACTERISTICS OF LABORATORY DATA

How do clinicians make a diagnosis (Sackett *et al.*, 1991; Kraemer, 1992; Bonnett, 1994; Kassirer, 1995)? Two approaches, the *hypotheticodeductive* and the *inductive* approaches are discussed. It is suggested that experienced diagnosticians, most of the time, use the hypotheticodeductive process (Kraemer, 1992). The history and presenting signs are used to establish a list of possible explanations (hypotheses). Each hypothesis is assigned a likelihood (probability), often at the subconscious level. Further clinical or paraclinical examinations (tests) are initiated. Tests are chosen that are expected to increase or decrease the probabilities for the hypotheses until one most likely explanation remains, or until further differentiation is unlikely to alter treatment or is uneconomical. The clinical information, and the experience of the clinician, establish the likelihood of a disease being present (prior probability). If a test is used with established characteristics of accuracy (diagnostic sensitivity (Sn) and specificity (Sp)), the post-test probability of disease can be determined. Diagnostic sensitivity is defined as a positive test result when the animal has the disease; diagnostic specificity is a negative test result when there is no disease. For a test to be useful, the results must *increase*, or *decrease*, the post-test probability of the disease being present, i.e. have a high positive or negative predictive value, respectively.

Predictive values of tests incorporate diagnostic sensitivity, diagnostic specificity and disease *prevalence*. Disease prevalence has a significant effect upon test predictive values. The clinician determines when a test will be used. Is the test being used to support or rule out suspected disease or is it being used to screen all individuals for possible disease, irrespective of whether there is suspicion of disease? Where and how the clinician uses the test will affect the *apparent* prevalence of the disease and thus will greatly alter the predictive value of tests when test diagnostic sensitivity and specificity remain the same. For example, the predictive value of serum bile acid observations will be higher when obtained from dogs with suspected liver disease than when observed from routine chemistry profiles for all sick dogs.

Encouragingly, there are an increasing number of clinical evaluations reporting test diagnostic sensitivity and specificity. When test diagnostic sensitivity and specificity are determined for decision limits (cut-off-point(s)) between diseased and clinically healthy animals, high estimates of diagnostic sensitivity and specificity are obtained, e.g. 95%, which make the test look very good. The cut-off points used in such studies are usually the laboratory reference limits. If the clinician is asking whether the patient value is similar or different from a healthy animal, these test diagnostic characteristics are valid.

More often, the clinician wants to differentiate between diseases that may present with similar clinical signs. This is a very different question. In this setting, the test diagnostic sensitivity and specificity are usually much lower and more closely approximate expected clinical usefulness. Diagnostic characteristics such as sensitivity and specificity have been developed for many serological tests but the user must examine each report to confirm whether the cut-off point used was between sick and healthy individuals or between sick individuals with similar signs but different diseases.

Test predictive values can be calculated using multiple decision limits and presented as likelihood ratios or as differential positive rates (Sackett *et al.*, 1991; Jensen, 1994). Alternatively, test receiver operating characteristics can be determined and presented in a graph to provide a visual explanation of the effects of increasing of decreasing the decision limit, or cut-off point, on test diagnostic sensitivity and specificity (Sackett *et al.*, 1991; Jensen, 1994). Test diagnostic characteristics are being studied in increasing numbers of clinical settings. Clinicians should become familiar with the significance of these various test diagnostic characteristics in order to interpret laboratory data well.

Another approach to diagnosis used by many clinicians is inductive. A database is developed that incorporates all information obtained from the history, clinical examination and the laboratory tests. The number of tests used may vary greatly, i.e. haematology and clinical chemistry profiles. Diseases are considered, or rejected, after considering the total database. Additional information (tests) may be required. The laboratory data are interpreted utilizing test diagnostic characteristics such as predictive values, if known. More often there is heavy reliance upon the laboratory 'normal' values and the experience of the clinician. The logic used may be confusing, especially to inexperienced clinicians who may erroneously assume that test results outside reference limits must be associated with patient abnormality and thus disease, or, alternatively, are in error and should be ignored.

The primary objective of the clinician is to identify and to differentiate disease. To do this the clinician must be familiar with both the analytical and diagnostic characteristics of laboratory tests in order to make informed decisions regarding test selection and interpretation.

REFERENCES AND FURTHER READING

Bonnett BN (1994) Proper interpretation of diagnostic tests. In: *Proceedings of the VI Congress of the International Society for Animal Clinical Biochemistry*, ed. JH Lumsden, pp. 19–21. University of Guelph, Guelph

Glick MR, Ryder KW and Glick SJ (1991) *Interferographs: User's Guide to Interferences in Clinical Chemistry Instruments. 2nd edn.* Science Enterprises, Inc., Indianapolis

Jacobs RM, Lumsden JH and Grift E (1992) Effects of bilirubinemia, hemolysis, and lipemia on clinical chemistry analytes in bovine, canine, equine, and feline sera. *Canadian Veterinary Journal* 33, 605–608

Jensen AL (1994) *Methods for the evaluation of laboratory tests and test results.* Thesis: The Royal Veterinary and Agricultural University, Denmark

Kassirer JP (1995) Teaching problem-solving – how are we doing? *New England Journal of Medicine* **332**, 1507–1509

Kraemer HC (1992) *Evaluating Medical Tests.* Sage Publications, Newbury Park

Kringle RO (1994) Statistical procedures. In: *Tietz Textbook of Clinical Chemistry, 2nd edn*, ed. CA Burtis and ER Ashwood, p. 441. WB Saunders, London

Little CJL, Gettinby G and Irvine D (1997) Rarity indices for clinical chemistry data based upon distrubutors found in a large veterinary hospital database. In: *Proceedings of the VI Congress of the International Society for Animal Clinical Biochemistry*, ed. JH Lumsden, p. 25. University of Guelph, Guelph

Lumsden JH and Mullen K (1978) On establishing reference values. *Canadian Journal of Comparative Medicine* **42**, 293–301

Lumsden JH (1989) Clinical chemistry: in-clinic analysis, quality control, reference values, and system selection. *Veterinary Clinics of North America: Small Animal Practice* 19: 875–897

Sackett DL, Haynes RB, Guyatt GH and Tugwell P (1991) *Clinical Epidemiology: A Basic Science for Clinical Medicine, 2nd edn.* Little, Brown and Co., London

Solberg HH (1994) Establishment and use of reference values. In: *Tietz Textbook of Clinical Chemistry, 2nd edn*, ed. CA Burtis and ER Ashwood, pp. 454–484. WB Saunders, London

Young DS (1990) *Effects of Drugs on Clinical Laboratory Tests.* AACC Press, Washington

CHAPTER THREE

Basic Haematology

Elizabeth Villiers and John K. Dunn

INTRODUCTION

This chapter describes the various methods of performing blood cell counts and measuring red blood cell indices that are required to produce a haemogram. All the reference values quoted in this chapter are from Central Diagnostic Services, Department of Clinical Veterinary Medicine, University of Cambridge, unless otherwise stated.

A haematology profile should always include examination of a blood smear, since morphological abnormalities, such as toxic neutrophils or spherocytic red blood cells, provide vital information about the underlying disease process. Techniques for making and examining blood smears are described.

Abnormalities in cell number, such as anaemia, neutrophilia and neutropenia, are discussed. The clinicopathological approach to disorders of blood coagulation and the common coagulopathies are considered. Finally, techniques for sampling and cytological evaluation of the bone marrow are described.

HAEMOPOIESIS

Haemopoiesis is the process by which blood cells are formed; it takes place primarily in the bone marrow. In neonates all bones are involved, but as the animal reaches maturity haemopoiesis becomes restricted to the marrow of the flat bones such as the sternum, ribs, pelvis and vertebrae, and the proximal end of the long bones, in particular the humerus and femur. All types of blood cell are produced in the bone marrow but lymphocytes are also produced in the peripheral lymphoid tissue (the lymph nodes, spleen and thymus). The liver and spleen are sites of haemopoiesis in the fetus; these organs retain the capacity to produce blood cells in the adult but extramedullary haemopoiesis only takes place in response to chronic hypoxic stimulation in anaemic animals.

The haemopoietic cells of the bone marrow consist of three groups of cells: pluripotent stem cells (Figure 3.1); differentiating progenitor cells; and mature blood cells. The most primitive stem cells have the potential

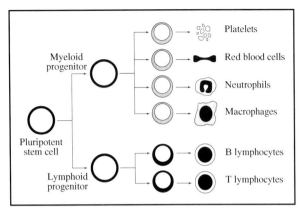

Figure 3.1: The haemopoietic cells of the bone marrow. The pluripotent stem cell gives rise to myeloid and erythroid progenitor cells which, in turn, give rise to committed CFUs.

to develop into any type of blood cell and are capable of self-renewal. They divide to form two types of committed stem cell: lymphoid stem cells and myeloid stem cells. Myeloid stem cells, capable of developing into all blood cells except lymphocytes, divide to form committed colony-forming units (CFUs) or burst-forming units (BFUs). Monocytes and neutrophils derive from the CFU-GM, megakaryocytes from the CFU-megakaryocyte, eosinophils from the CFU-Eo, basophils from the CFU-Baso, and red blood cells from the BFU-E.

Red blood cells

The fundamental stimulus for production of red blood cells (erythropoiesis) is erythropoietin, a glycoprotein produced by the kidneys in response to renal tissue hypoxia. Other hormones, such as corticosteroids, thyroid hormone and androgens, stimulate the production or release of erythropoietin but have no intrinsic erythropoietic activity.

BFU-Es divide and differentiate into CFUs and then into proerythroblasts under the influence of erythropoietin. Proerythroblasts continue to divide and differentiate into early normoblasts; these develop into intermediate and then late normoblasts. The late normoblast has a pyknotic nucleus and is incapable of cell division. A reticulocyte is formed when the nucleus is extruded. Reticulocytes remain in the bone marrow for 24–48 hours before they are released into the blood, where they reach full maturation after 24–48 hours. Reticulocytes are larger than mature red blood cells (erythrocytes) and show poly-chromatophilic (bluish-pink) cytoplasm with Romanowsky staining. The marrow transit time (proerythroblast to reticulocyte) in the dog is approximately 7 days. Haemoglobin synthesis takes place in immature red cells, including reticulocytes; mature red cells cannot synthesize haemoglobin. If the rate of haemoglobin synthesis is reduced, for example in iron deficiency, the marrow transit time is prolonged and additional cell division results in the production of smaller (microcytic) cells. The average

lifespan of a circulating erythrocyte is 110–120 days in the dog and 68 days in the cat. Aged or damaged red cells are removed primarily by macrophages in the liver, spleen and bone marrow.

Neutrophils

The production of neutrophils, eosinophils and basophils is termed granulopoiesis. In the production of neutrophils, CFU-GMs are stimulated to divide and differentiate, under the influence of colony stimulating factor (CSF), to form myeloblasts. The myeloblast divides and differentiates into promyelocytes (with distinctive primary granules) which, in turn, divide into myelocytes (in which the granules are no longer visible; Figure 3.2) and then metamyelocytes. After this stage there is no further cell division. Between 16 and 32 metamyelocytes are produced from one myeloblast. The metamyelocyte differentiates into a band cell and then finally into a mature neutrophil. These last three stages of the cells constitute the 'storage pool'. This acts as a reserve should there be a sudden demand for neutrophils; it contains about 5 days' supply of cells. A myeloblast can develop into a mature neutrophil in about 4 days. Mature neutrophils remain in the bone marrow for an additional 2 days, although they can be released earlier on demand. In an increased demand for neutrophils there is a lag phase of 3–4 days before an increased rate of granulopoiesis occurs, although bands and neutrophils may be released from the storage pool within hours of the causative insult.

The neutrophils in the bloodstream either circulate freely (the circulating pool) or adhere to the vascular endothelium (the marginal pool). In the dog the marginal pool and the circulating pool are approximately equal in size, whilst in the cat the marginal pool is two to three times larger than the circulating pool. There is a continual exchange of cells between these two pools. The half-life of circulating neutrophils is only 6–14 hours, after which time they leave the circulation and pass into the tissue pool. The circulating time is shortened during acute infections as neutrophils pass to the

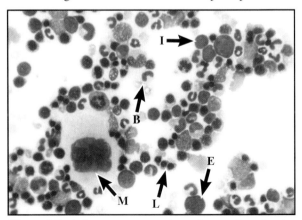

Figure 3.2: A bone marrow aspirate from a dog showing normal haematopoiesis. B = band neutrophil; E= early normoblast; I = intermediate normoblast; L = late normoblast; M = megakaryocyte. May-Grünwald Giemsa.

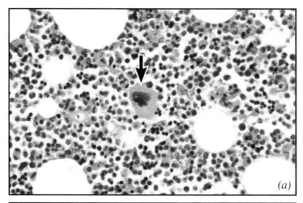

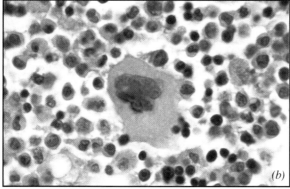

Figure 3.3: *(a) A histological section of normal femoral bone marrow from an adult cat, showing fat spaces and a megakaryocyte (arrowed) in addition to normal blast forms. (b) Higher power view of the megakaryocyte. H&E.*
Courtesy of Dr R.W. Else.

site of infection in the tissues. The main function of the neutrophil is the phagocytosis of pyogenic bacteria.

Monoblasts share a common precursor (the CFU-GM) with neutrophils. They have fewer maturation steps and divide and differentiate into promonocytes and then monocytes. After circulating in the blood for a few hours to several days, the monocytes enter the tissues, where they develop into mobile macrophages (e.g. pulmonary macrophages) and fixed macrophages (e.g. Kupffer cells) that can live for several weeks to months.

Lymphocytes

Lymphoid primitive stem cells divide and differentiate into pre-B lymphocytes and pre-T lymphocytes in the bone marrow. Pre-T lymphocytes mature and proliferate into T cells in the thymus. Pre-B cells proliferate in the bone marrow and migrate to peripheral lymphoid organs (spleen and lymph nodes) where further proliferation takes place.

Platelets

Platelets are produced from the cytoplasm of megakaryocytes (Figure 3.3). The megakaryoblast and its progeny undergo nuclear replication without cell division, resulting in the formation of very large cells, with 8–32 nuclei and abundant cytoplasm. Platelets are formed when the surface membrane of the megakaryocyte invaginates to form small islets of membrane-

bound cytoplasm. Megakaryocytes sit on the outside surface of vascular sinuses in the marrow and deliver platelets directly into the vascular lumen. Several thousand platelets are produced from each megakaryocyte. The entire process of megakaryocyte differentiation and maturation takes 3 days in dogs. The number of megakaryocytes is regulated by the circulating platelet mass; hence thrombocytopenia is normally followed by a rebound thrombocytosis, although there is a lag phase of approximately 3 days before increased platelet production is evident in the blood. Once in the circulation, platelets survive for 8–12 days. Up to 20–30% of circulating platelets can be sequestered in the spleen; the figure may be a high as 90% if there is splenomegaly. Old or damaged platelets are removed from the circulation by the spleen, liver and bone marrow.

ROUTINE HAEMATOLOGY

The complete blood count is an integral part of the diagnostic investigation of any systemic disease process. It consists of two components:

- A quantitative examination of the cells, including packed cell volume (PCV), total red cell count, total white cell count, differential white cell count, platelet count, mean corpuscular volume (MCV), mean corpuscular haemoglobin (MCH), mean corpuscular haemoglobin concentration (MCHC), and total plasma protein concentration
- A qualitative examination of blood smears for changes in cellular morphology.

For routine haematology, blood is collected into an EDTA tube (a commercially available tube containing a quantity of EDTA anticoagulant). The tube should be filled precisely to the level indicated, since underfilling may alter cell size and morphology and overfilling may lead to clot formation. Blood smears should be made soon after obtaining a blood sample, or cellular degeneration will impede interpretation. If a delay in processing is expected, the blood sample should be stored in the refrigerator and smears should be fixed in methanol for 3 minutes.

Quantitative examination

Packed cell volume
(Reference ranges: 0.37–0.55 l/l for the dog; 0.26–0.45 l/l for the cat.)

Anticoagulated blood is centrifuged in capillary ('microhaematocrit') tubes for 5 minutes at high speed (12,500–15,000 rpm). The red cells are concentrated at the bottom of the tube, with old or senescent cells at the bottom and young red cells at the top of the layer. The leucocytes (white blood cells) form a grey/cream layer on top of the red cells – the buffy coat. The platelets lie at the top of the buffy coat and may be discernible as a thin cream-coloured layer. The plasma is found above the platelet layer. The PCV is calculated by dividing the length of the packed red cells by the combined length of the packed red cells, buffy coat and plasma.

Examination of the microhaematocrit tube provides other useful information. Gross examination of the plasma detects icterus, haemolysis or lipaemia. A very broad estimate of the white cell count can be made by calculating the proportion of the sample occupied by the buffy coat (buffy coat depth divided by the combined length of the red cells, buffy coat and plasma). The first 1% equates to a concentration of 10×10^9 white cells per litre and each percent thereafter equates to 20×10^9 cells/l.

The interface between the buffy coat and the packed red cells should be clearly defined. If it is poorly defined and has a pinkish tinge this indicates the presence of increased numbers of reticulocytes and/or nucleated red cells.

Counting blood cells

Cell counts may be performed using an in-house manual haemocytometer. Automated haematology cell counters provide cell counts and also evaluate red cell indices and haemoglobin concentration.

Using a manual haemocytometer: A haemocytometer is a glass chamber which holds a thin suspension of blood cells that can be examined with a microscope. The Improved Neubauer haemocytometer has a chamber that is 0.1 mm deep and is divided into a grid precisely 3 mm x 3 mm (Figure 3.4). Blood is first diluted to a concentration suitable for the cells to be counted, using specific diluents supplied with the haemocytometer.

For counting red cells, the blood is diluted 200-fold; for platelets, the dilution factor is 100. Since there are fewer white than red blood cells in whole blood, the dilution factor for counting leucocytes is only 20. The white cell diluent lyses the red cells, facilitating rapid white cell counting.

To perform a total white cell count using the Improved Neubauer haemocytometer, the four corner squares of the chamber are used (marked W in Figure 3.4) and the total number of white cells counted is multiplied by the conversion factor 50, to give the white cell count per microlitre. (The conversion factors for red and white blood cells and for platelets are determined by the depth of the chamber, the area counted and the dilution factor.)

Since the red cell concentration is much higher, a smaller area is counted. The central square millimetre in the grid is subdivided into 25 smaller squares; five of these subdivisions are used (marked R in Figure 3.4) and the total number of red cells counted is multiplied by 1000 to give the red cell count per microlitre.

For platelets, two squares (one on each side of the

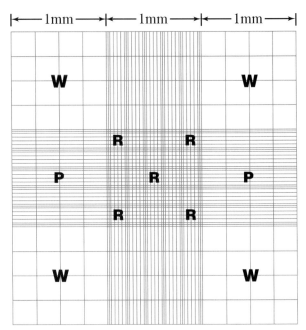

Figure 3.4: The haemocytometer grid. The squares marked W are used for estimating total white cells; those marked R are used for red cell counts and those marked P for platelets. See text for details.

central square) are used (marked P in Figure 3.4) and the total number of platelets counted is multiplied by 500 to give the platelet count per microlitre.

Cell counts should be performed in duplicate by using the grids on both sides of the haemocytometer. If the two counts vary by >10% for white cells and >20% for red cells the test should be repeated.

Commercial kits are available to provide a standardized procedure for pipetting and diluting whole blood and have the advantage that they do not involve pipetting by mouth.

Automated counters: Quantitative buffy coat (QBC) machines rely on the separation of red cells, granulocytes, monocytes and platelets into various layers. The cell counts are determined from the width of the layers. A two-part differential white cell count is produced, which gives a granulocyte count (neutrophils, eosinophils and basophils) and a combined lymphocyte/monocyte count.

Coulter counter machines count blood cells by measuring their electrical resistance as they pass through an aperture. The total white cell count, red cell count, platelet count, total haemoglobin concentration and mean red cell volume are measured, and the haematocrit (HCT), MCH and MCHC are calculated (see below).

Newer electronic counters provide differential white cell counts and measures of red cell distribution width (RDW, see below).

Laser cell counters use a laser detection system to measure the light scattered by cells. These machines provide a large amount of detailed information, including red cell count, total haemoglobin concentration,

	Dogs	**Cats**
Total red blood cells (x 10^{12}/l)	5.5–8.5	5.0–10.0
Haemoglobin (g/dl)	12.0–18.0	8.0–15.0
PCV (l/l)	0.37–0.55	0.26–0.45
MCV (fl)	60.0–77.0	39.0–55.0
MCH (pg)	19.5–24.5	12.5–17.5
MCHC (g/dl)	32.0–37.0	30.0–36.0

Table 3.1: Reference values for red cell indices.

HCT, RDW, total white cell count, differential white cell count, platelet count, and mean platelet volume. In addition, histograms are produced which illustrate: the distribution of red cells (according to cell size and haemoglobin concentration); the platelet population (according to size); and the various white cells (according to size, peroxidase content and nuclear density). These histograms give information about the whole cell population and may unearth subpopulations of cells; for example, a small number of microcytic (small) red cells might not be detectable from the MCV but would be seen on the histogram.

A blood smear should always be evaluated in conjunction with automated cell counts as part of routine quality control procedures and to assess red cell abnormalities, toxic neutrophils (see below), a left shift (see below), the presence of platelet clumps, or other alterations. If a QBC machine is being used, a blood smear will be needed to determine a more detailed differential white cell count, for quality control and also to examine for cell abnormalities.

Red cell indices

Knowledge of the MCH and MCHC are helpful in the evaluation of anaemia, particularly in the dog. Reference values for red cell indices are shown in Table 3.1. Individual laboratories may have different reference values.

Mean corpuscular volume (MCV): The MCV indicates the average size of the red blood cells. Normocytic cells have normal MCV; macrocytic cells have increased MCV; and microcytic cells have low MCV.

Increased MCV may be seen in:

• Regenerative anaemia (most common cause). Increased numbers of reticulocytes/immature red cells are present in the circulation. Since these cells are larger than mature erythrocytes, the MCV is elevated
• FeLV-related non-regenerative macrocytic anaemia
• Myeloproliferative disease (uncommon cause)
• Vitamin B12 and/or folate deficiency

(uncommon causes)
• Familial macrocytosis in the Poodle (rare) (Canfield and Watson, 1989).

Decreased MCV may be seen in:

• Iron deficiency due to chronic blood loss (most common cause). Iron is required for the synthesis of haemoglobin. Degeneration and extrusion of the nucleus in the maturing red cell is triggered when a critical concentration of haemoglobin has been reached. In iron deficiency, haemoglobin synthesis is slower and so nuclear degeneration is delayed. The red cell undergoes extra cell divisions, resulting in the formation of a microcyte
• Congenital portosystemic shunts in dogs
• Familial microcytosis without anaemia in the Akita.

The MCV may be measured accurately using automatic haematology instruments or may be calculated as follows, with units shown in parentheses:

$$\text{MCV (fl)} = \frac{\text{PCV (l/l)} \times 1000}{\text{total red cells (x } 10^{12}\text{/l)}}$$

Mean corpuscular haemoglobin (MCH): The MCH indicates the amount (weight) of haemoglobin per average red blood cell and is affected by both the size of the red cells and their average haemoglobin concentration. Falling MCH may give an early clue of impending iron deficiency, since MCH falls before MCV.

The MCH may be calculated as follows:

$$\text{MCH (pg)} = \frac{\text{total haemoglobin (g/dl)} \times 10}{\text{total red blood cells (x } 10^{12}\text{/l)}}$$

Since these calculations depend upon the accuracy of the red cell count and, for MCH, the haemoglobin concentration, they are less reliable than automated measurements and may be subject to considerable variation between serial samples.

Mean corpuscular haemoglobin concentration (MCHC): The MCHC indicates the average concentration of haemoglobin per red blood cell. Decreased MCHC is indicated by hypochromasia.

Decreased MCHC occurs in:

• Regenerative anaemias, where the larger, immature red cells and reticulocytes contain relatively less haemoglobin per cell than normal-sized red cells
• Iron-deficiency anaemia.

Elevated MCHC may occur:

• As an artefact due to haemolysis

	Dogs		Cats	
	Percentage	Absolute value (x 10⁹/l)	Percentage	Absolute value (x 10⁹/l)
Total white cell count (x 10⁹/l)	n/a	6–17	n/a	5.5–19.5
Band neutrophils	0–3	0– 0.3	0–3	0– 0.3
Neutrophils	60–77	3–11.5	35–75	2.5–12.5
Lymphocytes	12–30	1–4.8	20–55	1.5–7
Monocytes	3–10	0.2–1.5	1–4	0–1.5
Eosinophils	2–10	0.1–1.3	2–12	0–1.5
Basophils	rare	rare	rare	rare

Table 3.2: Reference ranges for total and differential white blood cell counts.

- If large numbers of spherocytes are present (e.g. in immune-mediated haemolytic anaemia) where fragments of cell membrane have been lost from the cell without loss of haemoglobin.

The MCHC may be calculated as follows:

$$\text{MCHC (g/dl)} = \frac{\text{total haemoglobin (g/dl)}}{\text{PCV (l/l)}}$$

This calculation has a better reproducibility than MCH because the variability in red cell count is not a factor.

Red cell distribution width (RDW): The RDW describes the variability in red cell size. It is more sensitive than the MCV. A relatively large number of cells must have altered size before the *mean* value (MCV) is altered. The RDW considers the size distribution of the entire population of red blood cells rather than giving one average value.

Differential white cell counts

The differential white cell count is performed by counting 200 leucocytes in a blood smear. The cells are counted along the long edge of the smear, using the battlement meander method: four high-power fields are counted in one direction, then four more in a direction at right angles to the first, and so on, following the shape of a battlement. The percentage of each type of cell is determined. This percentage is then multiplied by the total white cell count to obtain an absolute count for each cell type. The absolute count, rather than the percentage, should always be considered when evaluating the leucogram (white cell count). Reference values for the total and differential white cell counts are shown in Table 3.2. In both the dog and the cat the predominant leucocyte is the neutrophil, but the cat has a lower neutrophil:lymphocyte ratio than the dog because there are relatively more lymphocytes present. Abnormalities in white blood cell numbers are discussed below.

Plasma protein concentration

(Reference range: 60–80 g/l for the dog and cat)

Total plasma protein is measured using a refractometer. The capillary tube is scored and broken above the buffy coat layer and a few drops of plasma placed onto the prism of the refractometer. Most refractometers have scales calculated for plasma protein and urine specific gravity. If the scale is graduated only for refractive index, a conversion chart is necessary. Values may be falsely increased in hyperlipaemia, haemolysis and hyperbilirubinaemia. Plasma protein may also be measured using a biochemical analyser.

Total plasma protein (TPP) and PCV should be interpreted together. Recent or ongoing external haemorrhage results in reductions in both PCV and TPP, though TPP does not fall as much with internal haemorrhage. A low TPP with a normal PCV usually indicates hypoalbuminaemia (e.g. chronic liver disease, glomerulonephropathy). A high PCV and increased TPP are seen with dehydration. A high TPP with normal or low PCV is seen with myeloma and some B cell lymphomas. Evaluation of albumin and globulin concentrations and, in some cases, protein electrophoresis are indicated to investigate persistently low or high TPP.

Qualitative examination of a blood smear

A blood smear should always be evaluated when automated cell counts are made or when in-practice instrumentation is limited to a centrifuge for PCV.

Preparation of a blood smear

A small drop of blood is placed on one end of a glass slide, using a capillary tube. A spreader slide (made by breaking off the corner of another slide, after scoring it with a glass cutter or diamond writer) is placed on to the slide holding the blood drop, in front of the drop and at an angle of 20–40°. The spreader slide is slid backwards until its short edge comes into contact with the blood drop which then spreads out along the width of the spreader slide. The spreader slide is narrower than the sample slide, so the blood will not go over the edge. The spreader slide is then advanced forward smoothly and rapidly, producing a smear with a feathered edge. Slides should be air-dried and then fixed in methanol for 3 minutes before staining with Wright's stain or May–Grünwald Giemsa.

The technique for making blood smears is further discussed and illustrated in Chapter 7.

Cells adjacent to the long edge of the smear should be examined using the oil immersion x100 objective.

Evaluation of red cells

The canine erythrocyte has a wide rim of haemoglobin and an area of central pallor. The feline RBC is smaller and has minimal central pallor. Evaluation of the red cells should include an assessment of colour, size and shape. The cells should be evaluated for various types of inclusions and, in the cat, for the parasite *Haemobartonella felis*.

Colour: Polychromatophilic cells are larger than erythrocytes and stain blue-grey with Giemsa or Wright's stains. They may not be visible if rapid dunking-style staining kits are used. These cells equate to canine reticulocytes and feline aggregate reticulocytes. Normally only the occasional polychromatophilic cell is seen. Increased numbers of polychromatophilic cells, described as polychromasia (Figure 3.5), indicates increased release of immature red cells from the bone marrow. The degree of polychromasia is graded on a scale of occasional to 4+, according to the number of polychromatic red cells seen in each high-power field (hpf) (Table 3.3). Polychromasia is seen less frequently in cats since the red cells tend to remain in the marrow until they are only weakly polychromatophilic.

Pale-staining red cells contain reduced amounts of haemoglobin and are termed hypochromic. They are seen in iron deficiency (e.g. due to chronic haemorrhage) and are often also microcytic. Reticulocytes also have reduced amounts of haemoglobin (synthesis is not yet completed), but these are not pale staining; their characteristic blue-grey appearance is due to increased amounts of ribosomal RNA.

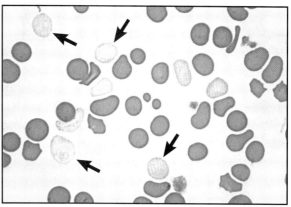

Figure 3.5: *Peripheral blood smear from a dog with anisocytosis and polychromasia of red cells. Larger blue-staining polychromatic cells are seen (arrowed). Leishman.*
Courtesy of Dr D.L. Doxey.

Size: Anisocytosis refers to a variation in cell size and may be due to the presence of macrocytic cells (usually reticulocytes) or microcytic cells (e.g. due to iron deficiency). Macrocytosis is graded according to the degree of enlargement of the macrocytes and the number of macrocytes per hpf (Table 3.3).

Shape: Poikilocytosis describes an alteration in red cell shape and may be indicative of abnormal erythropoiesis or specific organ dysfunction. There are a number of characteristic morphological changes:

- Leptocytes (target cells) (Figure 3.6) are thin, flexible cells with increased surface area. They have a dark rim of haemoglobin with a wider area of central pallor in which a small circle of haemoglobin is seen. They are seen in liver disease and in anaemias associated with chronic inflammation or neoplasia
- Acanthocytes (spur cells) (Figure 3.7) have rounded projections of variable length and may be seen in several disorders, including liver disease and splenic haemangiosarcoma
- Spherocytes (Figure 3.7) are small, round, densely staining cells that lack central pallor. They represent cells whose membranes have

Grade	Polychromasia in dogs	Polychromasia in cats	Macrocytosis (dogs and cats)
occasional	<1 cell per hpf	<1 cell every other hpf	slightly larger cells; <1 cell per hpf
1+	1–2 cells per hpf	<1 cell per hpf	slightly larger cells; 1–2 cells per hpf
2+	2–4 cells per hpf	1–2 cells per hpf	slightly larger and larger still cells present; 3–5 cells per hpf
3+	4–8 cells per hpf	3–5 cells per hpf	large cells present; 5–10 per hpf
4+	>8 cells per hpf	>5 cells per hpf	large cells present; >10 per hpf

Table 3.3: *A grading system for polychromasia and macrocytosis in dogs and cats. This grading is somewhat subjective and will also depend on the thickness of the smear and the total number of cells per high-power field (hpf). Grading systems may vary slightly between laboratories. (Values for polychromasia in cats taken from Loar (1994); other values from the University of Cambridge.)*

been partially phagocytosed by macrophages and are characteristic of immune-mediated haemolytic anaemia. They are difficult to identify in feline blood because normal feline erythrocytes are small and have minimal central pallor

- Schistocytes (Figure 3.7) are red cells that have been cleaved or fragmented following passage through a meshwork of fibrin filaments in the microvasculature. They are a feature of disseminated intravascular coagulation (DIC), haemangiosarcoma, congestive heart failure, and glomerulonephritis
- Crenated red cells have numerous short, evenly spaced surface projections of uniform dimension. Crenation is an artefactual change that occurs if there is a delay in making smears or if the drying time of the blood smear is prolonged (e.g. if the smear is too thick). It also occurs if the EDTA tube is underfilled, creating a relative excess of anticoagulant. Markedly crenated cells are sometimes seen in uraemia. Crenated cells must be differentiated from acanthocytes, which have irregular projections.

Inclusions: A variety of inclusions may be found in red blood cells:

- Howell–Jolly bodies are remnants of nuclear material, seen as small single refractile blue bodies. Cats frequently have significant numbers of Howell–Jolly bodies without anemia. Increased numbers are seen in regenerative anaemias and in splenectomized animals
- Heinz bodies are round refractile inclusions lying along the inner surface of the red cell membrane. They are best demonstrated with new methylene blue staining. Large numbers indicate exposure to oxidant chemicals or drugs, e.g. paracetamol toxicity, onion toxicity in dogs, or zinc toxicity following ingestion of nuts and bolts or coins (Luttgen *et al.*, 1990). Heinz body formation following oxidative damage results in haemolytic anaemia as the cells are phagocytosed by the mononuclear phagocytic system. Normal cats may have Heinz bodies in up to 10% of their red cells, not associated with anaemia
- Basophilic stippling (Figure 3.8) is visible with Romanowsky staining as multiple, small, dark blue punctate aggregates within the red cells. It is seen in highly regenerative anaemias and in lead poisoning (Morgan *et al.*, 1991)

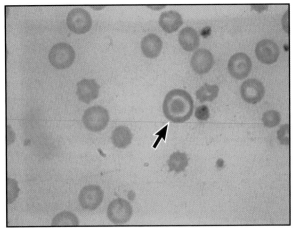

Figure 3.6: *Peripheral blood film from a dog, with a leptocyte (target cell) (arrowed). Leishman.*

Courtesy of Dr D.L. Doxey.

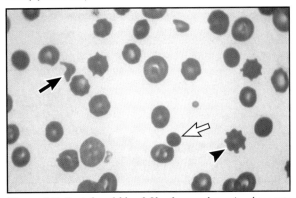

Figure 3.7: *Peripheral blood film from a dog. A spherocyte (open arrow) is small and lacks central pallor. A schistocyte (closed arrow) is an irregularly shaped fragment of a red cell. An acanthocyte (arrowhead) has irregular surface projections. May–Grünwald Giemsa.*

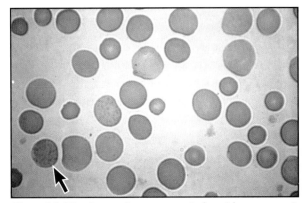

Figure 3.8: *Blood smear from an anaemic dog with macrocytosis and basophilic stippling (arrowed) of red cells. Leishman.*

Courtesy of Dr R.W. Else.

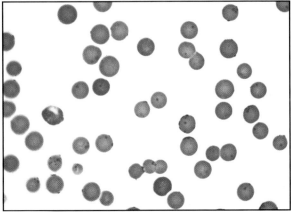

Figure 3.9: *Peripheral blood film from a cat with* Haemo-bartonella felis *infection. May–Grünwald Giemsa.*

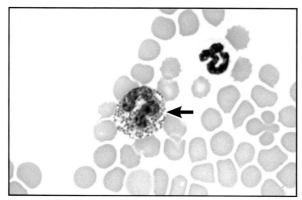

Figure 3.10: Peripheral blood smear from a dog, showing a mature neutrophil and a normal eosinophil (arrowed).

Courtesy of Dr D.L. Doxey.

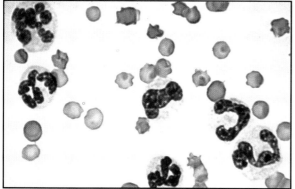

Figure 3.11: Peripheral blood smear from a bitch with pyometra showing an increased number of neutrophils, some of which show toxic change with vacuolated blue-pink cytoplasm. Leishman.

Courtesy of Dr R.W. Else.

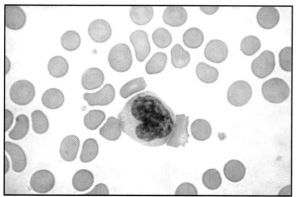

Figure 3.12: Peripheral blood smear from a healthy dog, showing a monocyte with blue cytoplasm and a band-shaped nucleus. Leishman.

Courtesy of Dr R.W. Else.

• *Haemobartonella felis* organisms can usually be identified with Romanowsky staining (Figure 3.9) but are more easily seen with acridine orange stain. They are very small coccoid organisms and may be located on the edge of or within the cells. They may occur singly or in chains. *Haemobartonella* may be easily confused with stain precipitate. Identification of chains of organisms, or so-called ring forms (with a dark outer rim and a pale interior) helps to confirm the

diagnosis. If *Haemobartonella* is suspected, smears should be made from fresh blood rather than blood submitted in EDTA tubes, since the anticoagulant may dislodge organisms from the red cell surface. The organisms are present only sporadically and smears may have to be examined for several days to detect organisms (Van Steenhouse *et al.*, 1993).

Leucocyte morphology

Neutrophils: Mature neutrophils have an irregularly lobed nucleus and pale cytoplasm which contains diffuse indistinct pale granules (Figure 3.10). Band neutrophils have a smooth horseshoe-shaped nucleus without any indentations or lobulations. Only small numbers of band neutrophils are present in normal blood.

Toxic change may be seen in neutrophils and bands in severe toxaemic states such as severe bacterial infection (Figure 3.11). The cytoplasm stains bluish-pink (distinguished from monocyte cytoplasm which is a darker blue) and with severe toxaemia may be extensively vacuolated. Darker blue, round or angular cytoplasmic bodies known as Döhle bodies may be seen.

Eosinophils: Eosinophils contain a bilobed or segmented nucleus and numerous pink-staining cytoplasmic granules (Figure 3.10). In the cat these granules are rod-shaped, whilst in the dog they are rounder. The granules usually fill the cytoplasm. In the Greyhound, eosinophils have vacuolated cytoplasm.

Basophils: Basophils are rare in normal blood. In the dog they have blue-grey cytoplasm with sparse red-purple cytoplasmic granules. In the cat the cytoplasm is full of pinkish-grey granules or sometimes darkly stained purple granules. Increased numbers of basophils are often seen in association with an eosinophilia.

Monocytes: A monocyte has a nucleus that is pleomorphic (variable in shape and size) and blue-staining 'ground-glass' cytoplasm which may contain numerous small vacuoles (Figure 3.12) . The nucleus is very variable in shape: it may be broad and irregular, without lobulation; or it may resemble the nucleus of a band neutrophil but with (in dogs) enlarged knob-like ends. Monocytes may be distinguished from neutrophils by their relatively darker-staining bluish cytoplasm, larger average size and nuclear morphology.

Lymphocytes: A small lymphocyte has a round nucleus that almost fills the cell, with a narrow rim of pale blue cytoplasm (Figure 3.13). Some have a small nuclear cleft. Lymphocytes are slightly bigger than erythrocytes and smaller than neutrophils. Small numbers of reactive lymphocytes may be seen in healthy animals; these are larger cells, with increased amounts of basophilic cyto-

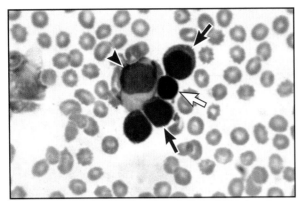

Figure 3.13: Peripheral blood from a dog with lymphoma. A small lymphocyte (open arrow), prolymphocytes (closed arrows) and a lymphoblast (arrow head) are seen. May-Grünwald Giemsa.

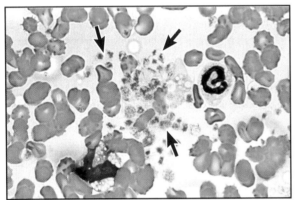

Figure 3.14: Peripheral blood smear from a cat, showing a cluster of platelets (arrowed). Leishman.
Courtesy of Dr R.W. Else.

plasm. Increased numbers of circulating reactive lymphocytes mat be seen after antigenic stimulation or vaccination. Lymphoblasts are two to three times bigger than erythrocytes, and have multiple prominent nucleoli and more basophilic cytoplasm. Lymphoblasts are not found in normal blood but are seen in acute lymphoid leukaemia and, occasionally, small numbers may circulate in association with lymphoma.

Evaluation of the platelets

Morphology: Platelets are small (about one-third the diameter of an erythrocyte), roundish 'packets' of megakaryocyte cytoplasm containing scattered or central pink granules (Figure 3.14). The cell membrane may be smooth or may have fine thread-like projections. Platelet clumping may occur as a result of venepuncture following tissue trauma. The platelet clumps tend to collect towards the feathered edge of the smear. If platelet clumping is observed, then the automated platelet count is invalid and a second sample should be submitted, ensuring that venepuncture is performed smoothly.

Number: Normal reference ranges are 200–500 x 10⁹/l in dogs, and 200–800 x 10⁹/l in cats.

The platelet count may be very roughly estimated by counting the number of platelets in 10 high-power oil immersion fields (x100 magnification) and calculating the average number per field. Each platelet in a single hpf represents approximately 15 x 10⁹ platelets per litre (Mackin, 1995). An average of 10–30 platelets per hpf corresponds to a normal platelet count; < 3 platelets per hpf indicates a marked thrombocytopenia. In a patient with a bleeding disorder, a count of 3 or more platelets per hpf suggests that thrombocytopenia is not the cause of bleeding. Platelet clumping lowers the estimated platelet count and the smear should be scanned, particularly near the feathered edge, to check for clumping.

Size: Large ('shift') platelets indicate increased synthesis of platelets and an active bone marrow. Small platelets (microthrombocytes) with MCV <5.4 fl may be seen in early immune-mediated thrombocytopenia (Northern and Tvedten, 1992). Microthrombocytes are analogous to spherocytes seen in immune-mediated haemolytic anaemia, arising due to phagocytosis of part of the platelet membrane.

ANAEMIA

Anaemia is characterized by an absolute decrease in red cell count, haemoglobin concentration and PCV. Decreased numbers of circulating red cells may be a result of haemorrhage, or of excessive destruction (haemolysis) or inadequate production of red cells.

Regenerative *versus* non-regenerative anaemia

Regenerative anaemias are caused by either haemorrhage or increased haemolysis. In response to the loss of red cells, increased numbers of immature cells are released from the bone marrow. Therefore the characteristics of a regenerative anaemia are polychromasia, macrocytosis with corresponding reduced MCHC, and

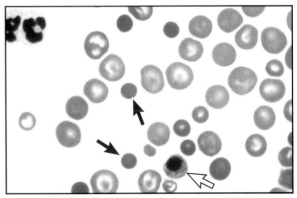

Figure 3.15: Peripheral blood smear from a dog with immune-mediated haemolytic anaemia, showing macrocytic red cells, spherocytes (closed arrows) and an early normoblast (open arrow). May-Grünwald Giemsa. Reproduced from Dunn (1991) with permission.

Morphological classification	Possible aetiology
Macrocytic, hypochromic	Haemorrhage or haemolysis
Normocytic, normochromic	Non-regenerative anaemia or following acute blood loss before erythroid regeneration occurs
Microcytic, normochromic	Iron-deficiency anaemia due to chronic external blood loss
Macrocytic, normochromic	FeLV, myeloproliferative disease, vitamin B12 and/or folate deficiency

Table 3.4: Classification of anaemia according to red cell morphology.

increased numbers of reticulocytes and nucleated red cells (late normoblasts) (Figure 3.15).

It should be noted that an increased number of nucleated red cells does not necessarily indicate a regenerative response. An *inappropriate red cell response* is one where the number of nucleated red cells exceeds the number of reticulocytes; it may occur with damage to the bone marrow stroma (e.g. in myeloproliferative disease or myelofibrosis), with lead poisoning, with decreased splenic function or in response to chronic hypoxia associated with congestive heart failure.

Non-regenerative anaemias may result from a primary failure of haemopoiesis (e.g. aplastic anaemia); such anaemias tend to be severe and, depending on the cause, may be accompanied by other cytopenias. Alternatively, reduced haemopoiesis may be secondary to an underlying metabolic or inflammatory disease. With the exception of renal failure, secondary failure of erythropoiesis tends to result in a mild to moderate anaemia. There is no increase in the number of immature red cells in the circulation and so non-regenerative anaemia is generally normochromic and normocytic, with no increase in the reticulocyte count.

Chronic external blood loss initially results in a moderately regenerative response, but when iron stores become depleted the anaemia becomes poorly regenerative, microcytic and hypochromic.

A macrocytic, normochromic non-regenerative anaemia is occasionally seen in association with feline leukaemia virus (FeLV) infection, myeloproliferative disease (e.g. erythremic myelosis) and vitamin B12 and/or folate deficiency (uncommon in dogs and cats). This type of anaemia is known as nuclear maturation defect anaemia.

Table 3.4 shows the possible aetiology of various types of anaemias, classified according to cell size and MCHC.

Evaluation of the MCV and MCHC, and the presence or absence of polychromasia and anisocytosis, help to distinguish regenerative and non-regenerative anaemias, but the most reliable way of evaluating the bone marrow's response is by measuring the reticulocyte count.

Reticulocyte number

Increased numbers of reticulocytes reflect increased erythropoiesis. Virtually all polychromatophilic red cells are reticulocytes, but not all reticulocytes are polychromatophilic; thus, while polychromasia gives some indication of erythropoietic activity, the reticulocyte count is a much more accurate way of assessing the marrow's response to anaemia. In normal blood, reticulocytes make up 1–2% of the red cells. Following acute haemorrhage or haemolysis, increased numbers of reticulocytes are not evident for at least 72 hours, with maximal production after 7 days. In regenerative anaemias the greater the severity of the anaemia, the higher the reticulocyte percentage should be. For example, in the dog a mild anaemia (e.g. PCV 0.30 l/l) should result in a slight increase in reticulocyte count (e.g. 2–4%), whilst a severe anaemia with a PCV of 0.01 l/l should result in a much higher reticulocyte count (e.g. 20–50%). Haemolytic anaemias generally result in a more marked reticulocytosis than do haemorrhagic anaemias.

Since the reticulocyte percentage is a *proportion* of the total red cells, it needs careful interpretation. As the number of mature red cells falls, the ratio of reticulocytes to mature cells increases, even if the absolute number of reticulocytes remains static. Therefore, a correction for variation in mature red cell number should be made. The absolute reticulocyte count corrects for variation in red cell number, i.e. the degree of anaemia:

absolute reticulocyte count (x 10^9/l) = observed reticulocyte percentage (%)
x total red cell count (x 10^{12}/l) x 10

An absolute aggregate reticulocyte count of >60 x 10^9/l in the dog and of >50 x 10^9/l in the cat is evidence of a regenerative anaemia. Alternatively, the corrected reticulocyte percentage (CRP) can be calculated as follows:

$$CRP (\%) = \frac{observed\ reticulocyte\ percentage\ (\%)\ x\ measured\ PCV\ (\%)}{average\ PCV\ for\ species\ (\%)}$$

A CRP above 1% indicates active erythropoiesis.

With increasing severity of anaemia, reticulocytes spend less time in the maturation pool in the bone marrow and longer in the circulation (1.5–3 days) before maturing into erythrocytes. In the dog the average lifespan of the circulating reticulocyte increases by 12 hours for every 10% decrease in PCV. For this reason the measured reticulocyte percentage may overestimate the degree of erythropoietic activity in the bone marrow. Therefore the CRP should be corrected for changes in maturation time to produce the reticulocyte production index (RPI):

$$RPI = \frac{\text{corrected reticulocyte percentage}}{\text{maturation factor}}$$

The maturation factor depends on the PCV:

Maturation factor (days)	PCV (l/l)
1.0	0.45
1.5	0.35
2.0	0.25
2.5	0.15

An RPI of <1 indicates that the anaemia is non-regenerative; an RPI of 1-2 indicates active erythropoiesis (e.g. blood loss); an RPI of >2 indicates accelerated erythropoiesis; and an RPI of >3 is consistent with haemolysis.

To perform a reticulocyte count, equal parts of blood (in EDTA) and a 0.5% solution of new methylene blue in normal saline are mixed. The solution is left to stand for 10-20 minutes, mixed again, and a smear made. Between 200 and 300 red blood cells (erythrocytes and reticulocytes) are counted to calculate the percentage that are reticulocytes. In the dog all reticulocytes are aggregate reticulocytes, which have large dark-staining clumps of aggregated ribosomes.

Feline reticulocytes: In the cat there are two forms of reticulocyte: aggregate and punctate reticulocytes. The aggregate reticulocytes are immature reticulocytes that have a similar appearance to canine reticulocytes. These mature into punctate reticulocytes, which contain small dots of reticulin (Figure 3.16).

Normal feline blood contains very few aggregate reticulocytes (0-0.9%) and 10% punctate reticulocytes.

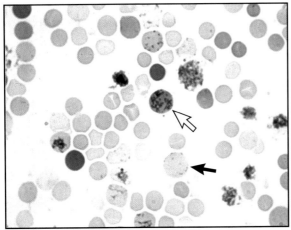

Figure 3.16: Peripheral blood film from a cat, showing aggregate (open arrow) and punctate (closed arrow) reticulocytes staining darkly with new cresol violet.
Courtesy of Dr D.L. Doxey.

Following acute severe loss of red cells the number of aggregate reticulocytes rises sharply, peaking within 4-7 days. Aggregate reticulocytes have a short lifespan and soon mature into punctate reticulocytes which have a much longer lifespan. Punctate reticulocyte numbers may remain elevated for up to 4 weeks following a single episode of blood loss. Therefore aggregate rather than punctate reticulocytes should be counted to assess the marrow's regenerative response following acute blood loss. Because of the varying lifespan of feline reticulocytes, the reticulocyte index is not generally used in the cat and the absolute aggregate reticulocyte count is thought to be the best way of assessing the marrow's regenerative response, with a count of >50 x 10^9/l indicating a regenerative response (Loar, 1994).

With mild anaemia, the punctate reticulocyte count is a more useful indicator of the marrow's regenerative response, since the marrow tends to hold on to the aggregate reticulocytes until they mature into punctate reticulocytes.

Acute haemorrhage

Acute haemorrhage may be due to trauma or surgery, bleeding gastrointestinal ulcers or tumours, rupture of a vascular tumour (e.g. splenic haemangiosarcoma), or a coagulopathy (e.g. warfarin toxicity). Immediately following acute haemorrhage the red cell parameters, including PCV, are normal because both red cells and plasma have been lost in proportion. Compensatory mechanisms such as splenic contraction may further offset any fall in PCV. The PCV falls when blood volume is replaced by interstitial fluid and so does not indicate the full magnitude of blood loss for at least 24 hours after the onset of haemorrhage. If the blood loss is external, the decrease in PCV is accompanied by a fall in plasma proteins. Following internal bleeding, total plasma protein concentration falls slightly but then may increase due to the release of acute phase proteins. After 3 days newly produced reticulocytes are released from the bone marrow and on a Giemsa-stained blood film there will be evidence of polychromasia, anisocytosis (with macrocytes) and, possibly, poikilocytosis. Acanthocytes may be visible following internal haemorrhage due to a process of autotransfusion. Increased numbers of Howell-Jolly bodies may be seen, especially in cats.

Acute blood loss is usually associated with a neutrophilic leucocytosis with increased numbers of band neutrophils, especially following haemorrhage into a body cavity. The presence of immature red cells and granulocytic precursors in the circulation is known as a leucoerythroblastic response. Immediately following haemorrhage there is a mild to moderate thrombocytopenia, reflecting increased loss of platelets; this is usually followed by a rebound thrombocytosis, with the production of large 'shift' platelets.

Following external blood loss the PCV rises quite rapidly and is usually low to normal within 2 weeks of a single haemorrhagic episode. The PCV rises more quickly following intracavitatory haemorrhage (assuming the haemorrhage has stopped), since some of the red cells may re-enter the circulation via the lymphatics.

The clinicopathological features of acute haemorrhage are:

- Anaemia: initially normocytic and normochromic; becoming macrocytic and hypochromic with increased reticulocytes
- Neutrophilia with left shift (see below)
- Thrombocytopenia, then rebound thrombocytosis
- Low plasma protein levels if blood loss is external
- Midly reduced, normal or mildly increased plasma proteins, if blood loss is intracavitatory.

Chronic haemorrhage

Chronic external blood loss (e.g. chronic gastrointestinal haemorrhage, renal or bladder neoplasia) initially results in a regenerative anaemia but gradually the anaemia becomes non-regenerative as the iron stores become depleted. Young animals become iron-deficient more quickly than adults following blood loss, partly because they have low iron stores and partly because their bone marrow is already very active producing red cells to match their growth rate and so has less capacity to increase its rate of haemopoiesis. True iron deficiency results in inadequate haemoglobinization of red cells and the release of microcytic, hypochromic erythrocytes into the circulation. Persistent thrombocytosis is a common feature of chronic haemorrhage.

The clinicopathological features of chronic blood loss and iron-deficiency anaemia are:

- Microcytosis (low MCV)
- Hypochromasia (low MCHC; pale-staining cells on blood smear)
- Low plasma protein levels
- Thrombocytosis
- Initially increased reticulocyte count, which falls as animal becomes iron-deficient.

Such findings should prompt a search for external blood loss. The source may be evident from the clinical history (e.g. melaena, haematuria). If not, urinalysis and tests for occult faecal blood should be carried out. The patient should be on a meat-free diet for at least 3 days before a faecal occult blood test is performed, since myoglobin (present in meat) will produce a false-positive result. Faecal analysis for endoparasites and/ or contrast radiography of the gastrointestinal tract or urinary tract may be useful in determining the site of blood loss.

Assessing iron stores may be useful in recognizing iron deficiency. A low level of iron in the serum is found in iron deficiency, but serum iron is also low in anaemia of chronic disease, acute inflammatory reactions and hypoproteinaemia, so this test is not specific. Non-heme iron is stored as haemosiderin (stored in the bone marrow) and ferritin (stored in the cells of the reticuloendothelial system). Haemosiderin stores can be assessed by staining a bone marrow aspirate with Prussian blue; if there is stainable iron in the bone marrow this rules out iron deficiency as a cause for anaemia (Stone and Freden, 1990).

Haemolytic anaemias

Most cases of haemolytic anaemia are immune-mediated. In the dog most cases of immune-mediated haemolytic anaemia (IHA) are primary (idiopathic) and are termed autoimmune haemolytic anaemia (AIHA). IHA may occur in association with: drugs (e.g. potentiated sulphonamides); lymphoreticular diseases (e.g. lymphoid leukaemia); systemic lupus erythematosus; or infections (e.g. *Babesia,* bacterial endocarditis). Primary IHA is much less common in the cat but secondary IHA may be induced by *Haemobartonella* or FeLV infection, lymphoproliferative diseases, and certain drugs.

Other causes of haemolytic anaemia include Heinz body anaemia (e.g. due to onion toxicity), acute leptospirosis and inherent metabolic defects (e.g. pyruvate kinase deficiency in Basenjis).

Immune-mediated haemolytic anaemia

Red cells are coated with IgG or IgM, with or without complement activation, and are subsequently removed from the circulation by phagocytosis in the spleen or liver (extravascular haemolysis) or by direct destruction in the circulation (intravascular haemolysis). Most cases of IHA involve extravascular destruction of red cells, which usually results in an anaemia of fairly insidious onset. The spleen and liver are the sites of red cell phagocytosis and this is reflected by hepatosplenomegaly.

Intravascular haemolysis results in a severe anaemia of acute onset. Haemoglobinaemia and consequent haemoglobinuria (which should be distinguished from haematuria) develops once the plasma haptoglobin system is saturated. Jaundice develops in both forms of haemolysis when the rate of bilirubin production from red cell damage exceeds the liver's capacity to conjugate it. Intravascular haemolysis usually has a higher rate of red cell destruction and so jaundice is more frequently seen.

The clinicopathological features of IHA are:

- Moderate to severe macrocytic, hypochromic anaemia (e.g. PCV 0.12–0.18 l/l)
- Marked reticulocytosis. Often the reticulocyte percentage is >25% and the absolute reticulocyte count is >500 x 10^9/l. The reticulocyte production index is generally >3

- Marked polychromasia (3+ or 4+)
- Spherocytes are usually seen (difficult to see in the cat); absence does not rule out IHA
- Marked anisocytosis due to the presence of large reticulocytes and small spherocytes
- Neutrophilia
- Plasma protein level normal to slightly increased
- Bilirubin and liver enzymes may be elevated, the latter being a reflection of hypoxic liver damage.

The diagnosis is confirmed by a positive Coombs' test and/or autoagglutination.

Coombs' test: This is used to detect the presence of antibody and/or complement on the surface of red cells. Coombs' reagent, which contains species-specific antiglobulin directed against IgM, IgG and complement, is incubated with the patient's washed red cells at 37 °C. The antiglobulin binds to antibodies or complement on the red cells, resulting in agglutination seen as small specks of clumped cells suspended in the test well. Both false-positive and false-negative results may occur. False-negative results may be due to technical problems, such as incorrect temperature, or to insufficient quantity of antibody on the red cell surface. False-positive results may occur if there is marked non-specific stimulation of the immune system, such as in chronic bacterial infection or if the animal has received a previous blood transfusion.

If haemolytic cold antibody disease is suspected, the Coombs' test should be performed at 4 °C. The 'cold' antibodies are activated at low temperatures and this rare disease manifests as intermittent haemoglobinuria associated with cold weather.

Autoagglutination: Large amounts of antibody on the red cell surface may result in spontaneous agglutination of red cells, seen grossly as red specks in an EDTA tube or on a glass slide. Autoagglutination must be distinguished from rouleaux formation. A drop of blood is diluted with one drop of saline on a glass slide and a coverslip placed over the mixture. The cells are observed with a microscope using the x40 objective. Rouleaux resemble organized stacks of coins, whereas autoagglutination results in random clumping of red cells, resembling bunches of grapes. The presence of autoagglutination negates the need for a Coombs' test and is itself diagnostic for IHA. Some dogs with autoagglutination will have a negative Coombs' test. Autoagglutination is associated with a severe anaemia of acute onset, often with jaundice and haemoglobinuria, and prognosis is usually guarded.

Intrinsic haemolytic anaemias
Inherent metabolic defects, most frequently deficiencies in red cell enzymes, have been reported in certain breeds. Red cell pyruvate kinase deficiency occurs in

Basenjis and has also been reported in a West Highland White Terrier (Chapman and Giger, 1990). The metabolic defect damages the cell membrane, with subsequent loss of potassium and cell dehydration. Affected red cells are removed from the circulation by splenic macrophages, i.e. extravascular haemolysis (Burman *et al.*, 1982). The disease is associated terminally with myelofibrosis and osteosclerosis.

Red cell phosphofructokinase deficiency has been reported in Springer Spaniels. Again the metabolic defect results in extravascular haemolysis. The PCV is generally at the low end of normal and reticulocyte counts are elevated. However, a haemolytic crisis may occur following exercise when hyperventilation leads to alkalaemia. The red cells show a marked alkaline fragility resulting in an increased rate of haemolysis (Jain, 1993).

Microangiopathic haemolytic anaemia
Red cells are damaged as they pass through abnormal vessels (e.g. in vascular neoplasms such as haemangiosarcoma) or through fibrin clots in disseminated intravascular coagulation (DIC). The cells are fragmented into variably shaped pieces (schistocytes) which are then phagocytosed by the reticuloendothelial system, resulting in anaemia. A regenerative anaemia with numerous schistocytes should prompt a search for a neoplasm such as haemangiosarcoma, and investigations such as radiography of the thorax and abdomen, and ultrasound examination of the liver and spleen are useful. A coagulation profile (see below) should also be obtained to investigate the possibility of DIC.

Primary bone marrow disorders
A bone marrow aspirate and/or core biopsy are mandatory in the investigation of primary bone marrow disorders. In most cases an aspirate gives sufficient material to make a diagnosis. In myelofibrosis, attempts at bone marrow aspiration result in a 'dry tap' and a bone marrow core biopsy is required for diagnosis.

Pure red cell aplasia
Pure red cell aplasia is characterized by selective depletion of erythroid precursors. This may be due to immune-mediated damage directed against the red cell precursors. Leucocyte and platelet production are unaffected.

Aplastic anaemia
Aplastic anaemia is characterized by a pancytopenia, i.e. anaemia, thrombocytopenia and granulocytopenia. Causes include infections (e.g canine parvovirus, feline panleucopenia virus, *Ehrlichia canis*); drug toxicity (e.g. phenylbutazone, oestrogens); and endogenous oestrogen toxicity due to Sertoli cell tumour. Thrombocytopenia results in a tendency to bleed and neutropenia predisposes to sepsis.

Myeloproliferative and lymphoproliferative diseases (leukaemias)

Leukaemia refers to neoplasia arising in the bone marrow. Any of the cell lines may undergo neoplastic transformation, but in the dog and cat most cases of leukaemia involve the lymphoid (Figure 3.17), erythroid and granulocytic lineages. Clonal proliferation of neoplastic cells (e.g. lymphoblasts in acute lymphoid leukaemia) result in crowding out of the bone marrow by the population of neoplastic cells. The neoplastic cells also compete for nutrients and release inhibitory factors. The result is a reduction in normal haemopoiesis, leading to anaemia, thrombocytopenia and neutropenia. The neoplastic cells are usually released into the circulation, often in very large numbers. For example, in acute lymphoid leukaemia there may be neutropenia, anaemia and thrombocytopenia, together with a marked leucocytosis due to many circulating lymphoblasts. The terms acute and chronic refer to the degree of maturation of the neoplastic cells. Hence in acute leukaemia the bone marrow contains numerous blasts which do not mature and differentiate, whilst in chronic leukaemia the marrow contains numerous well differentiated cells and their precursors.

Myelofibrosis

In myelofibrosis the normal haemopoietic tissue is replaced by fibrous tissue, resulting in reduced erythropoiesis and a marked non-regenerative anaemia but usually normal leucocyte and platelet numbers.

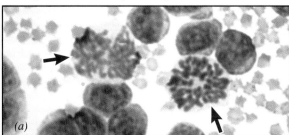

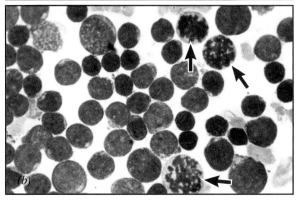

Figure 3.17: *(a) Peripheral blood smear from a dog with acute lymphoid leukaemia. Two mitotic figures are present (arrowed) with numerous large lymphoblasts. Leishman.*
(b) Bone marrow aspirate from a dog with acute lymphoblastic leukaemia. There are large numbers of abnormal lymphoid cells and several mitotic figures (arrowed). No normal haemopoietic cells are present. May-Grünwald Giemsa.

(a) Courtesy of Dr R.W. Else.

Secondary failure of haemopoiesis

Anaemia of chronic disease

Anaemia associated with chronic inflammatory disorders or malignant neoplasms is probably the most common form of anaemia in the dog and cat. The anaemia is mild to moderate (PCV 0.25–0.36 l/l in the dog, 0.18–0.26 l/l in the cat) and is usually normocytic and normochromic, although occasionally it is microcytic and hypochromic. There may be increased numbers of leptocytes and an inflammatory white cell picture. Anaemia of chronic disease is characterized by low serum iron levels, low or normal total iron-binding capacity, and normal to high marrow stores of iron. These factors help to differentiate it from iron-deficiency anaemia.

Anaemia secondary to renal failure is mainly due to decreased production of erythropoietin. In addition the red cell lifespan is shortened by uraemic toxins. The anaemia is normocytic and normochromic and there is minimal poikilocytosis. The anaemia is generally mild to moderate (PCV 0.20–0.30 l/l in the dog), but in long-standing cases may fall as low as 0.10 l/l.

Hepatic disease may result in a non-regenerative anaemia. The anaemia is frequently mild, normocytic and normochromic. Acanthocytes and/or leptocytes may be seen in blood smears. Mild anaemia may occur with hypothyroidism. Anaemia is a consistent finding with Addison's disease (hypoadrenocorticism). The anaemia is usually non-regenerative, normocytic and normochromic. The severity of the anaemia may be masked by haemoconcentration due to dehydration. Occasionally acute gastrointestinal haemorrhage occurs, in which case the anaemia is regenerative.

Anaemia and FeLV infection

Some 50–75% of anaemic cats are positive for feline leukaemia virus (FeLV) and/or feline immunodeficiency virus (FIV). In most of these cases the anaemia is non-regenerative. FeLV infection may cause a macrocytic non-regenerative anaemia, probably due to a direct myelodysplastic effect of the virus. FeLV may also be associated with aplastic anaemia and pure red cell aplasia, leading to a normocytic normochromic anaemia. FeLV- and FIV-related immunosuppression may lead to other infectious or inflammatory diseases which, in turn, may lead to anaemia of chronic disease. FeLV may also induce haemolytic anaemia by inducing the formation of antibodies directed against virus antigen on the red cell surface.

Diagnostic approach to non-regenerative anaemia

Anaemia of chronic inflammatory disease is the most common cause of non-regenerative anaemia. Usually the signs of the underlying disease are severe and the anaemia is an almost incidental finding. If the anaemia is more severe, iron deficiency or a primary bone marrow disor-

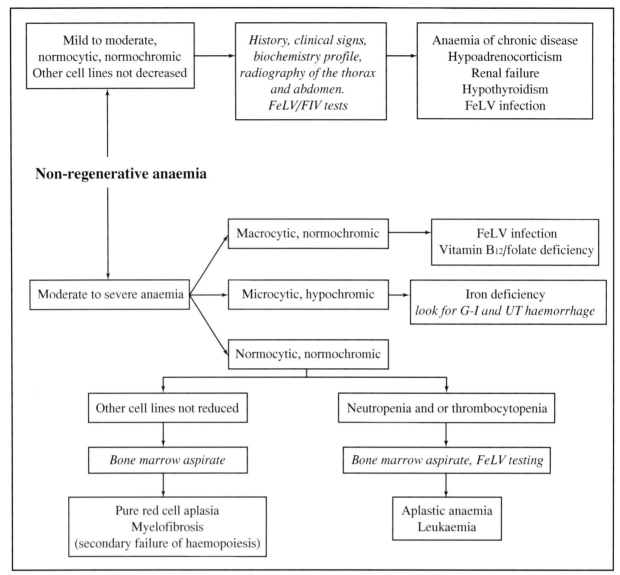

Figure 3.18: *Approach to non-regenerative anaemia.*

der should be considered (Figure 3.18). A microcytic hypochromic anaemia is indicative of iron deficiency and should prompt a search for external blood loss (faecal occult blood, urine analysis and contrast radiography may be useful). If there is nothing to suggest blood loss a bone marrow aspirate should be obtained. The technique for bone marrow aspiration is described below.

POLYCYTHAEMIA

Polycythaemia is characterized by increases in the red cell count, haemoglobin concentration and PCV. It can be classified as relative or absolute. Absolute polycythaemia may be primary (true) or secondary.

Relative polycythaemia is caused by disturbances in fluid balance, resulting in dehydration. The total RBC mass remains normal but the decrease in plasma volume results in an increase in total plasma protein.

Primary polycythaemia, also known as polycythae-

mia rubra vera, is a chronic myeloproliferative disease characterized by clonal proliferation of erythroid precursor cells, with maturation and differentiation into morphologically normal erythrocytes. This proliferation is not controlled by normal feedback mechanisms and is not driven by erythropoietin. Indeed, erythropoietin levels are often low or undetectable. The term polycythaemia implies that leucocytes and platelets are elevated as well as red cells and this is the case in humans with polycythaemia. However, in dogs and cats with primary polycythaemia usually only the red cell numbers are elevated; a neutrophilia is occasionally seen in dogs.

Secondary polycythaemia occurs in response to increased secretion of erythropoietin. The increased erythropoietin secretion may be an appropriate compensatory response to chronic hypoxia due to: chronic pulmonary disease; right-to-left cardiovascular shunting (e.g. patent ductus arteriosus; tetralogy of Fallot); or living at high altitude. Alternatively, the increased levels of erythropoietin may be present without systemic hypoxia (termed inappropriate secondary polycythaemia). This has been reported in conjunction with renal tumours (carcinoma, adenocarcinoma, fibrosarcoma and lymphoma) and is thought to be the result of local hypoxia within the kidney or secretion of erythropoietin by the tumour. Benign renal cysts and hydronephrosis have also been suggested as causes of inappropriate secondary polycythaemia. Extrarenal neoplasia is uncommonly associated with polycythaemia; one case report of polycythaemia in a dog with a nasal fibrosarcoma has been documented, in which the tumour was found to secrete erythropoietin (Couto *et al.*, 1989.

In the cat most cases of polycythaemia are primary, with secondary polycythemia only occurring occasionally in response to hypoxia (Watson *et al.*, 1994).

Diagnosis

In relative polycythaemia clinical examination usually reveals signs of dehydration. The PCV is mildly or moderately elevated and total plasma protein, urea and creatinine are elevated. The PCV returns to normal once the dehydration is corrected.

If relative polycythaemia can be ruled out, causes of secondary polycythaemia should be investigated. Arterial blood gas levels are useful in testing for hypoxia. Thoracic radiographs and echocardiography are used to assess the cardiopulmonary systems. An intravenous excretory urogram and renal ultrasonography are used to look for renal neoplasia. If secondary causes of polycythaemia can be ruled out, a presumptive diagnosis of primary polycythaemia is made. This diagnosis is confirmed if the serum erythropoietin concentration is low or undetectable. (This assay is not widely available but can be performed at Ninewells Hospital, Dundee.) Bone marrow aspiration is not helpful in distinguishing primary from secondary polycythaemia, since erythroid hyperplasia is present in both; the red blood cells and their precursors are morphologically normal.

DISORDERS OF WHITE CELL NUMBER

Neutrophilia

Neutrophils are distributed in the body among six pools (Figure 3.19). Once cells enter the tissue pool they cannot return to the circulation. There is no significant tissue pool in healthy animals, but neutrophils enter the tissues when there is inflammation or infection. The main function of neutrophils in tissues is the phagocytosis of pyogenic bacteria. The leucogram gives information only about the circulating pool.

Neutrophilia is defined as a neutrophil count of $>11.5 \times 10^9/l$ in the dog and $>12.5 \times 10^9/l$ in the cat.

There are numerous causes of neutrophilia (Figure 3.20).

In the bone marrow
Stem cell pool: CFU-GM
Proliferating pool: myeloblasts, promyelocytes and myelocytes.
Maturation/storage pool: metamyelocytes, bands and segmented neutrophils

In the bloodstream
Circulating pool: cells in the circulation
Marginating pool: cells adherent to vascular endothelium

In the tissues
Tissue pool: cells present at sites of inflammation/infection

Figure 3.19: The distribution of neutrophils in the body.

Physiological response (fear, excitement, exercise)
Stress/corticosteroid-induced
Acute inflammatory response:
    Bacterial infection (localized or generalized)
    Immune-mediated disease
    Necrosis, e.g. pancreatitis
    Neoplasia, especially with tumour necrosis
Chronic granulocytic leukaemia
Neutrophil dysfunction
Paraneoplastic syndromes

Figure 3.20: Causes of neutrophilia.

Physiological neutrophilia

Fear, excitement or exercise results in the release of endogenous adrenaline which causes increased blood flow. Neutrophils are washed out of the marginating pool into the circulating pool, producing a mild neutrophilia. The effect is more marked in the cat since this species has a larger marginating pool; the effect is not commonly seen in the dog. There is usually a concurrent lymphocytosis, which helps to distinguish this response from a stress/steroid-induced neutrophilia.

Stress/steroid-induced neutrophilia

'Stress', defined as pain, trauma, surgical procedures and severe debilitating disorders, causes the release of endogenous glucocorticoids. Neutrophils shift from the marginating pool and storage pool to the circulating pool and the circulating time of neutrophils is increased. The net effect is a mild neutrophilia without a left shift (see below). This is accompanied by lymphopenia and eosinopenia (due to steroid-induced movement of these cells to the marginating pool and the lytic effect of steroids on these cell lines) and, less frequently, by a monocytosis. This picture is known as the *stress leucogram.* A similar response is seen in dogs with hyperadrenocorticism (Cushing's disease) or following administration of corticosteroids.

Acute inflammatory response
This is characterized by a neutrophilia (usually >20 x 10^9/l) with a left shift (>1 x 10^9/l band neutrophils; see below). Bacterial infection is the most common cause for an acute inflammatory response, but there are numerous non-septic causes of acute inflammation, including tissue necrosis (e.g. pancreatitis), immune-mediated disease (e.g. haemolytic anaemia, poly-arthritis), and neoplasia (especially tumour necrosis).

Neutrophils migrate from the circulation to the site of inflammation in response to chemotaxis. This migration stimulates the release of colony-stimulating factor which, in turn, stimulates increased granulo-poiesis and release of neutrophils from the bone marrow. When this increased production and release exceeds demand, a circulating neutrophilia is observed. The increased granulopoiesis also causes release of immature neutrophils (band cells) into the circulation, and this is known as a left shift. The magnitude of the left shift tends to parallel the severity of the inflammatory process. The presence of metamyelocytes or younger neutrophil precursors indicates a severe left shift. The left shift may be regenerative – where both mature neutrophils and band forms are increased, or degenerative – where band forms are increased but the number of mature neutrophils is normal or decreased. A degenerative left shift is generally a poor prognostic indicator. Severe localized or systemic infections (e.g. pyothorax) result in toxic changes in the neutrophils (see above and Figure 3.11). The number of toxic neutrophils present parallels the severity of the inflammatory process.

The acute inflammatory response may progress to a steady state in which granulopoiesis equilibrates with tissue demand. This *chronic inflammatory response* is characterized by a neutrophilia with a variable left shift and a monocytosis (reflecting tissue necrosis). The neutrophilia may be relatively mild and the left shift tends to resolve with time.

Table 3.5 summarizes the different types of neutrophilic response.

Extreme neutrophilia
A very high neutrophil count (>50 x 10^9/l) is referred to as an inflammatory leukaemoid reaction and may be very difficult to distinguish from the neutrophilia observed with chronic granulocytic leukaemia. A leukaemoid reaction may be caused by a severe localized infection, such as closed pyometra, and in this context the neutrophilia is a poor prognostic indicator since the disease has not resolved despite the numerous neutrophils being released.

Extreme neutrophilia may be associated with immune-mediated diseases, especially immune-mediated haemolytic anaemia where the bone marrow is very active. Neutrophil dysfunction syndromes such as granulocytopathy syndrome in Irish Setters and neutrophil bactericidal defect in Dobermann

Type	Characteristics
Physiological neutrophilia	Mild neutrophilia + lymphocytosis
Stress leucogram	Mild neutrophilia + lymphopenia, eosinopenia, monocytosis
Acute inflammation	Moderate to marked neutrophilia with left shift

Table 3.5: *Evaluation of neutrophilia.*

Pinschers may result in a marked neutrophilia associated with concurrent chronic infections (Guilford, 1987). The skin, respiratory system and gastro-intestinal tract are common sites for infection. Extreme neutrophilia has also been reported in association with a renal carcinoma (Lappin and Latimer, 1988) and a metastatic fibrosarcoma (Chinn *et al.*, 1985). The neutrophilia was thought to be due to release of a colony stimulating factor-like substance from the tumour.

Causes of extreme neutrophilia are:

• Severe localized or generalized infections (e.g. pyometra)
• Immune-mediated haemolytic anaemia and other immune-mediated diseases
• Paraneoplastic neutrophilia
• Immunodeficiency syndromes characterized by neutrophil dysfunction.

Chronic granulocytic leukaemia
It can be very difficult to distinguish chronic granulocytic leukaemia (CGL) from an inflammatory leukaemoid reaction. Other causes of neutrophilia should first be ruled out. CGL often results in splenic or hepatic infiltration with neoplastic neutrophils and their precursors; a biopsy of the liver or spleen is therefore often helpful in confirming CGL. Maturation of neutrophils may appear disorderly in bone marrow aspirates, though this is not a consistent finding.

Pelger–Heut anomaly
An apparent left shift is seen with the Pelger–Heut anomaly. This is a rare inherited disorder reported in various breeds of dogs and in Domestic Shorthair cats, in which the nuclei of granulocytes, especially neutrophils, fail to mature into normal segmented nuclei. The neutrophils are functionally normal, the total white cell count is not increased and the syndrome is usually an incidental finding (Guilford, 1987).

Neutropenia

The three main causes of neutropenia are:

- An overwhelming demand for neutrophils
- Reduced production of neutrophils in the bone marrow
- Defective neutrophil maturation in the bone marrow.

An overwhelming demand for neutrophils may occur with peracute bacterial infections, especially Gram-negative sepsis and endotoxaemia. Other possible causes include peritonitis, pyometra, aspiration pneumonia and canine parvovirus infection. There is usually a severe degenerative left shift and numerous toxic neutrophils.

Reduced granulopoiesis may be associated with:

- Aplastic anaemia (which results in a pancytopenia)
- Myeloproliferative and lymphoproliferative diseases
- Infections (e.g. canine parvovirus, feline panleucopenia, FeLV)
- Cancer chemotherapy (e.g. cyclophosphamide)
- Endogenous or exogenous hyperoestrogenism
- Other idiosyncratic drug reactions.

Defective neutrophil maturation occurs when the maturation of neutrophil precursors is arrested. This is seen in acute myeloid leukaemia (AML), where neoplastic clones of myeloblasts do not mature and differentiate into neutrophils. Myelodysplastic syndrome (MDS) may cause neutropenia, anaemia and thrombocytopenia, in different combinations. Morphological abnormalities and a maturation arrest are seen in one or more of the cell lines, commonly the neutrophil series. The disease progresses slowly and in cats may terminate in an acute leukaemia (usually AML). In the cat, MDS is often associated with FeLV infection. Blue *et al.* (1988) found that 71% of a group of 20 cats with MDS were FeLV-positive.

Rare causes of neutropenia

Cyclic neutropenia is an inherited disease of Grey Collies in which defective stem cell proliferation leads to asynchronous cyclic fluctuations of all cell lines. The fluctuation in neutrophil numbers is the most dramatic, resulting in episodes of severe neutropenia lasting 2–4 days, occurring every 12 days (Campbell, 1985).

Immune-mediated neutropenia is very uncommon in the dog and cat and anti-neutrophil antibody testing is not routinely available.

Eosinophilia

Eosinophils are distributed in the body among various pools in a similar way to neutrophils, although the bone marrow storage pool is minimal. Eosinophils circulate in the bloodstream for only a few hours before entering the tissues, where they may live for several days. Their two main functions are to kill parasites and to regulate allergic and inflammatory reactions. Causes of eosinophilia are listed in Figure 3.21.

The hypereosinophilic syndrome is a rare disorder of cats, characterized by a circulating eosinophilia together with infiltration of eosinophils into numerous organs, including the intestine, liver, spleen and bone marrow. The syndrome is not thought to be neoplastic and may result form a severe uncontrolled reactive process (Harvey, 1990).

Eosinopenia

Eosinopenia in combination with lymphopenia occurs following stress, administration of corticosteroids and in spontaneous hyperadrenocorticism (Cushing's syndrome). There is also usually a neutrophilia (without a left shift), i.e. the stress leucogram. Eosinopenia may also be seen in acute inflammation or infection.

Basophilia

Basophils contain inflammatory mediators such as histamine and heparin and function in a similar manner

---

Skin disorders:
   Flea-allergic dermatitis
   Atopy
   Pemphigus foliaceous
   Ectoparasite infestation
   Eosinophilic granuloma complex (cats)
Respiratory disease:
   Feline asthma
   Canine pulmonary infiltrate with eosinophils
   Lungworms (e.g. *Aleurostrongylus* and *Oslerus osleri*)
   Chronic rhinitis and sinusitis in the cat
Gastrointestinal disease:
   Eosinophilic enteritis
   Endoparasitism e.g. hookworms, *Toxocara*
Neoplasia:
   Mast cell tumours (mast cells release chemotactants for eosinophils)
   Other tumours may occasionally be associated with an eosinophilia, e.g. lymphoma, basal cell tumours in cats, ovarian tumours.
   Eosinophilic leukaemia (very rare)
Canine panosteitis (especially German Shepherd Dogs)
Eosinophilic myositis
Oestrus may sometimes be associated with eosinophilia in bitches
Hypoadrenocorticism
Infectious diseases
   Feline infectious peritonitis
   Toxoplasmosis
Hypereosinophilic syndrome in cats

Figure 3.21: Possible causes of eosinophilia.

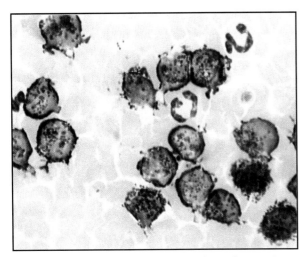

Figure 3.22: A buffy coat smear from a dog with systemic mastocytosis. Numerous mast cells with purple-staining granules are present. May-Grünwald Giemsa.

to mast cells in hypersensitivity reactions. Basophilia is rarely observed without a concomitant eosinophilia.

Mastocytosis

Mast cells are round cells with round nuclei and numerous purple granules which may obscure the nucleus. In healthy animals they are absent from blood and are rarely seen in the bone marrow. Circulating mast cells may be seen in animals with systemic mast cell neoplasia (systemic mastocytosis, Figure 3.22) which most commonly arises in the spleen and/or liver. In the cat systemic mastocytosis occurs independently from cutaneous mast cell tumours, whilst in the dog it almost always arises following tumour metastasis from a primary cutaneous lesion. Since only small numbers of mast cells may be seen in the blood of affected animals, examination of a buffy coat smear is recommended. Blood is spun in a microhaematocrit tube and the buffy coat is obtained by scoring and breaking the tube in the appropriate place. A smear is made and stained with Romanowsky stain. Primary cutaneous mast cell tumours may also metastasize to the bone marrow. This may result in a circulating mastocytaemia and extensive marrow infiltrates may result in variable anaemia, thrombocytopenia and neutropenia due to a reduction in normal haemopoiesis.

Monocytosis

There is no storage pool for monocytes in the bone marrow; they are produced and released on demand. After a short period in the circulation they migrate into the tissues to become macrophages. Their main function in the tissues is the phagocytosis of dead cells, microorganisms and foreign particles.

Causes of monocytosis are listed in Figure 3.23. In chronic inflammation, the monocytosis is usually accompanied by a mild to moderate neutrophilia, with a variable left shift.

Monocytopenia is not clinically significant.

Chronic inflammation, especially pyogranulomatous inflammation Tissue necrosis (e.g. large tumours with a necrotic centre) Immune-mediated disease (e.g. IHA) Stress Glucocorticoid therapy Hyperadrenocorticism Monocytic or myelomonocytic leukaemia

Figure 3.23: Causes of monocytosis.

Lymphocytosis

B and T lymphocytes cannot be distinguished morphologically with the light microscope but an average blood smear contains approximately 70% T cells, 20% B cells and 10% null (non-B, non-T) cells. Lymphocytes recirculate, i.e they pass from the blood through lymph nodes, tissues and bone marrow, and then back into the blood. T cells and memory B cells have a long lifespan (years), whilst non-memory B cells are short-lived.

The causes of lymphocytosis are listed in Figure 3.24. In chronic lymphocytic leukaemia (CLL) the lymphocytosis may be very marked. Acute lymphoblastic leukaemia (ALL) generally results in the release of abnormal lymphoblasts into the circulation.

Physiological lymphocytosis, with concomitant neutrophilia, in response to excitement (especially cats) Strong immune stimulation (e.g. in chronic infection, viraemia or immune-mediated disease) Chronic lymphocytic leukaemia Hypoadrenocorticism (lymphocytosis may be associated with an eosinophilia) Increased numbers of large reactive lymphocytes ('immunoblasts') may occur transiently following vaccination Young animals have a higher lymphocyte count than adult animals

Figure 3.24: Causes of lymphocytosis.

Lymphopenia

Causes of lymphopenia are listed in Figure 3.25.

Stress Glucocorticoid therapy Hyperadrenocorticism Chylothorax (loss of lymphocytes into the pleural space) Lymphangiectasia (loss of lymphocytes into the gut) Acute phase of most viral infections (e.g. canine distemper, parvovirus, FeLV) Septicaemia/endotoxaemia

Figure 3.25: Causes of lymphopenia.

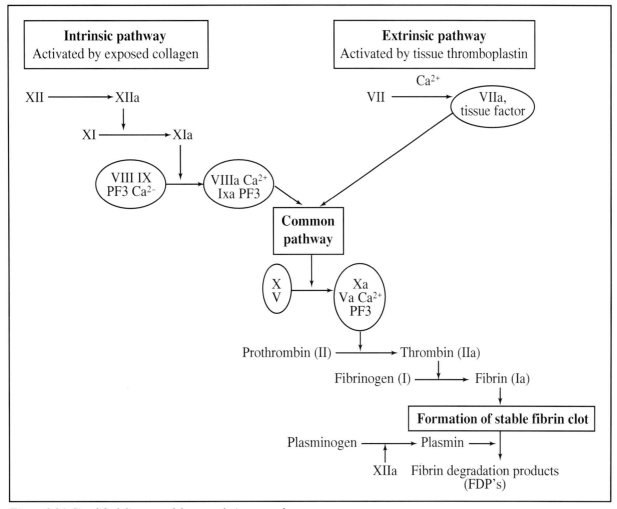

Figure 3.26: Simplified diagram of the coagulation cascade.

	Platelet count	**BMBT**	**OSPT**	**APTT**
Thrombocytopenia	decreased	increased	normal	normal
von Willebrand's disease	normal	increased	normal	normal or slightly increased
Warfarin poisoning	normal	normal*	increased	increased
Intrinsic pathway defect (e.g. haemophilia A)	normal	normal*	normal	increased
Extrinsic pathway defect (e.g. factor VII deficiency)	normal	normal	increased	normal
DIC	decreased	increased	increased	increased

Table 3.6: *Coagulation test results in various diseases. (*Stops in normal time but rebleeds if clot disturbed.)*

HAEMOSTASIS

The clotting process

Following vascular injury platelets adhere to exposed collagen, a process mediated by von Willebrand's factor. Platelets are then activated and release numerous chemotactic factors which attract additional platelets. Hence the primary platelet plug is formed and temporarily repairs the vessel defect. This is known as primary haemostasis. This primary plug is unstable, however, and activation of the coagulation cascade is required to strengthen it. The coagulation factors are activated by exposed collagen at the site of vascular injury, by tissue thromboplastin released from damaged cells and also by platelet factor 3 (PF3) which is released from platelets. The end result of the coagulation cascade (Figure 3.26) is the formation of polymerized fibrin which intertwines between the platelets and stabilizes the platelet plug.

This is known as secondary haemostasis.

The fibrin clot is broken down under the action of plasmin into fibrin degradation products (FDPs). Plasmin is derived from plasminogen which is activated by various molecules, including tissue plasminogen activator and factor XIIa. FDPs act as anticoagulants, interfering with polymerization of fibrin and platelet aggregation. Natural inhibitors in the circulation such as anti-thrombin III and protein C limit clot formation.

Laboratory assessment

Tests to assess primary haemostasis include:

- Platelet count
- Bleeding time
- Clot retraction.

Tests to assess secondary haemostasis include:

- Whole blood clotting time (WBCT)
- Activated clotting time (ACT)
- Activated partial thromboplastin time (APPT)
- One-stage prothrombin time (OSPT)
- Thrombin time (TT).

Table 3.6 shows the alterations in some of these parameters in various diseases.

Platelet count

The platelet count may be determined from a blood film or measured using an automated counter (see above). If thrombocytopenia is detected, tests of bleeding time are unnecessary and may result in prolonged bleeding.

Bleeding time

Bleeding time is most accurately assessed using a spring-loaded device which makes two standard cuts in the buccal mucosa. The upper lip is folded up, exposing the mucosal surface, and tied in place with a length of gauze. The spring-loaded device is placed against the mucosal surface, away from large blood vessels. Once the cuts have been made, excessive blood is removed by blotting the area *adjacent* to the incision every 5–10 seconds using filter paper. Care must be taken to avoid disturbing any clot forming on the wound. The reference range for normal bleeding time in dogs is 1.5–3.5 minutes (Littlewood, 1997). The buccal mucosal bleeding time (BMBT) is prolonged in von Willebrand's disease, thrombocytopenia and thrombocytopathia. However it is not prolonged with coagulation defects since the platelet plug forms normally. The plug is not stabilized by fibrin, so if the clot is disturbed bleeding will recommence.

An alternative to the BMBT is the cuticle bleeding time (CBT). Under general anaesthesia a toenail is cut short with nail clippers. Blood is allowed to drip freely and the time to cessation of bleeding is recorded. The normal CBT is <6 minutes (Littlewood, 1997). CBT may also be prolonged with coagulation defects, since large vessels are disrupted and so the platelet plug may be washed out if it is not stabilized by fibrin. This test is less accurate and less sensitive than the BMBT.

Clot retraction

This is a crude test for platelet function. Once a clot has formed the platelets contract, squeezing serum out of the clot. Thus the contracted clot is visible in the tube, surrounded by serum.

Blood is collected into a glass tube and allowed to clot. The tube is kept at 37 °C (e.g. in a water bath or heating block) and inspected after 2–4 hours by which time the clot should have contracted to approximately 50% of its original volume. Poor clot retraction occurs with thrombocytopenia or abnormal platelet function and in von Willebrand's disease.

Whole blood clotting time (WBCT)

Blood is collected into a prewarmed glass tube and kept at 37 °C. The tube is tilted every 30 seconds and examined for the presence of a clot. Normal WBCT is <6 minutes (Littlewood, 1997). This test evaluates the *intrinsic* pathway but is very insensitive. The clotting time is only prolonged if a clotting factor is severely deficient (<5% of normal). It may also be prolonged in severe, prolonged thrombocytopenia due to a deficiency in PF3. The test is also influenced by other variables such as the size of the tube, temperature and the PCV.

Activated clotting time (ACT)

This is a modified version of the WBCT. Blood is collected into commercially prepared tubes which contain a chemical activator of the intrinsic pathway. The tubes are prewarmed and the test is performed at 37 °C. Normal ACT is 60–100 seconds in dogs and <60 seconds in cats (Tvedten, 1989). This test is more sensitive than the WBCT but the ACT is only prolonged if a coagulation factor is reduced to <5% of normal. As with the WBCT, the ACT is prolonged in severe thrombocytopenia due to a deficiency in PF3.

Activated partial thromboplastin time (APTT)

This test evaluates the intrinsic and common pathways, i.e. factors XII, XI, IX, VIII, V, II and I. The intrinsic pathway is activated under controlled conditions in the presence of phospholipid (which equates to PF3) and calcium. Thus, apart from the coagulation factors, all the 'ingredients' for the intrinsic coagulation cascade are provided and the test is not influenced by variables such as the platelet count and PCV. The test is therefore much more reliable and sensitive than the WBCT and ACT.

APTT is prolonged if an individual coagulation factor is reduced to <50% of normal. Normal APTT is approximately 15–25 seconds but values vary between laboratories and so the results should always be compared to those for the control sample. An APTT prolonged by >20–25% of the control value is considered abnormal.

One-stage prothrombin time (OSPT)

This test evaluates the extrinsic and common pathways, i.e. factors VII, X, V, II, and I. Plasma is incubated with tissue thromboplastin and clotting is initiated by adding calcium. As with the APTT, this test is not influenced by variables such as the platelet count. The OSPT is very sensitive to factor VII deficiency since this has a very short half-life.

The OSPT is prolonged if an individual coagulation factor is reduced to <50% of normal. The normal OSPT is 7–10 seconds but values vary between laboratories and so the results should always be compared to those for the control sample. An OSPT prolonged by >20–25% of the control value is considered abnormal.

Thrombin time (TT)

This test measures the speed of conversion of fibrinogen to fibrin and therefore evaluates the common pathway. TT is prolonged in hypofibrinogenaemia and also by the presence of substances which inhibit the action of thrombin on fibrinogen, e.g. heparin or FDPs (elevated in DIC).

Assays for specific factors

Factor VIII and von Willebrand's factor can be assayed at the Animal Health Trust, Newmarket.

Sample handling for APTT, OSPT, TT and specific factor assays: Blood should be collected from the patient and from a control animal into tubes with sodium citrate, ensuring that the tubes are filled exactly to the right levels. The blood should be mixed thoroughly (>20 tube inversions). The samples should be spun down and the plasma separated from the cells within 30 minutes of blood collection. The samples should be mailed to the laboratory as soon as possible. If a delay is envisaged, the sample should be stored or mailed on ice.

Fibrin degradation products (FDPs)

The concentration of FDPs can be assayed using a latex agglutination test. The test kit provides special tubes which bind the remaining fibrinogen, thus preventing the formation of FDPs in the tube.

FDPs are elevated in DIC and in major vessel thrombosis.

Disorders of haemostasis

Disorders of primary haemostasis may result from thrombocytopenia, von Willebrand's disease (a deficiency of von Willebrand's factor) and platelet malfunction (thrombocytopathia) e.g. due to aspirin.

Disorders of secondary haemostasis may result from an inherited deficiency in a coagulation factor (e.g. haemophilia A is caused by a deficiency of factor VIII) or acquired deficiencies of one or several coagulation factors (e.g. warfarin toxicity results in deficiency of the vitamin K-dependent factors II, VII, IX and X).

Immune-mediated thrombocytopenia (ITP):
  Primary or idiopathic
  Induced by drug reaction (e.g. potentiated sulphonamides)
  Induced by neoplasia (e.g. lymphoma, solid tumours)
  Manifestation of SLE
  Secondary to immune-mediated haemolytic anaemia

Reduced platelet production due to a primary bone marrow disorder:
  Myeloproliferative/lymphoproliferative disease
  Aplastic anaemia
  Chemotherapy
  Idiosyncratic drug reaction (e.g. oestrogens, phenylbutazone)

Increased platelet consumption or sequestration
  Disseminated intravascular coagulation
  Sequestration of platelets in splenic masses or splenic torsion
  Acute severe haemorrhage may result in a transient mild thrombocytopenia

Figure 3.27: *Causes of thrombocytopenia.*

In general, disorders of primary haemostasis result in small haemorrhages (petechial and ecchymotic haemorrhages in the skin, mucous membranes and sclera, or epistaxis and melaena) since only a small amount of blood leaks out from the site of injury before a fibrin clot is formed. In contrast, coagulation cascade defects prevent fibrin stabilization of the platelet plug which rapidly breaks down, resulting in more severe haemorrhage. This may manifest as intracavitatory bleeding, large haematomas or haemarthrosis. Both primary and secondary disorders of haemostasis result in excessive haemorrhage following surgery.

Thrombocytopenia

Thrombocytopenia is the most common acquired bleeding disorder in the dog. Spontaneous bleeding may occur if the platelet count is $<50 \times 10^9/l$, although clinical signs of bleeding may not be present in animals with platelet counts as low as $10 \times 10^9/l$.

Causes of thrombocytopenia are listed in Figure 3.27.

Approach to thrombocytopenia: The diagnostic approach to thrombocytopenia includes the following considerations.

- The degree of thrombocytopenia: severe thrombocytopenia ($<50 \times 10^9/l$) would lead to spontaneous bleeding, whereas a mild thrombocytopenia (e.g. $>110 \times 10^9/l$) is more likely to be the result of haemorrhage rather than the cause

- The patient's recent drug history: e.g. oestrogens, potentiated sulphonamides
- A complete blood cell count: a concurrent anaemia and leucopenia suggest a marrow disorder (e.g. oestrogen toxicity results in a pancytopenia); a strongly regenerative anaemia with spherocytes and thrombocytopenia and many 'shift' platelets tends to suggest concurrent IHA or immune-mediated thrombocytopenia (IMT)
- Platelet size: microthrombocytes (small platelets) may be seen in blood smears from early IMT; 'shift' (large) platelets suggest a regenerative marrow response
- Anti-platelet antibodies: may be detected by an enzyme-linked immunosorbent assay (ELISA) or platelet immunofluorescence assay. These tests can produce both false-positive and false-negative results. A true positive result indicates IMT, which may be primary or secondary
- Screening radiography of the thorax and abdomen: may reveal underlying neoplasia
- A bone marrow aspirate: increased numbers of megakaryocytes with numerous immature forms suggests increased platelet production and is typical of IMT; occasionally IMT may result in immune-mediated destruction of megakaryocytes which are therefore reduced in number or may have foamy vacuolated cytoplasm. An anti-megakaryocyte antibody test may be performed on the bone marrow sample; absence of megakaryocytes is a poor prognostic indicator
- DIC: if suspected, OSPT, APTT, fibrinogen and FDPs should be evaluated.

Thrombocytosis

Mild to moderate thrombocytosis may occur transiently following acute haemorrhage and is often a persistent finding in iron-deficiency anaemia. A marked thrombocytosis (e.g. >1200 x 10^9/l) occurs in the rare myeloproliferative disease essential thrombocythaemia, which is characterized by recurrent episodes of spontaneous bleeding (due to platelet dysfunction) and/or thromboembolic episodes.

Thrombocytopathia

Non-steroidal anti-inflammatory drugs, such as aspirin and phenylbutazone, impair platelet function. This does not usually result in spontaneous bleeding but may cause bleeding in an animal with a pre-existing coagulation disorder. Other disorders known to impair platelet function include von Willebrand's disease (see below), severe uraemia and hypergammaglobulinaemia (e.g. in plasma cell myeloma). High concentrations of FDPs in animals with DIC may also impair platelet function. Rare inherited thrombocytopathias have been described in Otterhounds and blue-smoke Persian cats.

von Willebrand's disease

This inherited disease is characterized by reduced concentrations of von Willebrand's factor (vWF). Since vWF is required for normal platelet function, a deficiency leads to signs of platelet dysfunction. Factor VIII binds to vWF in plasma. If vWF levels are reduced, factor VIII is less stable and factor VIII levels are reduced to approximately 40% of normal (Thomas, 1996). In affected animals the bleeding time is prolonged but the platelet count, WBCT, ACT and OSPT are normal. APTT is usually normal or may be slightly prolonged due to reduced levels of factor VIII. Diagnosis is confirmed by demonstration of low concentrations (<50%) of vWF.

Congenital coagulation defects

Haemophilia A: The X-linked inherited deficiency of coagulation factor VIII occurs in many breeds of dog but is less common in the cat. APTT is increased in haemophilia A; OSPT and BMBT are normal. Diagnosis is confirmed through a specific assay for factor VIII. In the severe form of the disease, factor VIII levels are <1% of normal (Littlewood, 1997) and spontaneous bleeding is common (haematomas, haemarthrosis, or bleeding into a body cavity). In the moderate form, factor VIII levels are 1–10% of normal and spontaneous bleeding occurs only occasionally, although severe bleeding follows surgery or trauma. In the mild form, factor VIII levels are 10–20% of normal and bleeding occurs only after major trauma or surgery (Littlewood, 1989.) Heterozygous carrier females have factor VIII levels that are 50–60% of normal.

Haemophilia B (factor IX deficiency): This is much less common than haemophilia A, occurring in several breeds of dog and in British Shorthair and Siamese cats. APTT is prolonged and diagnosis is confirmed by specific assay.

Other inherited coagulopathies: These include: factor XI (dogs) and factor XII (cats) deficiencies, both resulting in a prolonged APTT and normal OSPT; and factor VII deficiency, which results in a prolonged OSPT and normal APTT.

Acquired coagulation defects

Vitamin K antagonism: Coagulation factors II, VII, IX and X are produced in the liver in an inactive form and are then activated by vitamin K. Anticoagulant rodenticides such as warfarin block the action of vitamin K, resulting in deficiencies of the active forms of these factors. OSPT, APTT, ACT and WBCT are markedly prolonged.

Factor VII has the shortest half-life and so becomes deficient first. Since this factor is part of the extrinsic coagulation cascade, the OSPT becomes prolonged before the APTT. The diagnosis of rodenticide toxicity may be confirmed by measuring the OSPT every 6–8 hours for 1–2 days after starting vitamin K1 therapy. The OSPT should fall progressively to normal. Second-generation rodenticides have a much longer half-life than warfarin. For example, with brodifacoum bleeding may persist for as long as 30 days. In view of the varying half-lives of different rodenticides, it is important to evaluate the patient after treatment has stopped to ensure that vitamin K antagonism is no longer occurring. The OSPT should be measured 2–3 days after cessation of treatment. If treatment has been stopped prematurely the OSPT will be increased and further treatment is indicated.

A more sensitive test that can be used to recognize vitamin K antagonism is the PIVKA (Proteins Involved in Vitamin K Antagonism) test. Briefly, the patient's plasma is added to a test plasma from which factors II, VII and X have been removed. Calcium is added and the clotting time evaluated. A prolonged clotting time indicates that the patient is deficient in factors II, VII and X, confirming vitamin K antagonism. If clotting occurs normally, the patient's plasma must contain factors II, VII and X and vitamin K antagonism can be ruled out.

Liver disease: Severe diffuse liver disease (e.g. acute hepatitis, cirrhosis, neoplastic infiltration) and portosystemic shunts may result in coagulation disorders due to decreased synthesis of coagulation factors. There may also be an associated thrombocytopenia. OSPT and APTT may be prolonged, but these tests are not very sensitive and patients with liver disease in which coagulation times are normal have the potential to haemorrhage following liver biopsy.

Disseminated intravascular coagulation (DIC): This may be triggered by a wide variety of diseases, including endotoxaemia, neoplasia (especially haemangiosarcoma), acute infections (e.g. infectious canine hepatitis), haemolytic anaemia, pancreatitis and heat stroke. The extrinsic pathway is activated by the release of tissue factor from damaged cells into the circulation. The intrinsic pathway is activated following endothelial damage, resulting in exposed collagen. Thus coagulation takes place within vessels. The natural anticoagulants antithrombin III and protein C are consumed, potentiating a hypercoagulable state. Once the supply of platelets and coagulation factors is exhausted, spontaneous bleeding occurs. The fibrinolytic system is activated, resulting in increased concentrations of FDPs which exacerbate the bleeding tendency by inhibiting fibrin formation and platelet aggregation. Thus a combination of intravascular coagulation and spontaneous bleeding occur simultaneously.

The clinicopathological features of DIC are:

- Thrombocytopenia
- Increased OSPT/APTT
- Elevated FDPs
- Low fibrinogen
- Schistocytes in the blood film.

All of the above parameters may be present, but since new platelets and clotting factors are continuously produced the parameters may fluctuate widely and some may be normal at a given time.

SAMPLING THE BONE MARROW

Indications for examination of the bone marrow include:

- Cytopenias (e.g. non-regenerative anaemia, thrombocytopenia, neutropenia, pancytopenia)
- Unexplained leucocytosis, polycythaemia or thrombocytosis
- Excessive numbers of circulating immature red cells or white cells, or cells with atypical morphology (e.g. myeloproliferative disease)
- Staging of multicentric lymphoma
- Unexplained hypercalcaemia
- Monoclonal hypergammaglobulinaemia
- Multifocal lytic bone lesions.

The bone marrow may be evaluated by two methods: cytological evaluation of a bone marrow aspirate; and histological evaluation of a core biopsy. Both sampling procedures are usually performed under sedation and local anaesthesia.

Bone marrow aspiration

The aspirate is obtained using a Klima needle, which has an interlocking stylet. The usual site for aspiration in the dog is the iliac crest (Figure 3.28a). In very small dogs and in cats the iliac crest is rather narrow and the trochanteric fossa of the femur is then the preferred site.

To obtain a sample from the iliac crest, the animal is positioned in sternal recumbency with the hindlimbs tucked up alongside the trunk. The skin over the iliac crest is aseptically prepared. A small amount of lignocaine is infiltrated into the skin and subcutis over the iliac crest and the needle of the anaesthetic syringe is then advanced on to the bone, which should feel hard. Mild pressure is applied to the needle and 1–2 ml of lignocaine infiltrated into the periosteum. A small stab incision is made in the skin and the Klima needle is introduced through the subcutis and on to the iliac crest which is stabilized between finger and thumb (Figure 3.28b). The needle is directed ventrally and slightly medially and is advanced into the bone cortex by rotating it to and fro whilst applying firm pressure. Once the Klima needle is through the bone cortex it will be firmly lodged in the bone. The stylet is removed (Figure 3.28c) and a 10 or 20 ml syringe is attached to the Klima needle. The marrow is then aspirated by

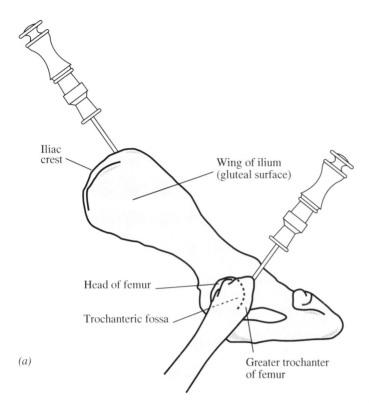

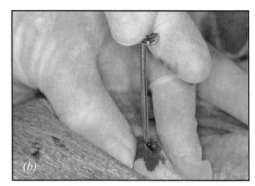

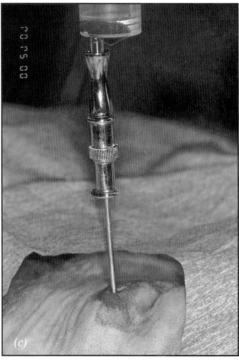

Figure 3.28: *Bone marrow aspiration. (a) The iliac crest is the usual site for bone marrow aspiration. (Adapted from Dunn, 1990 with the permission of* In Practice *(BVA Publications).) (b) The iliac crest is stabilized between the finger and thumb and the Klima needle advanced into the bone cortex. (c) The stylet is removed from the Klima needle and a syringe attached. The plunger is withdrawn briskly several times until marrow is seen entering the syringe.*

several quite forceful withdrawals of the plunger. The animal will show a transient pain response as the marrow is aspirated. The plunger is released as soon as bone marrow appears in the syringe and the needle and syringe are removed quickly, as one unit.

A drop of bone marrow is placed at the top end of several slides which are positioned at a near vertical angle. Blood runs down to the bottom of the slide, whilst the marrow spicules remain on the slide. A smear is made by placing a second slide flat over the first slide at right angles to it. This has the effect of crushing the marrow spicules. The upper slide is then drawn across the first slide in a horizontal plane and the smear is produced on the lower surface of the second slide (Figure 3.29). Smears should be made quickly as the marrow clots rapidly (usually within 30 seconds). To prevent clotting, 1 ml of 3% EDTA solution may be used as an anticoagulant in the barrel of the syringe.

If the Klima needle is not completely through the cortex, or if it has been pushed in too far and is lodged against the far cortex, aspiration will be unsuccessful. The stylet should be replaced and the needle withdrawn slightly before reaspirating. If aspiration if still unsuccessful the needle should be withdrawn and a second attempt made, directing the needle in a slightly

different direction, e.g. slightly obliquely, or at an alternative site such as the proximal shaft of the humerus. If aspiration is still unsuccessful a bone marrow core biopsy should be taken. Repeated 'dry taps' may be due to myelofibrosis, aplastic anaemia or packing out of the bone marrow by tumour infiltrate.

The smears are allowed to air-dry and should then be fixed in methanol for 3 minutes. A two-stage staining procedure using May–Grünwald and then Giemsa is used. Prussian blue (Pearl's) stain is used to demonstrate the marrow iron stores (haemosiderin deposits) which stain deep blue.

Cytological evaluation

The smear should first be examined under low power to assess whether the sample is of sufficient diagnostic quality. A good smear (Figure 3.30a) contains flecks (spicules) of haemopoietic cells that have spread out to form a monolayer. Excessive haemodilution results in poor cell morphology (Figure 3.30b). If no intact spicules are present interpretation is difficult or impossible.

The megakaryocytes are located in the marrow spicules and are assessed using low-power objectives.

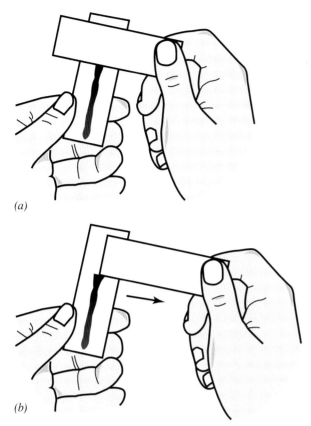

(a)

(b)

Figure 3.29: *A bone marrow smear is made by placing a second slide over the sample slide (a) and drawing the top slide over the sample slide (b). The smear is on the lower surface of the top slide.*

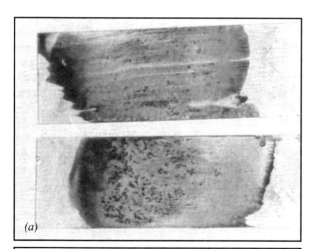

(a)

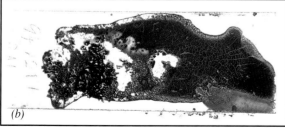

(b)

Figure 3.30: *(a) A good quality stained bone marrow smear with numerous marrow flecks, seen as dark particles. (b) A poor quality bone marrow smear which is very haemodiluted and has large clots. Reproduced from Dunn (1990) with permission of* In Practice *(BVA Publications).*

The number of megakaryocytes per fleck is variable, but normally 2-6 megakaryocytes are seen in a marrow fleck that occupies most of a low-power (x20) field.

The myeloid (granulocytic) and erythroid series are examined using high-power objectives. Myeloblasts and proerythroblasts are large cells with large round nuclei and a small amount of cytoplasm. The myeloblast cytoplasm is pale blue-grey whilst the erythroblast cytoplasm is deep blue. Promyelocytes are readily recognizable by their large pink cytoplasmic granules. These granules are no longer visible in the myelocyte, which has clear cytoplasm and a slightly indented nucleus. The nucleus becomes progressively bean-shaped (metamyelocyte) then horseshoe-shaped (band neutrophil) and finally segmented in the mature neutrophil.

Since one myeloblast gives rise to 16-32 neutrophils there should be more bands and neutrophils than myeloblasts and promyelocytes. Similarly, there should be more intermediate and late normoblasts than proerythroblasts and early normoblasts. Early normoblasts have very coarsely clumped chromatin and dark blue cytoplasm. The nucleus becomes progressively smaller and denser and the cytoplasm becomes progressively lighter through the intermediate to late normoblast stages. The late normoblast has a pyknotic nucleus and light blue-grey (polychromatophilic) cytoplasm. The myeloid:erythroid ratio is the ratio of myeloid cells to nucleated erythroid cells. This is usually estimated subjectively. The normal ratio is between 0.75:1 and 2:1 (Tyler and Cowell, 1989).

The bone marrow of normal dogs contains <15% lymphoid cells, which are mostly small lymphocytes, and <2% plasma cells. In the cat <20% of the cells are lymphoid cells and <2% are plasma cells. Small numbers of macrophages are present, which may contain phagocytosed cellular debris.

Bone marrow core biopsy

The site of choice is the iliac crest in medium to large dogs and the trochanteric fossa in cats and small dogs. A Jamshidi needle is inserted through the cortex. The stylet is removed and the needle is advanced a further 1-2 cm into the marrow cavity. The needle is then rotated vigorously in one direction to ensure the biopsy sample is completely cut at its base. The needle is removed from the bone and the core sample is expelled from the top of needle using a blunt probe. The sample should be fixed in buffered formalin. It must be decalcified for 24-48 hours prior to sectioning and staining. A core biopsy sample has the advantage that the architecture of the marrow can be evaluated and cellularity can be assessed accurately. Core biopsy is particularly useful in the diagnosis of aplastic anaemia and myelofibrosis.

REFERENCES AND FURTHER READING

Blue JT, French TW and Kranz JS (1988) Non-lymphoid haemopoietic neoplasia in cats: a retrospective study of 60 cases. *Cornell Veterinarian* **78**, 21-42

Burman SL, Ferrari L, Medhurst CL and Watson ADJ (1982) Pyruvate kinase deficiency anaemia in a Basenji dog. *Australian Veterinary Journal* **59**, 118-119

Campbell KL (1985) Canine cyclic haematopoiesis. *Compendium of Continuing Education for the Practising Veterinarian* **7**, 57-62

Canfield PJ and Watson ADJ (1989) Investigation of bone marrow dyscrasia in a Poodle with macrocytosis. *Journal of Comparative Pathology* **101**, 269- 277

Chapman BL and Giger U (1990) Inherited pyruvate kinase deficiency in the West Highland White Terrier. *Journal of Small Animal Practice* **31**, 610-616

Chinn RD, Myers RK and Matthews JA (1985) Neutrophilic leucocytosis associated with metastatic fibrosarcoma in a dog. *Journal of the American Veterinary Medical Association* **8**, 806-809

Couto CG, Boudrieau RJ and Zanjani ED (1989) Tumour-associated erythrocytosis in a dog with nasal fibrosarcoma. *Journal of Veterinary Internal Medicine* **3**, 183-185

Dunn JK (1990) Bone marrow aspiration and biopsy in dogs and cats. *In Practice* **12**, 200-206

Dunn JK (1991) Diseases of the haematopoietic system. In: *Canine Medicine and Therapeutics, 3rd edn*, ed. EA Chandler *et al.*, pp. 417-448. Blackwell Scientific, Oxford.

Guilford WG (1987) Primary immunodeficiency diseases of dogs and cats. *Compendium of Continuing Education for the Practising Veterinarian* **9**, 641- 648, 650

Harvey JW (1984) Canine bone marrow: normal haematopoiesis, biopsy techniques, and cell identification and evaluation. *Compendium of Continuing Education for the Practising Veterinarian* **6**, 909-925

Harvey RG (1990) Feline hypereosinophilia with cutaneous lesions. *Journal of Small Animal Practice* **31**, 453-456

Helfand SC, Couto CG and Madewell BR (1985) Immune-mediated thrombocytopenia associated with solid tumours in dogs. *Journal of the American Animal Hospital Association* **21**, 787-793

Jain NC (1993) *Essentials of Veterinary Haematology.* Lea & Febiger, Philadelphia

Jergens AE, Turrentine MA, Kraus KH (1987) Buccal mucosa bleeding times of healthy dogs and dogs in various pathologic states including thrombocytopenia, uraemia and von Willebrand's disease. *American Journal of Veterinary Research* **48**, 1337-1342

Lappin MR and Latimer KS (1988) Haematuria and extreme neutrophilic leucocytosis in a dog with a renal tubular carcinoma. *Journal of the American Veterinary Medical Association* **172**, 1289-1292

Littlewood JD (1989) Inherited bleeding disorders of dogs and cats. *Journal of Small Animal Practice* **30**, 140-143

Littlewood JD (1997) *Laboratory Investigation of Bleeding Disorders.* Lecture notes from: Advanced Course in Small Animal Medicine, University of Cambridge

Loar AS (1994) Anaemia: diagnosis and treatment. In: *Consultations in Feline Medicine,* ed. J.R. August, pp.469-487. Lippincott, Philadelphia

Luttgen PJ, Marlyn SW, Wolf AM and Scruggs DW (1990) Heinz body haemolytic anaemia associated with high plasma zinc concentration in a dog. *Journal of the American Veterinary Medical Association* **10**, 1347-1350

Mackin A (1995) Canine immune-mediated thrombocytopenia. Part II. *Compendium of Continuing Education for the Practising Veterinarian* **17**, 515-532

Morgan RV, Moore FM, Pearce LK, Rossi T (1991) Clinical and laboratory findings in small companion animals with lead poisoning: 347 cases (1977-1986). *Journal of the American Animal Hospital Association* **199**, 93-97

Northern J Jr and Tvedten HV (1992) Diagnosis of microthrombocytosis and immune-mediated thrombocytopenia in dogs with thrombocytopenia: 68 cases (1987-1989). *Journal of the American Veterinary Medical Association* **200**, 368-372

Stone MS and Freden GO (1990) Differentiation of anaemia of inflammatory disease from anaemia of iron deficiency. *Compendium of Continuing Education for the Practising Veterinarian* **12**, 963-966

Thomas JS (1996) Von Willebrand's disease in the dog and cat. *Veterinary Clinics of North America: Small Animal Practice* **26**, 1089-1110

Tvedten H (1989) Haemostatic abnormalities. In: *Small Animal Clinical Diagnosis by Laboratory Methods,* ed. MD Willard *et al.*, pp.86-102. WB Saunders, Philadelphia

Tyler RD and Cowell RL (1989) Bone marrow. In: *Diagnostic Cytology of the Dog and Cat,* ed. P.W. Pratt, pp.99-120. American Veterinary Publications, Goleta, California

Van Steenhouse JL, Taboada J and Millard JR (1993) Feline haemobartonellosis. *Compendium of Continuing Education for the Practising Veterinarian* **15**, 535-544

Watson ADJ, Moore AS and Helfand SC (1994) Primary erythrocytosis in the cat: treatment with hydroxurea. *Journal of Small Animal Practice* **35**, 320- 325

Willard MD, Tvedton H and Turnwald GH (1995) *Small Animal Clinical Diagnosis by Laboratory Methods, 2nd Edn.* WB Saunders, Philadelphia

Clinical Biochemistry

Joan Duncan

INTRODUCTION

The aims of this chapter are to aid the clinician in the selection of biochemical tests for the investigation of presenting clinical signs and to highlight the effect of sample quality (Figures 4.1 and 4.2) and drug therapy upon these parameters. The physiological and pathological states that produce alterations in the serum concentration or activities of the analytes are listed and outlined briefly. A detailed discussion of the clinical importance and role of these biochemical tests in the investigation of individual diseases is given in the organ-specific chapters of this manual.

The reference values stated are those proposed by Tennant (1997). Reference values not listed in the *BSAVA Small Animal Formulary, 2nd edition*, have been selected from the veterinary literature and the source documented. Each individual laboratory (or in-house analyser) may use a different assay time, temperature and concentration of substrate in the measurement of any given analyte. It is imperative that interpretation of data is made with regard to specific

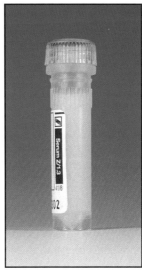

Figure 4.1: Opacity of serum due to the accumulation of triglyceride-rich lipoproteins (lipaemia). Lipaemia may interfere with the measurement of many analytes.

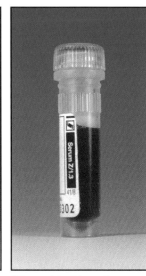

Figure 4.2: The red discoloration of the serum is caused by red cell destruction with leakage of haemoglobin (haemolysis).

reference ranges established for the methodology employed (see Chapter 2). This caveat is particularly true for the measurement of serum enzyme activities. 'Critical values' have been detailed for analytes in which a marked increase or decrease in serum concentration leads to life-threatening events.

SERUM PROTEINS

Total protein and albumin

Physiology
The circulating proteins are synthesized predominantly in the liver, although plasma cells also contribute to their production. Quantitatively the single most important protein is albumin (35–50% of the total serum protein concentration) (Kaneko, 1989). The other proteins are collectively known as globulins. The functions of proteins are many and varied but include maintenance of plasma osmotic pressure, transport of substances around the body (e.g. ferritin, caeruloplasmin), humoral immunity, buffering and enzyme regulation.

Indications for assay
The measurement of proteins is generally included in an initial health screen in all patients but especially where intestinal, renal or hepatic disease or haemorrhage is suspected.

Analysis
Protein concentrations can be estimated in serum, plasma, urine or body fluids with a refractometer or by spectrophotometry. Serum albumin levels are measured by bromocresol green dye binding and the serum globulin is calculated by subtraction of the albumin concentration from the total protein concentration.

Reference ranges

	Dogs	Cats
Serum total protein (g/l)	50–78	60–82
Serum albumin (g/l)	22–35	25–39
Serum globulin (g/l)	22–45	26–50

Neonates and very young animals have lower concentrations of albumin and globulins (due to minimal quantities of immunoglobulins). As the animal gains immunocompetence the protein concentrations rise to reach adult values. Physiological decreases in albumin may be noted during pregnancy (Kaneko, 1989).

Critical values
Marked hypoalbuminaemia (<15 g/l) is associated with the development of ascites and tissue oedema.

Accumulation of peritoneal fluid may occur at higher albumin concentrations if there is concurrent portal vein hypertension, e.g. in chronic liver disease.

Interfering phenomena
Lipaemia, haemolysis and hyperbilirubinaemia produce false increases in total protein concentrations.

Drug effects
Hormones have a marginal effect on plasma protein concentrations. Corticosteroids and anabolic steroids may increase the protein concentration due to their anabolic effects (Burkhard and Meyer, 1995) while the catabolic effects of thyroxine can cause a decrease (Kaneko, 1989).

Causes of hyperalbuminaemia
Haemoconcentration secondary to dehydration and a reduction in circulating fluid volume produces a rise in serum albumin concentration.

Causes of hypoalbuminaemia
Glomerular protein loss, protein-losing enteropathies and hepatic insufficiency are the most common causes of a serum albumin concentration below 20 g/l (Figure 4.3). Because of its small molecular size, albumin is selectively lost in renal and intestinal disease. Where intestinal lesions are more severe there may be a concurrent decrease in globulin concentration. The liver is the sole site of albumin synthesis and thus plasma protein concentration is a crude indicator of hepatic function. However, protein synthesis is one of the last hepatic functions to fail. In experimental studies, 80% of the liver mass must be surgically removed before hypoalbuminaemia develops (Hall, 1985). The differentiation of renal, intestinal or hepatic disease as a cause of marked hypoalbuminaemia may be made on the basis of clinical examination, history and additional laboratory tests. Glomerular protein loss is characterized by a normal globulin

---

Increased loss
Glomerular protein loss
Protein-losing enteropathy*
Cutaneous lesions, e.g. burns*
External haemorrhage*

Decreased production
Hepatic insufficiency
Malnutrition
Maldigestion
Malabsorption

Sequestration
Body cavity effusion

Figure 4.3: Causes of hypoalbuminaemia.
* Concurrent decrease in globulins may be noted.

concentration, proteinuria in the absence of an inflammatory urinary sediment, and an increased urinary protein:creatinine ratio. Where the hypoalbuminaemia is associated with liver disease there may be a normal or increased globulin concentration, variable liver enzyme changes and abnormalities of liver function tests. Intestinal protein loss is difficult to confirm as a cause of hypoalbuminaemia, but the clinical signs (including diarrhoea and weight loss) and a concurrent decrease in serum globulin concentration provide supportive evidence (see Chapter 8). Differential diagnoses include intestinal neoplasia (diffuse and localized), severe inflammatory bowel disease and lymphangiectasia.

The alterations in plasma proteins associated with nutritional changes are generally subtle but severe protein restriction results in hypoalbuminaemia and hypoproteinaemia. Other causes of hypoalbuminaemia should be excluded before dietary influences or maldigestion/malabsorption are incriminated as the sole cause of hypoproteinaemia.

Globulins

Analysis
Serum protein electrophoresis (SPE) on cellulose acetate gels allows fractionation of the proteins, depending predominantly on their charge and size. After staining for protein, the cellulose acetate strip is scanned by a densitometer which converts the relative intensities of the protein bands to percentages and generates a graph that demonstrates the protein fractions (albumin, α_1-globulin, α_2-globulin, β_1-globulin, β_2-globulin, γ-globulin).

Increased density of the globulin bands may be described as polyclonal or monoclonal gammopathy. Polyclonal gammopathies have a broad-based peak in the ß or γ region (or both) on the electrophoretic trace and are caused by the production of a mix of immunoglobulins and acute phase reacting proteins. This pattern is typically seen in chronic inflammatory conditions, hepatic disease or suppurative inflammation. Monoclonal gammopathies have a narrow-based spike which is generally present in the region and is the result of production of a single immunoglobulin class by a single plasma cell line. In dogs this pattern is most commonly associated with multiple myeloma but other differential diagnoses include Waldenström's macroglobulinaemia, lymphoma (malignant lymphoma, lymphosarcoma) and extramedullary plasmacytoma.

Reference ranges
Pathology laboratories performing SPE will provide reference ranges specific to the species sampled and the methodology employed. Interpretation of electrophoretic traces should be made with reference to these values.

Causes of hypoglobulinaemia
The most common pathological causes are haemorrhage and protein-losing enteropathies.

Causes of hyperglobulinaemia
In dogs, a marked rise in plasma globulins is most frequently noted with multiple myeloma while in the cat, feline infectious peritonitis (FIP) is a common cause of hyperglobulinaemia (globulins >60 g/l) (Figure 4.4). However, hyperproteinaemia (total proteins >78 g/l) is noted in only 55% of cases of effusive FIP and 75% of cases of dry FIP (Hoskins, 1991).

Confirmation of FIP requires histological evaluation of tissue samples but analysis of free peritoneal fluid, SPE and coronavirus titres often provide supportive evidence. A polyclonal gammopathy is most commonly noted on SPE but this is not pathognomonic for FIP. It has been suggested that the albumin:globulin ratio in free peritoneal fluid is helpful in establishing or excluding a diagnosis (Shelly *et al.*, 1988).

Multiple myeloma is the most common cause of a monoclonal gammopathy in dogs. Feline monoclonal gammopathies have rarely been described in the veterinary literature. The diagnosis of multiple myeloma depends on identifying at least two of the following criteria: radiographic evidence of lytic skeletal lesions, Bence–Jones proteinuria (i.e. the identification of immunoglobulin light chain dimers in the urine), infiltration of the bone marrow with plasma cells (>20%) and a monoclonal gammopathy (Dorfman and Dimski, 1992). Lytic skeletal lesions are often noted in the pelvis, vertebral column, ribs and long bones of the dog but are rare in feline myeloma (Hohenhaus, 1995).

Polyclonal gammopathy

Infections:
  Bacterial disease
  Viral disease (e.g. FIP)

Immune-mediated diseases:
  Systemic lupus erythematosus
  Rheumatoid arthritis
  Immune-mediated haemolytic anaemia
  Immune-mediated thrombocytopenia

Neoplasia, especially lymphosarcoma

Monoclonal gammopathy

Neoplasia:
  Multiple myeloma
  Macroglobulinaemia
  Lymphosarcoma

Feline infectious peritonitis (rare)

Figure 4.4: Causes of hyperglobulinaemia.

INDICATORS OF RENAL FUNCTION

Urea nitrogen

Physiology
Dietary proteins are hydrolysed in the intestines to their constituent amino acids which may, in turn, be degraded to ammonia by the action of gut bacteria. The ammonia and amino acids are transported to the liver via the portal circulation where they are utilized in the urea cycle. The urea formed in the hepatocytes is excreted via the kidney tubules. Urea plays an important role in concentrating the urine; the presence of high concentrations of urea and sodium chloride in the renal medullary interstitium creates an osmotic gradient for reabsorption of water.

Indications for assay
The urea nitrogen (urea) concentration is one of the tests used when screening renal function. It is often measured when the clinical signs include vomiting, anorexia, weight loss, polydipsia and dehydration.

Analysis
Urea can be measured in serum, plasma and urine by spectrophotometry. Stick tests for whole blood are also available.

Reference ranges

Dogs	3.0-9.0 mmol/l
Cats	5.0-10.0 mmol/l

Interfering phenomena
Gross lipaemia interferes with the analysis and produces variable effects depending on the methodology.

Drug effects
Increased urea and creatinine concentrations may be associated with corticosteroid therapy and the use of nephrotoxic drugs including non-steroidal anti-inflammatory drugs and aminoglycoside antibiotics (Figure 4.5). Aminoglycoside nephrotoxicity is the second most common cause of acute renal failure in the dog and cat (Chew and DiBartola, 1989).

Corticosteroids
Aminoglycoside antibiotics (e.g. neomycin, gentamycin)
Cisplatin
Ethylene glycol
Non-steroidal anti-inflammatory drugs (when there is pre-existing renal disease)
Frusemide

Figure 4.5: Drugs that may produce increased urea and creatinine concentrations.

Causes of reduced blood urea
Reduced dietary protein intake is associated with a low blood urea. In addition, patients with diffuse liver disease have an impaired capacity to synthesize urea and reduced hepatic production is noted in dogs with portosystemic shunts. Where hepatic disease is suspected, a complete biochemistry profile and a bile acid stimulation test are indicated.

The marked diuresis associated with some conditions, especially hyperadrenocorticism and diabetes insipidus, results in increased urinary loss of urea which, in turn, causes a reduction of the blood urea.

Causes of increased blood urea
Increased dietary protein intake produces a high level of urea in the blood (Finco, 1989). A moderate increase in dietary protein is not commonly associated with a notable rise in urea above the reference range, but high-protein diets can cause significant increases. A 12-hour fast is recommended before sampling for measurement of urea (Chew and DiBartola, 1989). Intestinal haemorrhage also results in an increased concentration which is reported to correlate with the severity of blood loss (Finco, 1989). Urea is freely filtered at the glomerulus and reabsorbed in the renal tubules. The rate of reabsorption is higher at slower urinary flow rates, e.g. in dehydrated patients. Blood urea is therefore not a reliable estimate of the glomerular filtration rate (GFR). Increased urea concentrations are associated with conditions other than parenchymal renal disease. These may be classified as prerenal disease (e.g. dehydration, cardiac failure) or postrenal disease (e.g. urethral obstruction, ruptured bladder). The presence of a concentrated urine sample (urine SG >1.030 in dogs, >1.035 in cats) supports the diagnosis of a prerenal azotaemia. It should be noted, however, that where other disease processes, such as hypercalcaemia and hypoadrenocorticism, interfere with the ability of the renal tubules to concentrate the urine, there may be a prerenal azotaemia without production of maximally concentrated urine.

Assessment of renal function, therefore, is best achieved by simultaneous measurement of blood urea and creatinine and urine specific gravity. Serial monitoring of the renal parameters during fluid therapy is a helpful means of establishing the reversibility of the azotaemia.

Creatinine

Physiology
Creatinine is formed from creatine in the muscles in an irreversible reaction. The quantity of creatinine produced depends upon diet (small contribution) and the muscle mass. Disease affecting the muscle mass may affect the daily creatinine production.

Both urea and creatinine are freely filtered at the renal glomerulus but urea is subject to tubular reabsorption and thus creatinine is said to be a better indicator of GFR.

Indications for assay

These are as for urea (see above).

Analysis

Creatinine can be measured in serum, plasma or abdominal fluid by spectrophotometric methods.

Reference ranges

Dogs   20–110 µmol/l
Cats   40–150 µmol/l

Interfering phenomena

False increases in serum creatinine concentrations are noted in lipaemic samples, while hyperbilirubinaemia has variable effects depending on the degree of icterus. Dry reagent methods may not be affected by hyperbilirubinaemia (reference should be made to the manufacturer's literature). Haemolysis may cause an increase or decrease in concentration depending on the methodology used.

Drug effects

Nephrotoxic drugs may cause an increase in serum creatinine concentrations (see Figure 4.5).

Causes of low serum creatinine

Since the daily production of creatinine is dependent upon the muscle mass of the animal, the body condition should be considered when interpreting serum creatinine concentrations. A poor body condition may be associated with low concentrations while minor rises in such cases may be more significant than in other individuals.

Causes of increased serum creatinine

Decreased glomerular filtration is the major cause of raised serum creatinine. However, approximately 75% of nephron function must be impaired before serum creatinine (and urea) is increased (Chew and DiBartola, 1989). Creatinine is considered a more reliable indicator of GFR than is urea nitrogen, since there are fewer factors which influence the serum concentration of creatinine.

MARKERS OF HEPATIC DISEASE

The biochemical parameters used to assess liver pathology may be divided into two classes: the hepatic enzymes that reflect liver damage and cholestasis, and the endogenous indicators of liver function (see Chapter 9). Alanine aminotransferase (ALT) is the most useful enzyme for identifying hepatocellular damage in dogs and cats but should not be used alone as a screening test for liver disease. The production of other enzymes, i.e. alkaline phosphatase (ALP) and gamma-glutamyl transferase (GGT), is increased secondary to intra- and extrahepatic cholestasis. These enzymes are markers of cholestatic disease. Bilirubin, serum albumin and serum bile acids are considered to be indicators of hepatic function (see Chapter 9). It is common for extrahepatic disease (e.g. pancreatitis, diabetes mellitus, hyperadrenocorticism and inflammatory bowel disease) to cause abnormalities of these biochemical parameters.

Alanine aminotransferase (ALT)

Physiology

ALT is found in the cytosol of hepatocytes and in muscle tissue in the dog and cat. Activities in the serum are elevated by leakage of the enzyme secondary to an increase in hepatocyte membrane permeability or cell necrosis. The former may simply be a consequence of hypoxia and need not reflect cell death. Increased serum ALT may be noted within 12 hours of an acute hepatic insult but can take 3–4 days to reach peak levels after experimental cholestasis (Hall, 1985). The degree of increase in enzyme activity correlates approximately with the number of hepatocytes affected but does not indicate the nature, severity or reversibility of the pathological process. ALT activity is not an indicator of hepatic function.

Indications for assay

Serum ALT is a useful aid in the diagnosis of hepatic disease and is measured where the clinical signs might suggest a hepatopathy, e.g. weight loss, anorexia, polydipsia, vomiting, diarrhoea, ascites and jaundice.

Analysis

The activity of the enzyme (in international units) is measured in serum or plasma by spectrophotometric methods under specified conditions.

Reference ranges

Dogs   <100 units/l
Cats   <75 units/l

The interpretation of data should be made with regard to specific reference ranges established for the methodology employed.

Interfering phenomena

Serum ALT activities are falsely increased with lipaemia and haemolysis.

Drug effects

Raised ALT may be associated with enzyme induction after administration of hepatotoxic drugs and glucocorticoids (Figure 4.6).

Causes of raised ALT activity

Guidelines for the interpretation of raised liver enzyme

Glucocorticoids
Phenobarbital
Primidone
Paracetamol
Barbiturates
Griseofulvin
Ketoconazole
Ibuprofen
Phenylbutazone
Salicylates

Figure 4.6: *Drugs that may cause increases in the serum activities of ALT, ALP, AST and GGT.*

activities in relation to liver diseases are given in Chapter 9. The majority of diseases that affect the liver could potentially cause an increase in serum ALT activity but those pathological processes that might cause a marked increase include parenchymal disease/ damage, cholangitis, cholangiohepatitis, chronic hepatitis, anoxia, cirrhosis and diffuse neoplasia, e.g. lymphoma (lymphosarcoma). However, in some cases these diseases may be accompanied by a negligible increase or no increase in serum ALT activity (Sevelius, 1995).

Causes of reduced ALT activity

An artefactual reduction in serum enzyme activities may result from substrate depletion. Dilution and repeat assay of the sample are necessary to exclude this phenomenon. Reduced ALT activities (below the reference range) are generally not considered to be of clinical significance, but the possibility of chronic liver disease and nutritional deficiencies (zinc or vitamin B6) should be considered (Meyer *et al.*, 1992).

Aspartate aminotransferase (AST)
(see also Muscle enzymes)

Physiology

AST is located in the mitochondria of the cell and is present in significant quantities in hepatocytes, erythrocytes and in muscle. AST is therefore not liver-specific but, like ALT, its activity in the serum is elevated by leakage of the enzyme from the cell.

Indications for assay

AST is included in diagnostic profiles for investigation of suspected liver disease or muscle disease.

Analysis

The enzyme activity is measured in serum and heparinized plasma by spectrophotometry.

Reference ranges

Dogs	7–50 units/l
Cats	7–60 units/l

The interpretation of data should be made with regard to specific reference ranges established for the methodology employed.

Interfering phenomena

Haemolysis and lipaemia may cause false increases in serum values.

Drug effects

Raised AST may be associated with enzyme induction after administration of hepatotoxic drugs and glucocorticoids (see Figure 4.6) .

Causes of raised AST

The most common causes of increased AST are hepatic disease, muscle disease (trauma, inflammation) and haemolysis. Concurrent measurement of other hepatic enzymes (ALT, ALP, GGT) and hepatic function indicators (albumin, urea, bilirubin, bile acids) are essential to establish the origin of the increased serum AST and to provide further information regarding liver damage and function (see Chapter 9). With respect to liver damage, the serum activity of AST tends to parallel that of ALT (Hall, 1985).

Alkaline phosphatase (ALP, SAP)

Physiology

In dogs and cats there are isoforms of ALP located in brush borders in the liver, placenta, intestine, kidney and bone. In the dog there is also a steroid-induced isoenzyme (SIALP), the origin of which has not been fully determined. The production of SIALP is increased by the administration of glucocorticoids (oral, parenteral or topical), by excessive production of endogenous glucocorticoids (hyperadrenocorticism) and in association with chronic disease (e.g. renal or hepatic). The liver isoenzyme is responsible for the serum activity in the normal adult dog and cat.

Indications for assay

Serum ALP is one of the tests commonly included in screening profiles for hepatic disease (cholestasis) and hyperadrenocorticism. It is therefore useful where the clinical signs suggest either of these diagnoses, e.g. weight loss, anorexia, polydipsia, vomiting, diarrhoea, ascites and jaundice.

Analysis

Serum ALP activity is measured in serum or heparinized plasma by spectrophotometry. SIALP can be measured by many commercial laboratories but is not suitable as a confirmatory test for hyperadrenocorticism.

Reference ranges

Dogs	<200 units/l
Cats	<100 units/l

The interpretation of data should be made with regard to specific reference ranges established for the methodology employed.

Interfering phenomena
Marked hyperbilirubinaemia, haemolysis and lipaemia may affect the enzyme activity. EDTA is not a suitable anticoagulant since it causes a falsely decreased result.

Drug effects
Raised ALP may be associated with the administration of anticonvulsants, glucocorticoids and drugs that cause cholestasis or enzyme induction (see Figure 4.6).

Causes of raised ALP
From a diagnostic viewpoint the most important isoenzymes in small animals are the bone, hepatic and steroid-induced forms. Increases in bone ALP causes raised serum activities in young growing animals, but values are rarely more than two-fold greater than the upper limit of the adult reference range (Dial, 1992). This physiological increase in serum ALP should be considered when interpreting results from immature patients.

Increases in the hepatic isoenzyme are commonly associated with cholestatic disease, which may be intrahepatic or extrahepatic. Causes of the latter include pancreatitis, pancreatic neoplasia and cholelithiasis. Choleliths are very rare in the dog. There is no correlation between hepatic function and the rise in ALP activity. The enzyme is generally included in profiles where it contributes to the diagnosis of hepatic disease (see Chapter 9). ALP should not be used alone when screening patients for evidence of liver disease.

In dogs, the increase in ALP associated with steroid administration varies depending on the patient, the drug used and the route of administration. In some individuals, drug administration (oral, parenteral or topical) can cause enzyme increases that persist for at least 6 weeks (Center, 1989). Although increased SIALP may be a consequence of hyperadrenocorticism, testing for SIALP does not differentiate between this endocrine disease and other diseases (see Chapter 17). SIALP is not recommended as the sole screening test for hyperadrenocorticism (Mack, 1994).

ALP in the cat has a very short half-life and the magnitude of increase noted in hepatic disease is generally less than that recorded in dogs (Meyer and Williams, 1992). Any increase in ALP is probably significant in a cat.

Gamma-glutamyl transferase (GGT)

Physiology
GGT is a cytosolic and membrane-bound enzyme found in highest concentrations in the brush borders of the renal and bile duct epithelium. Cholestasis and enzyme induction due to glucocorticoid therapy cause increased serum activities.

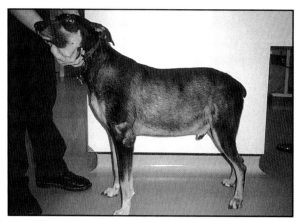

Figure 4.7: A 12-year-old crossbreed dog with hyperadrenocorticism. Classical biochemical abnormalities associated with Cushing's disease include raised serum ALP activity and hypercholesterolaemia.

Indications for assay
GGT is used in conjunction with ALP and other liver tests in the diagnosis and monitoring of hepatic disease. It is thought to be more useful than ALP in the cat and the serum activity in dogs does not appear to be affected by the administration of anticonvulsants (Meyer *et al.*, 1992.

Analysis
GGT activity is measured in serum and plasma by spectrophotometry.

Reference ranges

Dogs	0–8.0 units/l
Cats	0–8.0 units/l

The interpretation of data should be made with regard to specific reference ranges established for the methodology employed.

Interfering phenomena
Lipaemia may affect the measurement of GGT.

Drug effects
Raised GGT may be associated with the administration of glucocorticoids and drugs that cause cholestasis or enzyme induction (see Figure 4.6) .

Causes of increased GGT
Serum GGT is a marker for cholestatic disease in the dog and cat (see Chapter 9). In the cat it may be more useful than ALP in the diagnosis of cholestatic hepatic disease (Meyer *et al.*, 1992).

Bilirubin

Physiology
Bilirubin is derived from the catabolism of haemoproteins (predominantly haemoglobin) in the cells of the

reticuloendothelial system (see Chapter 9). The newly formed lipid-soluble bilirubin (unconjugated or indirect-reacting bilirubin) is then bound to albumin, which facilitates its transfer through the aqueous phase of the plasma to the liver. In the hepatocyte the bilirubin is conjugated with glucuronic acid, creating a water-soluble molecule (conjugated or direct-reacting bilirubin).

Indications for assay
Measurement of bilirubin is indicated where there is jaundice on clinical examination, visible icterus of the serum or plasma (Figure 4.8), or suspected hepatic disease. Clinical jaundice in the dog is detected when the bilirubin is at least 25–35 μmol/l (Center, 1989).

Analysis
The total serum bilirubin concentration (conjugated and unconjugated) is measured in serum or plasma by spectrophotometry.

Reference ranges

Dogs   0–6.8 μmol/l
Cats   0–6.8 μmol/l

Interfering phenomena
Severe haemolysis and lipaemia interfere with spectrophotometric methods of bilirubin measurement. Exposure of samples to fluorescent light and sunlight decreases the serum bilirubin concentration (up to 50% per hour).

Drug effects
Increased concentrations may be associated with drugs that induce hepatic necrosis or haemolytic anaemia, e.g. paracetamol.

Causes of hyperbilirubinaemia
Jaundice may be classified according to the underlying pathological process: prehepatic jaundice (increased production of bilirubin, e.g. haemolytic anaemia, and internal haemorrhage); hepatic jaundice (failure of uptake or conjugation of bilirubin); and posthepatic

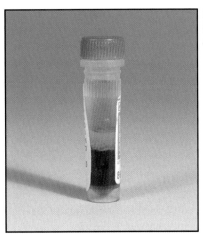

Figure 4.8: An icteric serum sample.

jaundice (obstruction of the biliary system). A full haematological profile is indicated in all jaundiced patients to exclude the possibility of prehepatic causes. Characteristic findings that may be noted in haemolytic anaemia include marked reticulocytosis (indicative of erythrocyte regeneration), autoagglutination of the red cells and the formation of spherocytes. The platelet count and serum proteins are commonly within the reference range for the species. The abnormalities of bilirubin associated with hepatic disease and cholestatic disease are discussed more fully in Chapter 9. Previously it was believed that the measurement of direct and indirect-reacting bilirubin would help to determine the cause of the jaundice. However, it is now clear that this is not the case in the dog and cat and that hepatic, haemolytic and biliary tract diseases produce variable increases in these fractions (Hall, 1985). Differentiation of prehepatic, hepatic and post-hepatic jaundice requires a full haematological and biochemical investigation (including measurement of red cell mass, examination of a blood smear and liver function tests) and may require examination of the biliary tract. Hepatic biopsy may also be necessary in some cases.

Bile acids

Physiology
The primary bile acids (cholic acid and chenodeoxycholic acid) are produced in the liver from cholesterol and are then conjugated to taurine or glycine. They are excreted into the biliary tree and stored in the gallbladder. Gallbladder contraction (stimulated by ingestion of food) releases the bile acids into the intestines where they facilitate the digestion and absorption of dietary lipid. The bile acids are efficiently reabsorbed in the ileum, resulting in very small faecal loss. The total pool of bile acids may undergo enterohepatic circulation two to five times during a single meal (Center, 1989).

Indications for assay
Inclusion of bile acids in a profile is indicated where there is suspicion of hepatic disease. Clinical signs in such patients might include hepatomegaly, microhepatica and abnormal central nervous system signs. The sensitivity of the bile acid assay may be increased by using a bile acid stimulation test (see below).

Analysis
Bile acids are measured in serum or plasma by radioimmunoassay, spectrophotometry and gas layer chromatography.

Reference ranges (fasted)

Dogs   0–15 μmol/l*
Cats   0–15 μmol/l*
*See Chapter 9

Interfering phenomena
Severe lipaemia and haemolysis of the sample may affect the measurement of bile acids.

Drug effects
Cholestyramine lowers serum concentrations by binding the bile acids in the intestine and preventing their reabsorption.

Causes of increased bile acids
The fasting serum bile acid concentration may be raised in association with primary or secondary hepatic disease. The assay facilitates identification of hepatic dysfunction but gives no indication as to the nature or reversibility of the liver pathology. Values exceeding 30 µmol/l are commonly associated with histological lesions and biopsy may be helpful in these cases (Center *et al.*, 1985). It is important to remember that the histological changes could still be associated with secondary hepatic disease even though the fasting bile acid concentration is >30 µmol/l, for example in hyperadrenocorticism.

The use of the bile acid stimulation test may improve the sensitivity of testing. For this, serum bile acid concentrations are measured in a sample collected after a 12-hour fast (fasting bile acid concentration) and 2 hours after a fatty meal (postprandial bile acid concentration) (see Chapter 9). In one study of 108 cats, the postprandial bile acid concentration was found to have the highest sensitivity of any single test for the diagnosis of feline liver disease (Center *et al.*, 1995).

Ammonia

Physiology
Dietary proteins are hydrolysed in the gut to amino acids which, in turn, may be degraded by intestinal bacteria, producing ammonia. Ammonia is transported to the liver where it is used as a precursor in the synthesis of urea. Increased blood ammonia concentrations are observed in some patients with diffuse liver disease (with a reduced capacity for urea synthesis) and in individuals with portosystemic shunts.

Indications for assay
Ammonia is used in the evaluation of hepatic function; the indications for measurement are the same as for bile acids (see above).

Analysis
Ammonia is measured in blood, serum or plasma by dry reagent and enzymatic methods. Samples should be collected into a chilled sample tube and stored on ice until analysis, which must be carried out within 20 minutes of collection (Willard *et al.*, 1994).

Reference ranges

Dogs	0–60 µmol/l
Cats	0–60 µmol/l

Interfering phenomena
Blood ammonia results are falsely increased where there is a delay in sample analysis. Use of fluoride or oxalate anticoagulants will also cause spurious increases.

Drug effects
The use of oral antibiotics (e.g. aminoglycosides), lactulose and enemas may decrease the ammonia concentration; increases are noted with diuretics (causing hypokalaemia).

Causes of increased ammonia
Increased ammonia concentrations are associated with feeding high-protein diets and with intestinal haemorrhage (due to the increased delivery of amino acids to the intestinal bacteria). Diffuse hepatic disease, resulting in the failure of conversion of ammonia to urea, and portosystemic shunts (congenital and acquired) will also produce increased serum ammonia concentrations.

PANCREATIC DISEASE

Amylase

Physiology
Amylase is a calcium-dependent enzyme, produced by the pancreatic acinar cells, which hydrolyses complex carbohydrates. The enzyme passes directly from the pancreas into the circulation where it is filtered by the renal tubules; the inactivated enzyme is reabsorbed by the tubular epithelium. Amylase activity in the tissues of the dog and cat is highest in the pancreas but is also found in the intestines and liver.

Indications for assay
Amylase should be measured when the presenting signs might suggest pancreatitis, e.g. vomiting, abdominal pain or icterus, or when there is free peritoneal fluid.

Analysis
Amylase activities may be measured in serum, heparinized plasma and abdominal fluid using spectrophotometric, amyloclastic, saccharogenic or chromogenic methods. Some saccharogenic methods are not validated for use in the dog. Amyloclastic methods, which measure the hydrolysis of starch, are suitable for use with canine serum or plasma.

Reference ranges

Dogs   400–2000 units/l
Cats   400–2000 units/l

The interpretation of data should be made with regard to specific reference ranges established for the methodology employed.

Interfering phenomena

The analysis of the enzyme is affected by sample lipaemia, which may cause a falsely low result, and by haemolysis, which produces a false increase.

Drug effects

The administration of glucocorticoids and some antibiotics (e.g. tetracyclines, sulphonamides) may play a contributory role in the development of pancreatitis or the exacerbation of existing disease (Willard *et al.*, 1994; Burkhard and Meyer, 1995) (Figure 4.9). In such cases the resulting pancreatic damage usually produces a characteristic increase in serum amylase activity.

Azathioprine
Oestrogens
Frusemide
Glucocorticoids (especially dexamethasone)
Metronidazole
Sulphonamides
Tetracycline
Thiazide diuretics
Calcium (via the production of hypercalcaemia)

Figure 4.9: Drugs that may be associated with the development of pancreatitis or the exacerbation of existing disease.

Causes of increased amylase

The tissue distribution of amylase is not restricted to the pancreas and therefore raised serum activities are not specific for pancreatitis. Reduced glomerular filtration (prerenal, renal, postrenal) is often associated with an increased serum amylase activity but in the author's experience this is commonly less than two to three times greater than the upper limit of the reference range. Serum activities above this level are suggestive of pancreatitis but the degree of increase does not correlate well with the severity of pancreatitis. If an azotaemic patient has an amylase activity two to three times the upper limit of the reference range then pancreatic disease must be considered. The simultaneous measurement of amylase and lipase in cases of suspected pancreatitis is advisable while additional tests of renal and hepatic function should also be included in the biochemical profile. Amylase is not a reliable indicator of pancreatitis in cats (Simpson *et al.*, 1994).

In cases that present with free peritoneal fluid, full analysis of the fluid (protein concentration, cell counts and cytological examination) and measurement of the serum and fluid amylase activities may be useful. The presence of a non-septic exudate with greater amylase activity than the serum may be associated with pancreatitis or bowel rupture.

Lipase

Physiology

Lipase is a digestive enzyme, produced by the pancreatic acinar cells, that hydrolyses triglycerides. The enzyme is cleared from the circulation by renal inactivation. As with amylase, lipase may originate from pancreatic or extrapancreatic sources. Pancreatic damage and inflammation results in the release of lipase into the surrounding gland and peritoneal tissue which may cause the development of necrosis in the peripancreatic peritoneal fat.

Indications for assay

Indications for the measurement of lipase are the same as for amylase. Amylase and lipase assays should be performed simultaneously in cases in which pancreatitis is suspected, but the increases in enzyme activities are often not parallel (marked increases in one enzyme may be associated with minimal increases in the other). The absence of raised serum amylase and lipase does not exclude spontaneous disease.

Analysis

Lipase activities are measured in serum, heparinized plasma and body fluids using turbidimetric methods.

Reference ranges

Dogs   0–500 units/l
Cats   0–700 units/l

The interpretation of data should be made with regard to specific reference ranges established for the methodology employed.

Interfering phenomena

Haemolysis, hyperbilirubinaemia and lipaemia may falsely decrease serum lipase activity.

Drug effects

Corticosteroids may cause an increase in serum lipase activity without histological evidence of pancreatitis, but the activity is often only slightly above the reference range (Parent, 1982). In addition, glucocorticoids and some antibiotics (see Figure 4.9) may be associated with exacerbation of existing pancreatic disease and a consequent rise in lipase activity (Willard *et al.*, 1994; Burkhard and Meyer, 1995).

Causes of raised serum lipase

Since lipase originates from both pancreatic and

extrapancreatic tissue, an increase in serum activity is not diagnostic of pancreatitis. Increased serum activity is also noted in azotaemic patients, although the values generally do not exceed two to three times the upper limit of the reference range. In addition, moderate elevations of lipase (up to 5-fold increases) have been reported in association with administration of dexamethasone without evidence of histological changes in the pancreas (Parent, 1982). A normal lipase activity does not preclude pancreatic disease.

Lipase has been reported to be persistently elevated in cats with experimentally induced pancreatitis (Kitchell *et al.*, 1986) but this is not a consistent finding in naturally occurring disease (Simpson *et al.*, 1994).

ELECTROLYTES

The water content of the body is distributed between two compartments: the extracellular fluid (ECF) and the intracellular fluid (ICF). Water passes freely between these compartments but the electrolyte composition of each is very different. Sodium, chloride and bicarbonate are the important extracellular electrolytes, while potassium, organic phosphates and proteins are important in the intracellular fluid. The concentration of sodium is high in the ECF and low in the ICF, while the converse in true for potassium. These concentrations are maintained by the energy-dependent sodium pump.

Sodium

Physiology
The volume of fluid in the vascular space (circulating volume) is related to the volume of the ECF which, in turn, varies with the total body sodium content. Decreases in the circulating volume are recognized by receptors in the cardiovascular circulation and kidney that activate the renin–angiotensin system and the secretion of aldosterone from the adrenal gland. Aldosterone promotes the reabsorption of sodium by the renal tubules while the osmolality of the ECF is maintained by the effects of antidiuretic hormone (which stimulates water reabsorption in the renal tubules) and by an increased water intake.

Indications for assay
Inclusion of serum electrolytes in a biochemical profile is indicted when clinical signs include vomiting, diarrhoea, polyuria, polydipsia, seizures or dehydration.

Analysis
Sodium concentrations are measured in serum or plasma by ion-specific potentiometry.

Reference ranges

Dogs	140–158 mmol/l
Cats	145–165 mmol/l

Drug effects
Hyponatraemia may develop during overzealous therapy with thiazides and frusemide. Hypernatraemia has been associated with fludrocortisone therapy or administration of sodium phosphate enemas in small dogs and cats.

Critical values
Neurological signs, including the onset of ataxia, seizures and coma, may occur at serum sodium concentrations below 120 mmol/l or above 170 mmol/l.

Causes of hyponatraemia
In simple terms, hyponatraemia is a consequence of movement of water into the ECF (from the cells), a retention of water in the ECF, loss of sodium from the ECF, or a shift of the electrolyte into the cells. The CNS signs associated with hyponatraemia are related more to the speed of onset of the abnormality rather than the severity of the resultant plasma osmolality (de Morais and Chew, 1992).

The most common causes of severe hyponatraemia (<135 mmol/l) in dogs and cats are vomiting, hypoadrenocorticism and congestive cardiac failure (Figure 4.10). Hypoadrenocorticism is caused by the reduced production of glucocorticoids and mineralocorticoids from the adrenal gland. Biochemical features of the disease include hyponatraemia and hyperkalaemia. The criteria for diagnosis is outlined below (see Causes of hyperkalaemia).

```
Gastrointestinal loss (vomiting, diarrhoea)
Hypoadrenocorticism
Congestive cardiac disease
'Third space' loss:
    Peritonitis
    Pancreatitis
    Uroabdomen (e.g. ruptured bladder)
    Pleural effusions (e.g. chylothorax)
Diabetes mellitus (secondary to hyperglycaemia)
Renal failure
```

Figure 4.10: Causes of hyponatraemia.

Causes of hypernatraemia
Hypernatraemia most commonly results from loss of body water in an excess of sodium. Such water loss may be associated with negligible loss of electrolytes (e.g. diabetes insipidus, heat stroke) or concurrent loss of electrolytes (e.g. vomiting, diarrhoea, chronic renal failure, diuretic therapy) (Figure 4.11). Hypernatraemia is most marked in patients with diabetes insipidus that are not allowed free access to fluids.

Pure water loss
Diabetes insipidus (central, nephrogenic)
Heat stroke, fever
Inadequate access to water
Adipsia (absence of thirst)

Hypotonic water loss
Intestinal (vomiting, diarrhoea)
Renal failure (acute and chronic, postobstructive
   diuresis)
Diuretic therapy
Diabetes mellitus (secondary to osmotic diuresis)

Figure 4.11: Causes of hypernatraemia.

Adipsia (absence of thirst) is commonly associated with hypernatraemia. Intracranial causes of adipsia include neoplasia (menigioma, glioma), trauma and inflammatory brain disease (Bagley, 1995).

Potassium

Physiology
Potassium is the major cation of the ICF. The serum concentration is under control by insulin, aldosterone and the sympathetic nervous system (de Morais and Chew, 1992). The intracellular electrolyte plays a role in the optimization of enzyme activity, the contraction of muscle and maintenance of a normal transmembrane electrical potential. Potassium is filtered freely by the renal glomeruli and then reabsorbed.

Indications for assay
Assay is indicated where intestinal or renal disease is suspected. Measurement is essential in patients with bradycardia and cardiac arrhythmia and where hypokalaemic myopathy is a differential.

Analysis
Potassium is measured in serum or plasma by ion-specific potentiometry.

Reference ranges

Dogs   3.8–5.8 mmol/l
Cats   3.6–5.8 mmol/l

Critical values
Serum potassium concentrations of <3.5 mmol/l are considered clinically significant (Willard, 1989) and concentrations of <2.5 mmol/l may cause muscle weakness. Marked hyperkalaemia (>7.5 mmol/l) is associated with cardiac conduction disturbances (Willard, 1989).

Interfering phenomena
Increased serum potassium concentrations in cats and dogs may result from a delay in separating samples with a marked leucocytosis (Henry *et al.*, 1996) or thrombocytosis (potassium is released from the platelets and white blood cells). The erythrocytes of the Japanese Akita contain high concentrations of potassium and haemolysis in a blood sample from this breed often results in a spurious hyperkalaemia. Contamination of a sample with potassium–EDTA can cause marked increases in potassium concentration. This most commonly occurs when the tip of the syringe containing the blood sample contacts EDTA in one container before ejecting the remaining blood into another tube.

Drug effects
Hypokalaemia may be a consequence of diuretic (frusemide, thiazides), mineralocorticoid or insulin therapy. Nephrogenic drugs, including cisplatin, may induce a hypokalaemia which is identifiable before the detection of azotaemia (Willard, 1989). Potassium-containing drugs and potassium-sparing diuretics may cause hyperkalaemia in the presence of other contributory factors (Chew and Carothers, 1989).

Causes of hypokalaemia
Hypokalaemia commonly results from increased renal or intestinal loss (Figure 4.12). In particular, moderate or severe hypokalaemia is associated with chronic vomiting, polyuric chronic renal failure and insulin therapy during the correction of ketoacidosis. Decreased intake of potassium may contribute to the development of hypokalaemia but is rarely solely responsible for a clinically significant decrease in serum electrolyte concentrations. Hypokalaemic myopathy has been described as the most common cause of rapid-onset generalized muscle weakness in the cat and is seen in animals with potassium depletion. The electrolyte abnormality is commonly a consequence of chronic renal failure in the cat (Dow *et al.*, 1989). Cats may present with acute life-threatening muscle weakness and paralysis or a less severe muscle weakness. Classically, there is cervical ventroflexion and a stiff gait. Affected individuals may collapse on exercise.

Gastrointestinal loss (vomiting of gastric
   contents, diarrhoea)
Chronic renal failure (especially in cats)
Renal tubular acidosis
Insulin therapy in diabetic patients
   (especially those with ketoacidosis or marked
   hyperglycaemia)
Alkalosis
Diuretic therapy (prolonged or excessively
   aggressive)
Decreased intake

Figure 4.12: Causes of hypokalaemia.

Causes of hyperkalaemia
Hyperkalaemia may arise secondary to diabetes

Hypoadrenocorticism
Urethral obstruction
Ruptured bladder/uroperitoneum
Diabetes mellitus
Tumour lysis syndrome (e.g. following chemo-
therapy for canine lymphosarcoma)

Figure 4.13: *Causes of hyperkalaemia.*

mellitus, acidosis and tumour lysis syndrome (Figure 4.13). However, life-threatening hyperkalaemia is most frequently a consequence of decreased urinary potassium excretion (urethral obstruction, ruptured bladder, ethylene glycol toxicity and hypoadrenocorticism).

Canine hypoadrenocorticism is usually associated with hyperkalaemia (with or without hyponatraemia) and a reduced Na:K ratio (<27:1). Diagnosis of the endocrine disease is made on the basis of a low or low/ normal basal cortisol followed by minimal stimulation after administration of tetracosactrin, an analogue of adrenocorticotrophic hormone (ACTH). In a recent study of canine hypoadrenocorticism a small number of dogs did not have hyperkalaemia at the time of presentation and the diagnosis of hypoadrenocorticism was made on the basis of an ACTH stimulation test alone (Peterson *et al.,* 1996).

Chloride

Corrected chloride concentration
Chloride is the major anion present in the ECF and plays an important role in acid–base regulation and maintenance of osmolality. Parallel changes in chloride ion and sodium ion concentrations result from changes in water balance, but primary changes in the chloride ion concentration may also occur. The patient's chloride concentration may be 'corrected' for changes in sodium concentration, allowing differentiation between changes in water balance and primary changes in the chloride concentration (de Morais, 1992). The following formulae may be used to calculate the corrected chloride concentration (de Morais, 1992):

For dogs: Cl^- (corrected) = Cl^- (measured) x [146/Na^+(measured)]

Reference ranges: Cl^- (measured) = 100-116 mmol/l*
Cl^- (corrected) = 107-113 mmol/l*

For cats: Cl^- (corrected) = Cl^- (measured) x [156/Na^+(measured)]

Reference ranges: Cl^- (measured) = 100-124 mmol/l*
Cl^- (corrected) = 117-123 mmol/l*

*Reference ranges may vary depending on the instrumentation used to measure the serum electrolyte concentrations.

Disturbances of the patient's measured chloride concentration may therefore be further classified as those associated with an increased or decreased corrected chloride concentration (corrected hyperchloraemia or hypochloraemia, respectively) or those associated with a normal corrected chloride concentration (artefactual hyperchloraemia and hypochloraemia). Artefactual hyperchloraemia and hypochloraemia secondary to changes in water balance are associated with abnormalities of the sodium concentration. In these cases the disturbances in the sodium ion concentration are generally given primary consideration.

Indications for assay
Chloride is measured concurrently with sodium and potassium and where the clinical signs include vomiting, diarrhoea, polyuria and polydipsia.

Analysis
The concentration of chloride is measured in serum, plasma and urine by ion-specific potentiometry and colorimetric methods.

Interfering phenomena
Icterus and haemolysis may produce falsely increased results when colorimetric methods of measurement are used.

Drug effects
Ion-specific electrodes measure other halides (e.g. bromide, iodide) as chloride. The serum chloride reading in animals receiving potassium bromide will therefore be spuriously increased. Frusemide potentially causes a decreased concentration (disproportionate loss of chloride relative to sodium).

Causes of hypochloraemia
The most common causes of corrected hypochloraemia are vomiting (of gastric contents) and aggressive diuretic therapy (frusemide, thiazides). In addition, experimentally induced chronic respiratory acidosis in dogs has been shown to produce increased urinary chloride excretion and a corrected hypochloraemia (de Morais, 1992). Approximately 50% of dogs with hypoadrenocorticism present with hypochloraemia (Peterson *et al.,* 1996).

Causes of hyperchloraemia
Causes of corrected hyperchloraemia include small bowel diarrhoea, fluid therapy (e.g. 0.9% NaCl), renal failure and renal tubular acidosis (deMorais, 1992). Patients with metabolic acidosis with a normal anion gap (e.g. diabetes mellitus) may also have a corrected hyperchloraemia.

Magnesium

Physiology
Magnesium is found in the highest concentrations in the ICF, particularly in bone and muscle. Mobilization of magnesium in young animals prevents hypomagnesaemia when dietary intake is low. In the adult animal,

however, the capacity for magnesium mobilization is small and continuous dietary supply is essential. The plasma magnesium concentration represents a very small percentage of the total body content and therefore may not reflect the environment in affected tissues and cells.

Indications for assay
It was previously assumed that disorders of magnesium metabolism were rarely of significance in cats and dogs. However, recent evidence suggests there is a high prevalence of hypomagnesaemia in critically ill dogs. The clinical manifestations of magnesium deficiency include cardiac arrhythmia, refractory hypokalaemia and hypocalcaemia, muscle weakness, ataxia and seizures.

Analysis
The concentration of magnesium is measured in serum and urine by spectrophotometry.

Reference ranges

Dogs	0.70–1.19 mmol/l
Cats	0.82–1.23 mmol/l

Interfering phenomena
Haemolysis may cause a false increase, while hyperbilirubinaemia could cause a false decrease in the magnesium concentration.

Drug effects
Therapy with cisplatin, aminoglycoside antibiotics and diuretics may cause hypomagnesaemia. Hypermagnesaemia has been associated with the administration of oral antacids (Nelson *et al.*, 1994) and progesterones (Burkhard and Meyer, 1995).

Causes of hypomagnesaemia
Diuretic (frusemide, thiazide) therapy is a potential cause of significant hypomagnesaemia (Cobb and Michell, 1992). A prolonged decrease in dietary intake may lead to hypomagnesaemia. The disease states that cause hypomagnesaemia in cats and dogs have not been studied extensively but it appears that critically ill patients, especially those with congestive cardiac failure treated with frusemide, are at risk (Martin *et al.*, 1995). Intestinal loss of magnesium secondary to enteropathies and bowel resection, and redistribution of the electrolyte associated with sepsis and trauma, have been reported as causes of hypomagnesaemia in man and may also occur in veterinary patients.

Causes of hypermagnesaemia
Hypermagnesaemia may be noted in dogs with hypoadrenocorticism and in those with renal failure receiving magnesium-containing drugs (Nelson *et al.*, 1994).

Calcium

Physiology
Calcium plays an essential role in the regulation of enzymatic reactions, blood coagulation, muscle function, neural activity and cell membrane permeability. The total blood calcium concentration is the most frequently used measurement and is composed of the protein-bound fraction, calcium complexes (citrate and phosphate) and ionized calcium. Ionized calcium is the biologically active form and its serum concentration is regulated predominantly by parathyroid hormone, calcitonin and vitamin D.

Indications for assay
Measurement is essential where the presenting signs could be compatible with hypercalcaemia (polydipsia, polyuria, lethargy, weakness) or hypocalcaemia (nervousness, seizures, hindleg cramping or pain, muscle tremors, intense facial pruritus). The clinical signs associated with hypocalcaemia in cats may be non-specific, e.g. lethargy and anorexia.

Analysis
The total calcium concentration (i.e. biologically inactive + biologically active) is measured in serum, plasma and urine by spectrophotometric methods. In the dog (but not the cat) it is possible to correct for the effect of the protein-bound calcium as follows (Meyer *et al.*, 1992):

$$\text{Corrected Ca (mmol/l)} = \{\, [\text{measured Ca(mmol/l)} \times 4] - [\text{albumin (g/l)}/10] + 3.5\} \times 0.25$$

Reference ranges

Dogs	2.20–2.90 mmol/l
Cats	2.10–2.90 mmol/l

Immature, large breed dogs (<12 months) may have serum calcium levels up to 0.25 mmol/l higher than adults (Nelson *et al.*, 1994).

Critical values
Marked hypocalcaemia (<1.65 mmol/l) is associated with the onset of tetany and seizures. Marked increases in serum calcium (>4.00 mmol/l) may result in the development of acute renal failure and cardiac toxicity.

Interfering phenomena
Serum calcium concentrations are falsely decreased by oxalate and EDTA anticoagulants and increased by the effects of dehydration (mild increase), lipaemia and haemolysis.

Drug effects
Hypocalcaemia may be a consequence of therapy with

anticonvulsants, glucocorticoids and phosphate-containing enemas. Raised serum calcium concentrations have been associated with excessive supplementation with vitamin D, cholcalciferol rodenticide toxicity and anabolic steroid therapy.

Causes of hypocalcaemia

Hypoalbuminaemia in the dog and cat may be accompanied by hypocalcaemia due to a reduction in the protein-bound calcium fraction. However, ionized calcium in these cases is generally within normal limits and therefore clinical signs consistent with hypocalcaemia do not develop. Acute pancreatitis in dogs and cats may also be associated with a mild hypocalcaemia, usually without clinical signs.

Symptomatic hypocalcaemia may be a consequence of puerperal tetany (eclampsia) and primary hypoparathyroidism in the dog and cat (Figure 4.14). However, in the cat, clinical signs of hypocalcaemia are most commonly recognized after bilateral thyroidectomy for the treatment of hyperthyroidism (Waters and Scott-Moncrieff, 1992). Idiopathic hypoparathyroidism is a rare condition of the dog and cat which may be suspected after exclusion of other causes of hypocalcaemia (Feldman and Nelson, 1987; Parker, 1991). The diagnosis can be confirmed by measurement of the serum parathyroid hormone (PTH) concentration (Torrance and Nachreiner, 1989).

Primary hypoparathyroidism*
Puerperal tetany (eclampsia)*
Renal failure (rarely causes clinical signs)
Ethylene glycol toxicity
Hypoalbuminaemia†
Acute pancreatitis†
Intestinal malabsorption (dog)†
Nutritional secondary hyperparathyroidism (rare cause of hypocalcaemia)†
Iatrogenic:
    Bilateral thyroidectomy for the treatment of hyperthyroidism (cat)
    Sodium phosphate enemas (cat)

* reported in dogs and cats but rarer in cats.
† not usually associated with clinical signs of hypocalcaemia

---

Figure 4.14: *Causes of hypocalcaemia.*

Causes of hypercalcaemia

Transient hypercalcaemia (3–3.25 mmol/l in dogs) may be noted in dehydrated patients (Chew and Carothers, 1989) but symptomatic hypercalcaemia in dogs and cats is most commonly associated with non-parathyroid neoplasia (Elliot *et al.*, 1991). The raised serum calcium concentrations may be a consequence of bone resorption caused by PTH-related peptides produced by the neoplasm or by local osteolysis. Canine lymphosarcoma is the most frequent neoplastic disease associated with hypercalcaemia (10–40% of cases present with increased serum calcium concentrations) (Chew

---

Immature animal
Dehydration
Malignancy:
    Lymphosarcoma
    Adenocarcinoma of the apocrine glands of the anal sac
    Multiple myeloma
    Mammary adenocarcinoma
    Nasal adenocarcinoma
    Soft tissue sarcoma (pulmonary)
    Squamous cell carcinoma (stomach, mammary glands)
Endocrine:
    Hypoadrenocorticism
    Primary hyperparathyroidism
Renal failure
Hypervitaminosis D

Figure 4.15: *Causes of hypercalcaemia.*

and Carothers, 1989). In the cat, hypercalcaemia has rarely been reported with lymphosarcoma and haemopoietic malignancies (Barber *et al.*, 1993). Other neoplasms associated with raised serum calcium concentrations have been reported (Figure 4.15). In patients with hypercalcaemia, identification of any underlying malignancy often requires survey radiography to identify discrete masses, lymphadenopathy and organomegaly. Biopsy of any identified masses or enlarged lymph nodes is usually necessary. The measurement of PTH in non-azotaemic animals allows differentiation between hypercalcaemia of non-parathyroid malignancy and primary hyperparathyroidism. However, in the azotaemic animal (with associated secondary renal hyperparathyroidism), the interpretation of PTH concentrations is more difficult and diagnosis may depend upon identification of the primary pathological process.

In one study, hypoadrenocorticism was identified as the second most common cause of hypercalcaemia in the dog (Elliot *et al.*, 1991). The mechanism of the abnormalities of calcium metabolism have not been elucidated.

Primary hyperparathyroidism is rarely recognized in the dog and cat and is characterized by overproduction of PTH by hyperplastic or neoplastic parathyroid glands. Functional adenomas have been identified as the major cause (Kruger and Osborne, 1994).

The importance of the identification of the cause of hypercalcaemia and therapy of the underlying disease (where possible) cannot be overstated. Hypercalcaemia is associated with the development of hypercalcaemic nephropathy which may lead to severe renal insufficiency. In a study of 12 dogs with lymphosarcoma and associated hypercalcaemia, all dogs had impaired renal function (Weller and Hoffman, 1992). Early cases of hypercalcaemic nephropathy may be reversible (to a degree which is

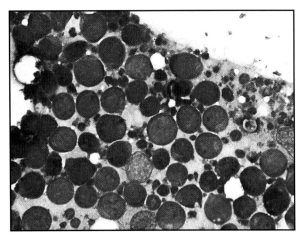

Figure 4.16: Canine lymph node affected by lymphosarcoma. Note the relatively homogeneous population of large lymphoid cells. Occasional small mature lymphocytes are present in this field. Hypercalcaemia may be associated with lymphosarcoma in the dog and, rarely, in the cat.

dependent on the extent of tissue mineralization and number of remaining functioning nephrons), but often the renal damage at the time of clinical presentation is advanced and associated with irreversible impairment of the renal function.

Inorganic phosphorus

Physiology
The serum inorganic phosphorus concentration is primarily regulated by renal excretion, mediated through the action of PTH. Although the phosphorus concentration has no direct effect on PTH regulation (which is controlled by the ionized calcium concentration) an increased serum phosphorus concentration will indirectly result in increased PTH secretion.

Indications for assay
The serum phosphorus concentration should be measured in patients with suspected renal insufficiency and disorders of calcium homeostasis. It is prudent to measure calcium and phosphorus concurrently in such cases.

Analysis
Inorganic phosphorus may be assayed in serum, heparinized plasma and urine by spectrophotometry.

Reference ranges

Dogs   0.5–2.6 mmol/l
Cats   1.1–2.8 mmol/l

Immature dogs and cats have higher phosphorus concentrations (dogs,1.3–2.9 mmol/l; Nelson *et al.*, 1994). These decrease to adult values by 12 months. In large-breed dogs the phosphorus concentration may remain elevated after 12 months of age (Dial, 1992).

Critical values
Serum phosphorus concentrations of <0.5 mmol/l are associated with haemolysis and the onset of neurological signs.

Interfering phenomena
Serum phosphorus concentrations are falsely increased by haemolysis.

Drug effects
Hypophosphataemia may be caused by diuretics and salicylates. Hyperphosphataemia is a potential consequence of the administration of phosphate-containing enemas in small dogs and cats.

Causes of hypophosphataemia
Hypophosphataemia is commonly noted with hypercalcaemia of malignancy, primary hyperparathyroidism (without renal failure) and in the early stages of therapy of diabetic patients with ketoacidosis (Figure 4.17). Mild hypophosphataemia without hypercalcaemia is generally not considered to be clinically significant.

Endocrine:
    Primary hyperparathyroidism
    Diabetic ketoacidosis
    Hyperinsulinism
Puerperal tetany (eclampsia)
Hypercalcaemia of malignancy
Respiratory alkalosis
Renal tubular defects (canine Fanconi syndrome)

Figure 4.17: Causes of hypophosphataemia.

Causes of hyperphosphataemia
In dogs and cats the most common cause of hyperphosphataemia is renal failure (renal secondary hyperparathyroidism) (Figure 4.18). The loss of functioning nephrons causes phosphorus retention but the glomerular filtration rate is generally reduced by at least 75% before persistent hyperphosphataemia is recognized (Yaphé and Forrester, 1994). Other manifestations of renal secondary hyperparathyroidism include decreased serum calcium concentrations and increased PTH concentrations.

Immature animal (<12 months of age)
Renal failure
Prerenal and postrenal azotaemia
Endocrine:
    Primary hypoparathyroidism
    Nutritional secondary hyperparathyroidism
    Hyperthyroidism
Hypervitaminosis D
Osteolytic bone lesions
Rhabdomyolysis (muscle trauma)

Figure 4.18 : Causes of hyperphosphataemia.

MUSCLE ENZYMES

Creatine kinase (CK)

Physiology
There are four isoenzymes of CK. They are dimers consisting of muscle (M) or brain (B) subunits and are numbered as follows: CK_1 (CK-BB), CK_2 (CK-MB), CK_3 (CK-MM), CK_4 (CK-Mt). In the dog, CK_3 is the dominant form found in cardiac and skeletal muscle. CK_4 is found in mitochondrial membranes. CK has a high activity in the brain but little is found in normal CSF. Raised enzyme concentrations in the CSF may be a non-specific but sensitive indicator of CNS disease.

Indications for assay
Measurement of serum CK activity is indicated where there is a suspicion of muscle disease or where the patient's presenting clinical signs include generalized weakness. CK is a sensitive indicator of muscle damage but displays poor specificity for individual disease processes.

Reference ranges

Dogs	0–500 units/l
Cats	0–600 units/l

The interpretation of data should be made with regard to specific reference ranges established for the methodology employed.

Causes of raised CK
Only large increases (>10,000 units/l) or persistent increases (>2000 units/l) in enzyme activity are considered of clinical significance (Willard *et al.*, 1994). Mild increases are noted with physical activity, restraint and intramuscular injections while moderate increases may be associated with convulsions, trauma and some neuropathies. Marked increases are observed with myositis, although feline lower urinary tract obstruction has also been associated with large increases in CK (the enzyme is present in the feline bladder). Causes of myositis include infectious disease (*Toxoplasma gondii*, *Neospora caninum*), immune-mediated disease (masticatory myositis) and endocrine disorders (hypothyroidism, hyperadrenocorticism). Significant muscle disease can occur without an increase in CK (see also Chapter 11).

Aspartate aminotransferase (AST)

Physiology
AST is located in the mitochondria of the cell. It is present in significant quantities in hepatocytes, erythrocytes and muscle.

Indications for assay
AST is included in diagnostic profiles for investigation of suspected liver disease or muscle disease.

Analysis
AST is measured in serum and heparinized plasma by spectrophotometry.

Reference ranges

Dogs	7–50 units/l
Cats	7–60 units/l

The interpretation of data should be made with regard to specific reference ranges established for the methodology employed.

Interfering phenomena
Haemolysis and lipaemia of the sample may cause false increases in AST activity.

Drug effects
Hepatotoxic drugs may cause an increased serum AST activity (see Figure 4.6).

Causes of raised AST
The most common causes of increased AST are hepatic disease, muscle disease (trauma, inflammation) and haemolysis. Measurement of AST activity alone is of little diagnostic value. Concurrent measurement of other hepatic enzymes (ALT, ALP, GGT), hepatic function indicators (albumin, urea, bilirubin, bile acids) and CK are necessary to identify the origin of raised serum AST activity.

CARBOHYDRATE METABOLISM

Glucose

Physiology
Glucose is the principal source of energy for mammalian tissues and is derived from the diet and hepatic gluconeogenesis. The blood concentration is controlled by hormones which regulate its entry into, and removal from, the circulation (insulin, glucagon, adrenaline, cortisol). In the kidney of the dog and cat, glucose entering the glomerular ultrafiltrate is reabsorbed by the renal tubules. However, the renal reabsorption of glucose is overwhelmed in the presence of blood glucose concentrations greater than 10–12 mmol/l, resulting in glucosuria (Feldman and Nelson, 1987).

Indications for assay
Measurement of blood glucose is essential where presenting clinical signs could suggest diabetes mellitus (polydipsia, polyuria, weight loss, cataract formation),

diabetic ketoacidosis (vomiting, diarrhoea, anorexia) or hypoglycaemia (weakness, collapse, seizures, disorientation, depression, blindness). In addition, the assay is included in general health screens where it may provide supportive evidence for other disease processes (hyperadrenocorticism, hepatic disease). Measurement of the blood glucose concentration is the ideal method of monitoring the stabilization of diabetic patients on insulin therapy and allows optimization of the therapeutic regimen. In such cases, glucose is measured in samples collected at 2-hourly intervals, allowing calculation of the duration of action and peak time of action of the administered insulin.

Analysis

Reagent strips: Rapid-analysis reagent strips require the use of whole blood with no anticoagulant.

Laboratory analysis: Spectrophotometric methods (enzymatic or chemical) are generally used for the measurement of blood glucose. Where in-house equipment demands the use of heparinized plasma, the sample must be separated immediately after collection. This prevents depletion of the plasma glucose by the erythrocytes. Collection of the blood into fluoride oxalate is the preferred method of preventing erythrocyte glucose utilization when a delay in analysis is anticipated, such as during transport to a commercial laboratory.

Reference ranges

Dogs   3.5–5.5 mmol/l
Cats   3.5–6.5 mmol/l

Critical values

Clinical signs associated with hypoglycaemia, including collapse and seizures, may be recognized at concentrations of <3.0 mmol/l. However, in chronic disease the concentration can fall below 1.65 mmol/l before the onset of clinical signs. Blood glucose concentrations of <0.5 mmol/l cause the onset of a coma.

The induction of a coma secondary to hyperosmotic diabetes mellitus is associated with marked hyperglycaemia (>55 mmol/l).

Interfering phenomena

Reagent strips: When using reagent strips the manufacturer's instructions must be followed with regard to timing. Excessive washing of the strips should be avoided. Inadequate coverage of the reagent pad has been associated with falsely low results, while a marked increase or decrease in packed cell volume (PCV) may also affect the glucose concentration. In general, these methods are less accurate at high glucose concentrations (>15 mmol/l).

Laboratory analysis: Haemolysis, icterus and lipaemia potentially interfere with the measurement of plasma glucose. Prolonged contact of the erythrocytes with the serum or plasma results in a decreased glucose concentration (approximately 10% per hour). Drug therapy (ascorbic acid, paracetamol and aspirin) produces falsely low results (glucose oxidase method), while azotaemia may cause a falsely high result when enzymatic methods of measurement are employed.

Drug effects

Hypoglycaemia may be caused by insulin and beta-blockers (e.g. propranolol). Salicylates and anabolic steroids have been reported to cause hypoglycaemia in diabetics (Nelson *et al.,* 1994).

Hyperglycaemia may be caused by glucocorticoid, progestagen or thiazide diuretic therapy. In the cat, megoestrol acetate can cause a transient or persistent rise in blood glucose. Less commonly, hyperglycaemia may be a consequence of administration of phenytoin and oestrogens.

Causes of hypoglycaemia

Marked hypoglycaemia (glucose <2 mmol/l) most commonly results from overproduction of insulin or excessive utilization of glucose by neoplastic cells. Insulin-secreting tumours of the pancreas (insulinomas) produce biologically active hormone which increases the uptake of glucose by the body tissues and impairs hepatic gluconeogenesis, resulting in hypoglycaemia. In one study of dogs with insulinomas the mean (±SD) plasma glucose concentration was 2.14(±0.82) mmol/l (Dunn *et al.,* 1993). Extrapancreatic tumours occasionally cause hypoglycaemia by secretion of an insulin-like substance or by increased utilization of plasma glucose.

Neoplastic:
    Insulin-secreting tumour of the pancreas
        (insulinoma)
    Hepatocellular carcinoma
    Leiomyosarcoma (liver)
    Haemangiosarcoma (liver, spleen)
Endocrine:
    Hypoadrenocorticism
Hepatic insufficiency:
    Congenital vascular shunts
    Acquired vascular shunts
    Chronic hepatic fibrosis (cirrhosis)
    Hepatic necrosis (e.g. hepatotoxins, bacterial
        infection, trauma)
Substrate deficiency:
    Neonatal hypoglycaemia
    Juvenile hypoglycaemia
    Hunting dog hypoglycaemia
    Glycogen storage disease
Sepsis

Figure 4.19: *Causes of hypoglycaemia in the dog. Cats may rarely be affected by insulinoma.*

Other causes of hypoglycaemia include impaired gluconeogenesis (hepatic disease), reduced dietary intake of substances necessary for gluconeogenesis, or a combination of these mechanisms such as in sepsis (Figure 4.19). The hypoglycaemia noted in canine hypoadrenocorticism is the consequence of a reduction in the hepatic production of glucose and an increased sensitivity of tissue cells to insulin (Feldman and Nelson, 1987).

Causes of hyperglycaemia
Hyperglycaemia commonly results from a relative or absolute lack of insulin. This leads to impaired tissue utilization of plasma glucose and an increase in the rate of gluconeogenesis.

Mild hyperglycaemia (6.7–10 mmol/l) in the dog may be noted as part of an adrenaline stress response or secondary to excessive secretion or administration of other diabetogenic hormones, in particular glucocorticoids and progesterone (Figure 4.20). The mild hyperglycaemia is a result of the hormonal antagonism of the actions of insulin. In addition, mild hyperglycaemia may be noted in the postprandial period in dogs fed a sugar-rich diet such as semi-moist foods.

A persistent, moderate to marked hyperglycaemia in the dog is consistent with diabetes mellitus. Such cases do not present with clinical signs (polyuria and polydipsia) until the renal threshold for glucose is exceeded, resulting in osmotic diuresis.

In the cat, an adrenaline-induced stress response may produce a moderate or marked increase in glucose concentration. The diagnosis of diabetes mellitus is often difficult in cats and confirmation requires documentation of persistent hyperglycaemia with compatible clinical signs.

Adrenaline stress response (especially marked in cats)
Postprandial
Diabetes mellitus
Hyperadrenocorticism (dogs and rarely cats)
Acromegaly (cats)
Acute pancreatitis (dogs and cats)
Renal insufficiency

Figure 4.20: Causes of hyperglycaemia.

Fructosamine

Physiology
Fructosamine is a glycated serum protein which is formed by the non-enzymatic reaction between a sugar and an amino acid. The total amount of fructosamine formed is proportional to the serum glucose concentration during the lifespan of the proteins. In dogs and cats, fructosamine has been found to be a useful parameter in the diagnosis and management of diabetes mellitus (Reusch *et al.,* 1993; Thorensen and Bredal, 1996).

Indications for assay
Serum fructosamine concentrations are useful in the diagnosis of diabetes mellitus and in identifying persistent hyperglycaemia during therapy (Thorensen and Bredal, 1996). Measurement of fructosamine may also be helpful in confirming the presence of persistent hypoglycaemia.

Analysis
Fructosamine is measured using a method based on the reducing ability of fructosamine in alkaline solution.

Reference ranges

Dogs   250–350 µmol/l*
Cats   150–270 µmol/l*

* See Chapter 18

Causes of low serum fructosamine
A low serum fructosamine concentration has been recorded in a dog with an insulin-secreting tumour of the pancreas (insulinoma) (Thorensen *et al.,* 1995). It has been suggested that the measurement of serum fructosamine in addition to glucose and insulin may be helpful in confirming the presence of insulinomas (Thorensen *et al.,* 1995).

Causes of raised fructosamine
Raised serum concentrations of fructosamine reflect persistent hyperglycaemia over the preceding 2–3 weeks. In dogs with diabetes the serum fructosamine concentration is significantly greater than in dogs with other diseases (Jensen, 1992). Fructosamine is also useful for confirming diabetes mellitus in the cat and can be helpful in identifying persistent hyperglycaemia after initial stabilization on insulin therapy (Reusch *et al.,* 1993; Thorensen and Bredal, 1996).

LIPID METABOLISM

Cholesterol

Physiology
Cholesterol is the most common steroid in the body tissues and acts as a precursor compound for steroid hormone and bile salt synthesis. It is also a major structural component of cell membranes and myelin sheaths. The majority of the body's cholesterol is synthesized by the liver, but the remainder originates from dietary sources. Excess cholesterol is excreted in the bile.

Indications for assay
Hypercholesterolaemia is often associated with endocrine disease in the dog and cat and is frequently measured as part of a general health profile in these species. Raised plasma cholesterol alone is not commonly responsible for the development of clinical

disease in the dog and cat. However, marked hyper-cholesterolaemia and hypertriglyceridaemia secondary to thyroid dysfunction in dogs have been associated with the development of peripheral vascular disease (Patterson *et al.,* 1985) and specific corneal lesions (i.e. arcus lipoides corneae; Crispin, 1993).

Analysis

Cholesterol concentrations are assayed in serum, heparinized plasma or EDTA plasma using spectro-photometric, chromatographic, automated direct and enzymatic methods.

Reference ranges

Dogs   2.7–9.5 mmol/l
Cats   1.5–6.0 mmol/l

Critical values

It was previously believed that raised serum cholesterol concentrations had no adverse effects on the health of pet dogs. However, hypercholesterolaemia (>30 mmol/l) in conjunction with moderate to marked hypertriglyceridaemia (>5 mmol/l) in hypothyroid dogs has been associated with the development of atherosclerosis (Patterson *et al.,* 1985).

Interfering phenomena

Icterus and possibly lipaemia are associated with false increases in cholesterol concentrations.

Drug effects

With the exception of hypercholesterolaemia secondary to glucocorticoid therapy, there are few drugs that produce recognized alterations in serum cholesterol concentrations (Figure 4.21). Phenytoin and thiazide diuretics may produce hypercholesterolaemia while azathioprine and oral aminoglycosides can lower the cholesterol concentration. The intravenous administration of dipyrone interferes with the assay, creating an artefactual hypercholesterolaemia.

Causes of hypocholesterolaemia

Hypocholesterolaemia is often associated with protein-losing enteropathies (Figure 4.22), particularly

---

Hypocholesterolaemia
Azathioprine
Oral aminoglycosides
Intravenous dipyrone *

Hypercholesterolaemia
Corticosteroids
Phenytoin
Thiazide diuretics

*interference with the methodology

Figure 4.21: Drugs that may affect cholesterol concentration.

Hypocholesterolaemia
Protein-losing enteropathy
Maldigestion/malabsorption
Hepatopathy (portocaval shunt, cirrhosis)

Hypercholesterolaemia
Postprandial hyperlipidaemia
Secondary hyperlipidaemia:
   Hypothyroidism
   Diabetes mellitus
   Hyperadrenocorticism
   Cholestatic disease
   Nephrotic syndrome
Idiopathic hyperlipidaemia
Hypercholesterolaemia of the Briard

Figure 4.22: Causes of alterations in plasma cholesterol concentrations.

canine intestinal lymphangiectasia, in which there is impaired lymphatic drainage and leakage of lymph into the intestinal lumen. Hypocholesterolaemia has also been observed with severe hepatic insufficiency (indicated by a marked increase in serum bile acids) and is commonly noted in dogs with cirrhosis and portosystemic vascular anomalies (Center, 1989).

Causes of hypercholesterolaemia

A marginal increase in the cholesterol concentration may be noted in samples collected in the postprandial period *versus* a fasted sample. This increased level generally does not exceed the reference range for the species (Watson and Barrie, 1993).

Hypercholesterolaemia in the dog and cat is most commonly associated with endocrine disease (diabetes mellitus, hypothyroidism, hyperadrenocorticism) (Figure 4.22). In each of these endocrine disorders there may be a concurrent increase in serum triglyceride concentration (Barrie *et al.,* 1993). Hypercholesterolaemia may also be noted in cholestatic disease and glomerulonephritis (Ford, 1977). A familial hypercholesterolaemia has been proposed in the Briard in the UK but the underlying defect of lipid metabolism has not been determined (Watson *et al.,* 1993).

Further specialist investigation (e.g. lipoprotein electrophoresis) may be necessary if no underlying systemic or endocrine disease can be identified and the hypercholesterolaemia is marked and persistent.

Triglycerides

Physiology

The triglycerides are the most abundant lipids in the body and their storage in adipose tissue provides an essential reserve of chemical energy for tissue requirements. They are derived from the diet and also synthesized *de novo* in the liver.

Indications for assay

Fasting hypertriglyceridaemia in the dog and cat is a pathological finding. The presence of large triglyceride-rich lipoproteins imparts a turbidity to the plasma or serum (lipaemia). Triglycerides should therefore be measured in all fasting blood samples that appear to be lipaemic. Clinical manifestations of hypertriglyceridaemia include recurrent abdominal pain, alimentary signs, lipaemia retinalis, lipid-laden aqueous humor and seizures (Crispin, 1993; Ford, 1993).

Analysis

The triglyceride concentration is measured in serum or EDTA plasma by spectrophotometric or enzymatic methods.

Reference ranges

Dogs   0.30–1.20 mmol/l*
Cats   0.30–1.20 mmol/l*

*Method: L/G kinase EP, no correction (IL Test™ Triglyceride; Instrumentation Laboratory Company). Grange Laboratories Wetherby, a division of Idexx Laboratories.

Critical values

Serum triglyceride concentrations of >5.00 mmol/l have been associated with the development of alimentary signs, including vomiting and abdominal pain. The latter often cannot be localized to a region of the abdomen. In some cases there may be enzymatic evidence of pancreatitis (raised serum amylase and lipase activities) but this is not a feature of many cases. It has also been proposed that hypertriglyceridaemia may be associated with the onset of seizures in some patients (Bodkin, 1992).

Interfering phenomena

Gross lipaemia often precludes an accurate measurement. Hyperbilirubinaemia, such as in cholestatic liver disease, may cause a spurious increase in serum triglyceride concentrations.

Drug effects

Hypotriglyceridaemia may be noted with ascorbic acid therapy and intravenous dipyrone (the latter interferes with the methodology). Glucocorticoids potentially raise the serum triglyceride concentration.

Causes of hypotriglyceridaemia

Hypotriglyceridaemia has not been consistently associated with any specific disease process although it has been reported in several cases of acute and chronic hepatic disease (Ford, 1977).

Causes of hypertriglyceridaemia

The most common cause of apparent hypertriglyceridaemia in the dog and cat is a failure to obtain a fasting sample (postprandial hyperlipidaemia). If hypertriglyceridaemia is documented in a sample collected after a 12-hour fast, endocrine and systemic disease should be excluded (diabetes mellitus, hypothyroidism, hyperadrencorticism, glomerulonephritis) (Figure 4.23). Many dogs with spontaneous acute pancreatitis have increased serum triglyceride concentrations (Schaer, 1979). The relationship between pancreatitis and hyperlipidaemia has not been fully elucidated but it appears that the increased triglyceride concentration may predispose patients to pancreatic pathology (Whitney *et al.*, 1987).

If underlying systemic disease has been excluded then consideration should be given to the possibility of familial hyperlipidaemias (e.g. idiopathic hyperchylomicronaemia of the Miniature Schnauzer; Ford, 1993) and familial hyperchylomicronaemia in the cat (Jones, 1993). Hypertriglyceridaemia without evidence of underlying disease (idiopathic hypertriglyceridaemia) has also been recognized in pedigree and crossbreed dogs (Barrie, 1993).

Postprandial hyperlipidaemia

Secondary hyperlipidaemia:
    Hypothyroidism
    Diabetes mellitus
    Hyperadrenocorticism
    Acute pancreatitis

Primary hyperlipidaemia:
    Idiopathic hyperchylomicronaemia of the
        Miniature Schnauzer
    Familial hyperchylomicronaemia in the cat
    Idiopathic hypertriglyceridaemia

Figure 4.23: Causes of hypertriglyceridaemia in the dog and cat.

MISCELLANEOUS TESTS

Iron

Physiology

Most of the body's iron is found in the erythrocytes in the form of haemoglobin, but iron is also stored in the tissues (especially the liver and spleen). Myoglobin, which is similar to a subunit of haemoglobin, is found in muscle where it acts as an oxygen reservoir. Iron deficiency results in impaired haemoglobin synthesis, anaemia and morphological changes of the erythrocytes (see below).

Indications for assay

Measurement is most commonly indicated to confirm that iron deficiency is the cause of a recognized anaemia. It may not be necessary in cases in which the morphological changes of the erythrocytes and the anaemia are pronounced.

Analysis

Iron is measured in serum by colorimetric methods or atomic absorption.

Reference ranges

Dogs   18.0–25.0 μmol/l*
Cats   12.0–22.0 μmol/l*

*Method: colorimetric ppt (IL Test™ Iron; Instrumentation Laboratory Company). Grange Laboratories Wetherby, a division of Idexx Laboratories.

Causes of decreased serum iron

Iron deficiency is commonly a consequence of chronic external blood loss secondary to external or intestinal parasites and bleeding intestinal lesions. It may also be seen in young animals where a milk diet provides insufficient iron for the rapid growth rate. Morphological changes, including microcytosis and hypochromasia, are noted in the erythrocytes secondary to impaired haemoglobin synthesis (Figure 4.24). The derived red cell indices — mean corpuscular haemoglobin (MCH), mean corpuscular volume and mean corpuscular haemoglobin concentration (MCHC) — are decreased in some affected patients. The presence of decreased serum iron is helpful in confirming iron deficiency, but it should be noted that chronic inflammatory disease can also cause a mild anaemia and decreased iron concentrations.

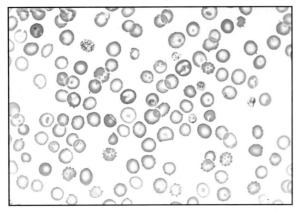

Figure 4.24: Microcytic hypochromic anaemia associated with iron deficiency in the dog. This is usually a consequence of chronic blood loss, such as intestinal blood loss, in adult dogs and cats.

Causes of raised serum iron

Increased iron concentrations may be associated with haemolytic disease and liver disease (Kaneko, 1989). Iron toxicosis in the dog may be a consequence of ingestion of iron supplements (Greentree and Hall, 1995).

Lead

Indications for assay

Lead poisoning may occur in all domestic animals. In the dog the clinical signs include anorexia, vomiting, constipation, behavioural changes and seizures.

Analysis

Lead concentrations are measured in whole blood by atomic absorption spectrophotometry.

Reference ranges

The reference range quoted for lead in the dog is 10–50 μg/dl. Concentrations of >30 μg/dl are supportive of lead poisoning, while >60 μg/dl confirms the diagnosis (Kaneko, 1989).

Zinc

Indications for assay

Toxicity may result from ingestion of objects or ointments that contain zinc. Ingested objects that cause clinical signs are often composed of at least 98% elemental zinc (Meurs and Breitschwerdt, 1995). The clinical signs in affected animals include anorexia, vomiting, diarrhoea and intravascular haemolysis.

Zinc-responsive dermatosis is a nutritional skin disease of dogs. Siberian Huskies, Alaskan Malamutes and Bull Terriers are affected. The disease may be a consequence of impaired absorption or metabolism of zinc and is an inherited (autosomal recessive) condition in the Bull Terrier. Rapidly growing large-breed dogs may also be zinc-deficient due to inadequate dietary intake. Currently the diagnosis of zinc-related skin diseases is made on the basis of history, clinical examination and histopathological examination of skin. Lowered plasma zinc concentrations have been reported in affected Bull Terriers but the concentrations may be difficult to interpret, especially where there is a mild deficiency (Willemse, 1992).

Analysis

Serum or plasma zinc concentrations may be measured to confirm a diagnosis. However, samples should be collected using syringes without rubber stoppers (which may be coated in material that contains zinc) and transferred to tubes designed for trace element studies.

Reference ranges

Meurs and Breitschwerdt (1995) state that serum zinc concentrations in normal dogs range from 0.7 to 2.0 μg/ml.

Copper

Indications for assay

Copper-associated hepatitis in the Bedlington Terrier is inherited as an autosomal recessive condition which is characterized by the accumulation of copper in the liver. The Dobermann Pinscher and West Highland White Terrier are also affected by apparently familial disorders that cause hepatic accumulation of copper. Intravascular haemolysis with severe jaundice has been noted in some affected Bedlington Terriers. In these individuals the serum copper concentrations have been high, but in cases with hepatic disease alone, the serum copper concentrations are not elevated.

Copper deficiency is more commonly recognized in lambs but may be associated with skeletal abnormalities in the dog (Kaneko, 1989).

Analysis

Copper may be measured in serum or plasma by colorimetric methods.

Reference ranges

Dogs   15.7–31.5 µmol/l*

*(Kaneko, 1989)

CHEMICAL PROFILES AND TEST SELECTION

On the initial presentation of an ill patient, a clinician formulates a list of differential diagnoses based on the history and clinical findings. Where the clinical findings are specific, e.g. pallor of the mucous membranes suggestive of anaemia, then steps are taken to confirm this suspicion and to elucidate the possible cause. A wider, more comprehensive investigation is necessary when clinical signs may be caused by many metabolic disorders; for example, polydipsia in the dog could be the result of endocrine disease, renal disease or hepatic disease. The selection of tests depends upon the differential diagnoses, the range of conditions that must be excluded, the availability of the tests, and the cost of tests. In the case of the polydipsic dog, a cost-effective profile is required to cover the possibility of organ failure (renal, hepatic), endocrine disease (diabetes mellitus, hyperadrenocorticism) and hypercalcaemia. Some of these differentials may be excluded or confirmed on the basis of individual tests (e.g. urea and creatinine for renal disease) but inclusion in a more comprehensive profile allows the simultaneous assessment and cost-effective exclusion of many other causes of polydipsia.

When the clinical signs are vague and a 'general health screen' is required, then it is necessary to select

Profile	Tests	Indications
Health screen	FBC†, TP, albumin, globulin, ALT, ALP, GGT, bilirubin, amylase, urea, creatinine, glucose, urinalysis	Routine screening
Pre-anaesthetic screen*	FBC‡, TP, albumin, globulin, ALT, ALP, bilirubin, urea, creatinine, glucose	Screen for existing disease prior to routine surgery
Extended** health screen	As health screen plus bile acids, electrolytes, cholesterol, CK, calcium, phosphorus	Gastrointestinal, endocrine disease and non-localizing signs
Polydipsia profile	FBC†, TP, albumin, globulin, ALT, ALP, bilirubin, bile acids, CK, cholesterol, urea, creatinine, glucose, calcium, phosphorus, electrolyte screen, urinalysis (SG, dipstick and sediment examination).	Polydipsia
Seizure profile	FBC†, TP, albumin, globulin, ALT, ALP, bile acids, urea, creatinine, glucose, calcium, CK, phosphorus, magnesium, electrolyte screen	Seizures, weakness, episodic collapse
Renal profile	PCV, TP, albumin, globulin, urea, creatinine, sodium, potassium, calcium, phosphorus, urinalysis (SG dipstick and sediment examination)	
Hepatic profile	TP, albumin, globulin, ALT, ALP, AST, GGT, bilirubin, bile acids, cholesterol	Monitoring hepatotoxicity

* Bile acids may be added as an additional indicator of hepatic function.
** Lipase may be added if vomiting is the predominant clinical sign (re pancreatitis). Serum protein electrophoresis may be added for pyrexia of unknown origin, lymphadenopathy, immune-mediated disease and feline infectious peritonitis.
† Full blood count including red cell indices, total white cell count and differential count, platelet count and smear examination.
‡ Full blood count including red cell indices, total white cell count and platelet count, but excluding a differential white cell count and smear examination.

Table 4.1: *A selection of profiles for use in small animal practice. FBC = full blood count; TP = total protein.*

a broad range of analytes which will reflect a number of common diseases or pathological states. The inclusion of tests that are not organ-specific but which provide general information regarding the hydration and essential homeostatic mechanisms is worthwhile, e.g. total proteins, albumin, electrolytes, glucose.

When considering which tests to include in a profile it is necessary to understand the significance of results outside the reference ranges. The quality of the results may be affected by many variables, including sample collection, patient preparation and sample storage (see Chapters 1 and 2). In addition, consideration must be given to the formulation and meaning of reference ranges. When interpreting the significance of abnormal results it is important to remember the origin of the reference ranges. Such ranges are generally determined by selecting an apparently healthy population and testing them for the chosen parameters. The results are statistically manipulated and the reference ranges determined. The range is usually reported as the mean, plus or minus twice the standard deviation. Therefore, even in a healthy population, only 95% of patients will have values inside the reference range. For a 15-test screen there is a 54% chance of finding one or more abnormal values in a healthy subject (Handelman and Blue, 1983). Results within the reference range have a high predictive value for 'non-disease' but further investigations should be considered to confirm suggestions of disease (Blackmore, 1988). It is of vital importance that all abnormalities are considered, together with the clinical presentation, the signalment of the patient and the knowledge of population variation.

The use of biochemical profiles allows selection of complementary tests that provide more information than tests performed in isolation. For example, raised alkaline phosphatase activity in a dog could be the result of drug therapy, hyperadrenocorticism, or hepatic or bone disease, but if the bilirubin concentration is also raised then hepatic disease would be a major consideration. In this way the inclusion of 'panels' of analytes may support a diagnosis and together provide valuable information which might be lost or overinterpreted if analytes were assayed alone. Such parallel screening provides maximum information, which then allows the selection of further diagnostic tests or procedures.

Where a disease has been confirmed and monitoring of therapy is required, individual tests or organ-specific profiles are a useful and cost-effective approach, e.g. blood glucose in the monitoring of diabetes mellitus, or a hepatic profile when checking for anticonvulsant hepatotoxicity.

A selection of profiles that may be useful for confirmation and monitoring of metabolic disease in the dog and cat is shown in Table 4.1.

REFERENCES AND FURTHER READING

Alleman AR (1990) The effects of hemolysis and lipemia on serum biochemical constituents. *Veterinary Medicine and the Small Animal Clinician* **85**, 1272-1284
Bagley RS (1995) Adipsia and the nervous system. *Compendium on Continuing Education for the Practising Veterinary Surgeon* **17**, 311-319
Barber PJ, Elliott J and Torrance AG (1993) Measurement of feline intact parathyroid hormone: assay validation and sample handling studies. *Journal of Small Animal Practice* **34**, 614–620
Barrie J (1993) *Hyperlipidaemia in the dog.* PhD thesis, University of Glasgow
Barrie J, Watson TDG, Stear MJ and Nash ASN (1993) Plasma cholesterol and lipoprotein concentrations in the dog: the effects of age, breed, gender and endocrine disease. *Journal of Small Animal Practice* **34**, 507-512
Bartges JW and Osborne CA (1995) Influence of fasting and eating on laboratory values. In: *Kirk's Current Veterinary Therapy XII*, ed. JD Bonagura, pp. 20-23. WB Saunders, Philadelphia
Blackmore DJ (1988) *Animal Clinical Biochemistry, The Future.* Cambridge University Press, Cambridge
Bodkin K (1992) Seizures associated with hyperlipoproteinaemia in a Miniature Schnauzer. *Canine Practice* **17**, 11-15
Burkhard MJ and Meyer DJ (1995) Interference with clinical laboratory measurements and examinations. In: *Kirk's Current Veterinary Therapy XII*, ed. JD Bonagura, pp. 14-20. WB Saunders, Philadelphia
Center SA (1989) Pathophysiology and laboratory diagnosis of liver disease. In: *Textbook of Veterinary Internal Medicine,* 3rd edn, ed. SJ Ettinger, pp. 1421-1478. WB Saunders, Philadelphia
Center SA, Baldwin BH, Erb HN and Tennant BC (1985) Bile acid concentrations in the diagnosis of hepatobiliary disease in the dog. *Journal of the American Veterinary Medical Association* **187**, 935-940
Center SA, Erb HN and Joseph SA (1995) Measurement of serum bile acid concentrations for diagnosis of hepatobiliary disease in cats. *Journal of the American Veterinary Medical Association* **207**, 1048-1054
Chew DJ and Carothers M (1989) Hypercalcemia. *Veterinary Clinics of North America: Small Animal Practice* **19**, 265-287
Chew DJ and DiBartola SP (1989) Diagnosis and pathophysiology of renal disease. In: *Textbook of Veterinary Internal Medicine,* 3rd edn, ed. SJ Ettinger, pp. 1893-1961. WB Saunders, Philadelphia
Cobb M and Michell AR (1992) Plasma electrolyte concentrations in dogs receiving diuretic therapy for cardiac failure. *Journal of Small Animal Practice* **33**, 526-529
Crispin SM (1993) Ocular manifestations of hyperlipoproteinaemia. *Journal of Small Animal Practice* **34**, 500-507
de Morais HSA (1992) Chloride ion in small animal practice: the forgotten ion. *Veterinary Emergency and Critical Care* **2**, 11-24
de Morais HSA and Chew DJ (1992) Use and Interpretation of serum and urine electrolytes. *Seminars in Veterinary Medicine and Surgery (Small animal)* **7**, 262-274
Dial SM (1992) Hematology, chemistry profile and urinalysis for pediatric patients. *Compendium on Continuing Education for the Practising Veterinary Surgeon* **14**, 305-308
Dorfman M and Dimski DS (1992) Paraproteinaemias in small animal medicine. *Compendium on Continuing Education for the Practising Veterinary Surgeon* **14**, 621-631
Dow SW, Fettman MJ, Curtis CR and LeCouteur RA (1989) Hypokalaemia in cats. *Journal of the American Veterinary Medical Association* **194**, 1604-1608
Dow SW and LeCouteur RA (1991) Potassium-depletion myopathy. In: *Consultations in Feline Medicine,* ed. JR August, pp. 519-522. WB Saunders, Philadelphia
Dunn JK, Bostock DE, Herrtage ME, Jackson KF and Walker MJ (1993) Insulin-secreting tumours of the canine pancreas: clinical and pathological features of 11 cases. *Journal of Small Animal Practice* **34**, 325-331
Elliot J, Dobson JM, Dunn JK, Herrtage ME and Jackson KF (1991) Hypercalcaemia in the dog: a study of 40 cases. *Journal of Small Animal Practice* **32**, 564-571
Feldman EC and Nelson RW (1987) (eds) *Canine and Feline Endocrinology and Reproduction.* WB Saunders, Philadelphia
Finco DR (1989) Kidney function. In: *Clinical Biochemistry of Domestic Animals,* 4th edition, ed. JJ Kaneko, pp 496-542. Academic Press, San Diego

Ford RB (1977) Clinical applications of serum lipid profiles in the dog. *Gaines Veterinary Symposium* **27**,12–16

Ford RB (1993) Idiopathic hyperchylomicronaemia in miniature schanuzers. *Journal of Small Animal Practice* **34**, 488–492

Greentree WF and Hall JO (1995) Iron toxicosis. In: *Kirk's Current Veterinary Therapy XII*, ed. JD Bonagura, pp.240-242. WB Saunders, Philadelphia

Hall RL (1985) Laboratory evaluation of liver disease. *Veterinary Clinics of North America: Small Animal Practice* **15**, 3–9

Handelman CT and Blue JT (1983) Laboratory data: read beyond the numbers. *Compendium on Continuing Education for the Practising Veterinarian* **5**, 687–695

Henry CJ, Lanerschi A, Marks SL, Beyer JL, Nitschelm SH and Barnes S (1996) Acute lymphoblastic leukemia, hypercalemia and pseudohyperkalemia in a dog. *Journal of the American Veterinary Medical Association* **208**, 1237–239

Hohenhaus AE (1995) Syndromes of hyperglobulinemia: diagnosis and therapy. In: *Kirk's Current Veterinary Therapy XII*, ed. JD Bonagura, pp.523-530. WB Saunders, Philadelphia

Hoskins JD (1991) Coronavirus infection in cats. *Compendium on Continuing Education for the Practising Veterinary Surgeon, European Edition* **13**, 231–245

Jensen AL (1992) Serum fructosamine in canine diabetes mellitus. An initial study. *Veterinary Research Communications* **16**, 1–9

Jones BR (1993) Inherited hyperchylomicronaemia in the cat. *Journal of Small Animal Practice* **34**, 493–500

Kaneko JJ (1989) Serum proteins and the dysproteinemias. In: *Clinical Biochemistry of Domestic Animals, 4th edition*, ed. JJ Kaneko, pp142–164. Academic Press, San Diego

Kitchell BE, Strombeck DR, Cullen J and Harrold D (1986) Clinical and pathologic changes in experimentally induced pancreatitis in cats. *American Journal of Veterinary Research* **47**, 1170–1173

Kruger JM and Osborne CA (1994) Canine and feline hypercalcaemic nephropathy. Part 1. Causes and consequences. *Compendium on Continuing Education for the Practising Veterinary Surgeon* **16**, 1299–1315

Mack RE (1994) Screening tests used in the diagnosis of canine hyperadrenocorticism. *Seminars in Veterinary Medicine and Surgery (Small Animal)* **9**, 118–122

Martin LG, Van Pelt DR and Wingfield WE (1995) Magnesium and the critically ill patient. In: *Kirk's Current Veterinary Therapy XII*, ed. JD Bonagura JD, pp. 128–131. WB Saunders, Philadelphia

Meurs KM and Breitschwerdt EB (1995) CVT update: zinc toxicity. In: *Kirk's Current Veterinary Therapy XII*, ed. JD Bonagura JD, pp. 238–239. WB Saunders, Philadelphia

Meyer DJ, Coles EH and Rich LJ (1992) (eds) *Veterinary Laboratory Medicine: Interpretation and Diagnosis*. WB Saunders, Philadelphia

Meyer DJ and Williams DA (1992) Diagnosis of hepatic and exocrine pancreatic disorders. *Seminars in Veterinary Medicine and Surgery (Small Animal)* **7**, 275–284

Nelson RW, Turnwald GH and Willard MD (1994) Endocrine, metabolic and lipid disorders. In: *Small Animal Clinical Diagnosis by Laboratory Methods, 2nd edn*, ed. MD Willard *et al.*, pp.147–178. WB Saunders, Philadelphia

Parent J (1982) Effects of dexamethasone on pancreatic tissue and on serum amylase and lipase activities in dogs. *Journal of the American Veterinary Medical Association* **180**, 743–746

Parker JSL (1991) A probable case of hypoparathyroidism in a cat. *Journal of Small Animal Practice* **31**, 470–473

Patterson JS, Rusley MS and Zachary JF (1985) Neurological manifestations of cerebrovascular atherosclerosis associated with primary hypothyroidism in a dog. *Journal of the American Veterinary Medical Association* **5**, 499–503

Peterson ME, Kintzer PP and Kass PH (1996) Pretreatment clinical and laboratory findings in dogs with hypoadrenocorticism: 225 cases (1979-1993). *Journal of the American Veterinary Medical Association* **208**, 85–91

Reusch CE, Liehs MR, Hoyer M and Vochezer R (1993) Fructosamine: a new parameter for diagnosis and metabolic control in diabetic dogs and cats. *Journal of Veterinary Internal Medicine* **7**,177–182

Schaer, M A (1979) Clinicopathologic survey of acute pancreatitis in 30 dogs and 5 cats. *Journal of the American Animal Hospital Association* **15**, 681–687

Sevelius E (1995) Diagnosis and prognosis of chronic hepatitis and cirrhosis in dogs. *Journal of Small Animal Practice* **36**, 521–528

Shelly SM, Scarlett-Kranz J and Blue JT (1988) Protein electrophoresis on effusions from cats as a diagnostic test for feline infectious peritonitis. *Journal of the American Animal Hospital Association* **24**, 495–500

Simpson KW, Shiroma JT, Biller DS, Wicks J, Johnson SE, Dimski D and Chew D (1994) Ante mortem diagnosis of pancreatitis in four cats. *Journal of Small Animal Practice* **35**, 93–99

Tennant, B (1997) *BSAVA Small Animal Formulary, 2nd edn.* British Small Animal Veterinary Association, Cheltenham

Torrance AG and Nachreiner R (1989) Intact pararthyroid hormone assay and total calcium concentration in the diagnosis of disorders of calcium metabolism in dogs. *Journal of Veterinary Internal Medicine* **3**, 86–89

Thorensen SL, Aleksandersen M, Lønaas L, Bredal WP, Grøndalen and Berthelsen K (1995) Pancreatic insulin-secreting carcinoma in a dog: fructosamine for determining persistent hypoglycaemia. *Journal of Small Animal Practice* **36**, 282–286

Thorensen SI and Bredal WP (1996) Clinical usefulness of fructosamine in measurements in diagnosing and monitoring feline diabetes mellitus. *Journal of Small Animal Practice* **37**, 64–68

Waters CB and Scott-Moncrieff JCR (1992) Hypocalcaemia in cats. In: *Feline Medicine and Surgery in Practice: The Compendium Collection*, pp.27–34. Veterinary Learning Systems, New Jersey

Watson P, Simpson KW, Odedra RM and Bedford PGC (1993) Hypercholesterolaemia in Briards in the United Kingdom. *Research in Veterinary Science* **54**, 80–85

Watson TDG and Barrie J (1993) Lipoprotein metabolism and hyperlipidaemia in the dog and cat: a review. *Journal of Small Animal Practice* **34**, 479–487

Weller RE and Hoffman WE (1992) Renal function in dogs with lymphosarcoma and associated hypercalcaemia. *Journal of Small Animal Practice* **33**, 61–66

Whitney MS, Boon GD, Rebar AH and Ford RB (1987) Effects of acute pancreatitis on circulating lipids in dogs. *American Journal of Veterinary Research* **48**, 1492–1497

Willard MD (1989) Disorders of potassium homeostasis. *Veterinary Clinics of North America: Small Animal Practice* **19**, 241–263

Willard MD, Tvedten H and Turnwald GH (1994) (eds) *Small Animal Clinical Diagnosis by Laboratory Methods, 2nd edn.* WB Saunders, Philadelphia

Willemse T (1992) Zinc-related cutaneous disorders of dogs. In: *Kirk's Current Veterinary Therapy XI*, ed. RW Kirk and JD Bonagura, pp. 532–534. WB Saunders, Philadelphia

Yaphé W and Forrester SD (1994) Renal secondary hyperparathyroidism: pathophysiology, diagnosis and treatment. *Compendium on Continuing Education for the Practising Veterinary Surgeon* **16**, 173–181

CHAPTER FIVE

Microbiological Testing

Irene A.P. McCandlish and David J. Taylor

GLOSSARY

CAV	Canine adenovirus
CCoV	Canine coronavirus
CDV	Canine distemper virus
CHV	Canine herpesvirus
COSHH	Control of Substances Hazardous to Health
CPIV	Canine parainfluenza virus
CPV	Canine parvovirus
ELISA	Enzyme-linked immunosorbent assay
FCoV	Feline coronavirus
FCV	Feline calicivirus
FeLV	Feline leukaemia virus
FHV	Feline herpesvirus
FIP	Feline infectious peritonitis
FITC	Fluorescein isothiocyanate
FIV	Feline immunodeficiency virus
HAI	Haemagglutination inhibition
HSE	Health and Safety Executive
IF	Immunofluorescence
PCR	Polymerase chain reaction
RIM	Rapid immunomigration
VI	Virus isolation
VN	Virus neutralization
VTM	Viral transport medium

INTRODUCTION

Advances in scientific techniques and increasing legislative control have revolutionized the use of microbiological tests in small animal practice. The development of easily stored 'kit' tests, based on enzyme-linked immunosorbent assay or rapid immunomigration techniques, has allowed the rapid in-practice identification of canine parvovirus, feline leukaemia virus and feline immunodeficiency virus. Similarly, the use of kit systems has simplified the identification of bacterial species, providing substrates for multiple enzyme and fermentation tests in immediately available and appropriate combinations, together with simple diagnostic keys.

In contrast, the introduction of COSHH regulations and guidelines for the disposal of potentially contaminated materials (Safe Disposal of Clinical Waste) (see also Chapter One) has meant that, for many practices, it is impractical to carry out isolation and sensitivity testing on material that may include potential human pathogens such as mycobacteria or *Chlamydia* spp. Complying with the legislation can be a daunting undertaking and may not be considered worthwhile for procedures that may be used infrequently, especially when good commercial diagnostic laboratory services are readily available.

The range of in-practice diagnostic tests is likely to expand as commercial companies develop the appropriate highly purified and specific microbial proteins, peptides and monoclonal antibodies that are required for tests against different infectious agents. Moreover, the advent and commercial application of newer techniques such as the polymerase chain reaction (PCR), means that even more sophisticated and sensitive laboratory-based tests will become available in future.

It is increasingly important that veterinary surgeons understand the basis of the various tests available to them, in order to select the most appropriate test in differing circumstances, and to appreciate the limitations and problems of interpretation that may arise. This chapter outlines the principles underlying commonly used practice-based and external laboratory tests and describes the application and interpretation of these aids to diagnosis.

LABORATORY SAFETY

As mentioned in Chapter 1, in-practice microbiology in the UK comes under a variety of legislative controls, in particular the guidelines of the Advisory Committee on Dangerous Pathogens. Work should take place in a Category 2 Laboratory of appropriate design, including an unpacking area, adequate benching, dedicated incubators and refrigerators, centrifuges, and handwashing basins. Specimens containing potential Category 3 pathogens, such as *Mycobacterium* spp. and *Chlamydia psittaci,* cannot be handled beyond reception unless there is adequate operator protection, e.g. a Class 1 safety cabinet. Any further work requires the agreement of HSE. Specimens should be treated as clinical waste and all laboratory waste must be made safe and disposed of by an appropriate and approved route (usually incineration). If a non-routine disposal route is used, the waste disposal chain must be followed to ensure that it is safe and that all legal constraints are met.

This Chapter describes the procedures to be followed where these conditions are met.

GENERAL METHODS OF MICROBIOLOGICAL INVESTIGATION

Many diagnostic techniques are common to both virological and bacteriological investigations.

Immunodiagnostic assays

All immunodiagnostic assays rely on the use of antibodies directed against microbial proteins. Polyclonal antisera, produced in laboratory animals by inoculation of whole organisms or partly purified extracts, have been replaced almost entirely by monoclonal antibody produced in cell culture and directed against individual microbial proteins. Monoclonal antibody has greatly improved the specificity, sensitivity and reliability of these assays and allowed their modification for in-practice use. False-positive reactions are relatively unusual, since the microbial epitopes that the tests identify are selected to be poorly cross-reactive with other agents or body components. False negatives can occur since the specific epitopes may not be produced in sufficient amounts to be detectable, or may not be available for reaction with the test antibody. For example, virus in secretions may be coated by antibody.

Immunofluorescence and immunocytochemistry

In immunofluorescence (IF) techniques (Figure 5.1), the antigen–antibody reaction is detected by labelling the antibody with fluorescent dye (usually fluorescein isothiocyanate, FITC). Suspect material, usually aspirates, mucosal scrapings or blood cells, is stained with the specific antibody. In direct IF tests, the primary antibody is itself conjugated with FITC. In indirect IF tests, the primary antibody is subsequently reacted with a secondary conjugated antibody directed against its Fc component. Indirect tests tend to be more sensitive but both sensitivity and specificity of IF tests are largely dependent on the quality of the antibodies. Use of monoclonal antibody increases the specificity of IF tests by eliminating many cross-reactions. IF is a rapid and sensitive technique but requires specialized fluorescence microscopy facilities and trained staff to interpret the results.

IF can also be used on fresh tissue samples collected at post mortem and this is frequently quoted as

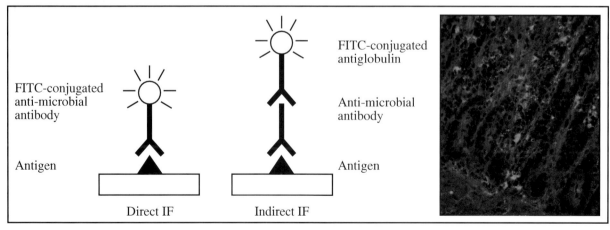

Figure 5.1: *(a) Direct and indirect immunofluorescence tests. Suspect material is placed on glass or plastic, then incubated with antibody to a specific microorganism. In direct IF, the antimicrobial antibody is conjugated to FITC. In indirect IF, an anti-globulin antibody conjugated with FITC is used in a second incubation phase. The presence of the microbe is detected by fluorescence under ultraviolet light. (b) Canine parvovirus in intestinal crypt epithelial cells, demonstrated by IF.*

a common diagnostic test. Frozen (cryostat) sections are cut and stained with FITC-conjugated antibody. Because fresh tissues deteriorate during transport, the technique is less commonly useful than might be thought. IF on post-mortem samples is largely being replaced by other immunocytochemical techniques such as immunoperoxidase staining. This can be performed on formalin-fixed paraffin wax-embedded tissues submitted for routine histological examination. Microbial antigen is exposed to enzyme-coupled specific antibody and a positive reaction is demonstrated by staining when the enzyme substrate is added (Figure 5.2). Once again, the value of the test is dependent on the availability of good specific antisera and the appropriate technology, but it is likely to become more widely used in the next few years.

ELISA

In ELISAs (Figure 5.3) antigen–antibody reactions are detected by labelling known antibody with an enzyme that, on reaction with its substrate, produces a visible colour change. The suspect material is adsorbed on to a carrier (glass, plastic or special membranes), and the specific antibody is added. This antibody may be directly conjugated with enzyme or a secondary enzyme-conjugated antibody may be added. Finally, the revealing substrate is added: the diagnostic colour change should only be seen where microbial antigen

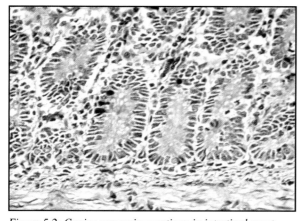

Figure 5.2: Canine parvovirus antigen in intestinal crypt epithelial cells, demonstrated by immunoperoxidase staining.

has initiated the chain of antigen–antibody–enzyme–substrate reactions. Thorough washing between the steps is essential to ensure that free antibody or enzyme do not produce false-positive reactions. In-practice ELISAs often incorporate automatic wash routines. Positive and negative controls must be included. ELISA technology is also used for detection of antibody where the test sample is reacted with known antigen.

Rapid immunomigration tests

In rapid immunomigration (RIM) tests, the revealing agent for the antigen–antibody reaction is an agent such as colloidal gold which has been bound to the specific antibody. The antigen–antibody–gold complex is allowed to migrate along a membrane and is trapped in a specialized matrix that concentrates the gold particles to produce a visible band. Appropriate control bands are included in kit tests. Binding the revealing gold particles to antigen allows the detection of antibody in samples.

Molecular biology assays

Modern molecular biology assays are dependent on the properties of DNA:

- Its resistance to degradation means that it remains unaltered in samples for long periods of time and can be manipulated without damaging its underlying structure
- Its complex nucleotide sequence allows it to be split into distinct identifiable fragments of different sizes (with a pattern unique to each organism) by special enzymes known as restriction endonucleases
- The complementary double-stranded structure permits precise identification of specific nucleotide sequences: known labelled single-stranded DNA sequences (probes) from specific microorganisms will only bind to (hybridize with) specific complementary sequences.

DNA hybridization

Microbial DNA of unknown type is broken down into fragments using restriction endonucleases; the frag-

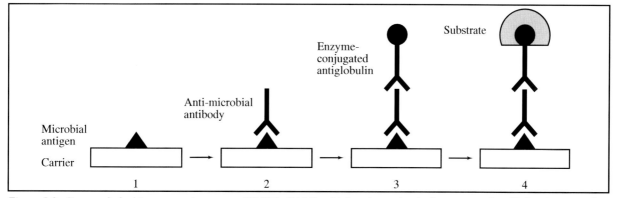

Figure 5.3: Enzyme-linked immunosorbent assay (ELISA). (1) Microbial antigen adsorbed on to a carrier. (2) Incubation with antibody to a specific microorganism. (3) Second incubation with enzyme-coupled antiglobulin. (4) Added substrate interacts with the enzyme to give a colour change visible with the naked eye or using a specialized reader.

ments are separated by electrophoresis and then identified by probing with known labelled sequences. Hybridization is increasingly used to identify different strains of bacteria. *In situ* hybridization, in which small amounts of microbial DNA are localized in tissue samples, offers great future potential for identification of persistent or very low grade infections, or organisms that would be hazardous or difficult to culture.

PCR

The PCR technique (Figure 5.4) produces massive amplification of very small amounts of DNA, even single copies of sequences. Basically, DNA in the test material is denatured to single strands. Known nucleotide sequences (primers) are attached at either end of the strands and, in the presence of a DNA polymerase and a suitable supply of nucleotides, new double-stranded DNA is produced. Repetition of the cycle (30–40 times) produces large amounts of DNA that can be analysed and identified using electrophoresis, hybridization and other techniques. For RNA viruses a variation of the technique, known as reverse transcriptase-PCR, is used. The extreme sensitivity of the PCR technique means that caution must be used in interpretation; the test may detect microbial material that is incidental to a current illness. In addition, precautions must be taken to avoid contamination of material with protein from external sources. However, as experience with this technology expands, it is likely to be used more frequently in diagnostic laboratories.

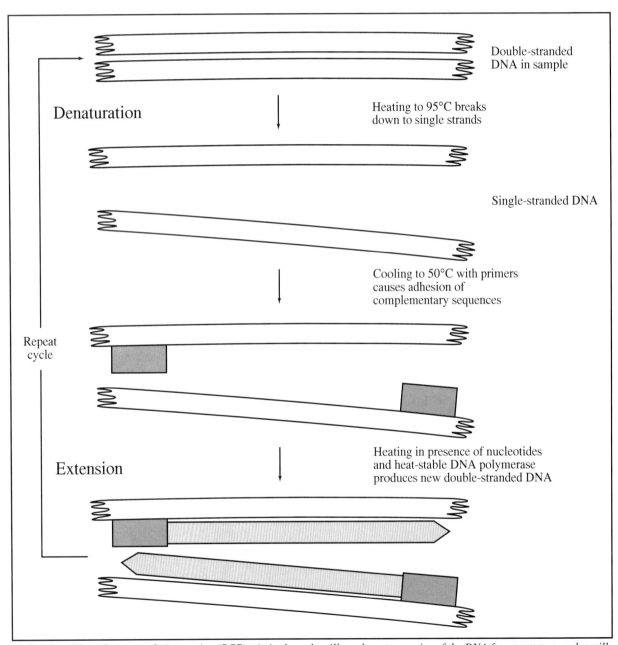

Figure 5.4: The polymerase chain reaction (PCR). A single cycle will produce two copies of the DNA fragment; two cycles will produce four copies, and three cycles will produce eight copies. After 30 cycles there will be approximately 10 million copies that can be identified by hybridization.

Serological assays

Demonstration of a serological response is often used in the diagnosis of microbial infections, especially where isolation or antigen detection is difficult, hazardous, unavailable, or time-consuming and expensive. Serology is also widely used in epidemiological investigations within kennels and catteries, in some control programmes (e.g. control of feline coronavirus) and in monitoring vaccine responses. Where animals have suffered from suspected vaccine-induced anaphylaxis, evaluation of their immune status can be useful in deciding whether they should receive further vaccination or not.

Antibody merely reflects exposure to either natural infection or vaccination and care must be taken in interpreting antibody titres, especially in relating them to current or recent illness. For example, in unvaccinated pups and kittens, a very high titre to canine or feline parvovirus can be taken as presumptive evidence of recent infection, whether clinical or subclinical. In older, even unvaccinated animals, high titres may have been present for months or years and may not be related to recent acute illness.

Classically, with recent infection, one should be able to demonstrate a 'rising titre', i.e. a 4-fold increase in antibody titre between an acute phase sample, taken when illness is first seen, and a convalescent sample, taken 3–4 weeks later. In practice, this is often difficult. First, the need for investigation may not be apparent on initial presentation, so that the first sample is not collected until disease is well established. Secondly, with some infections (e.g. canine parvovirus and adenovirus), titres rise very early in infection so that the required 4-fold rise is seldom seen even when the first sample is taken on initial presentation. A particular problem seen with canine distemper virus (CDV), is that clinically ill animals are usually immunosuppressed and develop only low antibody titres; animals that develop a good antibody response, with a rising titre, are usually subclinically affected.

A potential alternative to paired samples is emerging. Since IgM is produced in significant amounts only following primary exposure to antigen, determination of IgM and IgG specific titres can, in theory, differentiate between recent and past exposure: recently infected animals will have both IgM and IgG responses; past exposure will be associated with an IgG response. Differential IgG/IgM titres are difficult and cumbersome with the traditional serological tests such as virus neutralization (VN) or haemagglutination inhibition (HAI) but are easier with ELISA and IF tests. As these become more widely applied, differentiation of active infection should become easier.

The type of test used differs with the agent. Virus neutralization, despite the fact that it can be relatively laborious and slow (up to 5 days) is widely used for CDV and canine adenovirus (CAV) since it gives consistent and reliable results that correlate well with immunity. This is particularly important when evaluating immunity following vaccination. With canine parvovirus (CPV), neutralizing antibody also inhibits viral haemagglutination, and so HAI tests are commonly used since the difficulty of culturing CPV makes true viral neutralization impractical. HAI tests take only a few hours to obtain a result. IF antibody tests detect a broad spectrum of antibody and are used notably for feline coronavirus (FCoV) (Figure 5.5) and feline immunodeficiency virus (FIV).

ELISA tests are increasingly used and form the basis of in-practice kit tests. Most in-practice systems give only a positive or negative result but laboratory-based systems will often give specific titres. The basis of ELISA antibody tests is similar to that already described for antigen detection. Known amounts of microbial antigens are placed on a carrier and the test serum, or dilutions of it, is added, allowed to react and washed off. The presence of adherent antibody is then detected by addition of enzyme conjugated anti-immunoglobulin antibody followed by an appropriate substrate; a colour change occurs where viral-specific antibody is present. More complex competitive and sandwich ELISA tests may be also used. It is important to remember that the antigen used in ELISA tests is often a small epitope of the agent and that, since individual animals may produce antibodies to only some epitopes, an animal showing as negative on one ELISA test may prove positive with another. In addition, depending on the antigen, ELISA titres may not correlate well with neutralizing or protective antibody.

Serological tests for small animal bacterial infections are limited to diagnostic laboratories and are only available for a few organisms. The Rose Bengal plate test for *Brucella canis* is a non-quantitative test; quantitative agglutination tests are available in the USA and other countries where this is a significant infection. For detecting antibody to *Leptospira*, the usual test is the microscopic agglutination test (MAT). ELISAs are also used: examples include tests for antibody to *Borrelia burgdorferi* (using a 49kD recombinant flagellar antigen) in Lyme disease and to

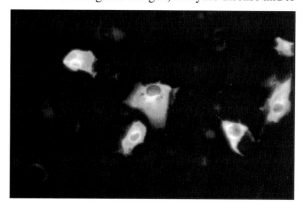

Figure 5.5: *IF test for antibody. Antibody to feline coronavirus detected by fluorescence of antibody attached to individual virus-infected cells.*
Courtesy of Dr D.D. Addie

Bordetella bronchiseptica (under development). Indirect IF is used to detect antibody to *Chlamydia*.

It is important to remember that an antibody titre obtained for any one sample can vary not only with the type of test employed, but also with the laboratory performing it. It is therefore essential that laboratories provide guidelines for interpretation. In most cases, interpretation of specific titres depends on clinical details, and a full history must be provided if the veterinary surgeon wishes the laboratory to give meaningful comments. Tests used for legislative reasons or international certification (e.g. *Leptospira* tests for export certificates) are performed at specified laboratories and are standardized against international standard sera. All commercially used antibody tests should be well defined and controlled in terms of sensitivity and specificity of the test.

Antibody may be detected in secretions, colostrum and milk as well as serum but, like the measurement of cell-mediated responses using lymphocytes from unclotted blood, this is a research procedure rather than a practical diagnostic technique.

VIROLOGICAL INVESTIGATION

Confirmation of viral infection is most important in kennels and catteries or when dealing with groups of animals, especially when control or eradication of disease depends on accurate identification of infected animals. Elimination of feline leukaemia virus (FeLV) from a group of breeding cats is a prime example of how assays can be used to identify and monitor infection in a group. Confirmation of viral infection may also be required in individual animals, especially when there is any question of potential legal problems or failure of vaccine response, such as the pup that develops suspected CPV infection within a few days of purchase or several weeks after vaccination. In live animals, virus isolation, demonstration of virus or viral antigen, and serological investigation are the mainstays of diagnosis. Histopathological examination is often useful, especially in fatal cases, and for some diseases is a faster, more reliable and cheaper method of confirmation. It is likely that an increasing number of rapid tests for viral antigens and antibodies based on ELISA or similar technology will become available in future. In addition to the immunodiagnostic assays, molecular biology techniques and serological tests mentioned above, virus isolation and electron microscopy are used for virus identification.

Sample collection and handling
The appropriate material for viral diagnosis varies depending on the virus concerned, the stage of disease, the reason for sampling and, last but not least, the tests available (see also Chapter 1). With in-practice kit systems, the requirements, whether serum, plasma, whole blood or faecal material, are well laid out in the literature that accompanies the kits. When dealing with referral laboratories, the samples will vary depending on laboratory facilities and the range of tests on offer. If in doubt, the laboratory should be contacted for advice; this will avoid unnecessary expense to the veterinary surgeon and client and optimize the chances of getting a definitive result.

For serological testing, clotted blood or serum is required. Separated serum is preferable since this avoids haemolysis which can interfere with some tests. Many practices now have small centrifuges, which makes production of well separated serum samples very simple. The amount of blood or serum required depends on how many tests are to be carried out and the type of test to be undertaken. Viral neutralization tests tend to need more serum than ELISAs. In general, 0.5 ml of serum (1 ml of clotted blood) is adequate for individual tests while 1–2 ml of serum (2–5 ml of clotted blood) is sufficient for a range of tests. Samples should be collected and processed aseptically.

With persistent infections such as FeLV, prolonged viraemia can be detected in a simple blood sample. In acute systemic (e.g. parvovirus) and superficial mucosal infections, viraemia is short lived or inapparent, and virus or viral antigen is most usually detected in secretions, whether respiratory, faecal or other mucosal sites.

For virus isolation, certain general principles should be borne in mind:

- Many viruses, particularly enveloped viruses, are labile and may be inactivated by heat (including normal room temperature) or drying, especially during transport
- Secretions, or swabs of them e.g. nasopharyngeal swabs, are best placed in a specialized viral transport medium (VTM) that contains serum proteins to help stabilize the virus and antibiotics to prevent overgrowth by normal bacterial commensals
- Dampening swabs with VTM before use helps prevent absorption of virus particles deep into the swab which can reduce recovery rates
- Use of gelatinous or charcoal-based bacteriological swabs is contraindicated since these materials can adsorb viral particles
- Tissue samples collected during post mortem should be collected as aseptically as possible and placed in VTM
- Samples should be refrigerated before posting. Inclusion of small ice packs in insulated boxes can be useful, especially for post-mortem tissue samples where tissue autolysis can interfere with cell cultures.

For IF tests, blood smears, mucosal smears or scrapings, and impression smears from post-mortem tissues are prepared on clear dry microscope slides. Smears and impressions are air-dried or fixed in acetone, depending on the test system; advice should be sought from the laboratory on the preferred method.

For electron microscopy and viral antigen detection in faeces, 2–5 ml of faeces is preferable to a swab; if a swab is submitted, it should be well coated with faeces.

Virus isolation

Pros:
- Definitive method
- Allows typing of isolates
- Identifies new viruses or variants

Cons:
- Restricted availability
- Time-consuming
- Often expensive
- Need viable virus in sample

Growth of virus from secretions or tissues is an obvious method of investigation but is the diagnostic method of choice in few infections. Virus isolation in cell culture is a labour-intensive, often expensive procedure, restricted to specialist, often research-based, laboratories. Viral growth in cell culture is identified

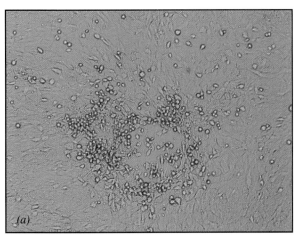

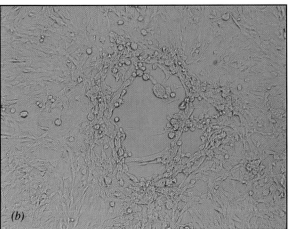

Figure 5.6: *(a) Feline calicivirus in cell culture; foci of cell rounding and aggregation. (b) Feline herpesvirus in cell culture; foci of cell degeneration and rounding.*
Courtesy of Prof. J.O. Jarrett.

by recognition of a cytopathic effect (CPE) within the cells, by electron microscopy, immunostaining or a combination of methods.

Different cell lines and conditions of culture are required for different viruses. Primary isolation from infected material may require repeated subculture and take several weeks. Depending on the agent and stage of infection, viable virus may no longer be present in secretions or tissues and inactivation of virus during transport can be a significant problem. In addition, some viruses, notoriously CDV and FCoV, are exceptionally difficult to grow in primary culture, even for laboratories working with them on a regular basis. Consequently, virus isolation as a routine diagnostic method is restricted to those agents, such as feline calicivirus (FCV; Figure 5.6a) or feline herpesvirus (FHV; Figure 5.6b), that grow well in specific cell lines under known culture conditions. With such agents, isolation can be carried out sufficiently rapidly and reproducibly to be practically and economically viable. Samples must be taken from appropriate sites and submitted in an appropriate viral transport medium. The golden rule for virus isolation is to contact the laboratory for advice before sending a sample.

Virus isolation and characterization is the essential method of diagnosis when clinical circumstances suggest the presence of a new virus or viral strain. Truly new viral diseases, such as the emergence of CPV infection in the late 1970s, are rare events, but variation in viral strains are more common. Only research laboratories are likely to have the facilities for such procedures.

Electron microscopy

Pros:
- Rapid

Cons:
- Restricted availability
- Need large amounts of virus
- Will only identify viral family

The consistent size and structure of different virus particles makes them easily recognized when examined using an electron microscope with negative contrast staining. However, large amounts of virus (10^8 particles/ml) must be present in order for the virus to be seen and generally only the virus family is identifiable. In small animal practice, electron microscopy is most frequently used to identify poxvirus (Figure 5.7a) in skin lesions in cats and when looking for viruses that are difficult to grow, such as rotavirus or coronaviruses (Figure 5.7b), that may be present in large numbers in diarrhoeic faecal samples early in infection. An electron microscope is an expensive piece of equipment and, consequently, tends to be limited to research laboratories.

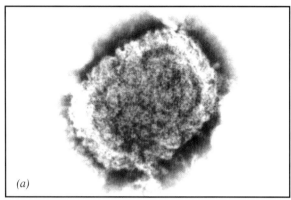

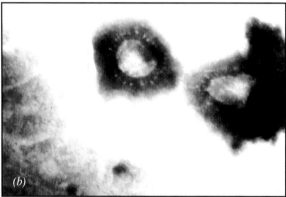

Figure 5.7: Negative-stain electron microscopy. (a) Typical poxvirus from a skin lesion in a cat. (b) Typical coronavirus particle in faecal sample from a pup with diarrhoea.
Courtesy of Prof. J.O. Jarrett.

Diagnosis of specific viral infections

Canine parvovirus (and feline parvovirus)

In-practice tests:

- Detection of CPV antigen in faeces or intestinal content
- CPV kit tests: may also detect FPV since the monoclonal antibodies used cross-react
- ELISA or RIM.

Interpretation: A positive result indicates free CPV (or FPV) antigen in the sample. Free virus is present in faeces for only a short time. By the time animals have been ill for a day or more, viral shedding may have stopped or virus in intestinal material may be coated by antibody and no longer detectable by these tests.

Laboratory tests:

- Isolation: very difficult
- Detection of viral haemagglutinin (Figure 5.8) (1–2 ml of faeces or intestinal content): FPV requires different conditions from CPV to demonstrate haemagglutination. Similar problems to in-practice tests, i.e. false negatives are common
- Electron microscopy: false negatives are common

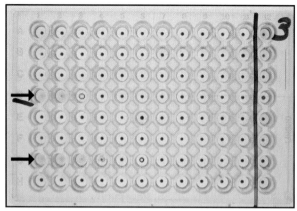

Figure 5.8: Detection of canine parvovirus haemagglutinin. Viral haemagglutinin causes the red blood cells to form a flat monolayer at the bottom of the wells rather than tight buttons. Samples are diluted out across the rows to give some quantitation of the amount of virus present; addition of anti-CPV antibody to the final column (an undiluted sample) abolishes viral haemagglutination. Samples in rows 4 and 7 are positive (arrows).

- Serology (1–2 ml serum): usually HAI test. The presence of high titres in unvaccinated animals confirms exposure to infection. Rapidly rising titres may prevent demonstration of the classic 4-fold rise in paired samples. Modern modified vaccines produce high titres that cannot be differentiated from active infection on titres alone. Use of IgG- and IgM-specific ELISA tests may allow differentiation between recent active infection and previous vaccination
- Histopathology: in fatal cases examination of small intestine (minimum of 3 different levels), mesenteric lymph node and thymus will reveal typical changes. If necessary, viral antigen can be detected by immunocytochemical and other more sophisticated techniques.

Canine distemper virus

Laboratory tests:

- Isolation: very difficult since established cell lines are resistant to CDV. Fresh canine alveolar macrophage cultures are more sensitive but are seldom available for routine diagnosis. The most effective method of CDV culture, direct growth of the suspect case's alveolar macrophages, lymphocytes or cerebellar tissue, is a technique justifiable only in exceptional circumstances
- IF: detection of viral antigen in conjunctival and tonsillar smears is frequently advocated but false negatives are common. Only small amounts of viral antigen may be intermittently present and secondary bacterial infection and autofluorescence of polymorphonuclear leucocytes may also interfere. Smears of bladder epithelial cells in spun urine samples may be less

contaminated. Check the laboratory has an appropriate antibody before submitting material

- Serology (1–2 ml of serum): usually neutralization test. Interpretation is often difficult. In unvaccinated dogs, a positive titre is consistent with exposure. Many dogs that succumb to CDV develop only low antibody titres and the classic 'rising titre' cannot be demonstrated. Detection of IgM-specific antibody (usually by ELISA) may differentiate between recent infection and previous vaccination. The presence of anti-CDV antibody in cerebrospinal fluid (CSF) samples (1 ml) is a reliable indicator of CDV encephalitis since CSF antibody is produced locally in response to infection and does not reflect response to vaccination. Blood contamination of CSF samples will interfere with interpretation
- Histopathology: in fatal cases examination will reveal changes, including lymphoid depletion and inclusion bodies, in a variety of tissues. Samples should include lymphoid (tonsil, lymph node, spleen), epithelial (bronchus, lung, gastric pylorus, intestine, urinary bladder) and nervous tissues (whole brain and cord where possible, but sections of cerebellum, medulla and midbrain are preferable to small portions of superficial cerebral cortex.) Immunocytochemical studies can confirm the presence of viral antigen. Biopsy and immunocytochemical analysis of footpads has been suggested as a pre-mortem diagnostic technique.

Canine adenovirus-1 (infectious canine hepatitis)

Laboratory tests:

- Isolation: CAV-1 is most readily cultured from oropharyngeal or tonsillar swabs early in infection. Virus is shed intermittently in urine in recovering animals but isolation from urine is not a reliable method of detecting 'carriers'. Liver (1 cm cube) in VTM may be submitted from fatal cases. CAV-2 in cases of respiratory disease can be isolated from nasal or oropharyngeal swabs
- Serology (1–2 ml serum): usually neutralization test. Ideally, paired serum samples 2–3 weeks apart will show a rising titre. Single samples from recovering animals are often diagnostic since active infection produces much higher titres than vaccination. Since current vaccines contain CAV-2, differential neutralization tests against CAV-1 and CAV-2 will show a higher titre to CAV-1 in infected animals.
- Histopathology: fixed samples of liver, mesenteric lymph node, kidney and intestine will be diagnostic in fatal cases of CAV-1 infection.

Canine herpesvirus

Laboratory tests:

- Isolation: in fatal systemic CHV infection in neonatal pups, small portions of liver, renal cortex, lung and spleen should be submitted in VTM. Attempts to recover virus from vaginal or preputial washings and swabs are almost invariably negative. Future development of DNA hybridization techniques may permit identification of carriers
- Serology: there is currently no readily available test for CHV in the UK. Virus neutralization and IF are available in some research laboratories and ELISA systems are likely to come into use.

Canine respiratory viruses

Laboratory tests:

- Isolation: nasopharyngeal or tonsillar swabs from dogs with kennel cough may reveal canine parainfluenza virus (CPIV), CAV-1, CAV-2, CHV or occasionally other agents such as reovirus. Swabs in VTM cannot also be used for isolation of *Bordetella bronchiseptica* since VTM contains antibiotic. In individual dogs, viral shedding has often stopped by the time a requirement for virus isolation arises. Isolation is most successful when samples are taken immediately on development of clinical signs in kennel outbreaks
- Serology: paired blood samples may show rising titres to CAV or CPIV by viral neutralization or haemagglutination inhibition. Samples are best taken a minimum of 3 weeks apart since the serum response to CPIV is slow. Titres to CPIV following natural infection are much higher than following vaccination.

Canine enteric viruses

Laboratory tests:

- Isolation: possible in theory for coronavirus, rotavirus and calicivirus, but seldom achieved or attempted due to technical difficulties
- Electron microscopy (2–5 ml of faeces): a wide range of agents may be identified. Enveloped viruses (e.g. CCoV) may deteriorate in transport
- ELISA (1–2 ml of faeces): canine rotavirus can be detected by tests designed for detection of group-specific antigens in calf diarrhoea
- Serology (1–2 ml of serum): IF tests may show rising titres to CCoV in paired samples.

Feline leukaemia virus

In-practice tests:

- Detection of p27 viral core protein from infected cells in blood or saliva
- ELISA or RIM assays.

Interpretation: A positive result indicates the presence of viral antigen in the sample. In a sick cat, this is very likely to reflect FeLV viraemia. In healthy cats, a positive result is best confirmed by virus isolation or IF. Up to 10% of healthy cats that tested positive will be negative by these other tests and most will become negative on all tests after 3–4 months. Very occasional sick cats that are negative by immunoassay will be positive by isolation or IF.

Laboratory tests:

- Isolation (1 ml of heparinized blood): virus should be recovered in cell culture within 7–10 days
- IF (1 ml of blood in EDTA or heparin, or unfixed air dried blood smears): viral antigen is detected in white blood cells. A rapid test that can be carried out within a few hours

Feline immunodeficiency virus

In-practice tests:

- Detection of antibody to purified FIV proteins or peptides, usually a transmembrane envelope protein (p41) or a viral core protein (p24). A higher proportion of cats may have antibody to p41 envelope protein
- ELISA or RIM assays.

Interpretation: A positive result indicates the presence of antibody due to permanent FIV infection. In a cat with appropriate clinical signs, these are likely to be due to FIV. Healthy FIV-positive cats may survive with few signs. Very occasional infected cats may be seronegative by a test to one specific protein. In suspicious cases, a negative result should be confirmed by test against another protein or by laboratory tests.

Laboratory tests:

- IF (1 ml of heparinized blood, plasma or serum): indirect IF test using FIV-infected cells as test antigen. Detects antibodies to all viral proteins. Tests results available in a few hours
- Immunoblotting (1 ml of heparinized blood, plasma or serum): also detects antibodies to all viral proteins. Results available in 48 hours

- Isolation: an expensive process that requires culture of lymphocytes from heparinized blood. Takes up to 3 weeks and used mainly as a research tool. PCR: detection of FIV being introduced.

Feline coronavirus (feline infectious peritonitis)

In-practice tests:

- Detection of antibody to FCoV in serum, plasma, ascitic or thoracic effusions. Tests can provide a simple positive or negative or a semi-quantitative result
- ELISA-based systems.

Interpretation: A positive result merely shows exposure to FCoV. It does not imply the cat has, or will develop, feline infectious peritonitis (FIP) nor that it is excreting virus or is a carrier. Useful as a screening test, e.g. for establishing the presence of infection in a cattery or in individual queens and studs prior to breeding.

Laboratory tests:

- IF (1–2 ml blood, serum or plasma): confirms the presence of antibody and gives a titre. High titres are common in dry FIP. Titres in wet FIP are more variable, with levels from low to high, and occasional cats with no detectable antibody due to complexing with viral antigen in blood or effusions. High titres may also occur in clinically normal animals. Diagnosis of FIP should never be based on serology alone but take into account clinical findings and other ancillary tests (albumin: globulin ratios, plasma α-1-acid glycoprotein, cytology, histopathology). However, monitoring of IF titres is useful in evaluating the progress of control programmes: cats with falling titres are unlikely to be excreting virus although cats may have to be kept in isolation for several months before titres start to fall
- ELISA and immunoblotting: can also be used to detect antibody
- PCR: viral RNA can be detected in blood, faeces or effusions. A very sensitive procedure but many healthy cats appear to carry the virus, giving similar problems in interpretation to those encountered with antibody tests
- Histopathology: samples of abdominal or thoracic organs, lymph nodes and other tissues (e.g. brain) may reveal changes typical or suggestive of FIP. Application of immunocytochemistry may confirm the presence of viral antigen in typical lesions, confirming the diagnosis.

Feline respiratory viruses

Laboratory tests:

- Isolation: oropharyngeal swabs in VTM will reveal virus within 3–5 days. Feline calicivirus is excreted continuously by infected cats, feline herpesvirus only intermittently, making detection of carriers difficult. FCV is widespread and some isolates are virtually non-pathogenic.
- Serology: VN tests can be performed but interpretation is difficult.

Orthopoxvirus

Laboratory tests:

- Isolation (portions of suspected skin lesions in sterile container): isolation should be achieved in 3–7 days
- Electron microscopy (portions of skin lesions): shows typical orthopox particles on negative staining
- Histopathology: eosinophilic intracytoplasmic inclusions are seen in epidermal stratum spinosum and follicular epithelium on standard H&E-stained sections.

Rabies virus

In the UK, all suspected cases of rabies must be notified to the Ministry of Agriculture, Fisheries and Food, who carry out all diagnostic tests; these are based on the detection of viral antigen in the central nervous system by IF or other tests.

BACTERIOLOGICAL INVESTIGATION

Identification of bacteria may be required for primary pathogens or secondary factors complicating other infectious or non-infectious disease processes. Appropriate antibiotic treatment is largely dependent on identification of bacterial type or specific antibiotic sensitivity testing. The immunodiagnostic assays described above are widely used in diagnostic laboratories to identify bacteria or bacterial products, such as clostridial toxins, in body tissues or secretions, but few are currently available for in-practice use. Molecular biology techniques are increasingly used in specialist laboratories to type bacteria and also, especially PCR, to identify small numbers of bacteria; results of such tests may now be encountered on laboratory reports and may be considered reliable.

The two other main techniques used in the identification of bacteria are direct visualization and bacterial isolation. Both methods depend on the presence of bacteria in the sample. The methods chosen to examine a sample are important and govern the quality of the

results obtained. Once antibody starts to develop, identification or isolation of initiating bacteria may become difficult.

Sample collection and handling

Samples should be collected into suitable sterile containers and examined as soon as possible. Samples should be stored in a refrigerator until they are examined, although examinations such as dark-ground examination of urine for *Leptospira* should be carried out immediately. Details of sampling methods are discussed elsewhere (see Chapters 1 and 15), but some kinds of sample limit the examinations that can be performed. A brief guide to the optimum sample types for the practice laboratory is given in Table 5.1. Samples from large portions of tissue must be taken using precautions that prevent infection of the operator and also prevent contamination of the inoculum for testing. They usually involve searing the surface of the tissue and then sampling aseptically through the seared area. The examinations to be performed may be qualitative or quantitative, depending on the origin of the sample and the history. Where it is thought that viable bacteria may no longer be present, samples may be submitted for detection of nucleic acid sequences or antigens which will confirm the presence of the agent or its products.

Direct detection

Pros:
- Methods usually rapid
- Minimal risk from live material
- Some methods specific
- Level of detection significantly higher than culture

Cons:
- Simple methods such as smears may not be specific
- No possibility of determining antimicrobial sensitivities
- No possibility of sending to reference laboratory

Bacteria may be seen by light microscopy in preparations made from pathological specimens. Simple examination can establish the presence of bacteria and may identify them.

Light microscopy of smears

Fixed blood films can be examined using general stains such as methylene blue to identify the presence of bacteria. The use of Gram staining allows the bacteria to be classified. Special staining methods allow identification to group level (e.g. mycobacteria are acid–alcohol fast with Ziehl–Neelsen stains) or reveal the bacteria more clearly (e.g. Giemsa for *Mycoplasma*). Blood smears viewed by light microscopy also contain neutrophils and other structures, the presence of which should be recorded as an aid to interpretation of results. It should be remembered that some Gram-positive bacteria can lose stain, leaving spots, and some Gram-negative bacteria may be difficult to identify if there is protein in the background. Neutrophils, macrophages and lymphocytes appear pink but details of the nucleus can be distinguished. Leptospires are too thin to be seen in smears without special stains. Some bacteria may be identified presumptively by their staining reaction and others by their morphology. *Campylobacter* spp., spirochaetes, streptococci, staphylococci, *Nocardia* and clostridia can all be identified tentatively in smears. Smears can be used to give rapid confirmation of the presence of bacteria in a sample and may give an idea of their identity.

Bacteria can be identified to species level in smears using IF or immunoperoxidase staining and specific antisera.

Dark-ground microscopy of urine

Urine may be examined for *Leptospira* organisms. In acute cases, leptospiruria may be seen with the naked eye as swirling pale clouds in the urine. The organisms may be identified by their characteristic hooked ends and gentle flexing movement. In old samples, those from animals which have received antimicrobial therapy, or those from animals that have developed some immunity, the organisms may round up and appear as small dots.

Urine contains a number of other long structures. Bacteria appear as thicker, sometimes motile rigid rods; sperm tails are larger but may move; and strands of fibrin appear thin and *Leptospira*-like but are less dense and do not have curved ends. Granular stiff rods represent casts from the renal tubules.

Bacterial isolation

Pros:

· Definitive method
· Allows identification of isolates locally or at a reference laboratory
· Allows determination of antimicrobial sensitivity
· May identify unsuspected bacterial involvement in a syndrome
· Speed of reporting if carried out in house

Tissue	Sample type	Comments
Blood for bacteraemia	Blood bottle (commercial)	Incubate and watch indicator; sub-culture/smear to identify; sensitivity
Urine	Dip slide (commercial) to indicate cystitis Urine alone in a sterile container	Antimicrobial sensitivity only by subculture Required for smear, identity and sensitivity
Skin	Plucked hairs for dermatophytes Toothbrushes Swab in transport medium for bacteria	Store at room temperature
Faeces	Faeces rather than rectal swab	Cannot smear rectal swab Heat faeces for clostridia Swab may be required for inclusion in *Salmonella*-selective culture
Tissue	In sterile container; seal to prevent drying	Large piece required if contaminated; if aseptic may be small
Tracheal washes/ bronchoalveolar lavages	In sterile container	May need centrifugation
Joint fluid	Can be taken in anticoagulant	Very thick when smeared; warm slide Sample, refrigerate and re-sample later
Cannulae, screws	In sterile container with saline or sterile broth	Must not dry out
Other lesions	Fluids in sterile containers Swabs with transport medium for orifices, surfaces	

Table 5.1: *Guide to samples for demonstrating bacteria.*

Cons:

- Costly facilities with a low throughput
- Requires skilled workers for best results
- Potential safety problems
- Depends on having viable bacteria in a sample

Choosing culture conditions

The choice of culture conditions may be limited by the range of facilities and media available. In this section it will be assumed that the veterinary practice has the following available:

- An incubator at 37 °C
- Blood agar
- MacConkey agar
- Sabouraud's agar or a similar medium (for fungi)
- Access to API biochemical strips for identification (or other identification methods)
- *Salmonella* agglutinating serum
- Antimicrobial discs.

Items considered important but which are not necessarily stocked by the general practice are a microaerophilic and an anaerobic capability (jars) and more media. Sheep blood agar is preferable to horse blood agar for general use and care should be taken to ensure that the blood has not lysed in storage. Procedures that may be difficult for a practice laboratory will be indicated below and, where the conditions for growth cannot be met, it must be assumed that the organism will not be cultured. It may be decided at that point to refer the sample to a commercial or other specialist laboratory.

Samples, their common bacterial flora and suggested culture conditions and media are set out in Table 5.2.

Interpreting the findings

This section is intended to act not only as a guide to the interpretation of the results of the practice laboratory, but also as a guide to the interpretation of reports from other laboratories.

Bacteria do not grow: They may be absent from the specimen or, if present, may have died or have been inhibited by the presence of antibody, antibiotic or other factors. The conditions for growth may not have been met (see Table 5.2). Handling the specimen with a too-hot bacteriological loop or vigorous searing may have killed the organisms.

Occasionally growth may occur only in the first streak if the organisms require a nutrient present in the inoculum but absent from the plate, e.g. urea for *Ureaplasma* spp. Growth may occur only in later streaks where inhibitors such as antimicrobials or antibody have been diluted out.

Bacterial contaminants: These may arise from the specimen; *Proteus* spp. are perhaps the most troublesome, as their growth on blood agar rapidly obscures any other bacteria. Some results may be obtained from a plate with MacConkey agar, and smears of the sample may reveal the presence of specific bacteria otherwise obscured by the contaminant. Where *Proteus* spp. are potential contributors to the syndrome from which they are isolated, the MacConkey agar plate indicates the true numbers of colonies.

Escherichia coli colonies may contaminate specimens and growth may occur in specimens such as urine taken by owners or without aseptic precautions. Other contaminants can arise from water contamination of the agar plate and appear as masses of flowing growth. Colonies may be present in the agar as deep or surface contaminants, and airborne contaminants may be located outside the sample streaks. Contaminant colonies may be picked up when streaking a plate and these contaminants have to be distinguished from the special nutrient effects described above.

Bacterial colonies from the specimen: The colonies present can be identified provisionally by their morphological characteristics after a standard period of incubation (often 18–24 hours) and the findings should be recorded. A smear should be made from colonies under investigation and examined and stained by Gram at this stage. The provisional identity of the organisms present on each type of plate and the numbers present should be recorded. Recording of bacterial numbers can only be approximate in qualitative bacteriology, but must be accurate in quantitative bacteriology. At this stage the significance of the findings must be assessed and decisions made about whether to report at this stage, confirm the identity of the organisms found, or carry out antimicrobial sensitivity testing. Decisions to continue with these examinations may extend the reporting period by 1 or 2 days (antimicrobial sensitivity testing) or much longer for identification. Commercial laboratories will often have isolation information or provisional results before they are ready to report.

The descriptions that follow are intended only as a guide to provisional identification and the reader is referred to a specialist bacteriology text (e.g. Quinn *et al.*, 1994) or to the commercial systems for more detailed identification. The identity of isolates should only be confirmed after subculture to ensure purity.

Confirmation of identity may be by the use of:

- Phenotypic characteristics such as colonial morphology and the appearance and staining reactions of the bacterial cells on non-selective, selective and indicator media
- Biochemical characteristics. These involve the fermentation of sugars and the demonstration of

Sample (species)	Bacterial flora	Culture conditions
Blood from fevered animal or one with local infected lesion (dog, cat, others)	Staphylococci Streptococci E. *coli* *Bacteroides*	Aerobic, BA, Mac Aerobic, BA, Mac Anaerobic BA*
Urine (dog, cat, others)	E. *coli* Staphylococci Streptococci	Aerobic, BA, Mac
Plucked hairs (dog, cat)	*Microsporum canis* *Trichophyton*	Aerobic, 30°C* moist chamber, 10 days, Sabouraud's agar
Skin lesions (dog, cat)	Staphylococci Streptococci *Malassezia*	Aerobic, BA, Mac Aerobic, BA, Mac Aerobic, 30°C*, Sabouraud's agar
Faeces (dog, cat)	β-haemolytic E. *coli* *Salmonella* *Campylobacter* *Clostridium perfringens* C. *perfringens* spores C. *difficile* Spirochaetes (*Serpulina pilosicoli*) (dog only)	Aerobic, BA, Mac Aerobic, BA, Mac, selective media* Microaerophilic* *Campylobacter* medium* Anaerobic*, BA Anaerobic*, BA (boil first) Anaerobic*, C. *difficile* agar* Anaerobic*, spectinomycin blood agar
Nasal swabs (dog, cat) also many throat swabs	*Bordetella bronchiseptica* *Pasteurella multocida* *Haemophilus felis* (cat) *Mycoplasma* Staphylococci Streptococci (*s.canis* in dog) *Aspergillus* *Cryptococcus* (cat)	Aerobic, BA, Mac Aerobic, BA, Mac 10% carbon dioxide (candle jar), heated blood agar*/staphylococcal streak Aerobic, BA, incubate 3-4 days Aerobic, BA, Mac Aerobic, BA, Mac Aerobic, 30°C*, Sabouraud's agar Aerobic, 30°C* Sabouraud's agar
Tracheal wash/ bronchoalveolar lavage (dog)	*Pasteurella* *Bordetella bronchiseptica* *Pseudomonas* *Acinetobacter*	Aerobic, BA, Mac Aerobic, BA, Mac Aerobic, BA, Mac Aerobic, BA, Mac
Skin (see also Chapter 15)	Staphylococci Streptococci *Malassezia* *Microsporum* *Trichophyton*	Aerobic, BA, Mac Aerobic, BA, Mac Aerobic, 30°C*, Sabouraud's agar Aerobic, 30°C*, Sabouraud's agar
Ears (dog)	Staphylococci *Pseudomonas* *Proteus* Streptococci *Malassezia*	Aerobic, BA, Mac Aerobic, BA, Mac Aerobic, BA, Mac Aerobic, BA, Mac Aerobic, 30°C*, Sabouraud's agar
Vagina (dog, cat)	*Streptococcus canis* (dog) *Streptococcus* *Staphylococcus* *Escherichia coli* *Pseudomonas* *Pasteurella* *Haemophilus* *Mycoplasma* *Bacteroides*	Aerobic, BA, Mac Aerobic, BA, Mac Aerobic, BA, Mac Aerobic, BA, Mac Aerobic, BA, Mac Aerobic, BA, Mac 10% carbon dioxide (candle jar), heated blood agar*/staphylococcal streak Aerobic, BA, incubate 3-4 days Anaerobic*, BA

Table 5.2: *Culture conditions for the bacteria to be expected in samples commonly examined from small animals. *Conditions may not be readily available in practice laboratories. BA = blood agar; Mac = MacConkey agar. (continued)*

Sample (species)	Bacterial flora	Culture conditions
Aborted fetus (dog, cat)	*Streptococcus canis* (dog) *Pasteurella* *Haemophilus* *Mycoplasma* *Brucella canis/abortus* (dog) *Campylobacter*	Aerobic, BA, Mac Aerobic, BA, Mac 10% carbon dioxide (candle jar), heated blood agar*/staphylococcal streak Aerobic, BA, incubate 3-4 days 10% carbon dioxide (candle jar), heated blood agar* for 4-5 days **Category 3, do not attempt in UK. Send to reference laboratory directly** Microaerophilic* *Campylobacter* medium*
Joint fluid	Staphylococci Streptococci *Erysipelothrix* *Borrelia burgdorferi*	Aerobic, BA, Mac Aerobic, BA, Mac Aerobic, BA, Mac Specialist laboratory only*
Thoracic fluid	*Pasteurella* Streptococci *Nocardia asteroides* *Haemophilus felis* (cat) *Mycoplasma* *Bacteroides* *Mycobacterium*	Aerobic, BA, Mac Aerobic, BA, Mac Aerobic BA (incubate 4 days) 10% carbon dioxide (candle jar), heated blood agar* Aerobic, BA, incubate 3-4 days Anaerobic*, BA **Category 3, do not attempt in UK. Send to reference laboratory directly**
Cannulae, screws and pins (sample should be plated directly and after incubation in broth, preferably with serum)	Staphylococci Streptococci *Pseudomonas* *Escherichia coli* *Bacteroides*	Aerobic, BA, Mac Aerobic, BA, Mac Aerobic, BA, Mac Aerobic, BA, Mac Anaerobic*, BA
Other samples including abscesses	Aerobes Anaerobes	Aerobic, BA, Mac 10% carbon dioxide (candle jar), heated blood agar*/staphylococcal streak Anaerobic*, BA

Table 5.2 continued.

products such as indole by testing for individual or multiple characteristics in commercial biochemical strips. The enzymes responsible may be identified directly by enzyme analysis. This is available for some genera (e.g. *Serpulina*) in the form of commercial strips. The combinations of enzymes possessed allow specific identification
• Antigenic analysis using specific antisera. These may confirm to genus (e.g. *Salmonella*), to species, to serotype (salmonellae) or to serovar (e.g. *Leptospira*). The tests concerned may use simple agglutination tests, in which organisms from culture are agglutinated by specific antisera directed against somatic antigens, or indirect means such as immunoperoxidase, IF or ELISA tests. ELISAs may also be used to detect bacterial toxins (e.g. clostridia and *Pasteurella*). Some of these tests are not readily available to practice laboratories

The above tests may be performed in routine laboratories, but those that follow are generally performed in specialized or reference laboratories.

• Phage typing. This is used to confirm species identity (e.g. *Bacillus anthracis* and *Brucella abortus*) and to identify phage types within species (*Staphylococcus aureus*) or serotypes (*Salmonella typhimurium*)
• Plasmid profiles
• Ribotyping
• Restriction endonuclease fragment analysis
• PCR using primers for sequences of 16S rRNA genes.

The identification of some bacteria may require the services of a specialist reference laboratory (salmonellae, campylobacters, mycobacteria). In the UK some bacteria must be reported to the Ministry of Agriculture Fisheries and Food on isolation (e.g. *Salmonella*).

Quantitative bacteriology

Quantitative bacteriology can be carried out in the practice laboratory. Most frequently it is used in clinical situations (e.g. 10^5 organisms per ml of urine confirm the presence of active cystitis), but a quantitative element is also used in assessing the results of qualitative cultures. Here the presence of growth on one, two, three or four streaks of a plate inoculated with a clinical specimen is used to gauge the number of organisms present.

For quantitative bacteriology, there must be a clear record of any dilution of the sample prior to or during transport and a clear idea of the organisms to be sought. The sample must be weighed or its volume measured upon arrival at the laboratory and uncontaminated material is then suspended in an appropriate diluent (phosphate-buffered saline), shaken or homogenized to give a uniform sample, and then diluted in 2-fold or 10-fold steps. A fixed volume of each dilution is then placed on the surface of a plate containing non-selective or enriched media for total viable counts and on selective or indicator media for individual species counts. In the pour plate technique, the dilutions are made in liquid agar which is then poured to make plates. The total number of colonies within each dilution can be recorded and the number of viable bacteria present per unit weight or volume can be expressed. The same process may be carried out mechanically by the use of systems such as spiral platers and approximately by the use of dip slides in samples such as urine. Rapid tests using inhibitors for other bacteria and enrichment and a substrate for the species under test can be used to detect metabolites within dilutions. It may be necessary to confirm the identity of the organisms present by means described below. The figures generated by these methods are of use in clinical situations (e.g. urine or milk samples) or in environmental monitoring (staphylococci or coliforms per square centimetre).

Settlement plates (exposed to the air) can give an idea of the number of organisms present in the air of parts of the practice and these can be recorded as organisms per square centimetre of surface per unit time.

Antimicrobial sensitivity testing

Isolates of bacteria and fungi can be tested for their sensitivity to antimicrobial agents in the practice laboratory using the Kirby Bauer method (zones of inhibition around an antimicrobial impregnated paper disc) or by broth dilution methods. Antimicrobial discs are commercially available and are used in conjunction with a suitable medium. This should be one of the sensitivity testing agars and may require the addition of blood for the growth of many veterinary pathogens. It is possible to measure the minimal inhibitory concentrations (MICs) of antibiotics against organisms under test by both methods, using plates of carefully standardized thickness and standardized inocula or commercially available broth dilution kits, but the techniques are rarely used in practice. Most practices measure resistance or sensitivity to antimicrobials by making a lawn of the organism under test on an agar plate, placing the discs under test on the surface, and reading the result after incubation (see Figure 1.3). Sensitivity is indicated by the presence of a wide zone of inhibition around the disc with no colonies within the zone of inhibition (Figure 5.9). Details of zone sizes which indicate resistance or sensitivity are given by Quinn et al. (1994); these vary with the antimicrobial and the organism under test.

Knowledge of the patterns of resistance and sensitivity of different organisms is essential for treating and controlling infection in small animal bacterial disease. The emergence of resistance and the infection of hospitalized animals with organisms of a particular resistance pattern makes the monitoring of resistance within a practice important, regardless of the source of the data. Such monitoring may lead to more effective prescribing practice and to an overall reduction in resistance to antimicrobials in a practice.

Bacteria isolated from small animal specimens

Gram-positive cocci
These are seen as round, purple-staining bacteria.

Staphylococci: These occur as clumps of Gram-positive cocci in smears and grow readily on blood agar as white 1–2 mm colonies. Some are haemolytic (clear the medium around the colony on blood agar). All grow on MacConkey agar (although not on the special MacConkey No.2 and No.3 agars; Quinn et al., 1994). They can be identified to species level using the criteria outlined by Quinn et al. (1994) or using a specific staphylococcal identification system.

It may be necessary to distinguish staphylococci from streptococci prior to biochemical identification and this can be done most conveniently using the

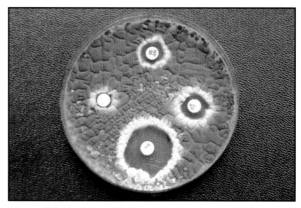

Figure 5.9: Antimicrobial sensitivity testing using discs. Aspergillus fumigatus *is sensitive to the bottom compound only.*

catalase test. The catalase test is carried out using a 3% solution of hydrogen peroxide, a clean slide, a thin glass capillary tube and a colony of the organism.

1. Bend the end of the tube in the edge of the flame of a Bunsen burner and allow to cool.
2. Place a drop of the hydrogen peroxide solution on the slide and then pick up some growth from a colony.
3. Place the material in the drop of hydrogen peroxide and look for the production of bubbles which confirm that the colony is that of a *Staphylococcus* not a *Streptococcus*.

Staphylococcus intermedius is the pathogenic species most commonly found in the dog, although *S. aureus* and *S. epidermidis* and other species may be present. *S. aureus* and *S. intermedius* are potential primary pathogens. In skin disease (e.g. pyoderma in the dog), pure and profuse cultures are most significant. Mixed cultures of several colony types suggest that the sample was not taken from the centre of the pustule or that the lesion is ageing. *S. aureus* and *S. intermedius* are also causes of otitis externa; pure cultures may indicate a primary role in the absence of yeasts, mites or physical factors. These species may also occur in septicaemias in pups, in osteomyelitis, in mastitis in bitches, and can localize in wound infections. The source of staphylococci in surgical wound infections is important: if the organism is identified as *S. intermedius*, it is likely to be of animal origin; the pathogen is only likely to be of human origin if identified as *S. aureus*. Unfortunately, commercial strip tests may not distinguish adequately between *S. aureus* and *S. intermedius* of canine origin and reliable methods of distinguishing between human and animal strains of *S. aureus* are not well developed or readily available. There is little evidence that dog staphylococci cause human disease. *S. intermedius* may be an incidental contaminant where samples are taken from the skin, nares or vulva and may indicate severe intestinal disturbance when present in the faeces.

The presence of *S. epidermidis* in samples is sometimes difficult to interpret. As this organism is a normal inhabitant of the skin, its presence is usually considered to indicate contamination. It has recently been found to colonize catheters, cannulae, screws and plates and may be significant if isolated in pure and profuse cultures from these sites.

Staphylococci are fully sensitive to heat and most disinfectants, but may be resistant to antimicrobial agents. 'Hospital' strains may occur in veterinary practices.

Streptococci: These occur in smears as chains of Gram-positive cocci and grow readily on blood agar as 1 mm, often transparent, circular colonies. Some species are haemolytic, and those that clear the medium completely are known as 'β-haemolytic streptococci',

usually *Streptococcus canis* in the dog. Identification can be confirmed to species level by biochemical tests. Information about Lancefield groups is not currently of much relevance to the clinician.

S. canis is found in wound infections and causes fading in neonatal pups, tonsillitis in older pups, and mastitis and infertility in breeding bitches. It may contribute to dermatitis, otitis externa and interdigital infections. Other species of *Streptococcus* are found in the same situations in cats.

Other streptococci occur in dogs and cats but are less clearly associated with disease. They may cause vegetative endocarditis, cystitis, mastitis and arthritis.

Streptococci are sensitive to heat and disinfectants. They are almost always sensitive to penicillin but less so to streptomycin. Enterococci found in wounds may be relatively resistant to antimicrobials.

Gram-positive rods

Bacillus: *Bacillus* spp. rarely cause disease in small animals but may be isolated from surface wounds. They possess spores and are destroyed by autoclaving but not by boiling. They are sensitive to most antibiotics and to many disinfectants, though these may not kill the spores. They are most important in practice bacteriology as contaminants on plates because of their rapid growth and large colonies (>5 mm).

Clostridium: *Clostridium* spp. are Gram-positive rods with large bulging spores; they only grow anaerobically and can be isolated in culture by practice laboratories with anaerobic facilities. They can be seen in smears made from samples, but they decolourize readily and may contain clear circles that represent unstained spores. The position of these spores may be important for identification.

Clostridium perfringens produces 3–5 mm circular β-haemolytic colonies on blood agar and can be confirmed as such using commercial strips such as the API anaerobe tests. If found in wound infections and gangrene it is likely to be a contributor to the lesions and may have initiated them following existing damage. Isolation from the gut requires more cautious interpretation. Profuse cultures of vegetative organisms may be isolated from some cases of haemorrhagic enteritis and bacterial overgrowth, where they may contribute to the disease or even cause it. In heated faecal samples, colonies that grow (Figure 5.10) are all spore-forming and may be enterotoxin-producing and therefore more likely to contribute to or cause enteritis.

C. difficile is the cause of post-antimicrobial enteritis and may be isolated from the faeces of animals with diarrhoea following prolonged antimicrobial treatment. The organism is most easily grown on *C. difficile* agar, where it forms 2–3 mm flat greyish colonies which sprawl along the streak line. The culture has a characteristic phenolic smell and fluoresces under ultraviolet

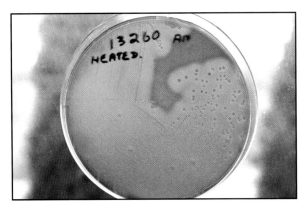

Figure 5.10: *Anaerobic culture of boiled dog faeces. Sporulating, enterotoxin-producing* Clostridium perfringens *has grown in the profusion.*

light. Gram-stained organisms are hairpin-like with a subterminal spore. Their identity can be confirmed using API anaerobe strips and their ability to produce toxin confirmed using latex agglutination tests for *C. difficile* toxins.

C. tetani, the cause of tetanus, is rarely isolated, but rods with a characteristic spore on the end may be seen in smears from the lesions responsible for the rare cases of tetanus in the dog.

C. botulinum, the cause of botulism, most commonly produces flaccid paralysis in hounds fed on contaminated carcasses. It is difficult to isolate and its isolation should probably not be attempted in a practice laboratory for safety reasons.

All clostridia can produce spores and these affect resistance to disinfectants and drying. The vegetative (non-sporulating) cells are killed easily by heat and disinfectants, but spores require autoclaving and are not easily destroyed by phenolic disinfectants. They are sensitive to penicillin and many other antibiotics but not to neomycin and its related compounds.

Listeria: *Listeria* is a small Gram-positive rod that does not form spores. It is an uncommon cause of disease in dogs and cats but can cause septicaemia, abortion and nervous signs. It is aerobic and forms opaque, 1 mm colonies on blood agar, often with a narrow ring of β-haemolysis. It is rapidly killed by heating and disinfectants. It has the unusual property of growing at room temperature or in a refrigerator and can therefore be present in stored animal foods. Cultures may be especially dangerous to pregnant women.

Erysipelothrix: This is a thin Gram-positive rod that forms small grey slightly haemolytic colonies on blood agar. It does not form spores and is rapidly killed by heat and disinfectants. It is a rare cause of arthritis and vegetative endocarditis in dogs and is always sensitive to penicillin.

Nocardia: This is a Gram-positive rod that breaks up into cocci. It is most frequently seen in taps from chronic pleurisy in dogs and may be associated with

wounds and chronic subcutaneous inflammation in rural dogs. It grows slowly on blood agar to produce 1 mm white crumbly colonies after 4 days which adhere strongly to the agar. The organism is sensitive *in vitro* to a number of antimicrobials which may be less effective *in vivo*.

Mycobacteria: *Mycobacterium* species are Gram-positive but do not stain very well. They are normally stained by Ziehl Neelsen's method and are acid-fast, appearing as thin red beaded rods on a blue ground. The organisms do not grow on conventional media and require media with egg and serum.

Mycobacteria found in tuberculous lesions in dogs and cats (tracheal washes, nasal and tonsillar secretions, and pleural fluids) and in skin tuberculosis of cats should be considered as Category 3 pathogens and after identification in smears stained by Ziehl Neelsen's method, the material (often lymph nodes or punch biopsies) should be sent to a mycobacterial reference laboratory for culture and sensitivity testing.

> **Mycobacteria are dangerous to handle and infectious to man. They should not be grown or handled in the practice laboratory.**

M. tuberculosis from infected owners often infects dogs and sometimes cats (occasionally *M. bovis*) and is in turn a risk to others including practice staff. Disease caused by *M. avium* in pigeons, ornamental fowl, parrots and budgerigars poses less risk to man but this species is also rated Category 3.

Gram-negative rods

Many families of these bacteria are involved in animal disease; only the most important are described here.

Escherichia: This is the genus to which the common gut bacterium *E. coli* belongs. It is present in the gut of normal animals and its isolation from other sites usually suggests faecal contamination. The organism may be seen in smears of infected tissue or samples as a short coccobacillus and is indistinguishable from most other members of its family. It is demonstrated by culture on blood agar (where some strains are β-haemolytic on sheep blood agar) and as a lactose-fermenter (pink colonies) on MacConkey agar. The colonies are 3–5 mm in diameter and circular. Its identity is confirmed biochemically by API; different strains and toxin types can be identified by antisera or using DNA probes and PCR. Some β-haemolytic strains cause enteritis in pups and sometimes in older dogs. Unfortunately, simple reagents are not yet available to identify pathogenic isolates in the practice laboratory and the isolation of these β-haemolytic colonies in pure and profuse culture may suggest that they are involved in the diarrhoea. In bitches other strains can be involved in pyometra and in both sexes *E. coli* causes cystitis. As the bacterium can multiply in urine, smears should always be checked for the presence of neutrophils and bacteria to confirm the presence of inflammatory change. *E. coli* can colonize abscesses and may invade inflammatory lesions such as otitis and interdigital cysts.

E.coli does not produce spores but survives drying for weeks or months. It is readily killed by almost all disinfectants at the recommended dilutions. *E. coli* is never sensitive to penicillin, but strains vary in their sensitivity to most other antimicrobials. 'Hospital' strains of *E. coli* may exist in some veterinary practices.

Salmonella: *Salmonella* is related to *E. coli* and is indistinguishable in tissue smears; however, it is non-lactose-fermenting and appears yellow on MacConkey agar. *Salmonella* is isolated directly from septicaemia and acute diarrhoea on blood agar or MacConkey agar, but when mixed in faeces or on surfaces, selective media such as tetrathionate are used, followed by plating onto *Salmonella*, *Shigella* or desoxycholate citrate agars, where the *Salmonella* colonies appear black or colourless. Suspect colonies can be identified biochemically by API or by slide agglutination tests using the *Salmonella* poly O and poly H agglutinating serum and emulsified colonies from a subculture. After this, isolates should be sent to a reference laboratory for identification of serotypes such as *S. typhimurium* or *S. heidelberg*. When confirmed in the UK, the veterinary authorities should be informed under the Zoonosis Order.

Salmonella is a major cause of enteritis and food poisoning in man, animals and birds and can cause septicaemia, especially in pups and kittens. As people can become infected from animals, the significance of isolation must be interpreted not only for the animal but also in terms of the risk to man. Pure and profuse cultures of salmonellae isolated directly from the organs of dead pups or kittens or from the faeces of diarrhoeic animals indicate the presence of clinical salmonellosis which should be treated and controlled. The overtly diarrhoeic animal is a risk to man and disinfection and hygiene is essential. Where small numbers of salmonellae are isolated from a continent dog or cat, the risk to man is less and may be minimal. The presence of salmonellae (demonstrated by culture in enrichment and selective media) in normal cat and dog faeces is not unusual and generally poses little risk to human health provided normal hygienic precautions are practised.

Salmonella is generally sensitive to heat, disinfectants and antimicrobials, although current (1998) infections of cats and dogs are often due to the multiresistant *S. typhimurium* phage type 104.

Proteus: *Proteus* is a genus of Gram-negative non-lactose-fermenting bacilli. Cultures of *P. vulgaris* and *P. mirabilis* 'swarm' over the whole agar plate. *Proteus* spp. can be distinguished easily from *E. coli* and *Salmonella* spp. on blood agar plate cultures because of its 'swarming' growth and foul odour, but it does not 'swarm' on MacConkey agar where it forms yellow colonies resembling those of *Salmonella*. *Proteus* is biochemically distinct and does not agglutinate with antisera to *Salmonella*. It is significant when found in profuse cultures (on MacConkey agar) in cystitis in dogs and cats, and in moist surface infections such as otitis and interdigital cysts. In smaller numbers it may be a contaminant. It is sensitive to heat, disinfectants and antibiotics.

Klebsiella: *Klebsiella* is like a rather mucoid *E. coli* and is found in chronic rhinitis. It can only be distinguished reliably by biochemical tests.

Yersinia: This produces small (1mm) non-lactose-fermenting colonies on MacConkey agar and grey colonies of similar size on blood agar. Identification is confirmed biochemically. The species most commonly found in dogs and cats is *Yersinia enterocolitica*, which may be the cause of enteritis if in profuse culture in the faeces. Both it and *Y. pseudotuberculosis* are much more important in rodents, where they cause not only enteritis but also abscesses. *Yersinia* spp. are a potential cause of human enteritis.

Pasteurella: Pasteurellae are Gram-negative rods or coccobacilli growing on blood agar to produce mucoid colonies 2–4 mm in diameter. *Pasteurella multocida* does not grow on MacConkey agar although some other species do. Identification can be confirmed by biochemical tests. Pasteurellae are found: in the respiratory tract, where they are associated with rhinitis, pneumonia and bronchitis; in the genital tract, primarily the vagina; in the mouth, especially in gingivitis in cats; in abscesses in cats and dogs, particularly those resulting from dog and cat bites; and in bite infections in man. Some species (e.g. *P. multocida* and *P. pneumotropica*) cause septicaemia in rodents. Pasteurellae are sensitive to heat, drying and most antimicrobials.

Bordetella: This is a slender Gram-negative rod. *Bordetella bronchiseptica* forms 1mm grey, slightly haemolytic colonies on blood agar after 48 hours and similar size yellow (non-lactose fermenting) colonies on MacConkey agar. It is identified biochemically. *B. bronchiseptica* is a cause of kennel cough and rhinitis in dogs and causes bronchitis and rhinitis in cats, rabbits and rodents. It is not the only cause of these syndromes, but when isolated in profuse culture is likely to be the cause. Its isolation from recovered animals or carriers has implications for the group and even when isolated in small numbers from tracheal washes it may be involved in any respiratory disease present. It is sensitive to heat but relatively resistant to drying and resistant *in vivo* to a number of antimicrobials.

Haemophilus: These are delicate slender Gram-negative rods. They require extra factors to grow on nutrient agar and sometimes on blood agar (X and V factors) and are therefore best cultured on blood agar with a staphylococcal streak or on heated blood ('chocolate') agar. The colonies are small (0.5 mm) and grow on blood agar near colonies of staphylococci but can grow independently on 'chocolate' agar. Identification to species level is a specialist task due to their delicacy, although enzyme patterns developed on a kit testing system can be used.

Haemophilus is found in the respiratory and genital tracts, sometimes in pneumonia, and sometimes in aborted and stillborn pups. It is of greatest significance when in pure or profuse culture. Recently *H. felis* has been found to cause upper respiratory tract disease and pneumonias in cats in the UK. Like other *Haemophilus* species, *H. felis* is so delicate that it may not be isolated unless samples are taken directly from the cat to the laboratory, cultured on 'chocolate' agar immediately and incubated in 10% carbon dioxide. *Haemophilus* is sensitive to drying, disinfectants and most antibiotics.

Brucella: *Brucella* is a tiny Gram-negative rod. It is absent from the UK except in tissues from seals. *B. canis* grows on blood agar to form 1 mm grey colonies after 48 hours. It causes infertility in dogs and abortion in bitches but is currently absent from Britain. It can infect man and is detected by serology or culture. Dogs and man may be infected by the related *B. abortus* from cattle, which requires 10% carbon dioxide for growth. These bacteria are Category 3 pathogens. If they are suspected, advice should be sought immediately and, in the UK, MAFF should be notified.

Bacteroides *and* Fusobacterium: These are anaerobic Gram-negative rods that can only be grown in anaerobe jars. They will grow on blood agar and are identified biochemically using special test strips. They are present in the gums and in the faeces of healthy animals, but when they occur in gum disease or in abscesses and pleurisy they may be important in the continuation of the disease. They die rapidly on exposure to air and are sensitive to most antimicrobials (including metronidazole) and to disinfectants.

Campylobacters: These are Gram-negative curved rods which look like seagulls on a smear (Figure 5.11). They grow only in reduced oxygen levels and are microaerophilic. Although they grow on blood agar they can only be isolated easily from faeces or the gut on selective media containing a special mix of antibiotics. *Campylobacter jejuni* can cause diarrhoea in cats and dogs and is then present in profuse culture; it can also occur in small numbers in recovered or healthy cats and dogs. It is a cause of painful but rapidly resolving diarrhoea in man and is a common cause of food poisoning; it can be transmitted to man from animal faeces. When animals are diarrhoeic and passing profuse numbers of the bacteria, stringent hygiene precautions should be taken and affected animals should be kept away from children. When the animal is continent, there is little risk as many normal dogs and cats carry the organism in small numbers. *Campylobacter* is sensitive to most disinfectants, heat, drying and to antimicrobials such as neomycin, tylosin and enrofloxacin.

Pseudomonas: This is a slender Gram-negative rod that grows readily on almost any medium but usually requires air. The colonies are grey and rough in appearance with a foul smell and may discolour the medium green. *Pseudomonas* produces non-lactose-fermenting colonies on MacConkey agar and its identity can be confirmed biochemically.

Pseudomonas is frequently isolated from contaminated wounds or chronic lesions, especially of the skin and ears. Where profuse cultures are isolated it is probably contributing to the lesions present and can cause conditions such as cystitis, otitis externa and chronic respiratory disease. Most isolates are identified as *P. aeruginosa*, but tracheal isolates from dogs and cats may include *P. maltophilia* and related species such as *Burkholdaria cepacea*.

Pseudomonas survives well in wet conditions, is killed by heat but is extremely resistant to antibiotics. Special antimicrobials such as gentamicin or enrofloxacin may have to be used. It is also resistant to disinfectants such as phenolics at low concentrations and will grow in quaternary ammonium disinfectants. Where present at low levels in the flora in a lesion, it may remain after antimicrobial treatment.

Leptospira: Leptospires are very thin tightly curled Gram-negative bacteria that end in hooks and are weakly motile. They can only be seen by light microscopy when stained with silver or when viewed by dark-ground microscopy. Identification is by dark-ground microscopy and by serology. Isolation is very difficult and a matter for specialist laboratories only. *Leptospira canicola* is the cause of canine interstitial nephritis and the urine of infected dogs contains the organisms. They live for weeks in cold water but die

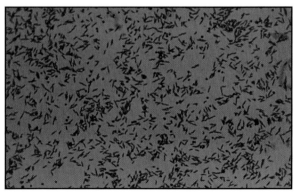

Figure 5.11: *Campylobacters from a culture. Note the characteristic shape. Gram stain.*

rapidly in the presence of soaps or disinfectants and are very sensitive to antibiotics. *L. icterohaemorrhagiae* can infect dogs but is difficult to see in canine urine. *Leptospira* spp. are potential causes of zoonotic infections and both staff and clients should observe strict hygiene precautions.

Borrelia: These are large (10 µm long) spirochaetes. *Borrelia burgdorferi*, the cause of Lyme disease in dogs and man, appears to be present in the UK. Diagnosed only on serology, the organism has not yet been isolated in UK from dogs or cats.

Serpulina: These are large anaerobic spirochaetes. *S. pilosicoli* and *S. innocens* have been identified in the faeces of diarrhoeic dogs and are present in some kinds of colitis in the dog. Their isolation on spectinomycin blood agar in anaerobic conditions or identification in smears from diarrhoeic faeces may suggest their involvement in such a colitis.

Other bacteria

Mycoplasms: Mycoplasms are pleomorphic Gram-negative tiny rods, cocci or coccobacilli. They are almost impossible to see in clinical specimens from dogs and cats, even when smears are stained with Giemsa. Isolation is generally a task for the specialist laboratory, but a few species may grow on blood agar after 3–4 days incubation in moist conditions. They appear as tiny dust-like colonies and may be slightly haemolytic. The organisms can be seen in Giemsa-stained smears from the cultures. They can be isolated from respiratory disease, especially rhinitis in cats, and can be found in aborted fetuses. They are delicate, rapidly killed by drying and sensitive to lincomycin, tylosin and enrofloxacin. They are killed by all disinfectants and also by alcohols.

Ureaplasmas: These resemble mycoplasms but require urea for growth. They may be present as tiny colonies on the urine-soaked initial streaks of urine samples or vaginal samples from infected bitches.

Chlamydia: *Chlamydia* spp. are seen inside cells with stains such as Koster's stain, appearing as red dots on a blue ground. They can be demonstrated in smears of tissue by fluorescent antibody but this is not carried out in the practice laboratory. They only grow in tissue culture and culture should *not* be attempted in practice.

One strain of *C. psittaci* infects cats and another more severe strain causes psittacosis in parrots, other birds and man, and is a Category 3 pathogen. PCR or culture in a reference laboratory may reveal the presence of the organism. The antigen may be detected in samples using commercial 'clearview' tests.

Chlamydia can survive drying in faeces and secretions and can occur in aerosols. They can be destroyed readily by boiling but may be difficult to kill with disinfectants when in pus. Those from parrots and other psittacines are a risk to human health.

MYCOLOGICAL AND OTHER INVESTIGATIONS

Yeasts
Yeasts are single-celled fungi with a rigid cell wall rarely forming either spores or hyphae (the name for fungal filaments). They reproduce by budding and grow in a similar way to bacteria on suitable media, where they form whitish opaque colonies 1–3 mm in diameter. The cell walls are Gram-positive and about 3–6 µm in diameter. The colonies are often oval in shape and may have buds if actively dividing.

Candida
These are oval yeasts that are Gram-positive and form buds. They grow readily on Sabouraud's agar and form 1 mm opaque white colonies with a fruity smell. They can be identified to species biochemically using the API AUX system. *Candida* may be isolated from wet lesions on skin, vulval lesions and chronic lesions in the gut and sometimes the ears. When present in profuse culture, they may prolong or exacerbate the lesions in which they are found. *Candida* are sensitive to heat, disinfectants and antifungal agents such as nystatin and econazole, but may survive drying.

Malassezia
Malassezia is a bottle-shaped Gram-positive yeast that grows more slowly than *Candida* and very rarely on blood agar. It is found in ears and on skin (see Chapter 15) where it is involved in skin disease and otitis (*M. pachydermatis*). *Malassezia* is sensitive to most skin antiseptics (including cetrimide and hexachlorophene) and to most antifungal agents.

Cryptococcus
This is a thick-walled yeast that will grow in culture to produce mucoid colonies. It is present in chronic rhinitis in dogs and cats and in pigeon droppings and is potentially infective to man.

Dermatophytes
Dermatophytes (fungi that infect skin; see Chapter 15) survive drying so well that they may be submitted for examination dried in paper or on hair and can be stored at room temperature. They form white-grey colonies on Sabouraud's agar, with characteristically coloured undersides. They may be identified by the appearance of the colony and by the microscopic appearance of the hyphae and associated structures. In hairs they may be detected by dissolving the sample in 10% potassium hydroxide and viewing under the microscope. The fungus contains chitin which is not broken down like the hair and allows the organism to be distinguished.

The hyphae break up into spores which are relatively resistant and can survive drying in the environment and may be resistant to disinfectants, particularly when in organic material. They are relatively rapidly killed by quaternary ammonium compounds, especially when these are formulated with soaps. Clinical treatment is with antifungal agents such as griseofulvin and ketoconazole. Antifungal treatment or the use of skin disinfectants may delay the appearance of the dermatophytes in culture for several days and the colonies that result may be unusually small.

Microsporum

Microsporum is the genus most commonly encountered in dogs and cats, and *M. canis* is the most important species. The hyphae fluoresce under a Wood's lamp (a source of ultraviolet light) both on the animal and when individual plucked hairs are viewed. Colonies on Sabouraud's agar are white in the centre and have rays of growth which become clear or brownish towards the edge of the colony; the underside is a tan colour. Lactophenol cotton blue-stained crush preparations on slides demonstrate the hyphae and the small microconidia (spores), but macroconidia are rare on this medium and require special media for demonstration. Other species such as *M. gypseum* have abundant boat-shaped macroconidia. *Microsporum* can infect man and therefore should be handled with care.

Trichophyton

Trichophyton occasionally causes disease in dogs and cats. It does not fluoresce under the Wood's lamp but can be identified in culture and in plucked hairs. The colonies may be more evenly white than those of *Microsporum* and the macroconidia are club-shaped. Species include *T. mentagrophytes* and *T. erinacei*.

Other fungi

Aspergillus

Aspergillus is a common mould which occasionally invades chronic lesions in the respiratory tract. It invades tissue by means of hyphae, producing granulomas and green fruiting bodies where these reach the airspace. *A. fumigatus* and *A. niger* are most common. Both species can cause considerable mortality in birds and can kill hatching eggs. In dogs, *A. fumigatus* may occur in chronic rhinitis (Figure 5.12). The sporangia may be visible in smears that have been cleared with potassium hydroxide, but culture on Sabouraud's agar is usually successful in isolating the organism. The presence of the fungus in small numbers in the airways may not be significant, but even small numbers of colonies are significant if any granulomatous lesions are present.

Toxoplasma and Neospora

Infection with the protozoan parasite *Toxoplasma gondii* is an uncommon cause of death in young pups and

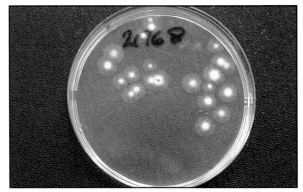

Figure 5.12: Sparse but significant growth of Aspergillus fumigatus *from a case of canine rhinitis.*

kittens, presumably due to heavy congenital infection, and a rare cause of illness in older, usually immunocompromised, dogs and cats. Most infections are asymptomatic. The cat is the definitive host for the parasite and produces infective oocysts in faeces, which are a risk to other cats and other species, including man. Like the dog, man is an incidental intermediate host and acquires infection either from vegetable material contaminated by infected cat faeces or from eating undercooked meat (usually lamb) that contains infective forms of the parasite. *Neospora caninum*, a more recently recognized protozoan parasite, like toxoplasmosis in older pups, also causes encephalomyelitis with hindlimb ataxia.

A variety of in-practice and laboratory-based tests for antibody to *T. gondii* have been developed. Tests that detect any class of antibody merely confirm exposure. Tests detecting IgM are indicative of recent infection, with a potential risk of oocyst shedding in cats. Identification of oocysts in faeces is possible (see Chapter 8), but is seldom attempted as shedding is uncommon in ill cats and the period of oocyst shedding is short (1–2 weeks). IF tests for neosporosis are available.

REFERENCES AND FURTHER READING

Addie DD and Jarrett JO (1995) Control of feline coronavirus infections in breeding catteries by serotesting, isolation and early weaning. *Feline Practice* **23**, 92–95

American Association of Feline Practitioners/Academy of Feline Medicine (1997a) Recommendation for feline leukaemia virus testing. *Compendium on Continuing Education for the Practising Veterinarian* **19**, 1105–1106

American Association of Feline Practitioners/Academy of Feline Medicine (1997b) Recommendation for feline immunodeficiency virus testing. *Compendium on Continuing Education for the Practising Veterinarian* **19**, 1106–1107

Appel MJ (1987) *Virus Infections of Carnivores.* Elsevier, New York

Castro AE and Heuschele WP (1992) *Veterinary Diagnostic Virology: A Practioner's Guide.* Mosby Year Book, St. Louis

Greene CE (1990) *Infectious Diseases of the Dog and Cat.* WB Saunders, Philadelphia

Quinn PJ, Carter ME, Markey B and Carter GR (1994) *Clinical Veterinary Microbiology.* Wolfe, London

Quinn PJ, Donnelly WJC, Carter ME, Markey BKJ, Torgerson PR and Breathnach RMS (1997) *Microbial and Parasitic Diseases of the Dog and Cat.* WB Saunders, London

Schochetman G, Ou C-Y and Jones WK (1998) Polymerase chain reaction. *Journal of Infectious Diseases* **158**, 1154–1157

Tenover FC (1998) Diagnostic deoxyribonucleic acid probes for infectious diseases. *Clinical Microbiology Reviews* **1**, 82–101

CHAPTER SIX

Immune-Mediated Diseases and Immunological Assays

Michael J. Day

CHAPTER PLAN

Introduction

**Laboratory tests for autoimmune and
immune-mediated diseases**

    Immune-mediated haemolytic anaemia

    Immune-mediated thrombocytopenia

    **Systemic lupus erythematosus and
related diseases**

    Immune-mediated arthritis

    Hypothyroidism

    **Immune-mediated skin, kidney
and joint diseases**

    Tests for other autoantibodies

Laboratory tests for hypersensitivity

    Type 1 hypersensitivity

    Other assays for hypersensitivity

Laboratory tests for immunodeficiency

    Serum immunoglobulin concentration

    **Complement concentration and
function testing**

    **Neutrophil and macrophage
function testing**

    Lymphocyte phenotyping

    Lymphocyte function testing

Laboratory tests for lymphoid neoplasia

    Phenotyping neoplastic cells

    Identification of paraproteins

Tissue and blood typing

References and further reading

GLOSSARY

AIHA	autoimmune haemolytic anaemia
ANA	antinuclear antibody
C3	complement factor 3 (classical and alternative pathways)
C4	complement factor 4 (classical pathway)
CD	clusters of differentiation, refers to leucocyte surface molecules that can be used to define particular cell populations
CD4	molecule expressed by the 'helper' subset of T lymphocytes
CD8	molecule expressed by the 'cytotoxic' subset of T lymphocytes
CH_{50}	total haemolytic complement (measures function of classical and terminal complement pathways)
CIC	circulating immune complexes (in serum)
DELAT	direct enzyme-linked antiglobulin test (diagnosis of AIHA)
DLA	dog leucocyte antigen system, the canine major histocompatibility complex
dsDNA	double-stranded DNA
EDTA	ethylamine diethyl tetra-acetic acid
ELISA	enzyme-linked immunosorbent assay
FACS	fluorescence-activated cell sorter, used to distinguish immunolabelled cell populations from unlabelled cells
FeLV	feline leukaemia virus
FIV	feline immunodeficiency virus

FLA	feline leucocyte antigen system, the feline major histocompatibility complex
IEP	immunoelectrophoresis
IgA	immunoglobulin A (major immunoglobulin in mucosal secretions)
IgE	immunoglobulin E (mediator of type I hypersensitivity)
IgG	immunoglobulin G (major serum immunoglobulin)
IgM	immunoglobulin M
IL	interleukin, a soluble factor (cytokine) derived from one cell which can produce an effect on another (IL-1 to IL-18 are defined)
ITP	idiopathic thrombocytopenia purpura (autoimmune thrombocytopenia)
mRNA	messenger RNA
RIA	radioimmunoassay
RA	rheumatoid arthritis (erosive polyarthritis)
RF	rheumatoid factor (IgM autoantibody against IgG in serum or synovial fluid)
SRBC	sheep red blood cells
SRID	single radial immunodiffusion (for immunoglobulin quantification)
SLE	systemic lupus erythematosus (multisystem autoimmune disease)
ssDNA	single-stranded DNA
T3	triiodothyronine
T4	thyroxine
UV	ultraviolet light

INTRODUCTION

There are four major clinical manifestations of immune-mediated disease in small animals:

- autoimmunity
- hypersensitivity
- immunodeficiency
- lymphoid neoplasia.

It is possible for more than one of these to be expressed concurrently in an individual patient. Such diseases are characterized by: a chronic, relapsing/remitting history of non-specific clinical signs; occurrence in particular breeds or pedigrees; and being refractory to standard therapy. Immune-mediated diseases present a diagnostic challenge and the laboratory tests described in this chapter are an important part of the diagnostic process. It should always be remembered that immune-mediated diseases are rare. Over an 11-year period, such disorders comprised 2% of total accessions to a university referral hospital (Penhale *et al.*, 1990).

Although awareness of immune-mediated disease has increased in recent years, the availability of veterinary clinical immunology diagnostic laboratories remains limited. Appropriate species-specific reagents are now commercially available but immunological tests are time-consuming and expensive to perform and require careful interpretation to distinguish false-positive and false-negative results. Immunodiagnostic procedures are not easily adapted from being laboratory research tools to commercially available tests, but most universities and larger commercial laboratories will offer a limited range of immunodiagnostic tests to veterinary surgeons. It is inadvisable to submit samples to human laboratories, which will not have species-specific reagents or the expertise in interpretation required for veterinary patients.

The immunodiagnostic tests described in this chapter should be considered as useful adjuncts to primary laboratory diagnosis. For example, a Coombs' test should not be performed without appropriate haematological indicators of immune-mediated haemolytic anaemia, and immunohistochemistry should be used to support a tentative diagnosis following histopathological examination of a biopsy. The successful diagnosis of immune-mediated disease requires consideration of history, clinical signs, presentation and primary diagnostic procedures (e.g. haematology, biochemistry, biopsy, radiology) together with immunological procedures. Immunodiagnostic tests also have a role in long-term monitoring of such patients.

Some immunological tests have specific requirements for sample type and handling, so it is wise to telephone the laboratory before requesting a test. Discussing a case with a clinical immunologist may also help in appropriate selection of tests and in interpretation of the test results in light of the clinical history. In the case of immunodiagnostic tests, a complete clinical history is essential, particularly with regard to recent therapy which may affect test results. Drugs may be a causal factor in immune-mediated disease or be the cause of false-negative results in the case of corticosteroid therapy (it is advisable to withdraw corticosteroids for at least 4 weeks before immunodiagnostic testing). The relapsing-remitting nature of many immune-mediated diseases may warrant repeat testing in animals which are initially negative in a particular test.

This chapter describes the application, methodology and interpretation of the commonly available procedures that can be used in the diagnosis of immune-mediated diseases. The samples for performance of each test are listed in Table 6.1.

LABORATORY TESTS FOR AUTOIMMUNE AND IMMUNE MEDIATED DISEASES

Immune-mediated haemolytic anaemia

Coombs' test

Application: The Coombs' test (or direct antiglobulin test) is used to detect the presence of immunoglobulin or complement bound to the surface of red blood cells (RBCs). A positive test is confirmatory of a primary immune-mediated haemolytic anaemia in which the antibody is specific for an erythrocyte membrane antigen, or a secondary immune-mediated anaemia with an underlying infectious, drug or transfusion related cause; however, most cases of immune-mediated haemolysis in the dog involve primary autoimmunity.

A Coombs' test is indicated for a dog with acute or chronic primary haemolytic anaemia with no apparent underlying cause. Such cases will often be markedly anaemic (PCV < 20%) but the anaemia will generally be strongly regenerative (with an associated neutrophilia) unless the autoimmune attack is directed against bone marrow erythroid precursors. There may be macroscopic or microscopic evidence of erythrocyte agglutination or spherocytosis. Occasionally, there may be concurrent (marked) thrombocytopenia which is also likely to be autoimmune in nature (idiopathic thrombocytopenic purpura, ITP). The combination of autoimmune haemolytic anaemia (AIHA) and ITP is known as Evans' syndrome.

Performance of a Coombs' test is less frequently indicated in the cat. In the majority of cases of feline immune-mediated haemolysis an underlying cause can be identified (e.g. feline leukaemia virus (FeLV) or *Haemobartonella felis* infection); however, primary autoimmune anaemia does occur in the cat and the immunological dysregulation induced by FeLV may trigger autoantibody production.

Test	Sample required
Coombs' test	5 ml blood in EDTA
Antinuclear antibody	5 ml clotted blood
Rheumatoid factor	5 ml clotted blood or synovial fluid in EDTA
Anti-thyroglobulin autoantibody	5 ml clotted blood
Immunohistochemistry	Biopsy tissue sample; depending upon laboratory requirements: formalin-fixed, snap-frozen or in Michel's medium
Allergen-specific IgE or IgG	5 ml clotted blood
Circulating immune complexes	5 ml clotted blood
Serum immunoglobulin concentration	5 ml clotted blood
Complement testing	5 ml clotted blood, frozen rapidly
Phagocyte function testing	10 ml preservative-free heparinized blood from test- and age-matched controls
Lymphocyte function testing	10 ml preservative-free heparinized blood from test- and age-matched controls
Immunoelectrophoresis for serum paraproteinaemia	5 ml clotted blood
Cross matching	5 ml clotted blood and 5 ml blood in EDTA from recipient and each potential donor
Blood typing	5 ml blood in EDTA

Table 6.1: Samples required for immunodiagnostic tests.

Methodology: The Coombs' test is performed in a microtitre system (Figure 6.1) by incubating a suspension of washed patient erythrocytes with serial dilutions of a panel of reagents at both 4°C and 37°C. The reagents used are: polyvalent Coombs' reagent; anti-IgG; anti-IgM; and anti-complement C3. The test is based on the principle of agglutination whereby the antisera cross-link the molecules of immunoglobulin or complement bound to patient RBCs. The result is recorded as a titre, which is defined as the reciprocal of the last dilution of antiserum able to cause agglutination of the patient's RBCs.

Interpretation: The Coombs' test provides three important pieces of information: (1) the class(es) of immunoglobulin bound to the RBC and whether complement has been fixed; (2) the optimum temperature reactivity of these molecules; and (3) the titre of the reactions. Although there is no recorded correlation between titre and severity of disease, these data will indicate the mechanism of haemolysis in a particular case (intra- or extravascular), and in light of clinicopathological findings can be useful in formulating a prognosis. Canine AIHA often falls into one of two patterns of disease as indicated in Table 6.2, although these divisions are not absolute and individual cases may vary.

False-negative Coombs' tests have been reported in 10–40% of dogs with AIHA. The Coombs' test is also a useful means of monitoring the effectiveness of immunosuppressive therapy. Erythrocyte-bound antibody usually declines over a period of weeks and continued monitoring of such cases following withdrawal of therapy is advisable (Barker *et al.*, 1992; Day, 1996b).

Less information is available concerning interpretation of the Coombs' test in feline haemolytic anaemia. Some laboratories report low-titred positive reactions in normal cats, which may reflect the presence of a spontaneously occurring anti-IgM antibody in this species (Werner and Gorman, 1984).

Other related tests

In recent years canine AIHA has been investigated using an ELISA-based modification of the Coombs' test, the direct enzyme-linked antiglobulin test (DELAT) (Barker *et al.*, 1993). Although more sensitive, the DELAT is a time-consuming procedure, which is useful in a research context but impractical for routine diagnosis. Moreover, important information concerning the temperature reactivity of the erythrocyte-bound immunoglobulin is not provided by the DELAT. An alternative to the Coombs' test was the 'papain test' which involved enzyme degradation of patient erythrocytes before incubation with patient serum, but recent studies have shown that this test is unreliable. In this regard, animals do not have significant levels of circulating (i.e. unbound to RBC) erythrocyte autoantibody, so the performance of the indirect Coombs' test (incubating patient sera with normal dog RBCs) is not valid in veterinary species.

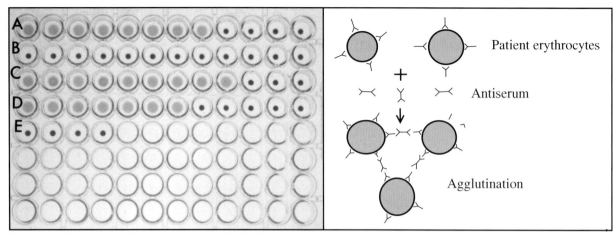

Figure 6.1: *Coombs' test: A suspension of washed patient erythrocytes is incubated with serial dilutions (from 1/5) of polyvalent antiserum specific for IgG, IgM and C3 (Coombs' reagent; Row A), anti-IgG (Row B), anti-IgM (Row C) and anti-C3 (Row D). Cells in saline (Row E) are a negative control. The antisera cause agglutination of immunoglobulin- or complement-coated erythrocytes and the test is performed in duplicate at 4°C and 37°C. In this plate (incubated at 4°C), there is a positive reaction with polyvalent Coombs' reagent (titre 640), anti-IgM (titre 1280) and anti-C3 (titre 320), indicating the presence of a cold-reactive, IgM antibody that fixes complement.*

	Intravascular haemolysis	**Extravascular haemolysis**
Autoagglutination	Positive	Negative
Coombs' reactivity	IgM and C3	IgG
Optimum temperature reactivity	4°C	37°C
Clinical features	Acute history and severe disease: jaundice, haemoglobinaemia and haemoglobinuria	Chronic history of weakness, lethargy and mucous membrane pallor
Prognosis	Poor to guarded	Guarded to good

Table 6.2: *Classification of canine AIHA*

Immune-mediated thrombocytopenia

This disease is not uncommon in the dog (usually autoimmune), but is rare in the cat and usually secondary to FeLV infection (Werner and Gorman, 1984). There is no readily available and universally accepted method of making a definitive diagnosis of this condition. Most dogs with ITP are severely thrombocytopenic (<10,000 platelets/µl) and it is not possible to isolate sufficient platelets from a blood sample to determine whether platelet-bound antibody is present. Dogs with ITP do not usually have significant circulating levels of antibody, which makes indirect testing, using normal dog platelets, difficult. Despite this, several approaches have been reported.

Platelet F3 test
In this test, serum from the thrombocytopenic dog is incubated with normal canine platelets, and normal dog serum incubated with a duplicate suspension of platelets as control. Serum autoantibody binds to and damages the platelets, causing release of platelet factor 3 which enhances clotting time compared to controls.

Direct testing
If sufficient platelets can be isolated from the blood of a thrombocytopenic dog, they may be incubated with antisera (as for the Coombs' test) and examined for evidence of microscopic agglutination. Alternatively, the platelets may be incubated with an antiserum conjugated to a marker which will fluoresce under ultraviolet light. Such direct immunofluorescence is evidence for platelet-bound antibody and may be assessed by microscopy or flow cytometry (Kristensen *et al.*, 1994b). The same technique has been applied to smears of bone marrow to detect megakaryocyte-bound autoantibody.

Indirect testing
Serum from the thrombocytopenic patient is incubated with normal dog platelets which are then used in the tests described above. Serum from dogs with ITP is able to inhibit the *in vitro* aggregation of normal platelets in the presence of activating substances (Kristensen *et al.*, 1994a). An ELISA for detection of serum anti-platelet autoantibody has been described. In this test normal dog platelets are incubated with test serum, before serial addition of an enzyme-linked anti-dog IgG reagent and the appropriate substrate (Campbell *et al.*, 1984).

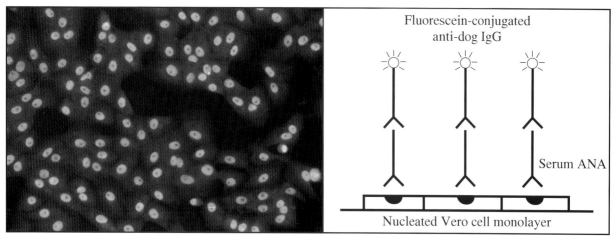

Figure 6.2: *Canine serum antinuclear antibody (ANA) detected by indirect immunofluorescence. Patient serum is incubated with a monolayer of Vero cells and binding of ANA is detected by anti-dog IgG conjugated to fluorescein isothiocyanate (FITC). Under UV light there is fluorescence of the cell nuclei when ANA is present.*

Systemic lupus erythematosus and related diseases

Antinuclear antibody test

Application: This test aims to identify whether a patient has significant levels of circulating autoantibody with specificity for one or more of a range of nuclear constituents (single-stranded or double-stranded DNA, RNA, histone and non-histone proteins). The presence of serum antinuclear antibody (ANA) is considered the definitive diagnostic criterion for systemic lupus erythematosus (SLE). It is now well recognized, however, that this is a non-specific autoantibody in the dog and cat and can occur in a wide range of inflammatory, neoplastic and immune-mediated diseases (Quimby *et al.*, 1980; Werner and Gorman, 1984; Bennett and Kirkham, 1987a). Approximately 10% of clinically normal dogs and cats will have a low titre of ANA. Despite this, the ANA test remains a useful and valid procedure for supporting a diagnosis of an autoimmune disease. The clinical indications for requesting an ANA test are where there is evidence of immune-mediated disease involving one or more systems (particularly the blood, skin, kidney or joints).

Methodology: The most frequently used method of detecting serum ANA involves screening on cell monolayers (Vero or Hep-2 cell lines grown on microscope slides divided into multiple compartments), or sections of rat liver (Schultz and Adams, 1978). Serum from the patient is serially diluted and each dilution is overlaid onto a separate monolayer. If the serum contains ANA, this will bind to the cell nucleus; this is visualized by a secondary antibody linked to a fluorescent label (for examination under UV light) or to an enzyme (for causing a colour change when incubated with substrate) (Figure 6.2).

Interpretation: The result of an ANA test will be presented as a titre (last serum dilution for positive nuclear staining) and pattern of nuclear staining. The important consideration with regard to interpretation of ANA is the titre. Those animals with non-immune disease or clinically normal animals with positive ANA generally have low titres of ANA. Therefore, a high titre of ANA in an animal with clinicopathological evidence of autoimmunity is likely to be significant and a useful piece of diagnostic information. The pattern of nuclear staining (homogeneous, nucleolar, speckled, rim) will also be recorded. In man, these patterns are associated with particular autoimmune phenomena but this has not yet been recognized in animals. Most animal ANA is of a homogeneous or speckled pattern. The ANA test may also be used to monitor the response to therapy of immune-mediated disease. ANA titre correlates well with clinical improvement on immunosuppressive treatment.

Other related tests

The fine specificity of serum ANA in the dog has also been examined using purified nuclear antigens in ELISA, radioimmunoassay (the Farr assay) or agar gel diffusion tests (Bennett and Kirkham, 1987a). Such tests are considered research tools and technical difficulties, such as non-specific binding of canine serum protein to double-stranded DNA makes interpretation difficult.

Immune-mediated arthritis

Rheumatoid factor

Application: Rheumatoid factor (RF) is an IgM autoantibody (sometimes IgA or IgG) with specificity for the Fc region of an IgG molecule. Rheumatoid factor is found in the circulation and synovial fluid of animals with immune-mediated polyarthritis, and deposition of immune complexes of RF and immunoglobulin presumably plays at least some part in the pathogenesis of disease. It is now well recognized that RF (like ANA) is a non-specific autoantibody and may be found in a variety of immune-mediated, inflammatory or neoplastic diseases (Bennett and Kirkham, 1987b; Chabanne et al., 1993), but performance of an assay for RF is still valid in cases of non-infectious, shifting polyarthritis of distal limb joints with appropriate radiographic changes and history.

The Rose–Waaler Assay
In this test, serum or synovial fluid levels of IgM RF are detected using as a 'target' sheep red blood cells (SRBC) coated with rabbit or dog antiserum specific for SRBC. The test serum is serially diluted in a microtitre system and the antibody-coated target cells added to each well. Positive and negative control sera are also included in the assay and as an additional control, the assay is repeated using SRBC without antibody ('unsensitized cells'). Where rheumatoid factor is present, the IgG 'sensitized' SRBC will be agglutinated and the end point is read as a titre (Figure 6.3).

Other related tests
An ELISA-based method for detection of RF has also been used in veterinary immunology. In this case, the 'target' IgG is bound to the plastic wells of microtitre plates rather than to SRBC, and binding of RF is determined by use of a secondary, enzyme-linked antibody (Bell et al., 1993; Chabanne et al., 1993). A test involving the agglutination of IgG-coated latex beads was popular at one time, but the results correlated poorly with traditional methods.

Interpretation: Historically RF has been thought of as diagnostic for rheumatoid arthritis (RA), however only 60–75% of dogs with RA will have demonstrable RF. Interpretation of the titre by the laboratory is important, as many ill animals will have low titres of serum RF. In cases of immune-mediated polyarthritis, it is always worth assaying for both ANA and RF, as there is considerable overlap in the occurrence of these autoantibodies; they are not restricted to SLE and RA, respectively. Seronegative cases should be retested one week later (if immunosuppressive therapy has not been instigated) because the presence of RF (as with other autoantibodies) may vary considerably from week to week. The titre of RF in synovial fluid is usually slightly lower than that of matched serum. It has recently been suggested that the presence of IgA RF may differentiate dogs with autoimmune polyarthritis from those with osteoarthritis (Bell et al., 1993).

Hypothyroidism

ELISA for anti-thyroglobulin autoantibody

Application: A large proportion of hypothyroidism in the dog is reported to reflect immune-mediated (autoimmune) thyroid pathology (see also Chapter 16). Although the majority of tissue destruction is likely to be mediated via lymphoid cytotoxicity, autoantibodies to a range of thyroid components may be generated. The best defined of these is autoantibody with specificity for thyroglobulin, the presence of which provides a useful adjunct to thyroid function testing in clinical diagnosis. Autoantibodies to T3 and T4 are rare in dogs.

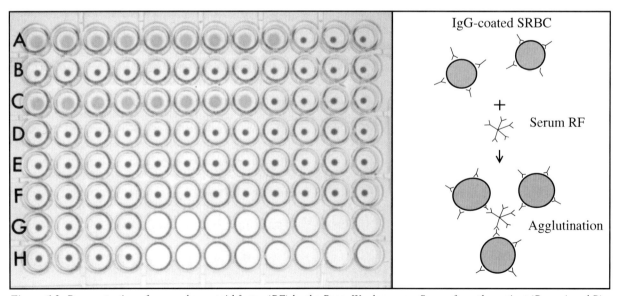

Figure 6.3: Demonstration of serum rheumatoid factor (RF) by the Rose–Waaler assay. Serum from the patient (Rows A and B), a positive control serum (Rows C and D) and negative control serum (Rows E and F) are serially diluted from 1/2 across the plate. Rows G and H contain saline (negative control). Sheep erythrocytes (SRBC) optimally coated ('sensitized') with IgG antibody are added to Rows A, C, E and G and control SRBC without antibody ('unsensitized') to Rows B, D, F and H. IgM RF causes agglutination of the sensitized SRBC in the test sample (Row A; titre 512) and positive control serum (Row C; titre 256).

Method: Anti-thyroglobulin antibody is generally assayed by ELISA. Purified canine thyroglobulin is coated on to plastic microtitre wells and serial dilutions of patient serum added. Binding of autoantibody to the antigen is demonstrated by subsequent addition of an enzyme-linked antiserum specific for canine IgG and the appropriate substrate. Autoantibodies to T3 or T4 are assayed by radioimmunoassay (RIA).

Interpretation: The result may be presented as a serum titre or numerical value depending upon the methodology used. In each case an interpretation of significance should be given by the laboratory. Between 50 and 70% of dogs with hypothyroidism will have anti-thyroglobulin autoantibody. Anti-T3 autoantibodies are less frequently recorded (0.2–38%) and anti-T4 autoantibodies are less common again.

Immune-mediated skin, kidney and joint diseases

Immunohistochemical detection of tissue-bound autoantibody

Application: Immunohistochemical staining will detect immunoglobulin (IgG, IgM or IgA) or complement (C3) molecules in tissue biopsies. The technique has a range of applications including the detection of autoantibodies bound to intercellular adhesion molecules in immune-mediated skin disease, and detection of deposited immune complex in immune-mediated skin disease, glomerulonephritis, vasculitis or arthritis. The most commonly used application is in the investigation of skin disease in animals characterized by vesiculobullous to crusting/ulcerated dermatosis of face, feet, ears, periorbital skin or mucosal surfaces where skin biopsy suggests an immune-mediated pathogenesis (Day *et al.*, 1993) (see Figure 6.4).

Methodology: The laboratory will have precise requirements for the sample required; however, it is possible to perform the technique on formalin-fixed tissue biopsy samples, such that a single biopsy will suffice for both routine light microscopic examination and immunostaining. For each sample submitted, a panel of reagents will be used in immunostaining. This will generally comprise antisera with specificity for IgG, IgM and C3. Where indicated, anti-IgA will also be employed. There are numerous immunostaining techniques, but each relies on demonstration of antiserum binding of tissue using a fluorescent (immunofluorescence) or enzyme (immunoperoxidase) marker (Vandevelde *et al.*, 1983; Figure 6.5).

Interpretation: Results are presented as a descriptive report indicating both the nature (i.e. immunoglobulin class) and distribution of positive staining. A comment

---

Systemic lupus erythematosus (rare in dog and cat)
Discoid lupus erythematosus (more often in dog than cat; rare)
Toxic epidermal necrolysis (rare in dog and cat)
Erythema multiforme (may be localized version of toxic epidermal necrolysis)
Dermatouveitis (Japanese Akita)
Dermatomyositis (Collie, Shetland Sheepdog)
Bullous pemphigoid (dog, rarely cat)
Pemphigus foliaceus (most common immune-mediated skin disease in dog and cat)
Pemphigus vulgaris (rare in dog and cat)
Pemphigus vegetans (rare in dog)
Pemphigus erythematosus (rare in dog and cat, may be overlap with systemic lupus)
Cutaneous vasculitis (rare in dog and cat, localized immune complex deposition)
Cutaneous drug eruption (may mimic any of the above)

Figure 6.4: Immune-mediated skin diseases of small animals.

will be made as to the significance of the result in light of clinical and histopathological data. Negative staining does not preclude the presence of an immune-mediated process if there is suggestive clinicopathological evidence. There are a number of reasons (e.g. immunosuppressive therapy, inappropriate biopsy site) why immunohistochemical staining may be negative. Similarly, false-positive reactions may occur for a variety of reasons and biopsy samples are best examined by an experienced immunopathologist (Day *et al.*, 1993).

Tests for other autoantibodies

Laboratory tests for detection of a range of other autoantibodies in the dog have been reported, but these may not be readily available other than by arrangement with a specialized laboratory. These include assays for antibody to type II collagen (Bari *et al.*, 1989) or heat shock proteins (Bell *et al.*, 1995) in rheumatoid arthritis, to retinal antigens in dermatouveitis of Akita dogs (Murphy *et al.*, 1991), to pancreatic beta cells in diabetes mellitus (Elie and Hoenig, 1995), to the acetylcholine receptor in myasthenia gravis (Garlepp *et al.*, 1984), to hepatocyte membranes in chronic liver disease (Andersson and Sevelius, 1992) and to spermatozoa in cases of infertility (Rosenthal *et al.*, 1984).

LABORATORY TESTS FOR HYPERSENSITIVITY

Type 1 hypersensitivity

In recent years serological diagnosis of type 1 hypersensitivity to a range of substances including indoor and outdoor environmental allergens, ectoparasites

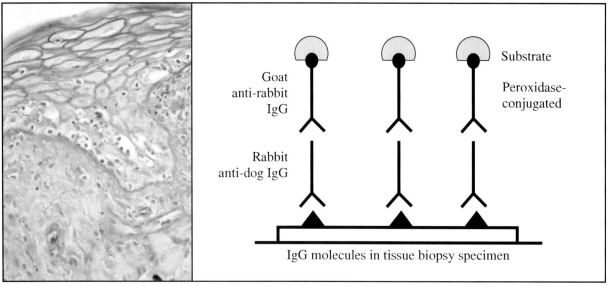

Goat
anti-rabbit
IgG

Rabbit
anti-dog IgG

Substrate

Peroxidase-
conjugated

IgG molecules in tissue biopsy specimen

Figure 6.5: Antibody binding to interepithelial adhesion molecules in the skin of a dog with immune-mediated dermatopathy. A wax/formalin-fixed biopsy section is incubated with rabbit anti-dog IgG, followed by anti-rabbit IgG conjugated to peroxidase. Bound antibody is detected as deposition of brown colour. Antisera specific for IgM and C3 are used on parallel sections from the same block.

and food has become widely available. There is ongoing controversy concerning the role of such *in vitro* tests in the diagnosis of hypersensitivity compared with the traditionally accepted methods of *in vivo* intradermal allergen provocation, ectoparasite control and elimination diets (e.g. Codner and Lessard, 1993).

Methodology: Assays are available for both the dog and cat that aim to demonstrate the presence of circulating, allergen-specific IgE antibody by ELISA. A strip test is marketed for use in the veterinary practice which incorporates various allergen groups and permits preliminary assessment of hypersensitive patients. In the full screen (usually performed by a laboratory), patient serum is incubated with a panel of antigens coated to plastic microtitre wells and binding is visualized using polyclonal antiserum to IgE which is conjugated to enzyme. An assay for allergen-specific IgG is also available for the dog.

Interpretation: The ELISA results are reported as a numerical score for each allergen tested and the laboratory will comment on likely significance. In general, there appears to be poor correlation between ELISA and intradermal testing as these assays measure different parameters: the presence of circulating as opposed to mast cell-bound IgE. False-positive results have been found in clinically normal or parasitized dogs. Some laboratories utilize the ELISA data to formulate a hyposensitization regimen incorporating the allergens to which the patient has been identified as being sensitized. The ELISA for allergen-specific IgG may be used to monitor such cases, as serum concentration of antibody of this class increases over the period of hyposensitization.

Other assays for hypersensitivity

The presence of circulating immune complexes (CIC) in the serum of animals with type III hypersensitivity diseases has been recorded. There are various methods of assaying for CIC, the simplest of which involves precipitation from serum by incubation with polyethylene glycol. T lymphocyte sensitization in Type IV hypersensitivity may be detected *in vitro* by stimulating mononuclear cells with antigen in tissue culture as described below.

LABORATORY TESTS FOR IMMUNODEFICIENCY

A range of laboratory tests exists for testing the function of the various arms of the immune system *in vitro*. These are most commonly used in the investigation of suspected primary immunodeficiency, for example in cases of unusual or chronic recurrent infections in young, littermate animals. Additionally, the tests are applicable to the investigation of any immune-mediated disorder in which normal function of the immune system may be impaired or excessively activated.

Serum immunoglobulin concentration

Measurement of the concentration of IgG, IgM or IgA in serum (or other fluids, e.g. tears) can be readily performed in dogs and cats, and serum IgE concentrations have been assessed in the dog (Hill and DeBoer, 1994). Serum concentrations of IgG subclasses have been measured in dogs (Mazza *et al.*, 1994).

Methodology: Immunoglobulin concentration can be measured using the principle of precipitation in the single radial immunodiffusion (SRID) test. Serum

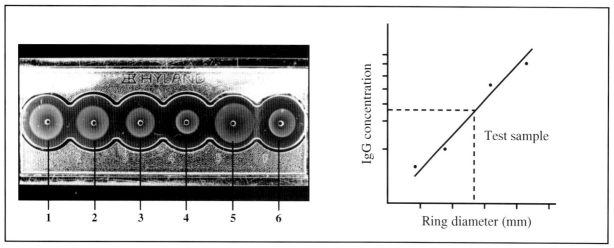

Figure 6.6: *Determination of serum IgG concentration by single radial immunodiffusion (SRID). The agarose gel contains antiserum to IgG. Standard samples of known IgG concentration (3–25mg/ml) are loaded into wells 1-4 and test serum from animals A and B to wells 5 and 6. During overnight incubation, the IgG diffuses from the well and forms a zone of precipitation where it interacts optimally with the antiserum in the gel. The diameter of the precipitin ring is proportional to the concentration of IgG and is determined using a series of standards for comparison.*

Sample	IgG (mg/ml)	IgM (mg/ml)	IgA (mg/ml)	IgE (µg/ml)
Dog	10 – 20	1.0 – 2.0	0.4 – 1.6	< 2 – 182
Cat	5.67 – 38.0	0.7 – 3.6	0.35 – 6.0	not defined

Table 6.3: *Serum immunoglobulin concentrations in dogs and cats. A summary of the most significant published studies.*

samples are loaded into wells punched into an agarose gel which contains an antiserum specific for the immunoglobulin to be measured (e.g. rabbit anti-dog IgG). The immunoglobulin diffuses out of the well and forms a zone of precipitation where it interacts with antiserum at the point of equivalence. The larger the diameter of precipitin ring formed, the greater the amount of immunoglobulin in the sample. A series of controls of known immunoglobulin concentration can be used to draw a standard curve (ring diameter *versus* immunoglobulin concentration) from which the test values can be interpolated (Barta, 1981; Figure 6.6).

A capture ELISA may also be used for determining immunoglobulin concentration. Microtitre wells are coated with an antiserum to an immunoglobulin that will 'capture' that immunoglobulin from the test serum. This interaction is recognized using a second enzyme-linked antiserum specific for that immunoglobulin.

Interpretation: Serum immunoglobulin concentrations may be compared with published known values, or reference values determined by the laboratory (Table 6.3). Concentration must be interpreted in light of the age of the animal to take into account passive transfer of maternal antibody. Low concentration of one or more immunoglobulins may suggest immunodeficiency but repeat testing is advisable in such cases. Other causes for depressed immunoglobulin

production should be eliminated. Increased levels may occur with polyclonal immune stimulation in chronic infectious or inflammatory disease, or monoclonal paraproteinaemia in myeloma.

Complement concentration and function testing

Testing of complement factors is only performed by specialist laboratories. Complement factors are heat labile, so serum samples must be frozen as soon as possible after collection. Serum levels of C3 and C4 have been measured by SRID in the dog (Day *et al.*, 1985) and the function of the classical and terminal pathways measured by the CH_{50} assay which assesses the ability of complement in patient serum to cause lysis of antibody-coated RBCs (Wolfe and Halliwell, 1980; Barta, 1981). Decreased complement concentration or function may indicate genetic deficiency or, alternatively, utilization of complement in the pathogenesis of disease (i.e. bound in immune complexes).

Neutrophil and macrophage function testing

These tests are available only from research laboratories. It is possible to isolate both neutrophils and macrophages from peripheral blood and to assess *in vitro* their ability to move along a chemotactic gradient, to phagocytose particles (e.g. latex beads, staphylococci), to kill intracellular bacteria or fungal spores or to release superoxide anions. Defective expression of adhesion molecules by canine leucocytes has been identified by functional studies and surface phenotyping using monoclonal antibodies. The laboratory will require samples from age-matched normal control animals and the functional parameters will be interpreted relative to those controls.

Lymphocyte phenotyping
With the availability of monoclonal antibodies specific for unique surface molecules of T and B lymphocytes (CD molecules), it has become possible to classify the relative numbers of T cell subsets and B cells in the circulation or in tissue (Cobbold and Metcalfe, 1994). Such assays however, are not yet readily available.

Lymphocytes can be isolated from blood and repeat aliquots of the cells incubated with different monoclonal antibodies. A secondary antibody conjugated to a fluorescent marker is subsequently added, and the cells processed by a 'flow cytometer' (fluorescence-activated cell sorter, FACS) which excites the marker with a laser beam and determines the number of positive cells in a sample of 10,000 cells counted. These antibodies may sometimes be used in immunohistochemistry (usually requiring frozen tissue) to identify lymphoid populations and assess their distribution in lymphoid tissue. Figures are available for the normal number of lymphocytes of various subsets in the blood of dogs and cats. Approximately 70% of blood lymphocytes are T cells and 20% B cells, with a small population of 'null' cells. CD4-positive T cells are generally in greater proportion than CD8-positive cells. Gross abnormalities in these ratios may suggest primary or secondary (e.g. FIV infection) immunodeficiency.

Lymphocyte function testing
These tests are only available from research laboratories and samples from control age-matched animals will be required. Mononuclear cells are isolated from blood and cultured *in vitro* in the presence of non-specific activators called 'mitogens'. Normal lymphocytes will be stimulated to proliferate by such substances; cell division is measured by the amount of radiolabelled thymidine that is incorporated into the DNA of dividing cells in the culture. After 48–72 hours of culture, the amount of radiolabel incorporated is measured by a beta counter (Barta, 1981; Kristensen *et al.*, 1982). Failure to proliferate adequately when compared to control samples may indicate a primary functional defect. Such assays have recently been extended to assess the ability of lymphocytes to respond *in vitro* to specific antigens and to determine whether the response has primary or secondary (memory) kinetics.

Another indicator of lymphocyte function is the ability to release specific cytokines when stimulated in culture. After a period of culture, supernates may be aspirated from the cells and the presence of cytokines measured by ELISA or bioassay. The latter tests the ability of the supernatant to support the growth of a cell line which has an obligate requirement for a specific cytokine. In this way, cytokines such as interleukin-1 (IL-1), IL-2, IL-6, tumour necrosis factor and γ-interferon have been assayed in the cat and dog (Fuller *et al.*, 1994; Lawrence *et al.*, 1995). Alternatively, stimulated lymphocytes may be examined by the polymerase chain reaction (PCR) for the expression of mRNA for a range of cytokines (Rottman *et al.*, 1995) or cytokine may be detected by immunohistochemical examination (Day, 1996a), but such technology is at present not routinely available.

LABORATORY TESTS FOR LYMPHOID NEOPLASIA

Phenotyping neoplastic cells
The techniques described above are applicable to the characterization of neoplastic as well as normal lymphocytes. Monoclonal antibodies can be used to determine the phenotype of neoplastic lymphocytes in blood (lymphoid leukaemia) or in tissue (lymphoma) (Day, 1995) Molecular techniques have been used to characterize rearrangements in T cell receptor and immunoglobulin genes (Rezanka and Neil, 1995). Although such studies are in their infancy, in the future it may be possible to formulate a prognosis for lymphoid neoplasia based on such parameters, for example a recent study suggests that T cell lymphoma in dogs carries a worse prognosis than B cell lymphoma (Teske *et al.*, 1994).

Identification of paraproteins
Neoplastic plasma cells in myeloma secrete large quantities of an altered immunoglobulin known as paraprotein. This can be identified on serum protein electrophoresis as a distinct spike in the gamma-globulin region. The technique of immunoelectrophoresis (IEP) can further characterize the molecule. Following electrophoretic separation of serum proteins, antisera specific for immunoglobulin heavy or light chains are added to troughs in the agarose gel cut parallel to the line of separated proteins. The antisera will diffuse from the troughs and form an arc of precipitation with identified protein (Schultz and Adams, 1978; Figure 6.7). The test will identify the class of immunoglobulin, and abnormality in the position or nature of the precipitin arc may be observed. Occasionally, free light chains (Bence–Jones protein) are secreted and may be released into the urine. These may be identified by IEP of a concentrated urine sample.

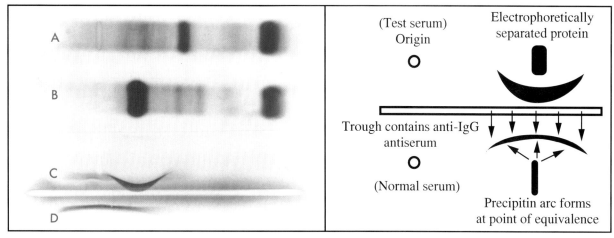

Figure 6.7: *Characterization of serum paraprotein in multiple myeloma by immunoelectrophoresis (IEP). Electrophoretically separated serum from a normal dog (Lane A) and a dog with paraproteinaemia (Lane B) demonstrating a monoclonal gammopathy. Serum from this dog (Lane C) and the normal dog (Lane D) are separated and antiserum to dog IgG loaded into a trough cut between the electrophoresed proteins. During overnight incubation, the antiserum diffuses from the trough and interacts with serum protein, forming an arc of precipitation. The nature of the precipitin arc in Lane C confirms that this is an IgG myeloma.*

Species	Blood group	Frequency of expression	Associated alloantibody
Dog	DEA 1.1*	Common	Rare
	DEA 1.2*	Common	Rare
	DEA 1.3		
	DEA 1 null		
	DEA 3	Rare	Rare
	DEA 4	Most dogs	None
	DEA 5	Less common	Rare
	DEA 6	Most dogs	Unknown
	DEA 7*	Common	Rare
	DEA 8	Common	None
Cat	A	Most common	May have weak anti-B
	B	Less common (but more prevalent in some pure-breds including British Short Hair, Rex and Birman)	Have high titres of anti-A
	AB	Rare	None

Table 6.4: *Blood groups in dogs and cats.*

* Most significant in producing clinical transfusion reactions.

TISSUE AND BLOOD TYPING

Characterization of the unique combination of molecules of the major histocompatibility complex expressed by blood mononuclear cells provides a means of closely identifying individuals at the protein or molecular level. Considerable knowledge of the molecules that make up the dog leucocyte antigen (DLA) and feline leucocyte antigen (FLA) systems has become available in recent years, but the complex methodology is still considered a research tool. The future potential for animal identification (e.g. in parentage disputes), for assessing transplantation compatibility or for predicting the onset of immune-mediated disease is an exciting possibility (Day and Penhale, 1987).

The dog and cat erythocyte antigen systems are well characterized (Table 6.4), and it is recognized that blood typing is of benefit prior to first transfusion in cats (due to the prevalence of spontaneously arising alloantibodies), or second or subsequent transfusion in dogs. Although blood typing is not routinely available, a simple, rapid and effective card test has recently become available for blood typing cats (A, B or AB blood groups) and dogs (DEA 1.1 only). As an alternative, cross-matching potential donors with the recipient is advisable. In the simplest cross-match, serum from the recipient is incubated with a suspension of washed RBCs from each potential donor and the presence of agglutination or haemolysis assessed relative to appropriate controls.

REFERENCES AND FURTHER READING

Andersson M and Sevelius E (1992) Circulating autoantibodies in dogs with chronic liver disease. *Journal of Small Animal Practice* **33**, 389–394

Bari ASM, Carter SD, Bell SC, Bennett D and Morgan K (1989) Anti-type II collagen antibody in naturally occurring canine joint disease. *British Journal of Rheumatology* **28**, 480–486

Barker RN, Gruffydd-Jones TJ and Elson CJ (1993) Red cell-bound immunoglobulins and complement measured by an enzyme-linked antiglobulin test in dogs with autoimmune haemolysis or other anaemis. *Research in Veterinary Science* **54**, 170–178

Barker RN, Gruffydd-Jones TJ, Stokes CR and Elson CJ (1992) Autoimmune haemolysis in the dog: relationship between anaemia and the levels of red blood cell bound immunoglobulins and complement measured by an enzyme-linked antiglobulin test. *Veterinary Immunology and Immunopathology* **34**, 1–20

Barta O (1981) Laboratory techniques of veterinary clinical immunology; a review. *Compendium of Immunological and Microbiological Infectious Disease* **4**, 131–160

Bell SC, Carter SD, May C and Bennett D (1993) IgA and IgM rheumatoid factors in canine rheumatoid arthritis. *Journal of Small Animal Practice* **34**, 259–264

Bell SC, Carter SD, May C and Bennett D (1995) Antibodies to heat shock proteins in dogs with rheumatoid arthritis and systemic lupus erythematosus. *British Veterinary Journal* **151**, 271–279

Bennett D and Kirkham D (1987a) The laboratory identification of serum antinuclear antibody in the dog. *Journal of Comparative Pathology* **97**, 523–539

Bennett D and Kirkham D (1987b) The laboratory identification of seurm rheumatoid factor in the dog. *Journal of Comparative Pathology* **97**, 541–550

Campbell KL, George JW and Greene CE (1984) Application of the enzyme-linked immunosorbent assay for the detection of platelet antibodies in dogs. *American Journal of Veterinary Research* **45**, 2561–2564

Chabanne L, Fournel C, Faure JR, Veysseyre CM, Rigal D, Bringuier JP and Monier JC (1993) IgM and IgA rheumatoid factors in canine polyarthritis. *Veterinary Immunology and Immunopathology* **39**, 365–379

Cobbold S and Metcalfe S (1994) Monoclonal antibodies that define canine homologues of human CD antigens: summary of the first international canine leukocyte antigen workshop (CLAW). *Tissue Antigens* **43**, 137–154

Codner EC and Lessard P (1993) Comparison of intradermal allergy test and enzyme-linked immunosorbent assay in dogs with allergic skin disease. *Journal of the American Veterinary Medical Association* **202**, 739–743

Day MJ (1995) Immunophenotypic characterisation of cutaneous lymphoid neoplasia in the dog and cat. *Journal of Comparative Pathology* **112**, 79–96

Day MJ (1996a) Expression of interleukin-1ß, interleukin-6 and tumour necrosis factor-by macrophages in canine lymph nodes with mineral-associated lymphadenopathy, granulomatous lymphadenitis or reactive hyperplasia. *Journal of Comparative Pathology* **114**, 31–42

Day MJ (1996b) Serial monitoring of clinical, haematological and immunological parameters in canine autoimmune haemolytic anaemia. *Journal of Small Animal Practice* **37**, 523–534

Day MJ, Hanlon L and Powell LM (1993) Immune-mediated skin disease in the dog and cat. *Journal of Comparative Pathology* **109**, 395–407

Day MJ, Kay PH, Clark WT, Shaw SE, Penhale WJ and Dawkins RL (1985) Complement C4 allotype association with and serum C4 concentration in an autoimmune disease of the dog. *Clinical Immunology and Immunopathology* **35**, 85–91

Day MJ and Penhale WJ (1987) A review of major histocompatibility disease associations in man and dog. *Veterinary Research Communications* **11**, 119–132

Elie M and Hoenig M (1995) Canine immune-mediated diabetes mellitus. *Journal of the American Animal Hospital Association* **31**, 295–299

Fuller L, Carreno M, Esquenazi V *et al.* (1994) Characterisation of anti-canine cytokine monoclonal antibodies specific for IFNγ. *Tissue Antigens* **43**, 163–169

Garlepp MJ, Kay PH, Farrow BR and Dawkins RL (1984) Autoimmunity in spontaneous myasthenia gravis in dogs. *Clinical Immunology and Immunopathology* **31**, 301–306

Grant CK (1995) Purification and characterization of feline IgM and IgA isotypes and three subclasses of IgG. In : *Feline Immunology and Immunodeficiency,* ed. BJ Willett and O Jarrett, pp. 95–107. Oxford Science Publications, Oxford

Hill PB and De Boer DJ (1994) Quantification of serum total IgE concentration in dogs by use of an enzyme-linked immunosorbent assay containing monoclonal murine anti-canine IgE. *American Jornal of Veterinary Research* **55**, 944–948

Kristensen AT, Weiss DJ and Klausner JS (1994a) Platelet dysfunction associated with immune-mediated thrombocytopenia in dogs. *Journal of Veterinary Internal Medicine* **8**, 323–327

Kristensen AT, Weiss DJ, Klausner JS, Laber J and Christie DJ (1994b) Comparison of microscopic and flow cytometric detection of platelet antibody in dogs suspected of having immune-mediated thrombocytopenia. *American Journal of Veterinary Research* **55**, 1111–1114

Kristensen F, Kristensen B and Lazary S (1982) The lymphocyte stimulation test in veterinary immunology. *Veterinary Immunology and Immunopathology* **3**, 203–277

Lawrence CE, Callanan JJ, Willett BJ and Jarrett O (1995) Cytokine production by cats infected with feline immunodeficiency virus: a longitudinal study. *Immunology* **85**, 568–574

Madewell BR, Hills DL and Franti CE (1980) Serum concentrations of immunoglobulins G, A and M in dogs with neoplastic disease. *American Journal of Veterinary Research* **41**, 720–722

Mazza G, Whiting AH, Day MJ and Duffus WPH (1994) Development of an enzyme-linked immunosorbent assay for detection of IgG subclasses in the serum of normal and diseased dogs. *Research in Veterinary Science* **57**, 133–139

Murphy CJ, Bellhorn RW and Thirkill C (1991) Anti-retinal antibodies associated with Vogt-Koyanagi-Harada-like syndrome in a dog. *Journal of the American Animal Hospital Association* **27**, 399–402

Penhale WJ, Day MJ, Lines AD and McKenna RP (1990) A review of cases submitted to Murdoch University for immunodiagnostic testing: 1978–1989. *Australian Veterinary Journal* **647**, 148–149

Quimby FW, Smith C, Brushwein M and Lewis RM (1980) Efficacy of immunoserodiagnostic procedures in the recognition of canine immunologic diseases. *American Journal of Veterinary Research* **41**, 1622–1666

Rezanka LJ and Neil JC (1995) The feline T cell receptor gene. In: *Feline Immunology and Immunodeficiency,* ed. BJ Willett and O Jarrett, pp. 65–83. Oxford Science Publications, Oxford

Rivas AL, Kimball ES, Quimby FW and Gebhard D (1995) Functional and phenotypic analysis of in vitro stimulated canine peripheral blood mononuclear cells. *Veterinary Immunology and Immunopathology* **45**, 55–71

Rosenthal RC, Meyers WL and Burke TJ (1984) Detection of canine antisperm antibodies by indirect immunofluorescence and gelatin agglutination. *American Journal of Veterinary Research* **45**, 370–374

Rottman JB, Freeman EB, Tonkonogy S and Tompkins MB (1995) A reverse transcriptase-polymerase chain reaction technique to detect feline cytokine genes. *Veterinary Immunology and Immunopathology* **45**, 1–18

Schultz RD and Adams LS (1978) Immunologic methods for the detection of humoral and cellular immunity. *Veterinary Clinics of North America* **8**, 721–753

Teske E, van Heerde P, Rutteman GR, Kurzman ID, Moore PF and MacEwan EG (1994) Prognostic factors for treatment of malignant lymphoma in dogs. *Journal of the American Veterinary Medical Association* **205**, 1722–1728

Vandevelde M, Hugi E, Isler A, Suter M and Pfister H (1983) Histological immunoenzyme techniques in canine tissues: evaluation of various methods and modifications. *Research in Veterinary Science* **34**, 193–198

Werner LL and Gorman NT (1984) Immune-mediated disorders of cats. *Veterinary Clinics of North America* **14**, 1039–1064

Wolfe JH and Halliwell REW (1980) Total haemolytic complement values in normal and diseased dog populations. *Veterinary Immunology and Immunopathology* **1**, 287–298

CHAPTER SEVEN

Cytopathology

Chris Belford and John H. Lumsden

INTRODUCTION

Cytology is the study of cell form and function. *Diagnostic* cytology refers to the procedures used to sample, examine and interpret cell morphology in order to assist making clinical diagnoses. Diagnostic cytology is used routinely in human and veterinary medicine. Representative cells are sampled from lesions, spread on glass slides, stained, and examined using a microscope. Detailed interpretation requires the training and experience of a cytopathologist. Basic inflammatory lesions and some characteristic tumours can be recognized by clinicians with adequate training.

The procedures used for obtaining samples of cells are simple, can be carried out rapidly and are relatively safe. The use of cytological examinations in selected cases is very cost-effective. Few resources are required to obtain representative cells from most lesions, usually without the use of general anaesthe-sia or even sedation. Because most samples can be obtained with minimal discomfort to the patient it is often possible to perform the procedure on the consulting room table. This may remove the need for hospitalization. When compared to surgical biopsies there is reduced risk, particularly in the geriatric or ill patient.

Surgical biopsy and histopathological examination may be required for lesions where cell exfoliation is poor, where architecture is a primary criterion for differentiating neoplasia, or where 'grading' for certain types of neoplasia is required.

Sampling and staining for cytology can be accomplished within minutes. Preliminary interpretation may be made in the clinic with final, or original, interpretation completed by a consulting cytopathologist. Although some interpretations are readily apparent, others require careful examination of several preparations by a qualified cytopathologist.

REQUIREMENTS FOR SUCCESS

Three primary factors determine the usefulness of cytology in the clinical setting. These are:

- The quality of the sample
- The reliability of the interpretation
- The amount of clinical information available to the interpreter.

Sample quality

The quality of the sample relies upon two distinct steps:

- The selection of suitable lesions and the use of appropriate techniques for harvest of representative cells
- The spreading of adequate numbers of representative intact cells, often called 'smears', on to glass slides.

Interpretation

Reliable interpretation depends upon:

- The use of, and familiarity with, appropriate staining techniques
- Access to a good quality microscope
- The training, knowledge and experience of the microscopist. Most clinicians rely upon the services of a qualified veterinary clinical pathologist for the final, if not the initial, interpretation. Examination of cytological preparations involves the assessment of individual cell morphology and this can be both a time-consuming and a demanding process.

Communication

Good communication requires:

- An accurate description of the lesion sampled, including duration, size, location and all relevant clinical details
- Labelling of each glass slide as to origin, especially if multiple sources are sampled
- The clinical differential diagnoses.

Although clinicians may prefer not to disclose their inital differential diagnoses, considering this to be the responsibility of the cytopathologist, including this information greatly increases the likelihood that a reliable interpretation will ensue. There are several logical reasons supporting this argument. The strength of the information obtained from the clinical history and during clinical examination is too valuable to be ignored when interpreting any type of laboratory data, including surgical and cytological biopsy samples. Description of the location and firmness of the lesion may help determine whether adequate representative

cells have been sampled. Many clinical differential diagnoses can be readily excluded or substantiated by examination of cytology submissions. In other cases, reliable interpretation may only be made if all pertinent clinical and cytological information is considered. Many types of therapy will alter cell morphology. For example, corticosteroids induce changes in lymphocyte and mast cell morphology and if this factor is not taken into account misinterpretation may occur. Similarly, bacteria may not be visible in septic lesions following administration of antibiotics.

GENERAL TECHNIQUES

Fine needle aspiration (FNA) biopsy

A 5 or 10 ml syringe with a 21–25 gauge needle should be used (Figure 7.1). Three to five clean glass slides are set out within arm's length on a clean area of the workbench. The needle is attached to the syringe. The needle tip is advanced into the lesion then the syringe plunger is withdrawn to apply 3–5 ml of vacuum, dependent upon the firmness of the tissue. Vacuum is maintained. The needle tip is moved forward and back a few millimetres while gently altering direction to include a fan-shaped area, as if attempting to infiltrate the lesion with local anaesthetic. A representative sample should enter the needle barrel within 1–2 seconds. Before allowing the needle tip to leave the lesion, the vacuum should be released by allowing the plunger to return towards the zero position. The needle is then removed from the lesion, the syringe detached and the plunger pulled out to fill the syringe with 3–5 ml of air prior to reattaching the syringe to the needle. The syringe plunger is depressed to push one drop of sample from the needle tip on to each glass slide. Direct smears are immediately prepared, as described below.

The procedure must be done quickly and gently. Unnecessary trauma induced by the needle tip will result in increased aspiration of blood and activation of clotting within a few seconds. A good distribution of well preserved cells cannot be expected if clotting of the sample occurs during aspiration or smear preparation. If clotting occurs, the aspiration should be repeated using clean equipment and a different sampling site. Aspirates from cats tend to clot more quickly than those from dogs, in the authors' experience.

Lesions must be of adequate size, preferably at least 1 cm in diameter, to allow reliable sampling of representative cells. Imaging techniques including radiography and ultrasonography are required to aspirate small internal lesions reliably. Since lesions vary in architecture and cell distribution aspirates should be obtained from multiple sites, especially for cystic or larger lesions, in order to increase the probability of harvesting representative cells. With cystic lesions it is necessary to obtain cells from both the outer wall and

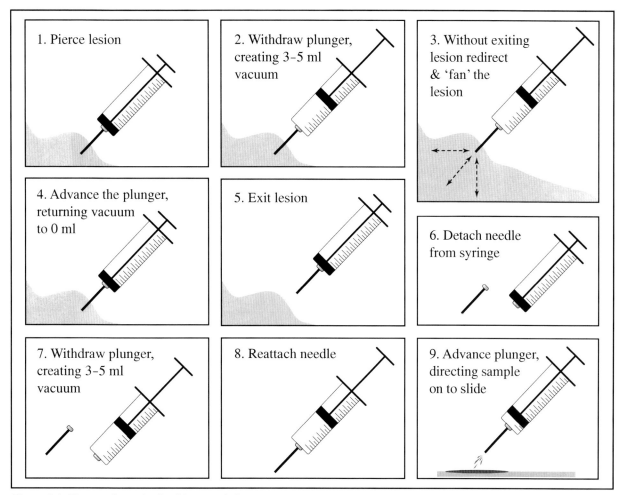

Figure 7.1: *Fine needle aspiration biopsy technique.*

the central cavity. Cystic fluid may contain few to no cells. When the patient has multiple masses a representative number of the lesions should be aspirated.

Soft lesions usually exfoliate readily. Less vacuum is usually required to obtain intact representative cells. This is of particular importance when aspirating lymph nodes or suspected lymphosarcomatous masses as lymphocytes, especially from cats, are very fragile.

Firmer lesions usually contain increased stromal cells which exfoliate less well resulting in decreased cell harvest. Increased vacuum and more vigorous movement of the needle tip may improve the cell sample. Use of a larger gauge needle is usually counterproductive. Larger gauge needles result in more blood contamination. Needles larger than 20 gauge tend to produce small core biopsies or cellular clumps which are unsuitable for cytological examination unless special fixation and staining techniques are used.

Pistol-grip syringe holders are manufactured that allow one to apply vacuum and direct the needle tip with one hand while the other hand is used to locate and immobilize the lesion. Syringe holders are very convenient to use but are not mandatory. Dexterity and practice are the primary requirements for consistently obtaining diagnostically useful fine needle aspirations.

Preparation of direct smears

Drawback and push away method
This is similar to the standard technique used for making blood smears (Figure 7.2). Larger cells and cell clumps tend to migrate to the feathered area of the smear. Consequently, the feathered tip of the smear must end within the working area of the glass slide. Too much material will result in loss of these important cells, especially if viscosity is low or an incorrect angle or speed is used for advancing the spreader slide.

Pull-apart method
A drop of aspirated material is placed upon one slide and a second slide is gently placed on top. Using only horizontal pressure, the slides are separated (Figure 7.3). Many cell types, especially if immature, rupture more readily when using this method. However, if the aspirate is mucinous or very viscous this method may be required to produce an adequate distribution of cells. Some authors recommend using two coverslips for this procedure to preserve fragile cells and improve cellular details. The labelling and staining creates an additional technical challenge due to the size and fragility of coverslips.

Four slides with representative smears are shown in Figure 7.4.

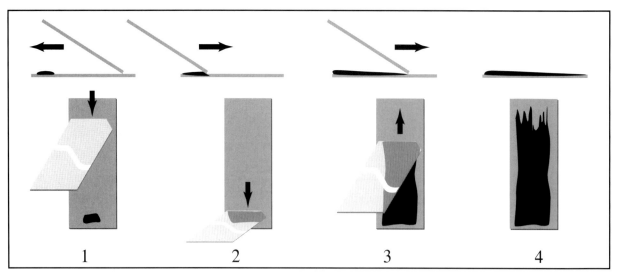

Figure 7.2: *Draw back and push away method for blood smears.*

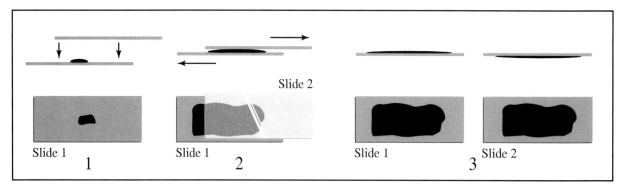

Figure 7.3: *Pull-apart method for blood smears.*

Scrapings

Cells may be scraped off surface lesions or surgical biopsy specimens using a scalpel blade. Most ulcerated surface lesions are covered with an exudate. The surface area should be cleaned and blotted dry using sterile gauze swabs prior to obtaining representative cells. In the case of surgical biopsies, a freshly cut

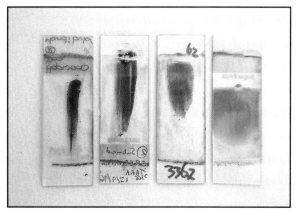

Figure 7.4: *Examples of good-quality aspirate smears. On three of the slides the edges and feathered tips remain within the working area. The slide on the right, containing mostly blood, might suffer from loss of important cells along one edge. Each slide has areas with a thin layer of cells necessary for adequate examination with a microscope.*

surface is exposed and blotted dry of plasma or serum prior to collecting cells.

A sharp edge such as a scalpel blade is held at a 90° angle and scraped across the surface vigorously several times. Scalpels with a rounded blade can be used like a paintbrush to gently transfer and spread a thin layer of cells over clean slides. In many areas of the smear the cell distribution will be too thick for routine cytological examination unless using wet fixation and trichrome stains. Peripheral areas should contain a single layer of intact cells which can be stained and examined using Romanowsky staining. A glass slide may be used as a spreader to distribute cells.

Impression smears

Impression smears may be made from superficial lesions or surgical biopsy specimens. If lesions are firm, few cells are likely to exfoliate using this technique; FNA biopsy or scraping techniques are usually more successful. Surfaces for impression smears should be prepared as for scrapings. In general, impressions produce less cellular samples than scrapings although morphology can be excellent. The surface must be dry otherwise only fluid is harvested. The slide should be gently touched to the lesion, using a slight rolling motion. If the slide is pushed directly on to the lesion and removed at a 90° angle from the surface there is a reduced cell harvest and cells may be distorted.

Swabs

Swab techniques are used primarily to obtain cytology samples from the nose, vagina and conjunctiva. A cotton bud or bacteriology swab is most often used. Cells are transferred to glass slides by rolling the swab over the clean surface.

FLUID AND BODY CAVITY SAMPLING

The preferred sampling location and approach varies with the species, the site of the suspect lesion and the operator. One or more commonly used procedures are described briefly here; additional procedures are described within the appropriate organ system chapters of this manual. Aseptic techniques should be used, including surgical preparation of the skin surface.

Sedation and local anaesthetics may be used but are often unnecessary.

The appearance of the aspirated fluid should be recorded. Colour and turbidity indicate the presence of pigments and cells, respectively. Lipids, from lymphatic leakage, can also create turbidity. Pink to red colour indicates haemoglobin, either free or within erythrocytes. If the haemoglobin is contained within intact cells, the supernatant will be clear following centrifugation. A brown appearance of peritoneal fluid warrants investigation of bile leakage. If there is contamination of the sample with blood during sampling, or if the fluid is clear initially but haemolysis occurs *in vitro*, the original appearance must be recorded for correct interpretation.

Fluid samples should be transferred into vials containing ethylene diamine tetra-acetic acid (EDTA) for cell counting and cytology examinations (Table 7.1). The EDTA anticoagulant binds calcium, thereby preventing clotting if fibrinogen is present. It also reduces

Source	Sample submission
Solid tissue (superficial or internal)	3-5 air-dried smears
Fluids:	
Thoracic, abdominal	EDTA vial Direct and sediment smears If tissue mass present, FNA as above
Synovial	Direct smears EDTA and plain vial if adequate volume
Cerebrospinal	Gravity sediment smear within one hour EDTA and plain vial EDTA + 2 drops of formalin if analysis delayed >1 hour
Peripheral blood	Direct smears (2) EDTA
Urine	Direct and sediment smears Plain vial for biochemistry plus a plain vial with a few drops of formalin in case analysis is delayed Sterile vial ± boric acid for culture
Cyst or abscess	3–5 air-dried direct smears each of fluid and FNA of adjacent tissue EDTA fluid Culture vials
Wash/flush/massage:	
Prostate; Bronchoalveolar; Tracheal; Nasal exudate/flush	Direct and sediment smears EDTA fluid Culture vial, if indicated
Eyes/ears/vagina	Swab or scraping smears Culture swabs/vial, if indicated

Table 7.1: Summary of sample submission

phagocytic cell activity, allowing differentiation of *in vivo* and *in vitro* phagocytosis of bacteria, erythrocytes and other nucleated cells. Other anticoagulants may be required for special tests.

Nucleated cells are counted using manual or automated methods. If there is a high cell count, i.e. >10 x 10^9 cells per litre, determined by counting or estimated from the degree of fluid turbidity, direct smears may be made for staining and examination. Otherwise cells should be concentrated by centrifugation and smears prepared from the sediment. This should be done as soon as possible to retain optimum cell morphology. If cells cannot be concentrated in the clinic or processed within hours in a referral laboratory, direct smears should be made immediately. This will provide the cytopathologist with a few freshly fixed cells to guide interpretation of the concentrated but less well preserved cells on the slides prepared at the referral laboratory. The special centrifuges designed for concentrating cells for cytological examination, cytocentrifuges, are usually found only in referral laboratories in view of their cost and specialist function.

Haemoglobin concentration, or packed cell volume (PCV), is used to estimate the amount of blood in cavity fluids. Protein concentration is determined using a refractometer or by chemical analysis. Increased lipid concentrations will interfere with both the spectrophotometric determination of haemoglobin and the refractometer determination of protein concentration. Samples for other clinical chemistry analyses should be placed in a vial without anticoagulant.

If clotting occurs in the vial without anticoagulant, this suggests that the fibrinogen concentration is increased, indicating an inflammatory response within the fluid.

Thoracocentesis

Thoracocentesis is performed while the animal is standing or in sternal recumbency. The usual site is the ventral third of the 7th or 8th intercostal space. (See also Chapter 10.) A 20-22 gauge needle is inserted close to the anterior edge of the rib to decrease the possibilities of injuring blood vessels and nerves located at the caudal border of each rib. Use of an over-the-needle catheter reduces the chance of lacerating the lungs. If there is excessive fluid to be drained, the use of a three-way valve will reduce the potential of creating a pneumothorax.

Abdominocentesis

Abdominocentesis is performed with the animal standing or in lateral recumbency. The usual site is 1-2 cm behind the umbilicus in the ventral midline. (See also Chapter 8.) A 20-22 gauge needle is selected, with a length capable of penetrating the estimated body wall thickness. The needle is inserted and fluid is collected by free flow. An over-the-needle catheter and three-way valve may be used.

Arthrocentesis

Needles of 20-22 gauge and adequate length to enter the joint space with syringes of 2-5 ml or larger capacity are used for arthrocentesis in dogs and cats. The location of the affected joint and the patient's temperament will influence the choice of positioning and restraint. Specific aspects of arthrocentesis are described in Chapter 11.

The synovial cavities of dogs and cats normally contain small volumes of fluid, i.e. one or two drops, which allow preparation of direct smears only. Only with disease, or from the largest cavities, can an adequate volume of fluid be aspirated for multiple analyses. If a significant volume of synovial fluid is obtained, it is placed into vials with, and without, anticoagulant. EDTA is preferred for cytology, whilst heparin is preferred for the mucin clot test (see below).

Cerebrospinal fluid (CSF)

Sampling techniques for CSF are described in Chapter 13. CSF normally contains a very low cell and protein concentration. Cells are very fragile in this environment. Routine techniques are unsatisfactory for concentrating CSF cells because of the low concentration of very fragile cells normally present. Simple gravity sedimentation methods are described (see Chapter 13) that can be used in the clinic. If the CSF protein concentration is increased, cells may be more stable.

CSF cells must be counted using manual techniques with a haemocytometer, due to the low concentration present in health and in most disease processes. Similarly, microtechniques are required for determining protein concentration. Urine dipstick tests can be used to identify an increase in CSF protein concentration, i.e. to >0.3 g/l (30 mg/dl), but the method is unreliable for quantitative determination and is generally more sensitive for measuring albumin rather than globulins.

Tracheal/bronchial lavage techniques

Bronchoalveolar lavage provides cytological information from alveolar areas and bronchi. (See also Chapter 10.) Other procedures may or may not provide cells representative of changes within the lung. Use of paediatric bronchoscopes is limited by the size of the endoscope and the patient.

Tracheal aspirates from healthy animals usually contain a mixed phagocytic population of cells, including bacteria, and this should not be over-interpreted or assumed to be indicative of lower airway disease. In contrast, fungi observed in tracheal aspirates are usually highly significant.

Respiratory tract lavage is described in Chapter 10.

Direct smears are prepared. If a centrifuge is available, the lavage fluid is gently spun (e.g. 3000 rpm for 3 minutes, depending upon size and angle of rotors) and smears made from the sediment. Samples for bacterial cultures should be taken before contaminating with non-sterile laboratory equipment. Smears from samples containing increased mucus are best made by the pull-apart method and waved rapidly in the air to increase the rate of drying. Special mucolytic agents, available through suppliers to human cytopathology laboratories, can be used to reduce mucus viscosity. Use of mucolytic agents will improve cell recovery but also require the use of alcohol fixation and H&E or trichrome stains.

The flush solution, and any fluid or sediment remaining following centrifugation and immediate slide preparation, is placed into vials containing EDTA for submission to a referral laboratory. Cell morphology tends to deteriorate more quickly when there is a low-protein environment or when bacterial toxins are present. Cell preservatives for use in fluids, such as alcohol, or on slides, require the use of special slide preparation and staining techniques. Their use should be prearranged with the referral laboratory. The morphology of cells on the smears made immediately in the clinic, usually the most representative of the *in vivo* environment, may have a great influence upon the interpretation of cells prepared later in the referral laboratory.

Bronchoalveolar lavage (BAL) techniques (see Chapter 10) allow cells to be obtained directly from specific bronchi, bronchioles and alveoli without being contaminated by cells and bacteria from the upper airway.

INTERNAL ORGANS

Aspirates can be obtained from most internal organs or lesions if palpable or outlined using imaging techniques. With experience, ultrasound-directed aspirates can be made from lesions as small as 0.5 cm. Greater success is expected when there are larger lesions or if there is diffuse organ involvement. A new sterile needle should be used for each repeat aspiration, especially if from vascular organs or lesions, otherwise thromboplastin activation will lead to immediate clotting. Activation of the clotting cascade including proteolytic enzymes interferes with the quality of the sample and the resulting cell harvest and morphology.

Prostate
Several methods have been described for cytological investigation of prostatic disease. The differential diagnosis determined from clinical examination, the equipment available and the experience of the clinician will direct the choice of technique to be used.

Prostatic massage/wash
Prostatic massage is recommended when prostatitis is the primary differential diagnosis. The bladder is catheterized, drained, then flushed with sterile saline. The last 10 ml of fluid is collected as a pre-massage sample. The tip of the catheter is partially withdrawn distal to the prostatic duct, and the prostate is massaged gently per rectum or via the abdomen for a minute or two. Sterile saline (20–30 ml) is injected. The catheter is advanced anteriorly and slowly into the bladder while gently aspirating.

The fluid recovered is placed in a tube containing EDTA. Since this fluid will have a low protein concentration, cells may be fragile. Direct smears should be made immediately if preparation of concentrated smears will be delayed more than a few hours.

Prostate samples may also be obtained by emptying the bladder, introducing a catheter to the level of the prostate and massaging the prostate per rectum whilst applying gentle suction with a syringe.

FNA biopsy
FNA biopsy is preferred when benign prostatic hyperplasia or neoplasia is suspected. If fluid is withdrawn, especially if it is turbid and suggestive of an abscess, the entire contents should be aspirated to reduce potential leakage of septic fluid into the abdomen or pelvic cavity. The technique for FNA biopsy is described above. An 80–150 mm spinal needle can be used for small to medium-sized dogs. A percutaneous caudolateral transabdominal approach is used to reach the prostate while an assistant positions the prostate cranial to the pelvic inlet, using an index finger inserted per rectum. Avoid entering the bladder. Special long guides and needles have been developed for per rectal prostatic aspiration in men. If available these can be adapted for use in larger dogs.

Direct smears are made of aspirated material.

Liver
Fine needle aspirations are obtained while animals are standing or in right lateral recumbency. A 35–80 mm 22 gauge needle is inserted, usually through the 12th to 13th left intercostal space into the liver. If a spinal needle with stillette is used, blockage of the needle prior to entering the liver is prevented. After the liver is entered and the stillette removed, several millilitres of vacuum are applied to the syringe while the needle tip is advanced and withdrawn relative to the body surface. Minimal lateral movement of the needle tip is used to reduce laceration to liver cells and blood vessels. The syringe vacuum is released before the needle tip is allowed to leave the liver. The syringe is filled with air and used to push small drops of aspirated material on to clean glass slides. Smears are made by the drawback and push away method. If samples are obtained using a needle only, the pull-apart method of making smears may be preferable.

Kidney
The kidney is immobilized by being held against the body wall. A 22–25 gauge needle is selected, with the

length determined by the thickness of the body wall. Care should be taken to avoid directing the needle tip into the vascular hilar area when aspirating cortex and medullary regions. If this occurs in error the event will usually be signalled by haemorrhage in the aspirated material followed by blood in voided urine. Direct smears are prepared using the drawback and push away method.

Spleen

General techniques for FNA biopsy are used. It is especially important to discontinue aspiration as soon as blood becomes visible in the tip of the syringe; otherwise, significant cells may become lost through dilution due to the vascularity of this organ. Insertion of a needle without attached syringe may improve the cell harvest. The smears are prepared from the initial material present in the barrel of the needle. Smears are made by the drawback and push away method.

FIXATION AND STAINS

Fixation

For routine Romanowsky staining, air drying without fixation at the time of sampling is all that is required. For wet fixation, required when using trichrome stains, slides are immediately dipped into alcohol or sprayed using a commercial fixative before air-drying of the cells has occurred.

Air-dried cells can be rehydrated in saline, fixed in methanol, and then stained using modified H&E or Papanicolaou staining techniques.

Each slide must be identified as to patient, lesion origin and date. Slides should not be refrigerated because the condensation which forms when they are returned to room temperature will result in lysis of many cells. Slides should not be allowed to contact formalin or formalin fumes as these create chemical changes that result in severe interference with most stains used for cytology.

Stains

Several groups of stains are available for use in the clinic or in the cytology laboratory:

- Romanowsky stains - modified Wright's; May–Grunwald–Giemsa; Leishman's
- Vital stains - new methylene blue; brilliant cresyl blue
- Rapid stains - multiple commercial preparations, e.g. Diff-Quik®
- Trichrome/H&E - Sano's; Papanicolaou; haematoxylin and eosin (H&E)

Most veterinary cytopathologists use one of the Romanowsky variations as the primary stain. Cytoplasm and nuclei are stained with excellent detail. Due to the density of nuclear staining only a single layer of cells can be examined satisfactorily. The stains are permanent. Different types and sources of Romanowsky stains vary in tinctorial properties and nuclear and cytoplasmic density. This will affect the appearance of some cells and blood parasites.

Vital stains, i.e. water-based, allow immediate staining of air-dried smears in the clinic. Nuclear detail is good. Cytoplasmic detail is poor except for fungal organisms and some parasites. The stained slides are not permanent.

Rapid stains are generally adequate for in-clinic use if the user is familiar with the staining characteristics of different cells within the species. Nuclear detail is usually less distinct. The rapid stains vary markedly in staining, especially for cytoplasmic inclusions such as mast cell granules and intracellular parasites.

Trichrome stains are used on cells that have been immediately alcohol-fixed, i.e. wet-fixed, either by dipping or spraying. This must be accomplished within fractions of a second or cell appearance and staining characteristics will be altered. Trichrome stains provide excellent nuclear detail. Cytoplasmic clearing and clumping of nuclear chromatin allow examination of cells at varying depths within dense clusters. Cytoplasmic inclusions are poorly stained but keratinization is readily apparent, assisting differentiation of squamous epithelial cells. Air-dried cells stained with H&E have poor nuclear and cytoplasmic detail. Variable success has been reported if air-dried cells are rehydrated, alcohol-fixed and stained using one of the H&E, Papanicolaou or even Diff-Quik® stains.

Cell diameter and nuclear:cytoplasmic ratio is altered significantly by the type of fixation. Thus, if air-dried cells are compared to the appearance of a fried egg, alcohol-fixed cells would be comparable to parboiled eggs, while histological sections would be as slices through a hard boiled egg. Descriptions of cell size and morphological changes must take into account the method of cell fixation.

All methods of cell fixation and staining create artefacts which may be apparent in cells or in the background. Stain precipitate, water and ruptured cell contents produce artefacts that can lead to serious misinterpretation by the inexperienced examiner. Use of clean glass slides, routine filtering of stains, adequate washing during staining procedures and fast drying following staining will prevent most common artefacts. Bacteria and fungi can contaminate and grow in some stains. Fungi can grow on slides stored in humid conditions. Strict adherence to the stain manufacturers' recommendations is advisable to avoid diagnostic disasters.

The cytologist must be familiar with the effects of fixation and staining on cell morphology in order to be able to identify origin of cells from different tissues and species and to be able to differentiate cell activity, i.e. whether benign or malignant.

CYTOLOGICAL INTERPRETATION

Microscopic techniques

A high quality, clean and properly adjusted microscope is mandatory. An integrated light source is recommended that can provide adequate light for examination of individual densely stained cells. A range of lenses are required which allow: low-power screening for areas of interest, e.g. 15–20X magnification; higher magnification for examination of cell types and morphology, e.g. 40–60X magnification; and a very high magnification for study of detail within cells, e.g. 100X magnification. Flat field lenses, especially for the high dry (40–60X) and oil magnifications (100X), allow the entire field to be viewed in the same focal plane. Correct adjustment of the condenser diaphragm is essential. If the condenser is lowered to examine urine sediment or faecal flotations, it is crucial that it is readjusted to the correct level when used to examine cytological or haematological preparations.

Coverslips must be used with high dry lenses to reduce light distortion and allow visualization of the smallest cellular details that can be detected by a light microscope. A drop of immersion oil, or permanent mounting medium, is placed upon the stained glass slide prior to applying the coverslip. Air bubbles should be removed by applying gently pressure to the coverslip. Also, immersion oil is placed between the coverslip and lens when using the oil objective (X100). The objective should be wiped gently to remove oil following use.

Labelled glass slides can be stored for reference purposes. Permanent mounting medium must be allowed to dry as directed by the manufacturer. Oil can be gently removed using a tissue prior to storage.

Principles of interpretation

Cytological interpretation will usually fall into one of the following categories:

- A definitive diagnosis, such as an abscess or a specific type of tumour
- A morphological diagnosis, such as mixed septic inflammation or poorly differentiated sarcoma
- Ruling out one or more accompanying clinical differential diagnoses
- No interpretation (e.g. because of an inadequate sample).

Either of the first three categories will provide clinical direction and possibly prognosis. Interpretation follows a sequential approach as per Figure 7.5. Knowledge of the cytological appearance of various cell types from normal tissues is necessary. Identification of cell origin is based primarily upon cytoplasmic morphology and less upon nuclear criteria. Immature cells, i.e. anaplastic cells, have less cyto-

plasmic differentiation, making identification of family origin more difficult. Epithelial cells tend to be round to oval, with distinct cytoplasmic outlines, and often have common adjoining borders. Epithelial cells of glandular origin contain cytoplasmic secretory vacuoles and may present as an acinar arrangement. Stromal cells tend to be elongated and have poorly defined cytoplasmic borders, e.g. spindle cells such as fibrocytes. Many cells contain pigments which assist identification of cell origin; commonly observed examples are melanocytes, melanophages, mast cells, granular lymphocytes, hepatocytes, macrophages with haemosiderin, lining cells in CSF, goblet cells, cells of glandular origin and squamous epithelial cells. With experience most of these cells can be readily identified. Special stains may be used to confirm initial impressions or may be required to differentiate the origin of some types of cell.

The cytopathologist and the clinician must understand the risks associated with false-negative and false-positive diagnoses. If a probability can be attached to a likely diagnosis, this information should be shared.

Inflammation

Examination and interpretation of the predominance, or mixture, of cells usually leads to the classification of a lesion as inflammatory or non-inflammatory. Inflammatory responses are classified according to the predominant cells, even though a mixture is usually present. If neutrophils predominate, various terms are used such as neutrophilic, purulent or suppurative inflammation. If monocytes and macrophages predominate, the term 'mixed mononuclear inflammation' may be used. The predominance and mixture of cells present provides an indication of the cytokine chemotactic influences present and thus potential aetiologies.

The terms active, chronic–active and chronic inflammation are also used by cytopathologists. Active inflammation is indicated by a predominance of neutrophils, chronic–active inflammation by an approximately equal mixture of neutrophils and monocytes/macrophages, and chronic inflammation by a predominance of macrophages. These classifications are intended to indicate the underlying process, *not* to reflect duration. These terms were initially borrowed from histopathology but are no longer used by many cytopathologists due to the marked differences in definition when used by histopathologists, cytopathologists and clinicians. Histopathologists require tissue architecture to diagnose chronic inflammation. This is unavailable to cytopathologists. Neutrophils may predominate in lesions present for weeks to months. The cytopathologist and clinician must be aware of the definition of terms used when writing and interpreting diagnostic reports.

When phagocytic cells predominate, especially if there is a supporting clinical history, careful examina-

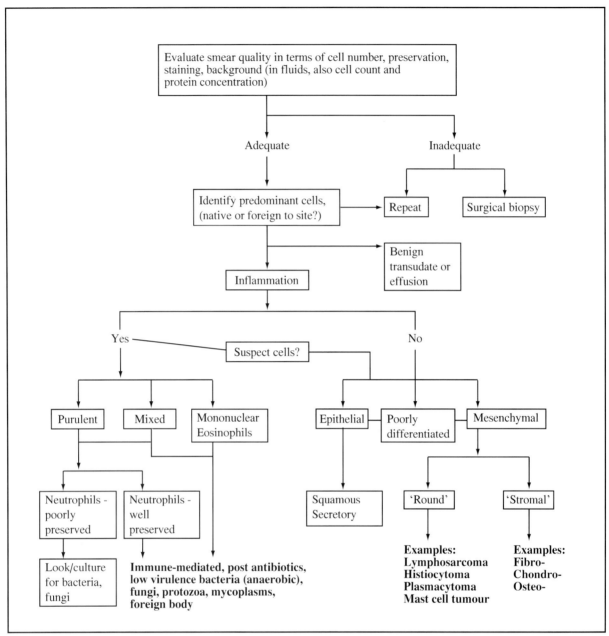

Figure 7.5: A basic approach to the interpretation of cytology smears.

tion is made for infectious agents (Figures 7.6 and 7.7). Most infectious agents induce cytokine production and chemotaxis of phagocytic cells. Different species of bacteria produce toxins with varying degrees of virulence. Nuclear degeneration occurs with normal ageing of neutrophils but is markedly enhanced in the presence of many bacterial toxins. When there is neutrophilic inflammation, the degree of nuclear degeneration is noted. The greater the degenerative changes, especially chromatolysis, the greater the effort indicated to determine whether bacteria are present. A marked mixed or neutrophilic response with only mild to moderate nuclear degeneration and the presence of many free and phagocytized pleomorphic bacteria requires investigation of anaerobic aetiology. Special techniques are required for transportation and culture of anaerobic bacteria.

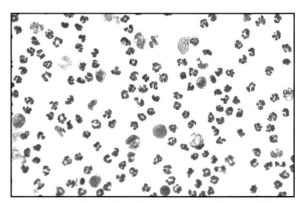

Figure 7.6: Sediment from CSF containing dense, mildly degenerate neutrophils and a few mononuclear cells. The apparent pleocytosis must be related to the concentration method used or, preferably, confirmed using a chamber count. Close examination and culture for infectious agents are required. Wright's.

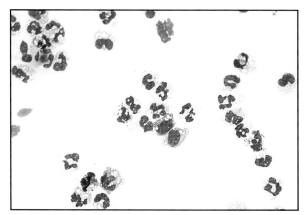

Figure 7.7: Higher-magnification view of a different area of the sediment smear in Figure 7.6. Cells are spread to a larger diameter on the glass. Neutrophil nuclei have lost the filaments separating their lobules due to chromatolysis, further indicating a need to search for infectious agents. Cytoplasmic vacuolation is a non-specific change observed frequently in cells within a fluid environment. Some monocytes/macrophages are present. A few indistinct bacteria are present indicating septic meningitis. Wright's.

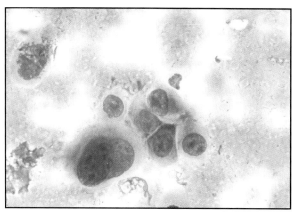

Figure 7.8: High-power view of squamous cell carcinoma. The cells have exfoliated in a small sheet and have well defined cell borders typical of epithelial cells. Perinuclear prekeratin is an important observation readily apparent with alcohol fixation and trichrome or H&E staining but not with Romanowsky stains. The prominent nucleoli in non-secretory epithelial cells and the marked anisokaryosis are important criteria supporting malignancy. Note the lysed cells in the background. Giemsa.

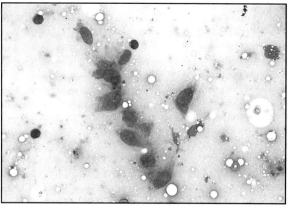

Figure 7.9: Single cells with round to elongated nuclei, prominent nucleoli and anisokaryosis, and basophilic, thin, irregularly shaped cytoplasm with indistinct borders, suggesting early spindle cells typical for poorly differentiated stromal/mesenchymal sarcoma. Wright's.

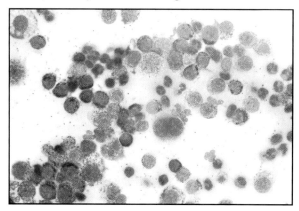

Figure 7.10: There is a mixture of intact and ruptured round cells. Even at this magnification (X400 objective), the low to moderate number of intracytoplasmic and free metachromatic granules identify many cells as mast cells. The sparse granulation, anisokaryosis and binucleation of a central cell would suggest a high-grade mast cell neoplasm. Trauma and corticosteroids will also reduce amount and appearance of granulation. Giemsa .

Inflammation may be reported as being non-septic, possibly septic, or septic, on the basis of neutrophil numbers, nuclear morphology and the presence of bacteria. If there is marked neutrophil predominance and nuclear degeneration without visible bacteria, the cytopathologist should recommend culturing for bacteria. *Mycoplasma* organisms generate a strong neutrophilic response with minimal nuclear degeneration. Prior use of antibiotics must be taken into consideration.

Inflammation and neoplasia may coexist. Hyperplasia and neoplasia may be very difficult to differentiate in the presence of infection.

Neoplasia

If inflammatory cells are not present, the origin of the most significant cell type is categorized as to family, apparent stage(s) of differentiation and whether indicative of hyperplasia, or benign or malignant neoplasia.

The primary objective, in addition to diagnosing the type of tumour, is to predict the expected biological behaviour or response to therapy. Most cell types can become benign or malignant tumours, although one will predominate usually for a species. The traditional nomenclature for benign tumours of epithelial or mesenchymal cells is to add the suffix 'oma' to the differentiated cell, e.g. adenomas for a benign tumour of epithelial cells. Malignant tumours of squamous or glandular epithelial cells are classified as squamous cell carcinoma (Figure 7.8) or adenocarcinoma, respectively. Malignant mesenchymal (stromal) cells are called sarcomas (Figure 7.9). Cytopathologists identify a group of readily differentiated tumours often categorized as 'round cell tumours'; most, but not all, are mesenchymal in origin. These include mast cell tumours (Figure 7.10), histiocytomas, lymphosarcomas (Figure 7.11), and transmissible venereal tumours.

If the cell type is adequately differentiated and characteristic nuclear changes are present, many tumours can be identified and classified using cytological techniques (Figure 7.12). For some cell types with early cytoplasmic differentiation, architecture may assist histopathological examination and classification. Poorly differentiated tumours, i.e. anaplastic cells, may require use of all available methods of examination for classification; cellular criteria for malignancy do not always correlate with biological behaviour. In canine mammary tumours invasion of tumour cells has a high predictive value of expected behaviour and metastases may be readily apparent in draining lymph nodes.

Nuclear criteria are used primarily to differentiate malignant from benign cells. The nuclear criteria expected for benign normal cells depend upon the cell type, stage of differentiation and cell division, growth or secretory activity. Nucleoli number, size and shape are noted. Chromatin patterns are observed and classified as fine, coarse or inapparent, depending upon cell activity. Nuclear moulding and nuclear:cytoplasmic ratio (n:c ratio) are noted. Artefactual effects of fixation and staining must be understood. Alcohol (wet) fixation creates characteristic artefacts that are not apparent when cells are air-dried. Each cell type has its own 'normal' appearance. Benign small lymphocytes have much higher n:c ratios than large lymphocytes. Nuclear size and n:c ratio decrease as normal squamous epithelial cells differentiate from parabasal,

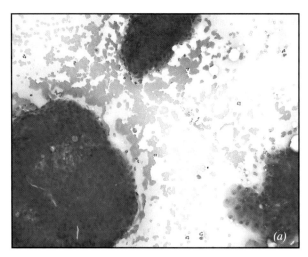

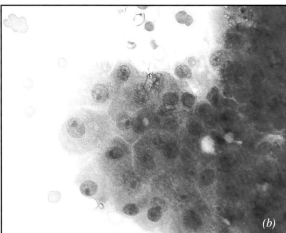

Figure 7.12: Large dense clusters of round cells are seen at low magnification (a). At higher magnification (b), individual round cells with large central nuclei, single prominent nucleoli and abundant pale, finely granular cytoplasm suggestive of hepatocytes are seen . These cells are typical for perianal (hepatoid) tumour. Wright's.

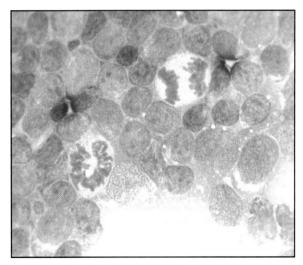

Figure 7.11: This high-power view of feline renal lymphosarcoma shows two mitotic figures surrounded by homogenous lymphocytes with high n:c ratios, prominent chromocenters and inapparent nucleoli. Lymphocyte size cannot be readily determined without the presence of erythrocytes in the field. Origin, homogeneity and appearance of lymphocytes strongly supports lymphosarcoma. No one morphological feature alone, including mitotic figures, is pathognomonic for neoplasia. Giemsa.

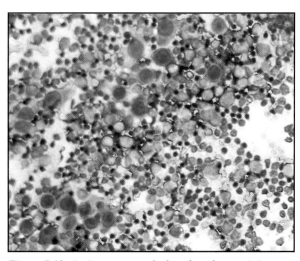

Figure 7.13: Aspirate smear of a lymph node containing pleomorphic lymphocytes and a prominent population of large round cells with large dark nuclei. These cells are obviously foreign to this location, i.e. non-lymphoid, and indicate metastasis. Wright's-Giemsa.

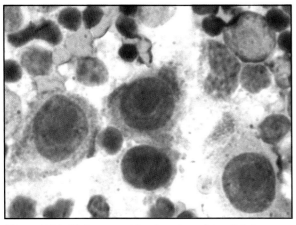

Figure 7.14: Higher-magnification view of the slide in Figure 7.13. There is a background of pleomorphic lymphocytes and red cells. The three very large angular cells, several erythrocytes in diameter, have abundant basophilic granular cytoplasm and very large hyperchromatic nuclei with prominent single nucleoli. Based upon the morphology at low and high magnification, these cells appear to be poorly differentiated epithelial cells and confirm metastasis of a probable carcinoma. A primary site should be investigated, if not already apparent to the clinician. Wright's–Giemsa .

through intermediate, to superficial stages. In comparison for each stage of differentiation, malignant cells tend to have larger and hyperchromatic nuclei, higher n:c ratio, larger, prominent, possibly multiple, variable sized nucleoli, and nuclear moulding.

Cell size can be an important criterion for diagnosis of neoplasia and is estimated most readily by comparison with erythrocytes. The observed cell size is compared with expected cell size.

SPECIFIC LESIONS AND SITES

Indications for the use of cytological techniques and the expected observations for common lesions are described below. Additional details regarding physical guidelines for sampling site and additional indications for cytological investigation are included in various chapters within this manual.

Superficial and subcutaneous masses
In dogs and cats, any discrete mass that is palpable or can be delineated on imaging is highly amenable to cytological diagnosis. Benign superficial lesions that are diagnosed with a high degree of reliability include seromas, haematomas, abscesses and inclusion cysts. Commonly encountered and readily diagnosed tumours include mast cell tumours, lipomas, histiocytomas, melanomas/melanosarcomas, secretory and non-secretory epithelial tumours, and many mesenchymal (stromal) tumours. The slides must contain an adequate number of well preserved representative cells. The reliability of the interpretation will then depend upon the experience of the microscopist as well as the

availability of history and the description of the lesion or differential diagnoses.

When lesions are ulcerated and infected, aspirates from within the mass are preferable to imprints and scrapings. Infected tumours may be difficult to differentiate from primary inflammatory lesions that have associated dysplastic cells.

Cytological investigation is particularly useful when investigating potential recurrence of tumours, both at primary and distant sites, as well as for metastasis to local lymph nodes.

Submandibular masses and swellings
Submandibular lesions most frequently involve the salivary glands, thyroid glands and lymph nodes. Salivary lesions are common in dogs. Aspirate smears from sialocoeles contain a characteristic amorphous blue material and medium to large mononuclear cells with low n:c ratios and variable degrees of cytoplasmic vacuolation. If infected, phagocytic cells and bacteria may be visible. Sialocoeles can be readily differentiated from thyroid masses. In highly vascular lesions, such as thyroid tumours, if the needle is inserted without using an attached syringe, there may be less dilution by blood of the principal cells. Thyroid adenoma aspirates appear very similar to well differentiated carcinomas.

Lymph nodes
Cytological examination of enlarged lymph nodes is usually very rewarding, leading to differentiation of inflammation, hyperplasia and the majority of primary and secondary neoplasias. Infectious agents are readily observed in some cases.

Good technique is required to obtain adequate intact representative cells, and when there is generalized lymphadenopathy multiple lymph nodes should be sampled. The cells usually exfoliate readily in fine needle aspirates but it is important that the needle tip is directed to sample both cortical and medullary regions of the node. The major technical challenge is to transfer the aspirated material and spread it in a thin layer on to a glass slide with a high percentage of intact cells. Cat lymphocytes are especially fragile. Use of minimal vacuum, gentle touch, speed and a trial of various spreading techniques may increase the percentage of intact cells. The pull-apart method, the 'showerburst' or gentle 'spraying' of cells on to the glass slide, and the coverslip method have all been recommended. It is important that the cells are air-dried immediately. Romanowsky-type stains are preferred for examination of lymph node aspirates.

Details of lymph node lesions are addressed in Chapter 12. An aspirate smear from a normal lymph node should contain a pleomorphic population of small, medium and large lymphocytes, very few macrophages and no neutrophils. Low numbers of plasma cells and mast cells may be seen in normal lymph nodes.

In dogs FNA biopsies are commonly and reliably used to identify the cause of enlarged lymph nodes. Lymphadenitis due to bacterial infection is rare in mature dogs but more common in younger animals. Cytologically it is characterized by an increase in neutrophils and/or macrophages. Lymph nodes in which benign hyperplasia is present contain pleomorphic lymphocytes, commonly with an increase in plasma cells. When lymphadenopathy is due to allergic skin disease, benign hyperplasia is commonly accompanied by eosinophilic lymphadenitis. Lymphosarcoma, which can reliably be diagnosed cytologically in dogs, is commonly associated with a monomorphic cell population as distinct from many other tissues in which other criteria of malignancy apply. In cases of generalized lymphadenopathy, multiple lymph nodes should be sampled, avoiding very soft lymph nodes which commonly contain necrotic areas as these have poor cell morphology. Corticosteroid lympholytic activity may lead to a reduction in size of lymph nodes and produce marked changes in lymphocyte morphology. It is important that the cytologist is informed of such treatment.

In cats FNA biopsies of enlarged lymph nodes are also a useful diagnostic procedure. However, the difficulty in obtaining quality samples together with subtle differences between the cytological appearances of some pathological processes makes diagnosis less straightforward.

Perianal lesions

Perianal lesions are readily palpable and accessible to aspiration biopsy. Perianal sac abscesses characteristically contain active inflammatory cells together with glandular debris. Benign hyperplasia and adenomas of the perianal (hepatoid) gland contain typical large cells resembling hepatocytes (see Figure 7.12) and a few small dark basal reserve cells. Differentiation of hyperplasia and adenoma is arbitrary on histopathology and may not be possible using cytology. Increased reserve cells, mitotic figures and prominence of nucleoli, and decreased differentiation of the hepatoid cells increases probability of carcinoma. Invasiveness, the only unequivocal criteria for perianal gland carcinoma, and many other types of carcinoma, can only be determined using histopathology.

Carcinoma involving the apocrine glands of the anal sac may contain cuboidal to columnar cells in tubular or acinar arrangements with increased mitotic figures. Anaplastic perianal gland carcinomas may be impossible to differentiate from solid apocrine carcinomas, even on histopathological examination. Serum hypercalcaemia or demonstration of parathyroid-like hormone immunohistochemistry would indicate apocrine carcinoma.

Cavity fluids

Sample collection, handling and the principles of interpretation are discussed above. Some additional procedures are described below for specific cavities. In each case cells are counted or estimated and examined on direct or concentrated smears and classified as to type and morphology. Inflammatory changes are observed with sepsis and with necrosis. Protein is estimated using a refractometer except where lipids are increased, as with a ruptured thoracic duct, or where concentration is expected to be very low, as in cerebrospinal fluid samples. Fluid is examined to determine if there is haemorrhage, inflammation (with or without infection), or if there are exfoliating tumour cells present.

Traditionally, abdominal and thoracic fluids without an increase in cells or protein concentration are called transudates. If either cells or protein are increased, the fluid is classified as a modified transudate. If both are increased the fluid is classified as an exudate. The increase in protein and the type of cells is used to estimate the degree of vascular damage or chemotactic stimulation and thus the extent and type of inflammation. This may suggest the aetiology. Transudates contain little to no fibrinogen. If clotting occurs when fluid is collected without anticoagulant, this suggests that fibrinogen is increased. The fibrinogen concentration will also be increased when inflammation or vascular leakage is present. Fluid must be submitted using the appropriate anticoagulant required for the method used in the referral laboratory.

Abdominal and thoracic fluid

Mesothelial hyperplasia is a very common response to fluid accumulation within the abdominal or thoracic cavity or when there is stimulation from an underlying tumour mass. Exfoliation of single cells and clusters is common. Many cytological criteria of malignancy, as used for most types of cells, are observed routinely in benign hyperplastic mesothelial cells, i.e. anisokaryosis, high nuclear:cytoplasmic ratio, hyperchromasia, multiple nuclei, multiple and large nucleoli, and increased mitoses. Hyperplastic mesothelial cells may often mislead inexperienced cytologists into diagnosing neoplasia. The morphological changes caused by hyperplasia require careful attention when using cytology to identify or differentiate benign and malignant mesothelial proliferations. Unexplained ascitic fluid with a marked increase in the number and arrangement of mesothelial cells alone may be the primary indicators of the rare mesothelial tumours observed *ante mortem*.

Total protein, albumin, globulin, creatinine, amylase, cholesterol and triglyceride concentrations may be helpful, depending upon differential diagnoses being considered. The ratio of abdominal fluid to serum concentrations of amylase and creatinine are useful indicators of pancreatitis and uroperitoneum, respectively.

Transudates are more commonly associated with hypoproteinaemia, cardiac or hepatic insufficiency and neoplasia in early stages.

Fluids are categorized as haemorrhagic if they have a typical red appearance or significant erythrocytes are present. Fluid can appear grossly similar to blood even if erythrocytes contribute less than 3% by volume. Packed cell volume (PCV) determination will identify the concentration of intact erythrocytes. If many red cells have lysed, haemoglobin concentration may be more reliable. Sediment smears may appear similar to peripheral blood following haemorrhage (Figure 7.15)

Turbid fluids require investigation for lipid content as an indicator of lymphatic leakage secondary to trauma, inflammation or neoplasia. These fluids do not become clear following centrifugation unless the turbidity is solely due to cells or chylomicrons. Fluids are categorized as being chylous or non-chylous, based upon the degree of lipid increase, i.e. whether triglyceride concentration is above or below 1 g/l (100 mg/100 ml). The term pseudochylous is no longer considered to be a useful category. There is considerable overlap in the lesions associated with non-chylous and chylous effusions. Cytological examination will indicate if inflammatory or neoplastic cells are present.

Direct or concentrated stained smears are examined for cell types and appearance. The degree of haemorrhage cannot be reliably determined from examination of concentrated cell preparations. This must be determined from the aspirated fluid since a background of erythrocytes will be present in most concentrated smears. Recent haemorrhage is indicated by the presence of erythrocytophagia. Macrophages containing diffuse blue-black to golden pigment indicate previous haemorrhage. Bile may appear as diffuse free or phagocytized tan to brown pigment. Haemoglobin and bile pigments may both be present if there is bile duct leakage and haemorrhage following abdominal trauma.

Inflammatory fluids are categorized as to degree and type, dependent upon the concentration of neutrophils and macrophages present. When neutrophils are significantly increased, nuclear morphology is examined for degenerative changes. Bacterial toxins are associated with increased nuclear lytic changes, especially if aerobic species are present.

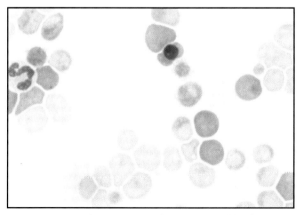

Figure 7.15: High-power view of a peripheral blood smear. Note the polychromatic and nucleated red cells in this responsive anaemia case. Giemsa.

Anaerobic bacteria induce marked mixed phagocytic cell chemotaxis but nuclear degeneration is less apparent. Bacteria are usually visible if they are the causative agents, although antibiotic therapy may reduce their concentration. Free bile and haemoglobin pigments are associated with chemotaxis of phagocytic cells.

A disappointingly low percentage of abdominal and thoracic tumours exfoliate into the corresponding cavity fluids. Differentiation of very hyperplastic mesothelial cells, mesothelioma and exfoliating carcinomas can be difficult and requires integration of all information obtained from ancillary examinations.

Synovial fluid

In dogs and cats the volume of synovial fluid limits the number of tests that can be performed. Routinely, two or three direct smears can be made from one or more drops of synovial fluid. Nucleated cell count and protein concentration are the next priorities. Synovial fluid from healthy joints contains a low concentration of nucleated cells; mean count <1 x 10^9 cells per litre, with an upper reference limit for larger joints of 3 x 10^9/l. The nucleated cells are predominantly mononuclear, usually with few neutrophils and no active macrophages. The upper limit for protein concentration depends upon whether determination is made using a refractometer, or using biochemical methods. The mucin clot test and fibrinogen concentration can be determined if there is sufficient volume of synovial fluid. The mucin clot test is used to estimate hyaluronic acid polymerization. One part of synovial fluid is added to 4 parts of 2.5% glacial acetic acid. In normal synovial fluid a tight clump is produced. With decreasing polymerization or concentration of hyaluronic acid, the clot is less tight or may be limited to loose flocculent material. Some referral laboratories can determine hyaluronic acid concentration.

Cytological examination can provide useful information to assist differentiation of haemorrhage, trauma, suppuration (with or without sepsis), degeneration and immune-mediated arthritis. Neoplastic lesions involving the synovial cavity are rare but if suspected the basic cytological diagnostic approach may be applied.

Haemorrhage associated with trauma is indicated by the presence of increased erythrocytes, active erythrocytophagia, and haemoglobin- or haemosiderin-containing macrophages depending upon the time interval. A marked increase in neutrophils, e.g. >30-50 x10^9/l, is indicative of either sepsis or immune-mediated disease. If septic, apparent nuclear degenerative changes and bacteria may be visible. With immune-mediated disease neutrophil nuclei will show ageing changes but are relatively well preserved. With degenerative lesions there is a mild to moderate increase in a mixed population of predominantly monocytes/macrophages, possibly with plasma cells and synoviocytes. Synovial cells may appear as single cells or in clusters, often poorly preserved, with continuous adjoining borders, i.e. in contrast to the appearance of aggregated macrophages that have 'windows' between adjoining cells.

Mammary lesions

Mammary lesions in dogs and cats can be readily aspirated, allowing cytological examination; even if the lesions are ossified or densely fibrous, a few representative cells can be harvested. Multiple aspirates should be obtained, especially where there are several or very large lesions. Both the fluid and surrounding walls of cystic lesions should be examined.

In the bitch, bacterial mastitis and focal abscesses are identified by a marked increased in neutrophils and bacteria. Cysts may be benign or associated with neoplasia and hence it is essential to sample adjacent solid tissue. The fluid may contain macrophages with blue-green cytoplasmic pigment.

Few studies have compared the histological and cytological classification of canine mammary tumours and hence prediction of their biological behaviour may be imprecise following FNA or surgical biopsies. A complete accompanying history and lesion description, combined with careful and experienced cytological examination, can be used to diagnose many mammary neoplasms with rare false-positive diagnoses if strict criteria are adhered to. However, the sensitivity and specificity of cytology is not as high for canine mammary neoplasms as it is for some other tumours such as canine lymphosarcoma.

Mammary tumours also occur in cats, with 80–90% being malignant. Fibroadenomatous hyperplasia appears following progesterone treatment, pregnancy or ovariohysterectomy and during pseudopregnancy. Together with a complete history, the cytological criteria usually allow reliable differentiation of hyperplasia from malignant tumours in cats.

On palpation, lesions of mammary glands can be confused with steatitis, *Mycobacterium* infection, inguinal lymph nodes and various tumours including lipomas, mast cell and skin tumours. Examination of cytological aspirates can be used to differentiate these lesions.

Internal lesions

Thoracic lesions

Thoracic lesions can be aspirated for cytological examination. Imaging should be used to guide the needle tip for aspirating small or focal lesions. Blind aspiration techniques are best reserved for large lesions or diffuse pulmonary pathology. Although FNA has a higher percentage of success than bronchoalveolar lavage for most lesions that can be outlined using imaging techniques, all potential methods may have to used before obtaining representative cells. If a general anaesthetic is used for obtaining a fine needle aspirate,

a bronchoalveolar lavage should be obtained at the same time.

Many inflammatory and neoplastic lesions can be diagnosed from cytology preparations but it is crucial that all pertinent clinical information is integrated into the final decision. A marked predominance of neutrophils, especially if accompanied by bacteria, or of eosinophils, is a characteristic observation for inflammatory lesions. Although small nodules may be difficult to aspirate and to interpret, some lesions can be identified with confidence. Primary tumours occur less frequently than metastatic tumours of the canine lung. Both may be identifiable as abnormal and, unless too anaplastic, may be classified as to cell type. Thymic lesions, in particular lymphosarcoma, may be diagnosed by direct FNA biopsy. General principles for the diagnosis of lymphosarcoma apply, as for lymph nodes.

Liver

Hepatic lipidosis and cholestasis are readily identified from fine needle aspirates. An increase in inflammatory cells, including neutrophils and plasma cells, suggests inflammatory disease but diagnostic sensitivity and specificity are relatively low. Architecture, required for identification of many types of liver lesions, cannot be assessed using cytology. Necrosis and nodular regeneration may be suspect from the heterogeneous appearance of hepatocytes combined with focal cholestasis and possibly inflammatory cells.

Diffuse metastatic tumours have a high probability for harvest and can be readily identified as abnormal for the location. For example, lymphocyte concentration and morphology allow ready identification of diffuse lymphosarcoma. Hepatocellular tumours are rare and not easily identified since the tumour cells have only subtle changes in morphology suggesting malignancy. Sampling success will limit the ability to identify focal neoplastic lesions.

Spleen

Normal splenic architecture and cell content must be considered when examining aspirate smears. Generalized splenomegaly is the primary stimulus for aspiration cytology examination. Extramedullary haemopoiesis, readily observed by the presence of increased nucleated erythrocytes, may be physiological or simulated by increased nucleated erythrocytes within vascular tumours such as haemangiomas/sarcomas. In cats, identification of increased mast cells and thus diagnosis of a visceral mast cell tumour is usually straightforward. Similarly, *Ehrlichia* and *Leishmania* organisms can be readily detected. Lymphosarcoma can usually be confirmed if representative cells have been harvested. As expected, diffuse or large tumours have increased probability of representative cell harvest. The ability to rule out an alternative diagnosis is high but the ability to confirm vascular tumours is low, in the experience of the authors.

Prostate

In prostatic abscesses large numbers of neutrophils and bacteria are present, while in cysts there is low to moderate cellularity with a mononuclear/macrophage predominance but no bacteria. As in other organs, cell size, n:c ratio and nuclear criteria are used in conjunction with all pertinent clinical information to differentiate benign from malignant cells.

Gastrointestinal lesions

Oral cavity lesions vary markedly in cell type, necessitating the use of different sampling techniques in order to obtain representative cells. Melanomas and carcinomas usually exfoliate adequately with FNA. Lesions containing well differentiated stromal cells, such as epulides, exfoliate very poorly. Scrapings may provide adequate cells from ulcerated lesions. Oral and extraoral eosinophilic lesions in cats are commonly diagnosed using cytology.

Gastric lesions may be investigated using cytological preparations made from gastric washes or brushings. Cellular constituents, including eosinophils, and the presence of organisms can be readily observed. To examine tissue architecture, surgical biopsy by endoscopy (see Chapter 8) and histopathology are required.

Intestinal masses may be aspirated using percutaneous FNA if they are palpable or can be outlined using imaging techniques.

Rectal scraping smears have been used to examine for the presence and types of inflammatory cells, for neoplasia and for estimating numbers of clostridial spores.

Musculoskeletal

FNA biopsies from bony lesions can be obtained directly or via holes drilled into the lesion (see Chapter 11).

Osteosarcomas, chondrosarcomas and fibrosarcomas each have characteristic cells but interpretation must consider sample quality and clinical information. Healing lesions, such as post-fracture callus formation, can be difficult to differentiate from changes of malignancy because of the morphological appearance of rapidly dividing and immature cells which are common to regenerating tissue. Aspirates should be obtained from multiple areas as focal necrosis within rapidly growing tumours may be difficult to distinguish from osteomyelitis.

Tumours of striated and smooth muscle are uncommon. Muscle cell origin can be readily identified but differentiation between hyperplasia and neoplasia may be difficult by cytology alone. Cell origin is identified by the presence of striations in elongated cells.

Body orifices

Nasal cavity

Cytological examination of nasal discharges or swabs from the nasal canal is commonly unrewarding. Septic inflammation may occur in association with neoplasia, foreign bodies and fungal infections. In fungal infections and neoplasia a positive finding is meaningful but negative cytology is of limited significance. Commonly more invasive biopsy techniques are required to diagnose neoplasia and ancillary tests needed to confirm mycotic infections.

Eye

Conjunctival discharges are recommended frequently in textbooks for cytological examination. Acquisition of swabs and scraping techniques have been described. These types of samples may be useful in early clinical stages of disease, e.g. where there is chlamydial infection. Most often, however, examination is initiated in later stages and following polypharmaceutical treatment. At this time, due to time and treatment effects, identification of primary disease or aetiology is frequently not possible.

Ear

Aural discharges are examined for inflammatory response and potential infectious agents such as *Malassezia* yeasts and bacteria. Fine needle aspirates are recommended to investigate discrete aural masses.

Vagina

Cytological smears may be used to investigate vaginal discharges and to assist in the staging of oestrus. Moistened swabs and a gentle rolling technique are used to transfer intact cells to the glass slide. If water, rather than isotonic saline, is used to moisten the swab, the hypotonic effects of water will lyse erythrocytes which may otherwise obscure significant cells, especially during pro-oestrus. There is increased use of serial hormone tests and decreasing use of vaginal cytology for staging oestrus in the bitch.

FURTHER READING AND REFERENCES

Cowell RL and Tyler RD (1989) *Diagnostic Cytology of the Dog and Cat.* American Veterinary Publications, Goleta, California

Duncan JR, Prasse KW and Mahaffey EA (1994) Cytology. In: *Veterinary Laboratory Medicine: Clinical Pathology, 3rd edn*, ed. JR Duncan *et al.*, pp 204–228. Iowa State University Press, Ames

Ettinger S J (1994) *Textbook of Veterinary Internal Medicine, 3rd edn.* W B Saunders, Philadelphia

Fournel-Fleury C, Magnol J-P and Guelfi J-F (1994) *Color Atlas of Cancer Cytology of the Dog and Cat.* Conférence Nationale des Vétérinaires Specialisés en Petits Animaux, Paris

Jacobs RM (1988) Diagnostic cytology. *Seminars in Veterinary Medicine and Surgery (Small Animal)* 3 (2), 83–182

Moulton JE (1990) *Tumours in Domestic Animals, 3rd edn.* University of California Press, Berkeley

Perman V, Alsaker RD and Riis RC (1979) *Cytology of the Dog and Cat.* American Animal Hospital Association, South Bend, Indiana

Rebar AH (1980) *Handbook of Veterinary Cytology.* Ralston Purina, St Louis

PART TWO

Solving Clinical Problems with Laboratory Investigations

CHAPTER EIGHT

Gastrointestinal System and Exocrine Pancreas

James W. Simpson

INTRODUCTION

Disorders of the alimentary tract are very common in small animal practice and range from life-threatening conditions, such as gastric torsions and haemorrhagic gastroenteritis, to chronic disorders, such as exocrine pancreatic insufficiency (EPI) and constipation. Consequently the clinician may be faced with the need to decide whether to instigate immediate treatment and/or carry out a more searching investigation. The inaccessability of the alimentary tract to detailed physical examination further frustrates the clinician in reaching a diagnosis and has led to the development of sophisticated non-invasive diagnostic procedures such as endoscopy, ultrasonography and dynamic tests.

In acute disease there is little time to carry out a thorough investigation as immediate symptomatic therapy is usually required. Where chronic disease is suspected, more time is required to permit a detailed investigation in order that a definitive diagnosis may be reached and specific therapy provided. Many of the new tests rely heavily on modern technology which permits the non-invasive collection of diagnostic information.

The aim of this chapter is to provide the clinician with information regarding the latest procedures that may be used in the diagnosis of alimentary tract disease; it will also review some older tests. Some of these new procedures may only be available at referral centres because of cost or technical difficulty, while others can easily be carried out in veterinary practices. The chapter has been approached from the point of view of procedures rather than disease. The types of test that may be of value for the common alimentary 'syndromes' are summarized in Figure 8.1. The reader can review the types of test recommended and then refer to the text for information on methodology and interpretation of test results.

Dysphagia and regurgitation
- Collect a history and conduct a thorough physical examination
- Complete a neurological examination
- Observe the patient eating, to assess the likely stage of the swallowing process affected
- Plain radiography of pharynx and oesophagus
- Possible contrast studies - barium swallow and fluoroscopy
- Examination of oral cavity and pharynx under general anaesthesia
- Endoscopic examination of pharynx and oesophagus

Vomiting
- Collect a history and conduct a thorough physical examination
- Characterize the vomitus produced
- Is the vomiting primary or secondary?

PRIMARY	*SECONDARY*
Haematology and biochemistry	Haematology and biochemistry
Plain radiography	Urinalysis
Contrast studies	Specific tests of organ function
Endoscopy/ exploratory laparotomy	

Diarrhoea
- Collect a history and conduct a thorough physical examination
- Physical examination of the faeces produced
- Is the diarrhoea primary or secondary?
- If primary, is the diarrhoea of small or large intestinal origin?

PRIMARY		*SECONDARY*
Small intestinal	*Large intestinal*	Urinalysis
Haematology/biochemistry	Faecal culture	Specific tests of organ function
Faecal culture	Worm egg count	
Worm egg count	Rectal examination	
Undigested food analysis	Plain radiography	
Serum folate/cobalamin	Endoscopy/biopsy	
Trypsin-like immunoreactivity		
Breath hydrogen assay		
Sugar permeability test		
Ultrasound scan		
Endoscopy/exploratory laparotomy		

Constipation
- Collect a history and conduct a thorough physical examination
- Rectal examination
- Neurological examination
- Orthopaedic assessment
- Plain radiography

Faecal tenesmus
- Collect a history and conduct a thorough physical examination
- Rectal examination
- Faecal culture and worm egg count
- Plain radiography
- Contrast studies
- Ultrasound scan
- Endoscopy/biopsy

continued ...

Figure 8.1: Possible diagnostic procedures for common alimentary symptoms.

Acute abdomen
- Collect a history and conduct a thorough physical examination
- Careful abdominal palpation
- Haematology and biochemistry
- Plain radiography
- Possibly contrast studies
- Paracentesis
- Ultrasound scan
- Exploratory laparotomy

Abdominal enlargement
- Collect a history and conduct a thorough physical examination
- Careful abdominal palpation
- Haematology and biochemistry
- Plain radiography
- Paracentesis
- Ultrasound scan
- Exploratory laparotomy

Figure 8.1: Continued.

FAECAL ANALYSIS

Physical appearance

Faecal examination can provide the clinician with very useful information regarding the causes of acute and chronic intestinal disorders. Figures 8.2 and 8.3 list the common causes of acute and chronic diarrhoea in dogs and cats. In addition to the many tests that can be carried out on faecal samples, simple physical examination of the sample may provide some information as to the location of the lesion.

Initial examination of a fresh faecal sample should concentrate on its physical appearance. In many cases of diarrhoea it is possible to decide whether it is associated with a small or large intestinal problem using the criteria shown in Table 8.1. Such a differen-tiation not only gives the clinician valuable informa-tion regarding the location of the lesion but conse-quently assists in the selection of further appropriate diagnostic tests (Figure 8.4). Unfortunately, not all diarrhoeas may be readily classified, and features of both small and large intestinal disease may be present. This may reflect a small intestinal problem which results in the abnormal presence of nutrients or other

Endoparasitism:
    Hookworms
    Whipworms
Giardiasis
Dietary indiscretions:
    Soiled foods
    Scavenging
    Over-eating
Viral infections:
    Feline panleucopenia
    Canine parvovirus
    Coronavirus
Bacterial infection:
    Salmonellosis
    Campylobacter infection
Intussusception
Haemorrhagic gastroenteritis

Figure 8.2: Major causes of acute diarrhoea in dogs and cats.

Small intestinal disease:
    Lymphocytic–plasmacytic enteritis
    Eosinophilic enteritis
    Gluten enteropathy
    Lymphangiectasia
    Lymphosarcoma
    Giardiasis

Exocrine pancreatic insufficiency (EPI)

Colitis:
    Lymphocytic–plasmacytic
    Eosinophilic
    Histiocytic
    Granulomatous
    Lymphosarcoma

Systemic disease:
    Hyperthyroidism (cats)
    Hypoadrenocorticalism
    Hypothyroidism (dogs)
    Chronic renal failure
    Hepatic disease
    FeLV, FIV and FIP

Figure 8.3: Major causes of chronic diarrhoea in dogs and cats.

Symptom/Sign	Small intestine	Large intestine
Faecal volume	Increased	Reduced
Faecal tenesmus	None	Present
Faecal blood	None or changed	Often present
Faecal mucus	None	Often present
Urgency	Rare	Often present
Dyschezia	Absent	Often present
Steatorrhoea	Often present	Absent
Vomiting	May occur	Occurs in 30% of cases
Weight loss	Present	Absent
Flatus/borborygmi	Present	Rare
Coat/skin condition	Poor	Normal
Appetite	Increased	Normal or reduced

Table 8.1: Characteristics of faeces passed in small and large intestinal diarrhoea.

Small intestinal disease
Faecal culture, worm egg count, undigested food
Haematology and biochemistry
Serum folate and cobalamin
Sugar permeability test
Breath hydrogen assay
Radiography and contrast studies
Endoscopy and biopsy

Large intestinal disease
Faecal culture, worm egg count
Haematology and biochemistry
Radiography and contrast studies
Endoscopy and biopsy

Figure 8.4: Procedures used in the investigation of small and large intestinal disease.

---

agents in the large intestine, thereby causing signs of large intestinal disease. Alternatively, it may reflect a condition that affects both the small and the large intestine equally. In either of these situations the clinician has no alternative but to carry out diagnostic tests to assess both small and large intestinal function.

Faecal blood

The physical assessment of faeces may reveal the presence of fresh blood. The extent of the blood loss often reflects the degree of damage to the intestinal mucosa, while the character of the blood in the faeces gives an indication of where the lesion is located. Fresh blood mixed through the faecal sample suggests it is of colonic origin, while fresh blood only on the surface of the faeces suggests a distal colon, rectal or anal origin.

It is important to emphasize the need to consider the whole patient and to interpret these findings in conjunction with the presence or absence of diarrhoea, constipation, tenesmus and dyschezia.

Melaena can be defined as the presence of changed blood in the faeces. The appearance of melaena will depend on the extent of bleeding and its location, but malaenic faeces normally appear black and tarry in consistency. This appearance is normally associated with bleeding into the small intestine, although melaena may originate from the stomach (with associated haematemesis) or from the oesophagus, pharynx, mouth or respiratory system. In the latter cases blood is swallowed and passes through the alimentary tract to appear as melaena, giving the impression of alimentary disease. Patients with clotting disorders may present with melaena, but again careful clinical examination should reveal bleeding from other locations, confirming a generalized disorder.

'Occult blood' refers to the presence of microscopic amounts of blood that can only be detected by laboratory analysis. Great care is required in interpreting a positive result in dogs and cats as they are often fed meat-based diets. The presence of haemoglobin or myoglobin in the diet will give false-positive results. It is therefore important to place the patient on a meat-free diet for a minimum of 3 days prior to testing for occult blood. Various commercial kits are available to detect occult blood and their instructions should be followed carefully. It is important to ensure the kit is not designed to detect only human haemoglobin as this may result in false results (either negative or positive). A true strong positive result indicates only that bleeding is occurring somewhere along the alimentary tract.

Environment:
    Available substrate
    Mucus layer
    Local IgA production
    Intestinal motility
    Gastric acid secretion
    Maldigestion, malabsorption

Diet:
    Fibre content
    Fermentable sugars
    Protein and fat content

Scavenging behaviour
Coprophagia

Figure 8.5: *Internal and external factors that influence whether small intestinal bacterial overgrowth (SIBO) may establish in an individual.*

Culture for bacteria

Normal flora

The small intestine lies between the almost sterile stomach (due to gastric acid) and the large bacterial population located in the colon. Bacterial numbers in the proximal small intestine are low but numbers increase in the ileum. The actual numbers present in any individual will vary depending on various internal and external factors (Figure 8.5). Many of the 'normal' flora are beneficial to the animal by producing vitamin K, biotin, folate and short-chain fatty acids (SCFAs). If the numbers of bacteria present in the small intestine increase, small intestinal bacterial overgrowth (SIBO) develops. Such a proliferation of bacteria can seriously damage the intestinal mucosa (see below). The point at which bacterial populations induce clinical signs of SIBO will vary with each individual and the genus of bacteria present.

The type of bacteria present also varies along the length of the small intestine and is different for dogs and cats. The numbers of anaerobes in the proximal small intestine is much greater in the cat than in the dog, since cats are obligate carnivores. In dogs Gram-positive aerobes predominate in the proximal small intestine, with few anaerobes present. However, in the distal small intestine the numbers of aerobes declines and the numbers of Gram-negative organisms and anaerobes increase, particularly *Bacteroides*, *Bifidobacter* and *Clostridium* spp. together with other Enterobacteriaceae. Coliforms are also more frequently found in the ileum than in the duodenum.

Pathogenic bacteria

Pathogenic bacteria may establish when there is interference with the normal physiological regulation of the resident flora. Bacterial properties that permit pathogens to establish include: the presence of flagellae;

production of enzymes such as proteases; the ability of bacteria to adhere to the mucosa; and production of factors that interfere with intestinal motility. The abilities to produce enterotoxin and to invade enterocytes significantly increase pathogenicity.

Potential pathogens include *Salmonella*, *Campylobacter*, *Yersinia* and *Clostridium* species and *Escherichia coli*. Recently, *E. coli* has been shown to have the ability to establish long-term colonization of the intestine by adherence to, or invasion of, the enterocytes. There has been a problem recognizing which *E. coli* subtypes are pathogenic and which are not. Faecal culture aims to identify potentially pathogenic bacteria. Enterotoxinogenic *E. coli* (ETEC) cause short-lived secretory diarrhoea due to the toxin's action on the intestinal mucosa. Enteropathogenic *E. coli* (EPEC) cause osmotic diarrhoea as they damage the microvilli and cause malabsorption. Enteroinvasive *E. coli* (EIEC) invade the colonocytes, causing significant mucosal damage and ulceration. Following the production of toxin, enterohaemorrhagic *E. coli* (EHEC) act in a similar manner to EPEC, but tend to affect the distal ileum and colon. Systemic effects are possible with these *E.coli* infections. Although clearly established as a cause of enteric disease in large animals, the role of *E. coli* in small animals is still to be clarified. Both EPEC and ETEC have been documented in dogs and cats. A further study suggested that EPEC and veratoxin-producing *E. coli* are important causes of enteric disease in dogs.

The presence of *Salmonella* spp. or *Campylobacter* spp. presents a significant public health risk and owners should be warned of the dangers, especially if children and elderly people live in the household. In both the dog and cat these organisms can be excreted by 'healthy' individuals showing no clinical disease. Equally, they can cause enteric and systemic signs of ill health. Diarrhoea associated with *Campylobacter* spp. can be acute, chronic or intermittent. Some strains produce enterotoxin and are locally invasive. Fortunately, diarrhoea is usually self-limiting; in many cases, although antibiotics reduce the shedding of organisms they do not alter the duration of ill health. *Salmonella* spp. may also result in acute, chronic or intermittent signs of enteric disease. Long-term shedding of organisms may occur, even after a clinical cure. Both *Salmonella* and *Campylobacter* are opportunistic and establish when there is some other underlying enteric problem such as EPI or small intestinal disease.

Bacillus piliformis may be associated with a fatal enteritis in kittens and is often evident due to the immunosuppressive effects of infection with FIV or FeLV. It has also been reported as causing chronic diarrhoea in dogs. *Yersinia* rarely causes a mild enteritis in cats, but may be a more frequent pathogen in dogs. The presence of *Clostridium perfringens* is not always of diagnostic importance unless enterotoxin is also detected. Fresh faeces can be analysed using a suitable commercial ELISA (enzyme-linked immunosorbent assay) test to detect enterotoxin. A positive test result is indicative of clostridial infection, while a single negative test result does not preclude infection as the toxin is only produced intermittently. In such cases, the assay should be repeated on at least two occasions before accepting a definitive negative result.

Persistent diarrhoea of unknown aetiology, or that results in pyrexia, leucocytosis or melaena or affects more than one animal in a group, should alert the clinician to a possible infectious cause. In such circumstances, faecal culture should be carried out on at least three fresh faecal samples over a week, as pathogens are frequently excreted intermittently. Actual faecal samples rather than faecal swabs should be submitted and they should be transported to the laboratory without delay. It is worth consulting the laboratory regarding the need for transport media for the culture of specific organisms. To avoid unnecessary contamination, faeces should be collected per rectum, using a gloved finger, and placed directly into a sterile container.

Duodenal aspirates

SIBO is not a diagnosis but rather a symptom of some other underlying disease state (Figure 8.6). In this condition, the small intestinal environment changes to permit bacterial proliferation. Normally bacteria are kept under control by gastric acid secretion, intestinal motility, limited intestinal substrate availability and bacteriostatic secretory factors. Failures in these protective mechanisms may lead to SIBO. The normal bacterial flora may be quantified by measuring the number of colony-forming units per millilitre of aspirate (CFU/ml). In dogs this is normally between 10^3 and 10^5 CFU/ml. Increases in both aerobic ($>10^5$ CFU/ml) and anaerobic ($>10^4$ CFU/ml) counts are considered significant in the dog. The normal level of bacterial flora in cats is higher than in dogs (up to 10^7 CFU/ml) and there is normally a greater proportion of anaerobes present, reflecting the obligatory carnivorous state.

Sampling for SIBO involves obtaining endoscopic aspirates directly from the duodenum. The patient requires a general anaesthetic. A flexible endoscope is

IgA deficiency
Achlorhydria
Stagnant loop syndrome
Paralytic ileus
Exocrine pancreatic insufficiency
Inflammatory bowel disease

Figure 8.6: Some underlying causes for SIBO. In a given case it is often difficult to determine the underlying cause, so symptomatic treatment is often the only method of relieving clinical signs.

passed through the stomach and into the duodenum, using as little air insufflation as possible. Once in the duodenum, a sterile endoscopic catheter is advanced through the endoscope biopsy channel and duodenal contents are aspirated. Samples are placed in sterile containers for aerobic and anaerobic culture. The number of colony-forming units per millilitre of duodenal fluid is calculated. Values above 10^5 CFU/ml are considered significant in the dog, while slightly higher values, $>10^7$ CFU/ml, are significant in the cat. Giardiasis may also be diagnosed from duodenal aspirates, by microscopic examination for trophozoites.

The problem with duodenal aspiration and culture is that it is not clear whether this truly reflects the flora present throughout the whole of the small intestine. It may, for example, be possible to have a normal duodenal floral culture but still have SIBO in more caudal regions of the small intestine. In this case duodenal culture will be normal and a diagnosis cannot be made.

Analysis for viruses

Canine parvovirus (CPV-2) infection usually results in an acute enteritis with secondary bacterial infection, involving especially *Salmonella* and *Campylobacter* spp. A definitive diagnosis of parvovirus infection requires collection of a fresh faecal sample for viral antigen detection. Ideally, samples should be collected within the first 2 days of infection when the largest number of virus particles are present. A commercial ELISA test kit is available for the detection of parvovirus antigen in faeces. Serology can also be carried out in order to detect a rising titre of antibody indicating recent parvovirus infection (see Blood tests, below).

A syndrome characterized by protruding nictitating membranes and chronic diarrhoea has been recognized for some time in cats. A high incidence has been reported in multiple cat households, suggesting an infectious cause. The disease is usually self-limiting, although clinical signs may persist for several weeks. Muir *et al.* (1990) isolated a torovirus-like agent from affected cats. Inoculation of kittens with the agent resulted in viral shedding in the faeces and a rise in serum haemagglutination-inhibiting antibody titre, indicating that the cats might be infected with the virus.

Endoparasites

Endoparasitic infection with roundworms (*Toxocara canis, Toxocara cati, Toxascaris leonina*) and tapeworms (*Dipylidium caninum, Taenia* spp. *and Echinococcus*) are, in the author's experience, very rare causes of diarrhoea in dogs and cats. However, *Echinococcus* and *Toxocara* both carry a significant public health risk and should be identified and treated whenever possible.

Infection with endoparasitic larvae, which invade and damage the intestinal mucosa rather than living free within the intestinal lumen, may present a clinical problem. This group consists of the hookworms *Ancylostoma* spp. (not in the UK) and *Uncinaria stenocephalus,* together with the whipworm *Trichuris vulpis.* Hookworms principally target the small intestine, whereas whipworms invade the colon. *Uncinaria* occasionally causes diarrhoea in dogs but is not a cause of diarrhoea in cats. *Uncinaria* does not suck blood, so the anaemia associated with *Ancylostoma* does not occur. However, *Uncinaria* is often associated with interdigital dermatitis due to larval penetration and migration. Although parasitic infections are rare, it is important to carry out at least two counts for worm eggs within one week (due to intermittent excretion) on the faeces of all dogs with chronic diarrhoea.

Giardiasis should also be considered in dogs and cats with either chronic diarrhoea or chronic intermittent bilious vomiting. The trophozoites appear to inhibit fat digestion by inactivating lipase, accounting for the frequent detection of steatorrhoea as well as diarrhoea. *Cryptosporidium* spp. are a rare cause of chronic diarrhoea in dogs but appear to be more common in the cat. Coccidia (*Isospora canis and I. felis*) most commonly affect puppies and kittens less than 1 year old that are housed in unhygienic conditions where they ingest a large burden of oocysts. Sporozoites are liberated in the small intestine and invade the enterocytes, resulting in bloody diarrhoea. These protozoans are difficult to detect because of the area they colonize and the small size of the cysts excreted in the faeces.

Examination of faecal samples for any of these parasites can be carried out relatively easily. The various methods available to detect eggs and cysts reflect the differences in the size and numbers excreted by the endoparasites and are detailed below. At least two separate faecal samples examined over a week should always be examined, as eggs and cysts are frequently excreted intermittently.

Faecal smears
Fresh faecal smears provide a quick and cheap method of examining faecal samples. However, as there is no concentration of ova it is easy to miss parasite eggs or cysts that are present in small numbers. A fresh faecal sample should be mixed with a small volume of physiological saline on a microscope slide. If protozoans are suspected, one drop of Lugol's iodine will highlight these parasites but will reduce their motility. A negative result may be accurate or may reflect the small numbers of parasitic eggs present, intermittent excretion, or the effects of agents such as barium sulphate, kaolin, pectin or enemas.

Faecal flotation
Faecal flotation is a more sensitive method than the faecal smear for the detection of parasite eggs and cysts because the technique concentrates their numbers into a small volume of solution. Several methods have been developed, but for the purposes of this chapter only two methods will be described. Faecal samples for detection of parasite eggs or cysts may be preserved by refrigeration at +4°C for up to 2 days prior to examination, but should *not* be frozen. Preservation of faecal samples may also be carried out using 1 part faeces to 3 parts preservative (1.5 g sodium acetate, 2 ml glacial acetic acid, 4 ml 40% formalin plus 92.5 ml water).

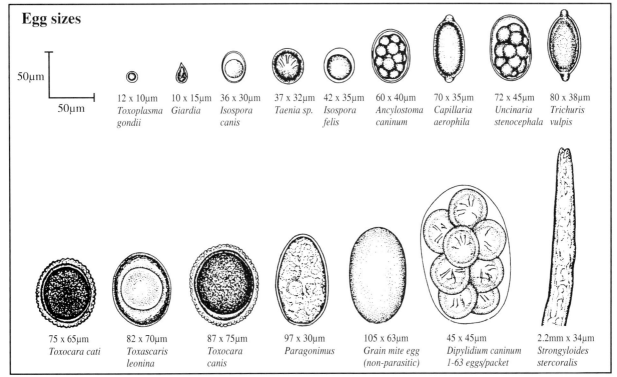

Figure 8.7: *Identification of protozoan cysts and worm eggs that may be found in the faeces of dogs and cats.*
By kind permission of Hoechst-Roussel-Agri Vet Company, USA.

The McMaster technique involves mixing 3 g of faeces with 42 ml of water and pouring the mixture through a 100 mesh sieve into a bowl (to extract gross debris). The filtrate is placed in two centrifuge tubes and gently centrifuged at 1500 rpm for 3 minutes. The supernatant is discarded and the deposit resuspended in an equal volume of saturated sodium chloride solution and mixed thoroughly. Using a Pasteur pipette, an aliquot of this suspension is placed on a McMaster slide and allowed to stand for 5 minutes before viewing under low power. All eggs and cysts can be identified (Figure 8.7) and counted within the chamber; the number per gram of faeces can be calculated by multiplying the number of eggs or cysts within a chamber by 50.

The zinc sulphate flotation test is essential for detecting *Giardia* spp. and *Cryptosporidium* spp. Three grams of fresh faeces are mixed with 42 ml of water and sieved into a bowl. The filtrate is placed in centrifuge tubes and centrifuged at 1500 rpm for 3 minutes; the supernatant is discarded. The tubes are filled with zinc sulphate solution (330 g/l in water) and centrifuged again at 1500 rpm for 3 minutes. The supernatant on the surface of the centrifuge tube is removed using a wire loop or glass rod and placed on a microscope slide. One drop of Lugol's iodine and a coverslip are applied before viewing. The number of cysts counted is multiplied by 20 and divided by the volume of solution used in the centrifuge tube to give the number of cysts per gram of faeces.

Giardiasis may also be detected by microscopic examination of duodenal aspirates collected by flexible endoscopy (as described above) or by faecal ELISA test for giardial trophozoite antigen. However, the majority of cases are diagnosed following detection of faecal cysts as described above.

The presence of eggs or cysts in a faecal sample should be considered as significant and treatment should be carried out immediately. Hookworms and whipworms may be difficult to eliminate and consideration must be given to contamination of the animal's environment and the risk of re-infection. Whenever parasitism is detected and treated, the patient should be reassessed to ensure that there is no other underlying disease present.

Proteolytic activity

Considerable importance has previously been placed on the measurement of faecal proteolytic activity or the 'trypsin digest test' in the diagnosis of EPI. However, this method of diagnosis is no longer acceptable for two reasons. First, there is a specific test available for the definitive diagnosis of EPI in both dogs and cats, namely the TLI (trypsinogen-like immunoreactivity) test (see Blood tests, below). Secondly, trypsin digest tests are very unreliable.

Where the TLI test is not available, proteolytic activity in faeces can be measured with reasonable accuracy using either the azocasein dye or radial diffusion tests. These tests, although subject to yielding false results on occasions, will give some indication of exocrine pancreatic function. They are not used routinely in the UK.

Undigested food residues

Faecal samples can be examined for the presence of undigested fat, starch and muscle fibres. This is a crude test but gives the clinician some indication of whether maldigestion exists; it will not detect malabsorptive states. The examination of faeces in this manner is no substitute for carrying out a TLI test to confirm the diagnosis. Clearly, all the nutrients must be present in the diet in adequate amounts and prior to the test there should be no history of recent or sudden dietary alterations. Barium sulphate, kaolin, pectin, mineral oil and castor oil administration, low-fat diets, azathioprine, aminoglycosides and cholestyrine will all influence the results.

To measure faecal fat in a semi-quantitative fashion, a small amount of fresh faeces is mixed with Sudan III on a microscope slide and heated gently. The slide is examined under low power for the presence of orange to red globules of fat (Figure 8.8a). Normal dogs and cats should have no evidence of fat in their faeces, while those with EPI or bile acid deficiency will have numerous fat globules per microscope field.

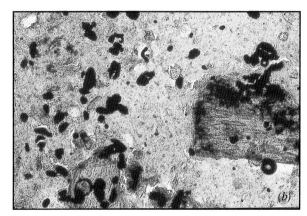

Figure 8.8: (a) A microscope field with numerous fat globules stained orange by Sudan III. (b) Starch granules (black) and muscle fibres in a fresh faecal smear stained with Lugol's iodine. Neither fat globules nor starch granules should be present in normal faecal smears; their presence suggests failure in the digestive process.

The detection of starch granules and muscle fibres can be made by mixing a small amount of fresh faeces with 2% Lugol's iodine on a microscope slide. Starch granules appear black, while muscle fibres have square ends and are reddish brown (Figure 8.8b). There should normally be no starch granules present in faeces and only occasional partially digested muscle fibres. The presence of more than four starch granules per low-power field is indicative of EPI. The presence of any undigested muscle fibres is also significant. It is essential that the patient is placed on a meat-based diet before this procedure is performed.

EXAMINATION OF VOMITUS

Vomiting is a common presenting complaint, and careful questioning of the client regarding the frequency, timing and character of the vomitus can be of considerable diagnostic value. In particular, a distinction must be made regarding whether the client has observed regurgitation or true vomiting and, in the latter case, whether this is primary or secondary (Figure 8.9). Vomitus may contain food, bile, white viscous fluid or blood, or it may be unproductive.

Food
It is important to determine when the food was vomited in relation to feeding and whether it was digested or undigested. Vomiting of undigested food can be associated with oesophageal retention and regurgitation, or a gastric disorder. The history should assist the clinician in making this distinction. Oesophageal disease should be investigated with the aid of radiography and contrast studies (see below).

If undigested food is vomited shortly after consumption, this suggests loss of receptive relaxation caused by increased intragastric pressure and is often associated with gastric inflammation. Loss of gastric motility is another indicator of inflammation. If the undigested ingesta is vomited many hours after consumption this suggests gastric stasis or outflow obstruction. The former is more likely, as outflow obstruction is usually associated with acute persistent vomiting.

Bile
Vomiting of bile is usually associated with persistent vomiting after the stomach has emptied. In acute inflammation, irritation of the stomach may lead to reflux of duodenal contents and vomition of gastric and intestinal secretions including bile. If the patient is vomiting bile it is reasonable to assume there is no gastric outflow obstruction.

White viscous fluid
This is commonly produced by anorexic dogs and cats that are vomiting persistently. It is associated with accumulation of saliva and gastric secretions. The material may be mixed with bile or, occasionally, with flecks of blood. It is not pathognomonic for any particular type of gastric disorder. White viscous fluid may also be produced by animals with mega-oesophagus, so it is important to ensure that the patient is vomiting and not regurgitating.

Blood
Haematemesis can be an indicator of serious gastric disease. The amount of blood produced and whether it

---

Regurgitation

A *passive* process whereby undigested food that has not entered the stomach may be re-presented shortly after ingestion.

It is usually associated with oesophageal disease:

> Mega-oesophagus: congenital or acquired
> Vascular ring anomaly
> Stricture formation
> Oesophageal foreign body
> Oesophageal neoplasia (very rare in the UK)
> Oesophagitis
> Oesophageal diverticulum
> Hiatus hernia

Vomiting

An *active* process where food is expelled from the stomach with the active participation of muscles of the diaphragm and abdominal wall.

Vomiting may be primary, associated with gastric disease, or secondary due to some systemic disease:

PRIMARY VOMITING:
> Acute gastritis
> Chronic gastritis
> Gastric foreign body
> Pyloric stenosis
> Gastric ulceration
> Gastric neoplasia
> Gastric motility disorder

SECONDARY VOMITING:
> Renal failure and azotaemia
> Hypoadrenocorticism
> Hepatic disease and hepatoencephalopathy
> Diabetes mellitus and ketoacidosis
> Pyometra
> Inflammation of abdominal viscera — pancreas, peritonitis, colitis

Figure 8.9: Many clients present their pet with a history of 'vomiting'. The clinician must determine whether the animal is actually regurgitating or truly vomiting. Even if vomiting is confirmed, this may be caused by primary gastric disease or may be secondary to some systemic disease.

is fresh or changed ('coffee grounds') are important factors. It is important to ensure that the patient is not bleeding from any other site, such as the nose or mouth, or into the urine or faeces, since generalized bleeding may indicate a clotting disorder rather than a gastric disease. In particular, haemorrhage from the nose, pharynx or oesophagus should be considered. Small flecks of blood are commonly observed in patients that are vomiting persistently. This is due to rupture of small capillaries in the stomach and is not serious. However, larger amounts of blood may indicate gastric ulceration or haemorrhagic gastroenteritis. Ulceration is commonly associated with gastric neoplasia but it is important to remember that absence of haematemesis does *not* rule out ulceration or neoplasia. The presence of changed blood in the vomitus results from the action of gastric acid over a period of time and is indicative of gastric stasis in association with gastric bleeding.

Unproductive vomiting

Occasionally the patient may vomit repeatedly without any vomitus being produced. This may simply indicate that the stomach is empty, or it may be a feature of gastric impaction or the presence of a foreign body lodged in the pylorus.

HELICOBACTER GASTRITIS

A group of microaerophilic, spiral, Gram-negative organisms has recently been found in the stomach of man and various other species. This group of bacteria belong to the new genus of *Helicobacter*. In man the organism isolated is *H. pylori*, while in dogs a large spiral organism known for some time as *Gastrospirillum hominis* has now been confirmed to be *H. heilmanii*. In the cat *H. felis* has been isolated from the gastric mucosa. In spite of this apparent species specificity, *Helicobacter* spp. may be zoonotic.

In man, *Helicobacter* infection is associated with gastric and duodenal ulceration, chronic gastritis and possibly adenocarcinoma and lymphoma. There is a need for much work to be carried out in the dog and cat to determine the importance of this genus in the aetiology of gastric disease. *Helicobacter* spp. has been associated with atrophic gastritis, lymphocytic plasmacytic gastritis and gastric adenocarcinoma in the dog and cat. Unfortunately, the organism may also be isolated from normal dogs and cats with no evidence of gastric disease. The author's own observations have revealed the presence of *Helicobacter* spp. in only 25% of dogs and cats presented with signs of gastric disease.

Helicobacter organisms are found in highest concentrations in the antrum of the stomach and this is the best site from which to collect biopsy samples for examination. The organism is a urease producer, converting urea to ammonia. It is this mechanism that allows the organism to make the environment more

| Hypoadrenocorticism |
| Feline hyperthyroidism |
| Hepatic disease |
| Renal disease |
| Heart failure |
| FIV infection |
| Feline infectious peritonitis |
| FeLV infection |

Figure 8.10: Systemic diseases that may be associated with chronic diarrhoea.

favourable for colonization. A diagnosis of *Helicobacter* infection cannot be made from visual examination of the gastric mucosa, as changes are at the microscopic level. Endoscopic biopsy samples should be collected and stained with either silver or Giemsa stains to demonstrate the organism. Culture of gastric juice or biopsy specimens for *Helicobacter* organisms can be very difficult, with some types failing to grow on any recognized media. There are several new tests being developed for man, including the urea breath test (which uses radiolabelled hydrogen) and a serological test for anti-*Helicobacter* antibodies in serum. The latter test is currently being evaluated in dogs by the author.

BLOOD TESTS

Although vomiting and diarrhoea are generally the hallmarks of primary alimentary tract disorders, they may be associated with systemic disease (Figure 8.10). For this reason, all patients presented with alimentary symptoms should receive a thorough clinical examination to determine whether there is evidence of systemic disease. Whenever systemic disease is suspected, blood samples should be collected for a routine haematology and biochemical profile.

Many of the conditions associated with the alimentary tract may also result in changes to blood parameters. Assessment of a routine blood panel will help the clinician determine the severity of alimentary disease, while more specialized tests, such as TLI, serum folate and cobalamin, will provide diagnostic information regarding the alimentary tract.

Serology for enteric viruses

Feline infectious enteritis, feline panleucopenia and feline parvovirus are all terms used to describe the viral enteritis associated with parvovirus infection. A faecal ELISA test is currently available commercially to detect the presence of viral antigen.

In both feline and canine parvovirus infections a profound fall in the white blood cell count is frequently detected, with values falling as low as $1-2 \times 10^9$ cells/l. This level of immunosuppression accounts for the ease with which secondary bacterial infections establish.

Feline infectious peritonitis (FIP) occurs most commonly in cats between 6 months and 2 years of age. It may present with very typical clinical signs, including ascites, or with vague chronic signs such as weight loss and chronic diarrhoea. Diagnosis of FIP is always difficult due to the close antigenic association between the FIP virus and feline enteric coronavirus (FECV) which itself can cause mild to moderate diarrhoea in cats. Serology therefore plays a minor role in the definitive diagnosis of FIP, as previous exposure to FECV will result in high serological antibody titres. A definitive diagnosis can only be obtained from a combination of typical clinical signs, the presence of yellow viscous high-protein ascitic fluid (see below) and histopathology of biopsy samples from the liver, intestine or peritoneum taken at laparotomy. An ELISA test for the detection of antibodies to FIP and other enteric coronaviruses is commercially available. A positive result in a kitten less than 12 weeks old may reflect the presence of maternal antibody. A negative result suggests that the cat has not been previously exposed to enteric coronavirus. Positive results must be interpreted in association with the clinical history and histopathology of biopsy samples.

Both feline leukaemia virus (FeLV) and feline immunodeficiency virus (FIV) infections may occasionally present with vague clinical signs associated with the alimentary tract, including stomatitis, weight loss and chronic diarrhoea. All cats presented with chronic alimentary symptoms should be checked for the presence of these viruses. ELISA tests are available for the detection of FeLV antigen and FIV antibody in serum.

Red cell parameters

The most commonly observed change to red cell indices occurs in patients with vomiting and diarrhoea who rapidly become dehydrated. The degree of elevation in their packed cell volume (PCV) and total serum protein levels reflects the severity of the dehydration. In some cases these changes may actually mask an underlying anaemia and hypoproteinaemia; it is very important, therefore, to monitor the change in these parameters following aggressive fluid therapy.

Anaemia is a much less common feature of alimentary tract disease but is observed where there is severe inflammation and subsequent ulceration. Chronic haemorrhage into the intestinal lumen will result in a regenerative anaemia characterized by a polychromasia and reticulocytosis in the peripheral blood. Very rarely an iron-deficiency anaemia will be observed, characterized as a microcytic hypochromic anaemia. Chronic haemorrhage may result in a mild increase in blood urea due to increased protein catabolism. If no visible evidence of haemorrhage exists in an anaemic animal with gastrointestinal signs, the faeces should be examined for the presence of occult blood.

White cell parameters

Marked leucopenia is a feature of both canine and feline parvovirus infection, where counts may fall as low as 1-2 x 10^9 cells/l. This is due to the marked immunosuppressive effects of parvovirus on the bone marrow. Rebound leucocytosis is frequently observed as the patient responds to therapy and immunosuppression declines, coupled with the effects of secondary infection. Systemic toxoplasmosis and FeLV infection may also cause leucopenia and alimentary symptoms.

A leucocytosis, neutrophilia and shift to the left (presence of immature neutrophils) are observed in some advanced cases of alimentary tract disease, especially where the mucosal integrity has been damaged or infection is present. In the author's experience such changes are most often observed in advanced inflammatory bowel disease (IBD), intestinal adenocarcinomas and granulomatous colitis. In many of these cases the owner will report the presence of melaena, further supporting the degree of damage to the mucosa. Melaena is rarely observed with enteric lymphoma but leucocytosis and lymphopenia (25-50% of cases) are frequently observed. Rarely, hypercalcaemia may be associated with enteric lymphoma, as may a markedly elevated lymphocyte count (50-200 x 10^9 cells/l). Lymphopenia may be observed in protein-losing enteropathies (PLE), especially lymphangiectasia, as well as in immunodeficiency states. A sustained eosinophilia (>2x 10^9 cells/l) is suggestive of intestinal parasitism, mast cell tumours, Addison's disease, eosinophilic gastroenteritis or hypereosinophilic syndrome in cats.

Acute pancreatitis will be suspected on clinical grounds and subsequent blood sampling will reveal a typical response to inflammation and pain, namely, a marked leucocytosis and shift to the left. With chronic pancreatitis the white blood cell response may remain high in spite of the reduction in severity of clinical signs.

Peritonitis results in a marked leucocytosis and shift to the left accompanied by a lymphopenia, eosinopenia and monocytosis. If the peritonitis is severe, this picture may change, due to sequestration of neutrophils in the peritoneum, to give a leucocytosis and degenerative shift associated with the presence of more immature than mature neutrophils in the circulation.

Feline hyperthyroidism sometimes presents with symptoms of alimentary tract disease, including weight loss and chronic diarrhoea and, occasionally, vomiting. These patients may also have a leucocytosis and neutrophilia.

Hypoadrenocorticism or Addison's disease frequently presents with chronic intermittent signs of vomiting, diarrhoea and weight loss, together with signs of other organ dysfunction. Although the white cell count may be within the normal range, some cases reveal a lymphocytosis and eosinophilia. The presence of other clinical pathology, such as an altered Na:K

Hypoproteinaemia
Malnutrition
Burns and haemorrhage
Sepsis
Protein-losing enteropathy
Protein-losing nephropathy
Hepatic disease

Hyperglobulinaemia
Feline infectious peritonitis
Cholangiohepatitis
Chronic inflammation/infection

Figure 8.11: Conditions causing alterations in serum protein levels.

ratio and ECG changes, should be checked for. If there is strong suspicion of Addison's disease, the diagnosis should be confirmed with an ACTH test, which will yield a flat response to ACTH.

Biochemistry

As part of a biochemical profile, serum alanine aminotransferase, alkaline phosphatase, bilirubin and bile acids can be used to assess liver damage, cholestasis and liver function (see Chapter 9). Elevations in serum alanine aminotransferase (SALT) may be observed in feline hyperthyroidism and hypocholesterolaemia may be observed in protein-losing enteropathy (PLE). Hypoglycaemia may be a feature of parasitism, neoplasia, liver disease or sepsis. Blood urea and creatinine assays, together with urinalysis, can be used to assess renal function. Both liver and kidney function require to be assessed even in patients with apparent intestinal disease because the hypoproteinaemia that accompanies advanced intestinal disease must be differentiated from that of hepatic and renal disease (see below).

Many patients with advanced alimentary tract disease present with marked weight loss. In spite of carrying out a careful clinical examination, no evidence of ascites, hydrothorax or subcutaneous oedema may be detected, even though the patient is hypoproteinaemic. This is because serum protein levels fall slowly, allowing compensatory changes to take place. It is therefore very important to check the serum protein levels in all cases where significant weight loss has occurred. Recognizing hypoproteinaemia reduces the list of differential diagnoses considerably (Figure 8.11). In general, hypoalbuminaemia is a feature of malnutrition, hepatic disease and protein-losing nephropathy. Protein-losing enteropathies (PLE) usually present with a fall in both albumin and globulin fractions. For this reason it is important to look not only at the total protein levels but also at the levels of different proteins. Having confirmed the absence of hepatic and renal disease using these parameters, a diagnosis of PLE can be made using ultrasonography, which identifies thickening of the

intestinal wall, by sugar permeability tests (see below) and by examination of biopsy samples from the intestine.

In addition to the examination of serum proteins for evidence of PLE, in cats serum proteins have another useful function. Cats presented with cholangiohepatitis and FIP may have significant elevations in globulins (>70 g/l). Although not always present, hyperglobulinaemia is supportive of these conditions and further reduces the list of differential diagnoses.

In dogs with gastrointestinal symptoms where hypoadrenocorticism is suspected, sodium and potassium levels should always be determined. The normal ratio of sodium to potassium should be >27:1; values below 25:1 are suspicious, while values below 20:1 are highly suggestive of Addison's disease. In such cases an ACTH test should be carried out to confirm the diagnosis. No increase in serum cortisol will be observed following injection of synthetic ACTH in animals with Addison's disease. Hyperkalaemia and hyponatraemia may occur rarely with *Trichuris vulpis* infection or salmonellosis.

Serum amylase and lipase values have traditionally been used to assist in the diagnosis of acute pancreatitis but are both unreliable indicators of this condition. Amylase is found in several tissues, including the liver, intestine and pancreas, and is normally excreted in the urine. Renal failure will elevate serum amylase values. Renal function should therefore be assessed and amylase values interpreted accordingly. Small intestinal obstructions and hepatic disease may also result in elevated serum amylase values.

The method of assay can significantly alter serum amylase values, with higher values being produced by the sacchrogenic method but more reliable values produced by the amyloclastic method (see Chapter 4). Serum amylase values increase in various pancreatic conditions, including acute pancreatitis, pancreatic neoplasia, pancreatic abscessation and pancreatic duct obstruction. Values should only be considered significant when they rise to more than three times the upper reference limit, while values just outside the reference range are very difficult to interpret. For example, serum amylase values one or two times the normal range may be associated with dehydration and poor renal perfusion. Serum amylase is of no diagnostic value in the cat.

Serum lipase is considered to be more reliable than amylase in the detection of pancreatitis. Unfortunately, lipase is found in the pancreas and the stomach, so conditions such as chronic gastritis and gastric neoplasia frequently result in elevations in serum lipase values. Lipase is degraded by the kidneys, therefore elevations may occur in renal failure. Lipase values may be elevated to as much as five times the normal level following administration of glucocorticoids or heparin prior to sample collection; this is due to activation of lipoprotein lipase by heparin. Haemolysis and jaundice may also elevate lipase levels; care is therefore required in collecting the blood sample and in the

Significance of trypsin-like immunoreactivity (TLI) testing for EPI in dogs

<2.5 µg/l:	Exocrine pancreatic insufficiency (EPI)
2.5 to 5 µg/l:	Inconclusive; ensure fasted samples collected; retest
>5.0 µg/l:	Normal exocrine function; check for malabsorption

Figure 8.12: The clinical signs of small intestinal disease and EPI are very similar. The clinician normally needs to carry out a series of different diagnostic tests in order to differentiate these two conditions. The TLI test is a definitive test for exocrine pancreatic function. If this value is normal, the clinician should investigate for small intestinal disease.

interpretation of results where liver disease may be a differential diagnosis. Serum lipase levels are, however, considered to be more reliable than serum amylase in detection of pancreatitis. Values in excess of three times the normal range should be considered diagnostic. The severity of pancreatitis, however, cannot be determined simply by the rise in serum lipase. Where the clinical signs suggest pancreatitis but lipase levels remain normal, the patient should be reassessed and a TLI test carried out.

Recent work has suggested that the serum TLI test (see below) is a more reliable and sensitive indicator of pancreatitis than measuring amylase or lipase. In general, a diagnosis of acute pancreatitis is not made from any single blood sample but from a careful assessment of the patient using a combination of test results such as serum amylase, lipase and TLI, together with changes observed on radiography and ultrasonography. In the future, trypsin activation proteins (TAP) in plasma and urine may provide a more specific marker for pancreatitis.

TLI test

The serum trypsin-like immunoreactivity test has now become the definitive test for diagnosing exocrine pancreatic insufficiency (EPI) in the dog and cat. Normally the pancreas releases very small amounts of trypsin into the circulation, where it can be measured; the normal range is 5–35 µg/l for dogs and 17–49 µg/l for cats. A definitive diagnosis of EPI can be made when TLI levels are <2.5 µg/l in dogs and <10 µg/l in cats. Canine serum TLI can be measured by several UK laboratories, but there is currently only one laboratory where feline TLI can be assayed (Dr D. Williams, Purdue University, USA). Malabsorption and EPI are indistinguishable clinically and the differentiation depends on the results of diagnostic tests of which TLI plays a major role (Figure 8.12).

As indicated above, TLI may also be used to assist in the diagnosis of acute pancreatitis. Serum TLI values >35 µg/l in dogs and >49 µg/l in cats are considered significant. It is important to collect fasted blood samples early in the course of the disease as TLI values fall sharply after the first 3 days.

Serum folate and cobalamin

Folate, a water-soluble vitamin, requires small intestinal mucosal deconjugase to increase its availability for carrier-mediated absorption specifically in the proximal small intestine. Very little is absorbed in the distal intestine. Cobalamin, another water-soluble vitamin, is selectively absorbed from the distal small intestine after a complex series of events. Ingested cobalamin must be complexed by gastric acid and enzymes before it is bound to R protein (secreted from the salivary glands and gastric mucosa). The cobalamin–R complex enters the duodenum where pancreatic proteases digest the R protein, releasing the cobalamin which then binds with intrinsic factor (secreted by the pancreas). It is this complex that is recognized by receptors in the ileum, where it is absorbed.

Serum values are labile, reflecting a balance between dietary intake (normally in excess), intestinal absorption and bacterial utilization and/or production. Measurement of serum levels of these two parameters has been used to detect the presence of small intestinal disease (malabsorption) (Table 8.2). Low serum folate occurs in proximal small intestinal disease and low cobalamin in distal small intestinal disease.

Condition	Serum folate	Serum cobalamin
SIBO	High	Low (occasionally normal)
Proximal small intestinal disease	Low	Normal
Distal small intestinal disease	Normal	Low
Diffuse small intestinal disease	Low	Low

Table 8.2: Values of serum folate and cobalamin in small intestinal diseases.

Reference ranges for serum folate: dog: 3.5–8.5 µg/l; cat: 13.4–to 38 µg/l
Reference ranges for serum cobalamin: dog: 200–500 ng/l; cat: 200–1680 ng/l

Hypoadrenocorticism (Addison's disease)
Focal myasthenia gravis
Lead poisoning
Hypothyroidism
Botulism
Systemic lupus erythematosus
Secondary to oesophageal obstruction

Figure 8.13: *Specific conditions that may be associated with acquired mega-oesophagus in the dog.*

Absorptive capacity is high and only after significant mucosal damage over a period of time will values fall significantly. In man low cobalamin leads to megalo-blastic anaemia and in dogs non-regenerative anaemia has been recorded. In the author's experience, only significant decreases in either parameter, with a serum folate of <1 µg/l and cobalamin of <100 ng/l, are indicative of small intestinal disease. Unfortunately, many factors may influence these parameters, which makes a diagnosis of SIBO or small intestinal disease difficult. It is therefore important to look at these parameters in conjunction with other diagnostic tests. Hereditory cobalamin deficiency has been reported in the Shar-Pei and Giant Schnauzer.

Gastrin assay

Gastrin is a hormone produced by the G cells of the pyloric antrum and duodenum and by the D cells of the endocrine pancreas. Gastrin secretion is stimulated by the sight and smell of food and by the presence of food in the mouth and stomach. An increased level of hydrogen ions in the duodenum reduces gastrin secretion. Gastrin stimulates gastric acid, pepsin and pancreatic secretions; it also promotes gastrointestinal motility.

Anorexia, chronic vomiting, diarrhoea and weight loss are abnormalities observed in the Zollinger–Ellison syndrome. This syndrome is associated with a gastrin-secreting tumour which may be located in the stomach, duodenum or pancreas. Although well documented in man and dogs, the syndrome has rarely been recorded in the cat. Canine fasted gastrin levels may become grossly elevated in this condition but the results are variable. Intravenous infusion of calcium salts normally stimulates gastrin secretion, but in Zollinger–Ellison syndrome an excessive response is observed. Blood samples must be collected after a 24-hour fast and the serum separated immediately after clot formation and deep-frozen prior to assay. Gastrin is usually measured by radioimmunoassay and the test is available from a limited number of specialist laboratories. The mean normal fasted gastrin value for dogs is 65 ± 17pg/ml, although values below 100 pg/ml are usually considered normal. Dogs with Zollinger–Ellison syndrome have gastrin values in the range 360–2700 pg/ml. Mean fasted values in cats are 40 ± 3 pg/ml. Cats with hypergastrinaemia have values above 300 pg/ml.

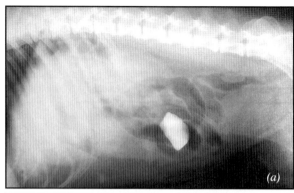
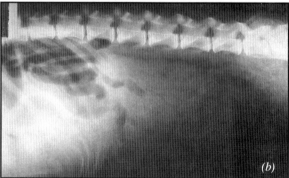
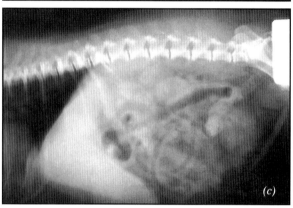

Figure 8.14: *Plain radiographs and contrast studies may sometimes be of diagnostic value in alimentary tract disease (although they are often of limited value). Radiographs showing: (a) a radiodense intestinal foreign body; (b) an intussusception; (c) gross hepatomegaly; (d) pancreatitis; (e) lymphosarcoma; and (f) BIPS.*

Antibodies to acetylcholine receptors

The majority of mega-oesophagus cases seen in the dog (>90%) are said to be 'idiopathic' and result from some failure in the sensory perception of a food bolus in the proximal oesophagus, rather than a defect in motor function. However, a minority of have a detectable underlying disease (Figure 8.13). Recent research has suggested that up to 25% of mega-oesophagus cases may be due to a focal form of myasthenia gravis. These dogs show no signs of systemic myasthenia and a diagnosis can only be made from detection of serum antibody to acetylcholine receptors. Currently this can only be carried out in the USA (Dr Shelton, University of California). Normal dogs have values up to 0.6 nmol/l, while dogs with focal myasthenia gravis have values of >0.6 nmol/l.

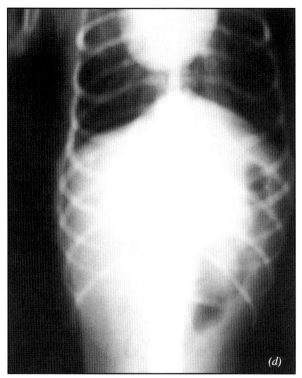

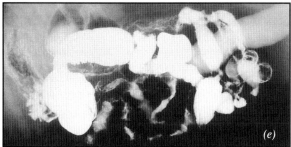

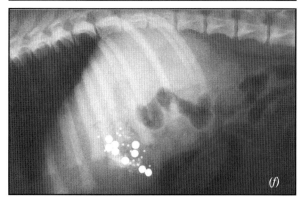

Figure 8.14: Continued.

IMAGING TECHNIQUES

Radiography

Survey radiographs are of value in the investigation of alimentary tract disease. They are useful for highlighting foreign bodies, tumours, and changes in organ position and size (Figure 8.14). Where motility disorders are suspected, contrast studies may be of greater value. Barium swallows, in conjunction with fluoroscopy, can be of particular value in the investigation of dysphagias. Where fluoroscopy is not

available, serial radiographs may still be of value. Contrast studies may prove useful in locating the presence of non-radiodense foreign bodies and filling defects (due to ulcers and neoplasms). Plain radiographs and contrast studies are of little value in the investigation of chronic diarrhoeas, as changes are usually at the microscopic level.

Contrast media used in gastroenterology include barium sulphate, which has traditionally been used to examine the alimentary tract but should not be used where perforation of the bowel is suspected or where aspiration into the respiratory tract is likely. In these situations barium sulphate is poorly resorbed and may cause local reactions. An iodine-based contrast medium may be used in situations where perforation may be present as it is readily resorbed from body cavities or the respiratory tract. The disadvantage of iodine contrast medium is that it is usually hypertonic and results in fluid movement into the bowel which may already be seriously compromised. It is therefore important to give careful consideration to the type of contrast medium used.

BIPS

Barium-impregnated polyethylene spheres (BIPS) are available for the detection of gastrointestinal obstructions and motility disorders. The BIPS have a similar radiodensity to food and are designed to be readily identifiable on plain radiographs (Figure 8.14f). Capsules containing 10 large BIPS (5 mm in diameter) and 30 small BIPS (1.5 mm in diameter) may be given on their own or with food, depending on the condition under investigation.

The small BIPS mimic the passage of food along the gastrointestinal tract, while the large BIPS are useful for the detection of partial and complete

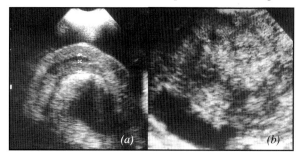

Figure 8.15: Abdominal ultrasonography can be useful in the diagnosis of disorders of the digestive tract, in particular for detecting thickening of the small intestine (a) and for examination of the liver (b).

obstructions. In particular BIPS may be used to determine gastric emptying time and gastrointestinal transit time. Various tables are provided by the manufacturer for average transit times in the dog and cat. The reader is recommended to review these data when interpreting the results of a BIPS investigation.

Retention of BIPS within the stomach suggest an outflow obstruction or gastric hypomotility, while bunching of the BIPS anywhere along the intestinal tract suggests a site of obstruction. Unopposed passage of the small BIPS along the intestine but bunching of the large BIPS suggests a partial obstruction. Scattering of BIPS throughout the intestine suggests paralytic ileus.

As the passage of BIPS can take many hours (>6 h) care is required in patient selection. Animals that are persistently vomiting and dehydrated may be compromised by the time required to carry out this investigation.

Ultrasonography

Ultrasonography has proved to be a useful tool in the investigation of alimentary tract disease. Loops of small intestine may be examined and the thickness of the intestinal wall assessed (Figure 8.15). The author has found this particularly useful in confirming the presence of protein-losing enteropathies and lymphosarcoma. Small volumes of ascitic fluid are more readily detected by ultrasonography than by radiography. The liver may also be scanned for changes in echogenicity, and ultrasound-guided biopsy is now commonly employed to reach a definitive diagnosis of liver disease (see Chapter 9). The pancreas may, with

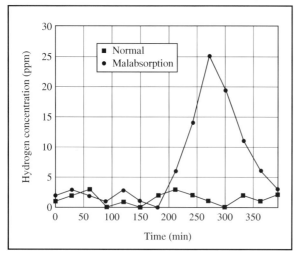

Figure 8.16: Breath hydrogen assay curve for a normal dog, together with a curve from a dog with small intestinal disease. The peak in exhaled hydrogen in the diseased animal occurs 3–4 hours after administration of the oral substrate.

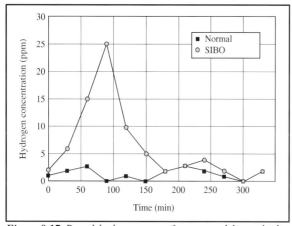

Figure 8.17: Breath hydrogen curve for a normal dog and a dog with SIBO. The peak in exhaled hydrogen in the dog with SIBO occurs within 2 hours of oral substrate administration.

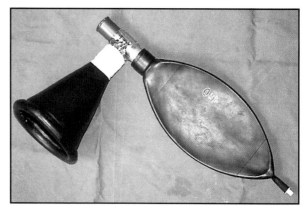

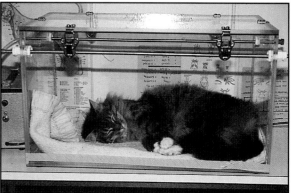

Figure 8.18: Collection of exhaled breath in dogs is carried out using a face mask, one-way valve and anaesthetic collection bag. In cats a perspex cage is used through which a constant flow of air is provided. Aliquots of air are sampled to produce a hydrogen curve.

some difficulty, be examined to assist in the diagnosis of pancreatitis, and the detection of pancreatic abscesses and tumours.

BREATH HYDROGEN ASSAY

When a normal dog or cat ingests a meal, the food is digested efficiently and absorbed from the small intestine, leaving a small residue of undigestible material (fibre) which enters the colon. Resident bacteria in the colon ferment the fibre to provide short-chain fatty acids and a mixture of gases, including hydrogen. Some of the hydrogen is absorbed into the circulation and transported to the lungs, whence it is lost in exhaled breath. The amount of hydrogen produced in this way by normal animals is low, usually <4 ppm. Recognition of any small elevation in breath hydrogen may be used to determine orocaecal transit time by feeding a substrate such as lactulose which will be readily fermented when it reaches the colon.

If an animal has a malabsorption syndrome, undigested carbohydrate from the small intestine will be delivered to the colon where resident bacteria will metabolize the carbohydrate as described above, producing large amounts of hydrogen. This can be assessed quantitatively by feeding xylose to the animal and collecting timed samples of exhaled

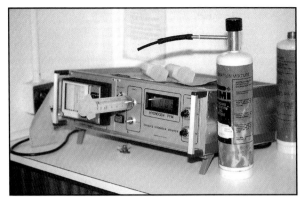

Figure 8.19: *The breath hydrogen analyser. The level of hydrogen, in ppm, is shown in the analyser window.*

breath. A peak in hydrogen production will occur between 3 and 4 hours after ingestion (Figure 8.16).

In SIBO there is an abnormally high bacterial population in the small intestine which competes for nutrients with the processes of digestion and absorption, resulting in an elevation in exhaled hydrogen levels. This can be measured by feeding either lactulose or xylose to the animal and detecting an early elevation in exhaled hydrogen of at least three times base levels between 60 and 90 minutes after ingestion (Figure 8.17). Although there is some confusion over the substrates used in the test and the subsequent values obtained, human studies suggest that the breath hydrogen test is a sensitive (93%) and specific (78%) test for SIBO. Accuracy figures for the dog and cat have still to be produced.

The test requires the collection of exhaled breath using an anaesthetic mask connected to a one-way valve and collection bag for dogs and a sampling chamber for cats (Figure 8.18). The breath hydrogen analyser uses a hydrogen cell to detect the presence of hydrogen in breath samples. Exhaled air should be collected in 50 ml syringes and injected into the analyser (Figure 8.19).

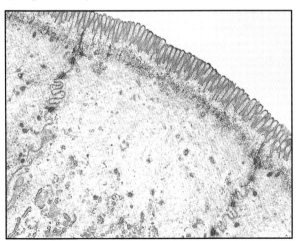

Figure 8.20: *Enterocytes line the villi of the small intestine and normally form an impermeable barrier to the passage of antigen. When the integrity of the tight junctions between these cells is damaged, macromolecules leak into the submucosa. Using sugar probes of different size allows the degree of 'leakiness' to be assessed.*

An immediate reading in parts per million will be provided by the machine. The patient should be starved overnight before the test. A suitable substrate is administered orally after collection of a resting breath sample. Further samples are collected at 15-minute intervals in cats and at 30-minute intervals in dogs and are read by the analyser. The test should continue for at least 4 hours. It is not necessary to own a hydrogen analyser as exhaled air samples are stable and may be safely collected in stoppered and labelled 50 ml syringes. These can then be taken to a local hospital for analysis, making a considerable saving in cost.

INTESTINAL PERMEABILITY AND SUGAR PROBES

Intestinal permeability is now thought to be an important cause and effect of small intestinal diseases. In a previous assay system, radiolabelled albumin was infused intravenously and the level of radioactivity determined in faecal samples. Orally administered [^{51}Cr]–EDTA has also been used but in this case radioactivity in urine is measured. These tests are limited to those centres where radioactive isotopes can be used.

In order to overcome this significant difficulty, the use of sugar probes has been developed. Normally, substrates such as xylose, glucose and rhamnose (which are monosaccharides) are absorbed by carriers on the surface of the enterocytes. Larger molecules such as lactulose (disaccharide) cannot enter these pores and may only be absorbed if the tight junctions between the cells (Figure 8.20) become porous or 'leaky'. Absorption by this route should not normally occur as it would expose the lamina propria to luminal antigen and induce an immune response. Such a response may cause further increases in permeability, leading to protein-losing enteropathy.

To assess intestinal permeability two sugar probes are required — one that normally enters through the enterocyte pores or carriers, and another that can only enter between the tight junctions when they are disrupted. By using two probes the effects of delayed gastric emptying or other motility disturbances are equalized as both sugars are treated similarly. The probes must not be metabolized in the small intestine or by the liver following absorption and must be excreted directly into the urine. Rhamnose and lactulose have fulfilled these requirements, as have cellobiose and mannitol.

The test is carried out following an overnight fast and the urinary bladder must be thoroughly emptied prior to administration of the sugar probes. An oral dose of rhamnose (1 g) plus lactulose (3 g) in 10 ml of water is administered. Five hours after oral dosing the urinary bladder is completely emptied and the total volume of urine measured. In the author's experience dogs will retain urine comfortably for 5 hours, but if this proves to be a problem repeated catheterization can be carried out. A 10 ml aliquot of urine preserved in thiomersal is sent to the laboratory for analysis, usually by high-pressure liquid chromatography. The percentage excretion of each sugar and the ratio of lactulose to rhamnose excretion are calculated. This ratio is considered to be of greatest diagnostic value. The lactulose: rhamnose (disaccharide: monosaccharide) ratio in normal dogs is 0.12 ± 0.05 (SD) while dogs with protein-losing enteropathy and significant intestinal permeability have ratios of 0.59 ± 0.37 (SD). Values are currently being assessed for dogs with other forms of intestinal disease. The test is a valuable diagnostic tool (Quigg *et al.*, 1993) but also has value in assessing response to treatment; repeating the sugar probe assay 2–4 weeks after initiating therapy allows the clinician to determine the degree of improvement that has occurred without resort to further intestinal biopsy.

ENDOSCOPY

Information obtained from the clinical examination and subsequent clinical investigation rarely permits more than a tentative diagnosis, indicating the region of the alimentary tract affected. A definitive diagnosis normally requires histological examination of biopsy samples collected from the suspect region. Until recently, biopsy samples could only be obtained by performing an exploratory laparotomy. However, the availability of flexible endoscopes now permits biopsy without resort to invasive surgery. Rigid endoscopes may be used for the same purpose but are restricted to use in the diagnosis and treatment of oesophageal, colonic and rectal disorders.

For details on the principles of endoscopy, the types of endoscopic equipment available, and biopsy interpretation, the reader is recommended to review the *BSAVA Manual of Canine and Feline Gastroenterology* (Thomas *et al.*, 1996).

Biopsy
The alimentary tract should be carefully examined for macroscopic changes as the endoscope is advanced; in this way iatrogenic changes induced by the endoscope will not be misinterpreted. Where lesions are detected, multiple biopsy samples should be collected, including material from surrounding 'normal' tissue. These samples should be placed in separate, carefully labelled containers in order to assist the pathologist in interpreting the significant changes present. Where no obvious macroscopic abnormality is detected, changes may still be present at the microscopic level, so it is important to collect multiple samples of the tissue being examined.

Endoscopic biopsy samples are small (2–3 mm). Biopsy forceps only collect mucosal samples by avulsion and deeper tissues are not collected. Therefore,

only lesions involving the mucosa will be detected, while those involving deeper tissues will be missed. The author has recorded several cases where endoscopy failed to confirm the presence of a lesion, necessitating an exploratory laparotomy in order to reach a diagnosis.

It is essential to collect multiple samples of any lesion or tissue under investigation, as some samples will be physically damaged no matter how carefully they are collected. Single samples are simply unacceptable and are unlikely to be of diagnostic value.

Biopsy samples may not be diagnostic for several reasons:

· Sampling parallel to the mucosa results in superficial samples, often containing only the tips of the villi
· Sample crushing may occur due to the action of the forceps closing or through rough handling of the sample after collection
· Splinting of the sample on card may distort the sample and make orientation difficult
· There may be a failure to collect representative samples of the lesion and of normal adjacent mucosa for comparison.

Once a lesion has been detected the endoscope should be oriented to provide the best possible perpendicular view of the lesion. The biopsy forceps (with jaws open) should then be advanced towards the lesion and pushed against the mucosa. While maintaining this 'tenting' force, the jaws are closed and the sample retrieved through the endoscope biopsy channel. The jaws of the forceps are then opened and the sample 'floated off' into formol saline. As a guide, where no gross lesion is detected, some eight to twelve biopsy samples should be collected from various sites within the stomach or intestine.

Preparation for upper alimentary endoscopy
For examination of the pharynx, nasopharynx, oesophagus, stomach and duodenum, the patient should be starved for at least 12 hours before the procedure, as endoscopic examination of the stomach is impossible when food is present. If gastric stasis is suspected, a lateral radiograph of the abdomen should be taken prior to carrying out the endoscopy. Following induction of general anaesthesia an endotracheal tube should be tied to the mandible and a gag *must* be placed in the mouth to prevent damage to the endoscope. This facilitates the passage of the endoscope into the pharynx and oesophagus without obstruction. An endotracheal tube is also essential to reduce the risk of aspiration of gastric secretions during endoscopic examination.

Oesophagus
Examination of the oesophagus is indicated for detection of diverticuli, strictures, foreign bodies (Figure

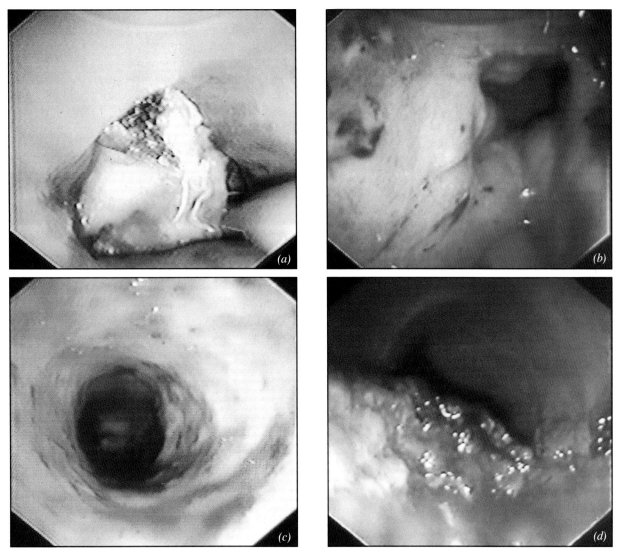

Figure 8.21: *Conditions of the oesophagus, stomach, duodenum and colon may be diagnosed using endoscopy: (a) oesophageal foreign body; (b) gastric neoplasia; (c) ulcerative colitis; and (d) rectal tumour.*

8.21a) and oesophagitis. These changes are usually visible, so biopsy samples are rarely required. The endoscope may be used therapeutically for the removal of oesophageal foreign bodies and for the dilation of strictures.

Stomach

Examination of the stomach is indicated in any patient presented with vomiting and especially where haematemesis is observed. In particular, endoscopy will yield valuable diagnostic information regarding the presence of non-radiodense foreign bodies, chronic inflammation, ulceration and neoplasia (Figure 8.21b). In some cases of chronic inflammation little may be observed macroscopically. All areas of the stomach should be carefully examined prior to collecting biopsy samples and great care should be taken not to over-inflate the stomach. Gastric dilation reduces blood flow to the heart, makes breathing more difficult, causes gastric mucosal ischaemia and makes biopsy collection more difficult, yielding superficial samples.

If a lesion is detected, at least six biopsy samples should be collected if it is safe to do so. It is *not* advisable to sample the craters of ulcers, as they are likely to perforate and usually only yield fibrous tissue that is of little diagnostic value. With ulcers, the periphery of the lesion should be sampled, together with apparently 'normal' tissue next to the lesion. Where no gross lesions are observed, multiple samples should be taken from the cardia, fundus, antrum and pyloric regions of the stomach.

Duodenum

Passage of the endoscope into the duodenum is probably the most difficult procedure undertaken by the endoscopist. This is due to the sharp angle formed between the stomach and the duodenum and because the endoscope 'reds out' (loss of vision) while carrying out this procedure. Great care is needed not to force the endoscope through the pylorus, as perforation of the bowel may occur. Overdistension of the stomach will also make duodenal intubation difficult.

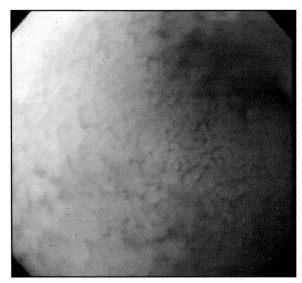

Figure 8.22: *Endoscopic view showing the appearance of the normal duodenum.*

The endoscope should be advanced towards the pylorus and allowed to be 'taken up' with an antral contraction, while applying gentle pressure. This gentle pressure should be maintained if the endoscope appears to be progressing through the pylorus. Once in the duodenum the lumen should be inflated with air to visualize the mucosa which will be readily recognized by the velvet-like appearance produced by the intestinal villi (Figure 8.22). Bile staining and the pancreatic papillae may also be observed. It is rarely possible to pass the endoscope further than the caudal duodenal flexure. The duodenal mucosa is easily sampled but care is needed to ensure that deep biopsy samples are collected and not villus tips. Most often inflammation and loss of the 'velvet' appearance is all that will be noted macroscopically, so multiple biopsy samples should be collected. Duodenal aspirates may be collected using endoscopic catheters for bacterial culture and for the detection of SIBO and giardiasis.

Preparation for colonoscopy

Careful preparation is essential if the colon, caecum, ileocaecocolonic junction and distal ileum are to be examined thoroughly. Patients should be fasted for at least 12 hours before the procedure and should receive a bowel cleanser on the afternoon prior to colonoscopy. In addition, on the morning of the colonoscopy warm water enemas should be administered until clear fluid is voided. Use of soaps or other agents should be avoided as they cause inflammation and interfere with the interpretation of endoscopic findings. Most dogs may be examined under the influence of acepromazine and buprenorphine. Cats should be examined under a general anaesthetic.

With the exception of the rectum, the large intestine should be examined as the endoscope is advanced, to avoid iatrogenic changes. The splenic and pancreatic flexures of the colon are clear landmarks to the endoscopist and the ileocaecocolonic junction is readily identified once the ascending colon has been traversed. Although the ileum cannot be visualized, it is possible to insert biopsy forceps into the ileum and carefully collect a 'blind' biopsy sample.

The most common colonic disorder in the author's experience is lymphocytic–plasmacytic colitis but eosinophilic colitis, granulomatous colitis, whipworm colitis and tumours have also been detected. As with upper alimentary endoscopy, all focal or diffuse lesions observed require biopsy. If no gross changes are identified, multiple samples from the ascending, transverse and descending colon should be taken. It is important to try and place the biopsy forceps perpendicular to the mucosa to ensure that the mucosa is sampled correctly.

The author finds examination of the rectum easier to carry out when gently withdrawing the endoscope from the colon. Air should be constantly infused or the anus pinched with gloved fingers to dilate the rectum. There is marked folding in the rectum, with many sensory receptors present that may cause the patient to strain during this part of the examination. Strictures, polyps and tumours are the most likely findings. In each case it is very important to obtain biopsy samples in order to determine the exact cause of any abnormality.

REFERENCES AND FURTHER READING

Batt RM, Rutgers, HC and Sancak, AA (1994) Enteric bacteria: friend or foe. *Proceedings of the Waltham Symposia.* European Society of Comparative Gastroenterology

Ludow CL (1995) Methods of testing small intestinal function. *Veterinary Medicine* **90,** 934–948

Kirkpatrick CE and Farrell JP (1982) Giardiasis. *Compendium of Continuing Veterinary Education* **4,** 367–374

Kruth SA (1991) Viral and bacterial associated diarrhoeas of the dog and cat. *Waltham International Focus* 1, 24–29

Muir P, Harbour DA, Gruffydd-Jones TJ, Howard PE, Hopper CD, Gruffydd-Jones EAD, Broadhead HM, Clarke CM and Jones ME (1990) A clinical and microbiological study of cats with protruding nictitating membranes and diarrhoea; isolation of a novel virus. *The Veterinary Record* **127,** 324–330

Neer TM (1991) Hypereosinophilic sydrome in cats. *Compendium of Continuing Veterinary Education* **13,** 549–555

Quigg J, Bryden G, Ferguson A and Simpson JW (1993) Evaluation of canine small intestinal permeability using the lactulose/rhamnose urinary excretion test. *Research in Veterinary Science* **55,** 326–332

Simpson JW, Burnie AG, Miles RS, Scott JL and Lindsay DI (1988) Prevalence of Giardia and Cryptosporidium infection in dogs in Edinburgh. *The Veterinary Record* **123,** 445

Simpson JW and Doxey DL (1988) Evaluation of faecal analysis as an aid to the detection of exocrine pancreatic insufficiency. *British Veterinary Journal* **144,** 174–178

Simpson JW and Else RW (1991) *Digestive Diseases of the Dog and Cat.* Blackwell Scientific, Oxford

Thomas DA, Simpson JW and Hall EJ (eds) (1996) *Manual of Canine and Feline Gastroenterology.* BSAVA, Cheltenham

Westermarck E and Sandholm M (1980) Faecal hydrolase activity as determined by radial enzyme diffusion: a new method for detecting pancreatic dysfunction in the dog. *Research in Veterinary Science* **28,** 341–346

Williams DA and Reed SD (1990) Comparison of methods for assay of faecal proteolytic activity. *Veterinary Clinical Pathology* **19,** 20–23

Zajac AM (1992) Giardiasis. *Compendium of Continuing Veterinary Education* **14,** 604–611

Hepatobiliary System

Edward J. Hall

INTRODUCTION

Diseases of the liver frequently present the small animal clinician with a diagnostic challenge; signs are often varied and vague and, despite a wide array of diagnostic tests of both hepatic damage and function, there is rarely a single test that identifies the problem definitively. For example, jaundice is often considered a cardinal sign of liver disease, yet can be caused by non-hepatic conditions (e.g. haemolysis, extrahepatic bile duct obstruction) as well as a range of different liver diseases. Conversely, significant liver disease can exist in the absence of jaundice. Nevertheless, following a thorough history-taking and careful physical examination, astute interpretation of a panel of laboratory tests in conjunction with radiographic and ultrasonographic imaging of the hepatobiliary system will often permit a presumptive diagnosis to be made. In most cases, however, with the exception of congenital portosystemic shunts (PSS), definitive diagnosis of primary liver disease will require histopathological examination of liver tissue.

One significant difficulty in the interpretation of laboratory tests is that results suggestive of liver disease can actually represent secondary effects of non-hepatic disease. Both primary hepatic disease and the liver's response to extrahepatic disease can cause hepatic test abnormalities and histopathological changes. Secondary liver involvement is problematic, as it mimics primary hepatic disease and diverts attention from the underlying disease. Extrahepatic disorders that can cause abnormal hepatic tests are listed in Figure 9.1.

It must always be borne in mind that the liver has great functional reserve capacity and remarkable regenerative capabilities and, therefore, signs often do not occur unless there is severe acute or widespread chronic damage. Yet the sensitivity of some laboratory tests enables detection of hepatic damage before

Acute pancreatitis
Diabetes mellitus
Exocrine pancreatic insufficiency
Extrahepatic bacterial infection
Hyperadrenocortisolism
Hyperthyroidism
Hypoadrenocorticism
Hypothyroidism
Immune-mediated haemolytic anaemia
Inflammatory bowel disease
Protein-losing enteropathy
Right-sided heart failure
Septicaemia
Shock

Figure 9.1: Some of the more common extrahepatic disorders that can cause abnormal liver test results.

Function	Abnormal laboratory test result associated with liver dysfunction
Carbohydrate metabolism: Glucose homeostasis	Hyper- or hypoglycaemia

Lipid metabolism:
    Cholesterol
    Fatty acids
    Lipoproteins
    Bile acids
	Hypo- or hypercholesterolaemia
	Hypertriglyceridaemia
	Lipaemia
	Elevated bile acids

Protein metabolism:
    Albumin
    Globulins
    Coagulation proteins
	Hypoalbuminaemia
	Increased acute phase proteins, immunoglobulins
	Coagulopathies

Vitamin metabolism	? Decreased folate, cobalamin Vitamin E, vitamin K may be reduced depending on the disease
Immunological functions	Hyperglobulinaemia Increased acute phase proteins
Detoxification	Hyperammonaemia Decreased urea Hyperbilirubinaemia

Table 9.1: Clinicopathological abnormalities associated with disturbances of hepatobiliary function.

obvious signs of liver disease are noted. Clinicopathological evidence of hepatic disease in a relatively healthy animal obligates the clinician to establish whether significant primary disease or secondary disease is present. For example, mild elevations in liver enzymes in an older patient may reflect a response to relatively innocuous periodontal disease, or herald the imminent onset of end-stage liver disease. It is only by a combination of tests (often ultimately including biopsy) that the significance of liver enzyme elevation can be determined. In the absence of serious signs, repetition of laboratory tests 2–4 weeks after institution of symptomatic therapy and/or withdrawal of potential hepatotoxins is warranted before attempts at definitive diagnosis are made.

NORMAL HEPATOBILIARY FUNCTION

The liver has a central role in a variety of metabolic functions, a fact reflected in the diverse biochemical abnormalities that may accrue from hepatobiliary dysfunction (Table 9.1). In addition, the liver is the largest reticuloendothelial organ of the body, having a crucial role in the immune system. Kupffer cells of the mononuclear phagocytic system (MPS) provide protection from gut-derived bacteria and toxins in the portal blood, and the liver is the source of complement, acute phase proteins and various cytokines. The liver can also be a major site of extramedullary haematopoiesis.

The acinar architecture of hepatic tissue (Figure 9.2) is the functional basis of the multiple biochemical processes of storage, synthesis, degradation and enterohepatic recycling. Nutrients and toxins are delivered to the liver by the dual arterial and portal venous blood supplies; hepatocytes are in intimate contact with blood constituents filtered through fenestrated sinusoids. Nutrient products of hepatic metabolism are distributed to the body by the hepatic veins, and wastes are excreted through the biliary system. Excess filtered plasma is returned from the space of Disse via lymphatics. Zones of hepatocytes between the portal area and central vein have different levels of oxygenation and different functions, and each is susceptible to different types of injury, such as hypoxia and poisons, that can result in characteristic patterns of test results.

The liver has a crucial role in central metabolism. It is the moderator of fat metabolism, being the site of: cholesterol synthesis, esterification and excretion; fatty acid oxidation and mobilization; triglyceride metabolism and storage; lipoprotein synthesis and release; and phospholipid metabolism. It is also intrinsically involved in carbohydrate metabolism: it enables glucose homeostasis through gluconeogenesis, glycogen storage and degradation, and metabolism of insulin, glucagon and growth hormone. Regulation of amino acid turnover is linked both to glucose and protein metabolism, and synthesis of conditionally essential amino acids, such as glutamine, occurs in the liver. The majority of serum proteins (albumins and α- and β-globulins), as well as carrier proteins (caeruloplasmin, transferrin) and the major coagulation factors, are synthesized in the liver. The liver is involved in the

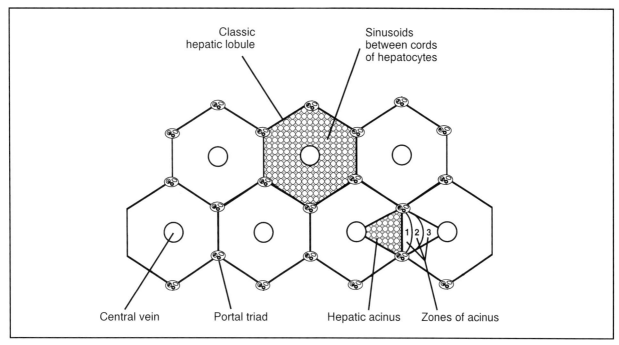

Figure 9.2: Functional acinar structure of the liver that corresponds to zonal distribution (1-3) of blood flow, hepatocellular functions and some histopathological changes.

storage and activation of both water-soluble and fat-soluble vitamins, and metabolic processes are also influenced by the liver's role in the metabolism of polypeptide and steroid hormones.

The urea cycle in hepatocytes is the site of the detoxification of ammonia (derived from muscle during exercise and intestinal bacterial fermentation) to urea for renal excretion. The formation and excretion of bile by the liver is crucial in the metabolism of haemoproteins to bilirubin and the liver is the site of metabolism and conjugation during the detoxification of various xenobiotics. Bile salts are synthesized in the liver and excreted in the bile, playing a crucial role in fat digestion and absorption before undergoing enterohepatic recycling.

CLINICOPATHOLOGICAL CHANGES IN LIVER DISEASE

Consequences of hepatobiliary dysfunction

The diverse functions of the hepatobiliary system are reflected in the diverse clinicopathological changes that can be found in liver disease (Figure 9.3). The defective metabolism and excretion of bilirubin, causing accumulation of circulating bilirubin and the development of jaundice, is often considered the hallmark of liver disease, but it is only one of many abnormal laboratory tests that may found in liver disease. Indeed, even hyperbilirubinaemia from biliary obstruction is usually associated with hypercholesterolaemia and elevations of cholestatic marker enzymes.

The central metabolic role of the liver is highlighted by the inability of the diseased liver to respond by storing substances in times of excess and releasing stores in times of need. Hypoglycaemia is seen in rare glycogen storage diseases and sometimes in end-stage liver disease because of reductions in glycogen stores, gluconeogenic potential, and insulin degradation. Hypocholesterolaemia and hypotriglyceridaemia may be found in congenital PSS and acquired hepatic dysfunction. Hypoalbuminaemia may be a reflection of decreased hepatic synthesis of albumin and may contribute to the development of ascites. Reduced clotting factor synthesis results in bleeding tendencies.

Hyperammonaemia, resulting from failure to detoxify ammonia and associated with accumulation of several other toxins, is a marker of the syndrome of hepatoencephalopathy. Defective urea production is considered to be one of the mechanisms, as well as failure to metabolize cortisol, causing the polyuria/polydipsia sometimes seen in liver disease. Failure to metabolize aldosterone may lead to sodium retention and contribute to ascites/oedema.

Depression, decreased appetite and lethargy
Stunting and weight loss
Vomiting, diarrhoea, and grey acholic faeces
Polydipsia and polyuria
Ascites
Icterus
Altered liver size
Bleeding tendency
Abdominal pain (rare)
Encephalopathy

Figure 9.3: Clinical signs of hepatobiliary disease. Adapted from Sevelius and Jönsson (1996).

Correlation with clinical signs

The clinical signs of liver disease are many and varied (Figure 9.3) and may be related to specific laboratory abnormalities. Signs are often vague and not apparent until there is significant hepatic dysfunction, which is why laboratory testing is helpful in detecting and characterizing early liver disease. However, it must always be remembered that equally abnormal tests may be secondary to a primary systemic disease. For example, fatty infiltration of the liver in diabetes mellitus can cause increases in serum activities of liver specific enzymes in both dogs and cats, and can result in jaundice in cats.

Depression and diminished appetite

These signs are reflections of disturbed metabolism in liver disease, but are not associated with specific laboratory test abnormalities. Anaemia of chronic disease may be present. Abnormal lipoprotein and cholesterol metabolism may occur. Hypoglycaemia is seen in end-stage disease and may be one of many factors producing the signs of liver failure usually attributed to accumulation of metabolic toxins.

Stunting and weight loss

Congenital PSS and juvenile hepatopathies are associated with stunting, but the biochemical disturbances responsible are multifarious. Hypoproteinaemia is often associated with muscle wasting.

Gastrointestinal signs

Grey, acholic faeces are seen in biliary obstruction, and are therefore associated with jaundice. Diarrhoea may be a reflection of hypoproteinaemia causing bowel oedema, although lack of luminal bile salts and portal hypertension are more likely causes.

Polydipsia and polyuria

These signs may be associated with low levels of serum urea, although other mechanisms, e.g. hypercortisolism, are involved in their pathogenesis.

Ascites

Hypoproteinaemia is a recognized cause of tissue fluid accumulation. However, ascites is more common than generalized oedema in liver disease, suggesting portal hypertension in acquired liver disease is also an important factor.

Icterus

Hyperbilirubinaemia causes jaundice, and may be due to prehepatic (haemolysis) or posthepatic (biliary obstruction, biliary leakage) disease as well as primary intrahepatic causes.

Liver size

Diseases causing altered liver size are listed in Figure 9.4, but there are no specific laboratory markers of

---

Microhepatica
Portosytemic shunts (especially in dogs)
Idiopathic hepatic fibrosis
Cirrhosis in dogs
Decreased perfusion (hypotension)
NB. Rule out ruptured diaphragm, peritoneo-pericardial-diaphragmatic hernia

Hepatomegaly

Generalized	*Localized*
Steroid hepatopathy	Primary neoplasia
Fatty infiltration:	Cysts
Diabetes mellitus	Abscess
Feline hepatic	Haematoma
lipidosis	
Congestion:	
Cardiovascular	
Biliary	
Inflammation	
Neoplasia:	
Metastatic	
Lymphosarcoma, myeloproliferative	
Hepatocellular and biliary carcinomas	
Nodular hyperplasia	
Severe anaemia	
Glycogen storage diseases	
Amyloidosis	

Figure 9.4: Differential diagnosis for altered liver size.

liver size and many diseases are not associated with abnormal liver size. Lipaemia may correlate with fatty infiltration of the liver.

Bleeding tendency

Coagulation times are usually abnormal if severe liver dysfunction causes bleeding. Generalized bleeding and haemorrhage from hepatic peliosis (cats) and vascular tumours, such as metastatic haemangiosarcoma, may result in regenerative anaemia.

Hepatoencephalopathy

This syndrome is caused by accumulation of toxins because of severe hepatic dysfunction and/or portosystemic shunting of blood. Hyperammonaemia is a sensitive and specific marker for the syndrome, although other metabolic disturbances are involved.

DIAGNOSTIC APPROACH TO LIVER DISEASE

In most cases, a tentative diagnosis can be deduced from the results of laboratory tests in conjunction with imaging techniques. However, the definitive diagnosis of primary liver disease usually depends ultimately on histological examination of liver biopsy specimens. Primary extrahepatic causes of secondary liver disease will hopefully be identified before biopsy is undertaken.

The age, sex and breed of the patient may help in making a list of differential diagnoses; for example, chronic hepatitis is more prevalent in middle-aged female Dobermann Pinschers (Sevelius and Jönsson, 1996). Acute diseases have a sudden onset, but chronic disease may also have an apparently sudden onset when the liver's reserve capacity is exhausted. Nevertheless, careful questioning of owners often elicits evidence of previous recurring low-grade illness. History of weight loss and ascites also suggests chronic disease.

Physical examination is important in identifying problems that may be causing secondary liver disease. For example, hyperadrenocorticism may produce cutaneous signs such as thin skin, comedones and calcinosis cutis, as well as secondary hepatic enlargement and elevated serum alkaline phosphatase. Indeed the importance of history and physical examination cannot be overemphasized, and any test results must always be interpreted in the light of these findings.

Thus a diagnostic approach to liver disease includes:

- Clinical history
- Physical examination
- Laboratory tests
- Examination of ascitic fluid
- Imaging:
    Radiography
    Ultrasonography
    Angiography
    Scintigraphy
- Liver biopsy.

Some acute hepatopathies may resolve with symptomatic treatment without the need for a definitive diagnosis, and the presence of a congenital PSS may be demonstrated by ultrasonography, scintigraphy and portovenography without resorting to biopsy. However, laboratory tests are still performed to identify an acute

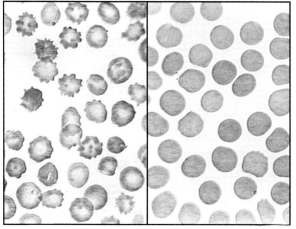

Figure 9.5: Blood smears from (left) a dog with a congenital PSS, showing anisocytosis, microcytosis, mild hypochromia, and several echinocytes (spur cells); and (right) a normal dog. Wright's Giemsa.

Courtesy of Miss M Graham.

hepatopathy or a suspected PSS, and are necessary to document chronic liver dysfunction before liver biopsy is performed.

The aims of laboratory testing are:

- To identify and characterize any hepatic dysfunction
- To identify possible primary causes of secondary liver disease
- To differentiate causes of icterus
- To evaluate potential anaesthetic risks
- To identify causes of anaemia of unknown origin
- To assess prognosis
- To assess the response to xenobiotics
- To monitor response to therapy.

There is a wide range of laboratory tests available for assessing liver status, but they can be conveniently divided into four classes:

- General screening tests
- Markers of liver damage
- Liver function tests
- Prognostic indices.

The tests routinely available to the practising veterinary surgeon and indications for their use will be discussed in detail, and more specialized tests mentioned only briefly.

GENERAL SCREENING TESTS

These tests include haematology, urinalysis, and measurement of serum biochemical parameters performed routinely as part of the minimum data base when investigating any sick animal.

Routine haematology

Red cell series
Mild to moderate anaemia (haematocrit >0.20 and <0.35) is not unusual in liver disease; it may be a reflection of chronic illness, or be associated with haemolysis, gastrointestinal bleeding or a coagulopathy. Profound anaemia (haematocrit <0.20) is typical of primary haemolytic disease, when jaundice may be expected, and otherwise is only seen in liver diseases that result in profuse haemorrhage, such as hepatic trauma, peliosis and vascular tumours like haemangiosarcoma. Microangiopathic haemolytic anaemia, with the presence of RBC fragments (schistocytes) as well as platelet consumption, is characteristic of inflammatory and neoplastic changes.

Microcytosis is a quite common finding in dogs with congenital PSS (Figure 9.5), but whether the mechanism involves abnormal iron metabolism is

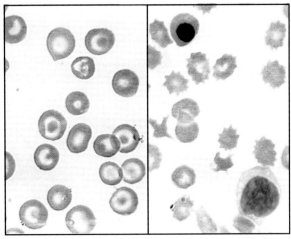

Figure 9.6: (Left) Blood smear fom a Cocker Spaniel with chronic hepatitis, showing slight anisocytosis, hypochromia and target cells. (Right) Blood smear from a German Shepherd Dog with hepatic haemangiosarcoma, showing large polychromatic RBCs and several echinocytes, with a single nucleated RBC (normoblast) and two acanthocytes. A large lymphocyte is also present. Wright's Giemsa.

Courtesy of Miss M Graham.

controversial. Chronic blood loss with iron deficiency anaemia is the major differential diagnosis.

Variable red cell shapes (poikilocytosis) with regularly (echinocytes) and irregularly spiculated erythrocytes (acanthocytes) may be seen in chronic liver disease (Figures 9.5 and 9.6) and are probably the result of changes in phospholipid metabolism.

White cell series
There are no WBC changes pathognomonic for hepatic disease. The total WBC count may be increased and an inflammatory differential count seen in acute infectious disease, e.g. leptospirosis, and sometimes in severe chronic inflammatory hepatopathies and metastatic liver disease with necrosis of tumour nodules.

Platelets
Moderate reduction in platelet numbers and abnormal platelet function are non-specific changes sometimes seen in severe liver disease.

Urinalysis
Orange urine may be the first indication to owners that their pet is jaundiced, but careful biochemical and microscopic examination of urine may provide the clinician with further information about liver dysfunction.

Specific gravity
The consistent presence of a low urine specific gravity (< 1.020) can provide evidence to confirm a history of polyuria/polydipsia in animals with liver disease.

Bilirubin
Circulating unconjugated bilirubin is bound to albu-

min and is not filtered at the glomerulus (Figure 9.7). Conjugated bilirubin is filtered, and bilirubinuria may be an early indication of liver disease in dogs before hyperbilirubinaemia develops. However, the presence of small quantities of bilirubin in urine is normal in dogs as there is a low renal threshold for conjugated bilirubin and the renal tubular cells in male dogs can also metabolize some haemoglobin to conjugated bilirubin. Thus, only a large total amount of urine bilirubin is significant. Semi-quantitative results must therefore be interpreted in light of the overall urine concentration; for example, 2+ bilirubin on a dipstick of isosthenuric urine is probably significant, but this reading is likely to be normal in a urine with 1.050 specific gravity. There is a high renal threshold for bilirubin in cats, which may be why cats are so prone to jaundice even with secondary hepatic disease, and feline bilirubinuria is always of note as it usually occurs in conjunction with jaundice.

Urobilinogen
The origin of urobilinogen (Figure 9.7) will be discussed below, but its presence in urine is normal. Increased amounts are associated with hyperbilirubinaemia, unless there is complete biliary obstruction, when it will be absent. Although the test is found on most urine dipsticks its usefulness is minimal.

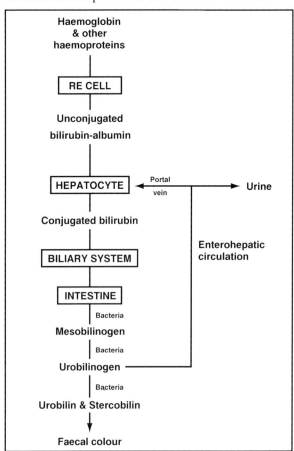

Figure 9.7: Schematic representation of normal degradation of bilirubin and metabolism of urobilinogen.

RE = reticuloendothelial

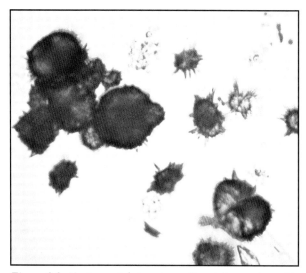

Figure 9.8: *Urate crystals in urine sediment from a dog with a congenital portosystemic shunt.*

Courtesy of Mr W Millard.

Urate crystalluria

Abnormal uric acid metabolism and hyperammonaemia in liver disease can result in precipitation of ammonium biurate crystals in the urine. Occasionally massive crystalluria causes obvious brown turbidity, but mostly characteristic crystals are found by microscopic examination of urine sediment (Figure 9.8). The shape of these crystals are described as resembling mites or thorn-apples. Urate crystals can be found on serial urinalyses in about two-thirds of dogs with congenital PSS.

Serum biochemistry

A number of electrolytes and serum biochemical constituents included in the routine minimum database are not specific indicators of liver disease, but are tested to aid recognition of diseases either mimicking the clinical signs of liver disease or actually causing secondary liver disease. For example, hypercalcaemia may be a marker of hepatic lymphosarcoma, and elevated amylase and lipase activities suggest that pancreatitis may be the cause of elevated liver enzymes.

Some tests routinely included in the minimum database, such as serum enzymes and bilirubin, can be liver-specific and will be discussed later. However, others test abnormalities that, as well as being significant in other diseases do offer a crude assessment of liver status, and they will be discussed here.

Cholesterol

Cholesterol is derived from the diet and hepatic synthesis, and undergoes enterohepatic recycling. However, the usefulness of serum cholesterol concentration as a marker of liver disease is limited as its concentration may be decreased, normal or increased, depending on the type of liver disease and the dietary intake. Hypocholesterolaemia can be found in cases of PSS, cirrhosis and liver failure as well as in

malabsorption. Hypercholesterolaemia may be present in major bile duct occlusion in dogs and cats, and is typically found in a number of metabolic diseases, including diabetes mellitus, hyperadrenocorticism, hypothyroidism, and hyperlipidaemia, as well as pancreatitis and nephrotic syndrome, which may all secondarily affect the liver.

Triglycerides

Abnormalities of lipid metabolism in canine and feline liver disease are not well characterized; although abnormal lipoprotein profiles have been identified in human liver disease, serum triglyceride concentration is likely to be the only test available to veterinary surgeons. Hypertriglyceridaemia is seen in biliary obstruction, and reduced concentrations may be seen in chronic hepatitis. Lipaemia is seen in a number of metabolic diseases that secondarily affect the liver, e.g. diabetes mellitus.

Glucose

Transient postprandial hyperglycaemia may occur in liver disease because of the failure of glucose homeostasis, but homeostatic mechanisms are so effective that significant fasting hypoglycaemia is only seen occasionally in massive hepatic necrosis, PSS and end-stage liver disease. Sepsis and large or diffuse tumours, such as hepatoma or lymphomas, may cause hypoglycaemia through excessive glucose utilization or release of insulin-like activities.

Congenital hepatic enzyme deficiencies, termed glycogen storage diseases, are very rare but may cause hypoglycaemia and hepatic engorgement with stored glycogen. Glycogenoses caused by deficiencies of glucose 6-phosphatase (type I – von Gierke's disease) and the debranching enzyme amylo-1,6-glucosidase (type III – Cori's disease) have been described very rarely in dogs. The differential diagnosis of hypoglycaemia in young dogs includes transient juvenile hypoglycaemia, hypoadrenocorticism and PSS. Hypoglycaemia in older dogs is most commonly caused by insulin-secreting pancreatic tumours (insulinomas).

Urea and creatinine

Azotaemia (increased serum urea and creatinine concentrations) indicates decreased glomerular filtration which is sometimes the consequence of primary hepatic disease. A disproportionate increase in urea compared with creatinine in a fasting sample may be seen in animals with gastrointestinal haemorrhage because of increased ammonia synthesis by intestinal bacteria. Coagulopathies and portal hypertension in liver disease can lead to occult gastrointestinal haemorrhage that may be detected by changes in the urea:creatinine ratio before haematemesis or melaena is noted.

Low serum concentrations of urea, relative to serum creatinine, are sometimes seen in animals with

Cause	Albumin	Globulin	Clinical signs	Confirmatory test
Liver disease	↓	Normal or ↑	Varied (includes diarrhoea & weight loss)	Liver function test
Protein-losing enteropathy	↓	↓	Diarrhoea & weight loss	None readily available ($[^{51}Cr]$-albumin excretion)
Protein-losing nephropathy	↓	Normal	Nephrotic syndrome & weight loss	Proteinuria (dipstick, urine protein:creatinine ratio)

Table 9.2: Differentiation of hypoproteinaemia.

PSS or severe liver dysfunction because of the failure to convert ammonia to urea. However, this is an unreliable marker because the normal lower limit for serum urea concentration is near the limit of the assay, and prolonged anorexia can produce very low urea concentrations.

Serum proteins
Serum total protein (reference ranges: dog 50–78 g/l; cat 60–82 g/l) and, especially, albumin concentrations can be considered crude markers of liver function as the liver is the source of all albumin and most globulins except γ-globulins. Their value as prognostic markers will be discussed below. The differential diagnosis of hypoproteinaemia includes liver disease and protein-losing enteropathies and nephropathies. These three classes of disease can often be distinguished by their clinical signs, their relative changes in albumin and globulin concentrations, and simple confirmatory laboratory tests (Table 9.2).

Albumin: (Reference ranges: dog: 22–35 g/l; cat: 25–39 g/l.) Mild decreases in albumin concentration are seen in anorexia, in inflammatory diseases as an acute phase response with down-regulation of synthesis (in an inverse relationship to an increase in serum globulin), and in ascitic animals because of the increased volume of distribution. Dogs and cats have a large reserve capacity for albumin synthesis, and profound hypoalbuminaemia in liver disease is usually only seen with PSS and severe disease. In end-stage liver disease there is both decreased albumin synthesis and dilution of serum by sodium and water retention. The half-life of albumin in dogs is variously reported to be between 1 and 3 weeks; whichever, significant reductions in albumin concentration develop relatively slowly and indicate the existence of chronic disease.

Globulins: (Reference ranges: dog: 22–45 g/l; cat: 26–50 g/l.) Hyperglobulinaemia is common in acquired liver disease not just because there may be an inflammatory aetiology, but also because of any acute phase response and decreased clearance of antigen by Kupffer cells resulting in a systemic immune response.

Thus most globulins are increased in inflammatory diseases; α- and β-globulins include acute phase proteins and increase in inflammation in parallel with immunoglobulins. The hyperglobulinaemia may be sufficient to mask hypoalbuminaemia if only total protein concentration is measured. Hyperglobulinaemia is particularly seen in cats with feline infectious peritonitis and lymphocytic cholangiohepatitis, two conditions that can cause jaundice and ascites.

ENZYME MARKERS OF LIVER DISEASE

Increased serum activities of liver-specific enzymes are considered markers of liver damage. However, increased activities are common and are not necessarily associated with clinically significant liver disease. Systemic disease and various drugs can cause misleading and potentially reversible increases in serum activities. Conversely, severe hepatic dysfunction without significant liver damage, such as with a congenital PSS, may be associated with no or minimal marker enzyme release. The difficulty clinicians face is deciding whether liver enzyme elevations are significant, and if so whether they represent primary or secondary liver disease. It is here where interpretation of results in light of the other aspects of the diagnostic investigation, and in particular the history and physical examination, is important. For example, feline hyperthyroidism causes secondary increases in liver enzymes, and measurement of thyroid function is indicated before liver biopsy in older cats with polyphagia, weight loss and increased enzyme activities.

Even when increased serum activities are associated with primary liver disease, it is a popular misconception that these are 'liver *function* tests'. It is important to recognize that these tests give little evidence of the type of lesion present, and no information concerning whether it is localized or diffuse, the overall functional state of liver, or the reversibility of the disease. The magnitude of the increase in activity is not necessarily important, although it may correlate with the number of cells involved; thus, mild elevations may either be of no consequence or may indicate loss of almost all hepatocytes in end-stage disease.

Serum enzyme activities depend on their total hepatic activity, their intracellular location and thus their tendency to leak from hepatocytes, their potential for induction by drugs and also their serum half-life. It has been postulated that occasional persistent elevations of liver enzymes in the absence of abnormal hepatic function and histopathology may reflect the presence of macroenzymes; large, antibody-bound complexes of enzymes are cleared slowly but have no clinical significance. However, persistently elevated liver marker enzymes usually indicate persistent, chronic disease.

Liver enzyme activities that can be measured in serum can be classified into two major types:

- Hepatocellular enzymes released by cell damage (leakage markers)

- Biliary enzymes whose synthesis is induced by drugs and retained bile (cholestatic markers).

A number of enzymes are available for measurement, but within a class one enzyme rarely offers greater diagnostic advantage over the others. Therefore, the routine biochemical profile usually only offers one or two enzymes within each class, and with which the clinician should become familiar. Reference values will vary between laboratories depending on the assay methodology.

Hepatocellular/leakage enzymes

Alanine aminotransferase
(ALT or serum ALT (SALT);
formerly SGPT = serum glutamate-pyruvate dehydrogenase)
Reference ranges: dog <100 units/l; cat <75 units/l[1]

This cytosolic enzyme is found in hepatocytes in concentrations 10,000-fold greater than in normal serum, and measurement of its release into serum is considered the test of choice for hepatocellular damage. ALT is considered to be liver-specific in dogs and cats, although small amounts are found in heart, kidney and muscle; ALT is negligible in horses and ruminants. The serum half-life of ALT in dogs is variously reported to be between 3 hours and 4 days. Nevertheless, the half-life is shorter in cats and therefore the normal reference range is lower in cats and smaller increases are as significant. Immediate increases in serum ALT activities are found following release either by hepatocyte necrosis or by 'leakage' because of altered cell membrane permeability and/or altered cell metabolism. Acute hepatopathies, such as infectious canine hepatitis or caused by toxins, may cause a rapid 100-fold increase in activity (Figure 9.9). Increases may not be as marked in chronic hepatitis but are persistent.

Measurement of ALT is *not* a test of function. Whilst the magnitude of the rise in ALT in acute liver disease is roughly proportional to the number of hepatocytes affected, it gives no information on whether the lesion is focal or diffuse, and does not directly reflect the severity of the disease, its reversibility or the prognosis. A common mistake in the interpretation of ALT is to give too much significance to the magnitude of the rise. ALT tends to increase more in acute than chronic disease, and indeed an end-stage liver may have activities within the reference range if there are only a few hepatocytes left to leak enzyme. Yet recovery from acute hepatitis is more likely than with chronic disease; it is the persistence of enzyme elevation that is often of more diagnostic and prognostic importance (Figure 9.9).

Whilst a fall in ALT activities can also be a bad prognostic sign if it reflects loss of hepatocytes, usually a gradual decline in ALT following an acute insult indicates a good prognosis; activities should fall by 50% every 3–4 days, and have returned to normal in 2–3 weeks (Figure 9.9). The fact that activities decline more slowly than would be predicted from the enzyme's short half-life has led to a recent suggestion that serum ALT is derived from regenerating hepatocytes as well as the initial leakage from damaged cells.

ALT rises immediately following acute hepatocyte injury, but increases occur more slowly in cholestatic liver disease (Figure 9.9). It often does not reach the magnitude of the increase in cholestatic marker enzymes (see below). Presumably bile stasis leads to secondary hepatocyte damage due to accumulation of toxic bile salts. Similarly cholangiohepatitis in cats causes a moderate (5–10-fold) increase in ALT. Rises in ALT activity are also seen in some but not all cases of primary and secondary hepatic neoplasia; any tumour-associated necrosis or leakage from tumour cells will cause the rise. It should be stressed again that in end-stage liver disease, when there are few remaining viable hepatocytes, activities of ALT may be in the reference range or only mildly increased.

Small increases in ALT can also be caused by microsomal enzyme induction after administration of hepatotoxic drugs. The rise in activity tends to be dose-dependent. Therapeutic doses of anticonvulsants such as phenobarbitone usually produce a 4–5-fold increase, whereas toxic doses can cause a 50-fold rise. Idiosyncratic reactions with the development of significant liver dysfunction are likely to be associated with greater rises in ALT. Glucocorticoids can also induce ALT activity; a very high dose of >4 mg/kg prednisolone can eventually cause a 10-fold rise in ALT, but the increase is usually disproportionately less than the induced rise in cholestatic enzymes (see below). Increased activity may persist for several weeks following a single dose of steroids.

[1]*Reference values will vary with assay method and laboratory.*

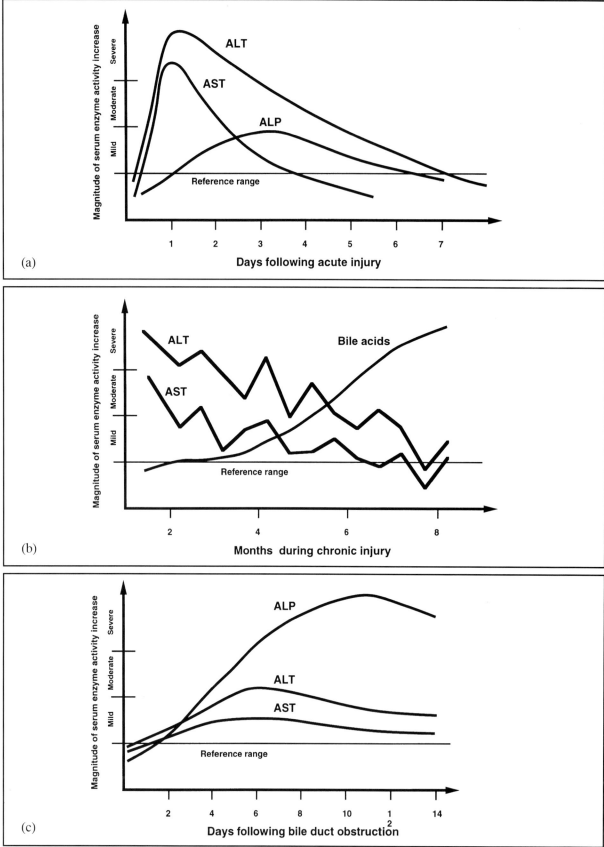

Figure 9.9: *Patterns of changes in serum liver enzymes following (a) an acute injury with resolution, (b) persistent injury and (c) cholestasis. In (a) note the parallel rise in ALT and AST but longer persistence of ALT because of its longer half-life and synthesis during hepatic repair. The rise in ALP lags behind ALT, may continue to rise for a period after resolution, and persists for longer. In (b) hepatocellular marker enzymes remain persistently elevated although there is a general decline with disease progression as assessed by increasing bile acid concentration. In (c) note the rise and plateau in ALP with lesser increase in ALT and AST.*

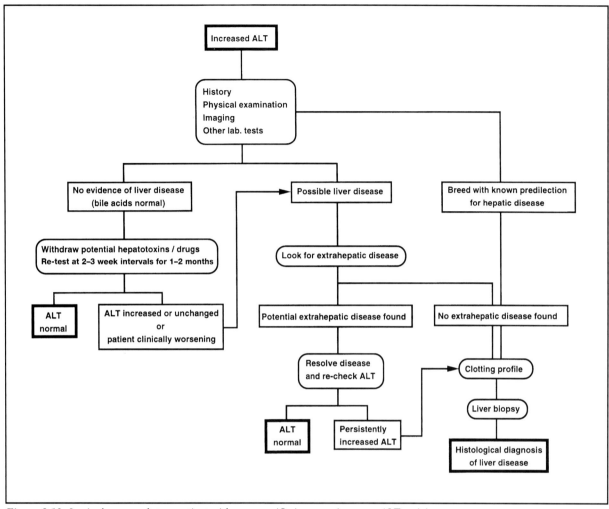

Figure 9.10: *Logical approach to a patient with non-specific increase in serum ALT activity.*

Another problem of interpretation of ALT activities is that the changes in activity are very sensitive to secondary and clinically insignificant hepatic disease. It is not unusual to see 5-fold increases in ALT in dogs with primary gastrointestinal disease. Liver biopsy is not indicated in most of these cases as liver function tests (see below) are normal but, if performed, histological changes are mild or absent. It is believed that release of cytokines by activated Kupffer cells results in mild hepatocyte damage. The author has seen dogs with exocrine pancreatic insufficiency with 10-fold increases in ALT that reverse with treatment of the primary disease.

When a clinician is faced with a patient with apparently non-specific increases in ALT, found either on a routine biochemical screen or during illness, a logical approach to be taken is shown in Figure 9.10.

Increased ALT is usually expected secondary to fatty infiltration in diabetes mellitus, but the unwary may be distracted from the primary problem when they find some increase in ALT in haemolytic anaemia, secondary to hypoxic damage. The liver can also be considered a large lymph node, and reaction with increased ALT may be seen in response to sepsis and endotoxaemia from any site. Thus, since even

periodontal disease can cause mildly elevated serum ALT activities, the careful clinician usually checks at least one other liver enzyme and performs a liver function test before embarking on liver biopsy. Persistent elevation of ALT over 1–2 months is indication for further investigations such as liver biopsy even if clinical signs are not yet apparent.

Aspartate aminotransferase
(AST or serum AST (SAST);
formerly SGOT = serum glutamate-oxaloacetate transaminase)
Reference ranges: dog 7–50 units/l; cat 7–60 units/l

This is another hepatocellular enzyme that is released by cell damage, but unlike ALT it is also found in significant quantities in other tissues, most notably the heart and skeletal muscle. However, skeletal muscle inflammation is relatively uncommon in the dog and cat, and measurement of a muscle-specific enzyme such as creatine kinase (CK) can define any muscle damage. In liver disease, rises in AST usually parallel ALT, and an increase in AST and CK but not ALT probably indicates muscle damage.

Since AST appears to have no advantage over ALT as a marker of hepatocyte damage in terms of liver-specificity, it is not valued by some workers.

However, because some of the hepatocellular AST is mitochondrial-bound rather than all free in the cytosol, its release depends more on cell necrosis than just a leaky membrane. Release of AST often lags slightly behind ALT, but its half-life is shorter and therefore its presence probably suggests more profound or persistent injury than if just ALT is increased. It therefore can be a more specific marker of significant liver damage than ALT as it is not so susceptible to minor insults. For example, AST is only minimally increased by glucocorticoids. In human beings differentiation of the cytosolic and mitochondrial isoforms of AST has prognostic implications, but this level of sophistication is not currently available in veterinary medicine.

Increases in AST in acute hepatitis parallel increases in ALT although they are rarely more than 50-fold. Although they decline over several weeks they usually normalize before ALT; persistently elevated AST is a poor prognostic sign (Figure 9.9). Smaller increases in AST are seen in chronic hepatitis and cholestatic disease. Once again, the plasma AST half-life of 1 hour in cats is less than in dogs (5 hours) and therefore smaller increases are as significant, and it has been suggested that AST is a more sensitive marker of significant liver disease in cats.

Others

In most cases ALT, and perhaps AST, are the only hepatocellular marker enzymes that need to be measured. However, there are a number of other candidate markers, developed primarily for ruminants (which have no ALT), that have been proposed for use in dogs and cats. None has been shown to have any significant advantage.

Arginase: Another liver-specific enzyme, arginase, is localized in the mitochondria, and therefore its release is less influenced by trivial damage. Leakage of arginase ceases during recovery unlike ALT and, therefore, persistent increases carry a poorer prognosis. The measurement of arginase has not yet become routine, because of difficulties in the past with the test methodology.

Glutamate dehydrogenase: The preferred enzyme marker of hepatocyte necrosis in ruminants, glutamate dehydrogenase (GD, GLDH) probably offers no advantage over ALT in dogs and cats. However, it is mitochondrial-bound, and therefore its release may indicate hepatocyte necrosis. Suggestions that the zonal distribution of GLDH differs from ALT and therefore can help differentiate different patterns of damage have yet to be substantiated.

Lactate dehydrogenase: Lactate dehydrogenase (LDH) is of very limited value as isoenzymes are found in heart and muscle as well as liver and other tissues, and isoenzyme quantification is not available in dogs and cats.

Sorbitol dehydrogenase, and ornithine carbamoyltransferase: Sorbitol dehydrogenase (SDH) and ornithine carbamoyltransferase (OCT) are two liver-specific enzymes that have no proven advantage over ALT. SDH is not stable in serum and must be assayed within hours.

Biliary/cholestatic marker enzymes

One or two membrane-bound enzymes that are released particularly in response to cholestasis are usually

Primary liver disease	Extrahepatic conditions

Cholestasis:
   Intrahepatic
   Extrahepatic
 Hepatic inflammation:
   Parenchymatous
   Cholangitis
 Nodular hyperplasia
 Neoplasia
 Corticosteroids (dogs):
   Iatrogenic
   Hyperadrenocorticism
   Endogenous (stress)?
 Anticonvulsants:
   Phenobarbital
   Primidone
   Phenytoin
	Bone metabolism:
	   Growth
	   Osteomyelitis
	   Fracture repair
	   Osteosarcoma
	   Secondary renal hyperparathyroidism
	 Gastrointestinal disease:
	   Gastroenteritis
	   Pancreatitis
	 Hyperthyroidism
	 Pregnancy
	 Right-sided heart failure
	 Sepsis:
	   Systemic infections
	   Pyometra
	 Urological disease:
	   Nephritis
	   Cystic calculi

Figure 9.11: Causes of increased ALP in dogs. Cats do not produce steroid-induced ALP isoenzyme, and increased activities are less notable in extrahepatic disease.

measured in a biochemistry profile in conjunction with ALT. However, their specificity for cholestatic disease is limited; increases are frequently seen in other diseases, and in the dog a corticosteroid-induced isoenzyme is a frequent complication which needs to be taken into account.

Alkaline phosphatase

(ALP, AP or serum AP [SAP])

Reference ranges: dog <200 units/l; cat <100 units/l

Alkaline phosphatase (ALP) is found in the microsomal and biliary canalicular membranes of hepatocytes and is normally secreted in bile. Increased amounts are released into the blood in response to cholestasis and drug induction. Cholestasis-induced increases do not represent just simple regurgitation, but also both *de novo* synthesis and solubilization from membranes by accumulated bile salts. After an acute hepatic insult ALP release is delayed compared with ALT because of the need for induction of synthesis. ALP is also usually the last enzyme to decline after an acute insult, as impairment of bile flow is usually the last functional disturbance to resolve and increased synthesis may persist beyond resolution of the injury (Figure 9.9).

After biliary obstruction ALP starts to rise after 8 hours, and increases 15-fold in 2–4 days. Peak activity of 100-fold above normal is reached in 1–2 weeks, and then activity reaches a plateau at a lower level. Extrahepatic bile duct obstruction by pancreatitis and pancreatic neoplasia causes a rise in ALP. However, intrahepatic cholestasis is also associated with increased ALP and can be caused not only by cholangiohepatitis but also by hepatitis with hepatocyte swelling occluding smaller biliary vessels. There is a tendency for periportal injury to cause greater increases in ALP than centrilobular damage; however, the level of ALP activity cannot be used to distinguish between intra- and extrahepatic cholestasis.

Fatty infiltration of the liver causes a rise in ALP in metabolic diseases such as canine diabetes mellitus and idiopathic feline hepatic lipidosis. Liver ALP is increased in hepatitis, presumably because inflammation and swelling cause intrahepatic cholestasis, and hepatocellular and biliary carcinomas have also been associated with increased ALP.

Unfortunately, the value of ALP as a test of cholestasis is limited by the presence of a number of isoenzymes, particularly in dogs. Indeed it is probably the most frequently abnormal test in serum biochemistry (Figure 9.11). The half-life of liver ALP in cats is only 6 hours compared to 3 days in dogs, and there is also a smaller total ALP activity in feline liver; therefore, what constitutes a significant rise in cats is less than in dogs. ALP probably has higher specificity in cats, but in both dogs and cats isoenzymes of ALP are found in the intestinal mucosa, kidney, placenta and bone.

The ALP activity of intestine is actually higher than liver but, because the plasma half-life of the intestinal isoenzyme (~6 minutes) is much shorter than the liver isoenzyme (3 days) and because it is lost into the intestinal lumen, raised serum activities of this isoenzyme are rarely seen. Increased serum ALP in primary intestinal disease is more likely the result of secondary hepatic damage than the presence of the intestinal isoenzyme. Renal ALP is excreted in urine and is of no significance when measuring serum ALP. Placental ALP is only detectable in pregnancy.

Bone ALP is released in response to osteoblastic activity. In young growing dogs the normal total serum ALP range is approximately twice the adult level because of the presence of the bone isoenzyme. In adult dogs with active bone lesions such as fractures, osteomyelitis and bone tumours and in secondary renal hyperparathyroidism, ALP increases are seen but are rarely more than 5-fold. If there is any confusion, assay of another cholestatic marker which has no bone isoenzyme will be helpful (see GGT).

In dogs most problems of interpretation arise because of the presence of a (cortico)steroid-induced ALP isoenzyme (CIALP or SIALP). To confuse the issue further, varying proportions of SIALP may be produced in primary cholestatic liver disease. The SIALP isoenzyme can be quantified by a number of chemical manipulations of the enzyme assay, of which levamisole inhibition assay is the most useful (Center, 1995), more easily than by electrophoretic separation. However, there is some controversy whether SIALP represents a truly novel isoenzyme. It has recently been proposed (Meyer, 1996a) that it is actually the intestinal isoenzyme that undergoes abnormal glycosylation by the liver, delaying its clearance from the blood by mononuclear phagocytes, rather than there being *de novo* synthesis by the liver. In this theory, instead of the circulating half-life of 6 minutes of the native intestinal isoenzyme, hyperglycosylation prolongs the half-life to the 3 days of the SIALP.

SIALP does not appear be a problem in cats, but in dogs the response to exogenous corticosteroids varies with the type of steroid, route of administration and dosage, and also between individuals, resulting in massive elevations in some patients. Furthermore, the increase may persist for 6 weeks after the administration of steroids is stopped. Thus, whatever its origin, SIALP complicates the interpretation of increases in total ALP as it may be induced by endogenous and exogenous steroids (oral, parenteral and topical), and perhaps even in response to endogenous steroids in 'stress', and so may be increased in many diseases. Normal dogs have <15 % SIALP, but after glucocorticoid administration this may rise to 85%. SIALP has also been found in primary hepatobiliary disease, diabetes mellitus, hypothyroidism and pancreatitis, and synthesis can also be induced by anticonvulsants. Hyperbilirubinaemia is not a feature of drug-induced increases in ALP, although sometimes bilirubinuria and slightly increased serum bile acid concentrations (see below) are found. The finding of increased total ALP in isolation (i.e. with no or minimal increase in ALT) is suggestive of hyperadrenocorticism, but increased ALP may also be seen in benign nodular hyperplasia of the liver, and a review of the clinical signs and/or evaluation of adrenal function (see Chapter 17) should be performed to distinguish the two conditions.

As hypercortisolism tends to induce SIALP, the absence of SIALP may help rule out Cushing's disease. However, ALP induction in spontaneous hyperadreno-corticism is variable, and its presence is an unreliable marker for Cushing's disease. Induction by steroids is unpredictable, and ultimately steroids may cause intra-hepatic cholestasis and increased liver isoenzyme as well. Equally important, SIALP may be expressed in other hepatobiliary diseases, diabetes mellitus, hypothyroidism and pancreatitis (Meyer, 1996a).

Gamma-glutamyl transferase (γGT, GGT)
Sometimes called γ-glutamyl transpeptidase, GGT is another microsomal membrane-bound glycoprotein associated with the biliary tree that increases in plasma in response to cholestasis. (Reference range for dogs and cats: 0-8 units/l.) It generally parallels rises in ALP activity, but is perhaps less influenced by hepatocyte necrosis. There are GGT isoenzymes in other tissues, notably kidney, pancreas, intestine, heart, lungs, muscle and RBCs, but most circulating GGT is presumed to be of hepatic origin. There is no bone isoenzyme and therefore increased GGT is not seen in growth or bone disease. However, colostrum and milk contain GGT and may cause an increase in nursing animals. As with ALP, steroid-induced enzyme also occurs, but synthesis is apparently less likely to be induced by anticonvulsants.

Differences in the distribution of GGT compared with ALP may influence the sensitivity of GGT in various diseases. GGT is also found in the lower biliary tree but, like ALP, GGT lacks complete specificity in differentiating cholestatic from hepatocellular disease. It has been suggested that measurement of ALP and GGT together increases their diagnostic value. In dogs it is probably more specific and less sensitive than ALP, but in cats the converse appears true. In cats, most cholestatic disease causes greater increases in GGT than ALP but in idiopathic hepatic lipidosis ALP increases in the absence of a significant rise in GGT. It has been postulated that this discordance reflects either delayed clearance of ALP or excess production.

In summary, measurement of ALP in dogs is generally preferred to GGT, with the converse in cats, but in some situations measurement of both enzymes may provide additional information.

LIVER FUNCTION TESTS

As stated earlier, increases in liver marker enzymes do not necessarily correlate with the degree of liver damage and do not distinguish localized from diffuse disease. They, therefore, do not offer any information on overall liver function, and in cases of congenital PSS may actually be normal. In these situations specific tests are available to measure liver function.

Liver function tests may be crude markers of overall liver function, e.g. bilirubin metabolism, or they may dynamically assess certain functional pathways in the liver, e.g. enterohepatic recycling of bile acids. The former are often adequate markers of significant liver disease whilst the latter are usually performed to prove the necessity of further investigation when clinical signs are unclear. In the presence of jaundice many

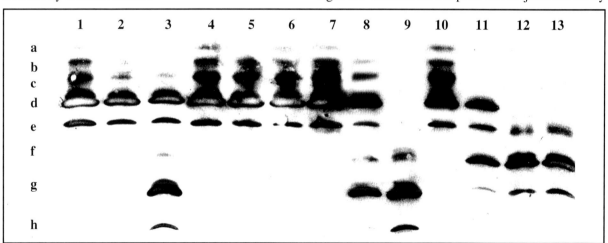

Figure 9.12: Immunoprint patterns of canine α1-antitrypsin phenotypes after isoelectric focusing. Depending on isoelectric mobility there are three phenotypes: F (fast), I (intermediate) and S (slow). They appear in either homozygous (FF, II, SS) or heterozygous (FI, FS, IS) forms. Each AAT phenotype comprises seevral fractions with different amount of sialic acid. The main fraction of the I-type is seen in band f. AAT of the I-type has a tendency to accumulate in hepatocytes leading to cell death and chronic hepatitis and/or cirrhosis.
Lanes 1, 2, 4, 5, 6, 7 and 10 = FF homozygous; 3 and 8 = FS heterozygous; 9 = SS homozygous; 11 = FI heterozygous; 12 and 13 = II homozygous

Characteristic	Transudate	Modified transudate	Exudate
Specific gravity (refractometer)	<1.017	1.017–1.025	>1.025
Total protein (g/l)	<25	>25	>25
Nucleated cells (x10⁹/l)	<5	>5	usually >50
Predominant cell types	Mononuclear Mesothelial	Lymphocytes Monocytes Mesothelial RBCs Neutrophils	Neutrophils Mononuclear RBCs
Bacteria	Absent	Absent	Variable

Table 9.3: *Physical characteristics of abdominal effusion used to differentiate transudate, modified transudate and exudate.*

Fluid	Commonest causes	Additional tests for fluid
Transudate	Hypoalbuminaemia Prehepatic portal hypertension	See Table 9.3

Modified transudate	Hepatic disease:
	    Idiopathic hepatic fibrosis
	    Chronic hepatitis / cirrhosis
	    Cholangiohepatitis (cats)
	Caudal vena caval obstruction
	Cardiac tamponade
	Right-sided heart failure
		See Table 9.3

Exudate	Feline infectious peritonitis Septic peritonitis (ruptured viscus) Pancreatitis Carcinomatosis	See Table 9.3 Cytology, culture Amylase, lipase Cytology
Chyle	Lymphangiectasia Ruptured cisterna chyli (trauma, malignancy)	Low cholesterol High triglyceride, cytology
Bile	Ruptured biliary tract	Bilirubin, cytology
Blood	Traumatic organ rupture Ruptured haemangiosarcoma	PCV Cytology
Urine	Ruptured lower urinary tract	Creatinine (not urea), cytology

Table 9.4: *Characteristics of abdominal fluids.*

dynamic liver function tests (e.g. bile acid assay) will invariably be abnormal and are therefore redundant. In this circumstance, assuming haemolytic jaundice has been ruled out, evidence of hyperbilirubinaemia is a specific marker of hepatobiliary dysfunction.

Markers of liver function

Serum proteins and albumin

Total concentrations of albumin and globulin offer crude indices of liver function, as discussed above. Serum protein electrophoresis offers prognostic information (see below) and may be helpful in identifying increased synthesis of acute phase proteins associated with inflammatory hepatopathies and perhaps production of abnormal proteins in certain liver diseases. The fetal liver-derived protein, α-fetoprotein, is not usually synthesized by normal adult liver, but it is released into serum when hepatic regeneration takes place; its presence is found in a number of liver diseases but the assay is not routinely available. Similarly, chronic hepatitis caused by α_1-antitrypsin accumulation can be characterized by demonstration of abnormal isoforms by isoelectric focusing (Figure 9.12). In contrast copper hepatotoxicosis cannot be identified by assay of plasma caeruloplasmin.

Liver autoantibodies (e.g. antinuclear antibody, anti-mitochondrial antibody) develop in human liver disease, and have been noted in canine chronic hepatitis. Their significance is not clear, and their routine measurement is not undertaken.

	Dogs	Cats

Prehepatic	Haemolytic anaemia:
	    Autoimmune haemolytic anaemia
	    Babesia (not in UK)
		Haemolytic anaemia:
		    Haemobartonella
		    Autoimmune haemolytic anaemia

Primary liver disease	Acute hepatitis:
	    Drugs, leptospirosis,
	    infectious canine hepatitis
	Chronic hepatitis and cirrhosis:
	    Copper, α_1-antitrypsin, anticonvulsants
	Cholangiohepatitis:
	    Suppurative
	Neoplasia:
	    Carcinoma
		Acute hepatitis
		Chronic hepatitis and cirrhosis
		Cholangiohepatitis:
		    e.g. lymphocytic–plasmacytic type
		Idiopathic hepatic lipidosis
		Neoplasia:
		    Lymphosarcoma

Secondary liver disease	Septicaemia and endotoxaemia	Feline infectious peritonitis Diabetes mellitus *Toxoplasma* Paracetamol (acetaminophen) Hyperthyroidism (rarely)

Posthepatic disease	Extrahepatic biliary disease:
	    Common bile duct or gall bladder rupture
	    Pancreatitis
	    Pancreatic carcinoma
	    Biliary carcinoma
		Extrahepatic biliary disease:
		    Chronic pancreatitis

Table 9.5: Common causes of jaundice in dogs and cats.

Ascites

The accumulation of free fluid in the peritoneal cavity can be indicative of liver disease. Diagnostic abdominocentesis, and measurement of the protein and cellular content of any fluid aid differentiation of the exact cause. Classification of the fluid as transudate, modified transudate or exudate can be helpful (Table 9.3). The presence of a protein-rich cellular exudate, or the presence of significant amounts of blood, chyle or urine, suggests extrahepatic diseases (Table 9.4).

A pure, low-protein transudate will accumulate if there is hypoproteinaemia (see Table 9.2). Liver disease usually causes ascites through a combination of hypoalbuminaemia and portal hypertension resulting in a modified transudate. The term 'modified transudate' is perhaps an unfortunate misnomer in liver disease, as it is usually not 'modified' after formation. Whilst modification by infection and inflammation can occur, ascitic fluid in liver disease is usually simply a transudate from the liver. However, as hepatic sinusoids are highly permeable and the hepatic tissue fluid normally entering the space of Disse contains approximately 80% of serum proteins, any ascites in liver disease has the characteristic protein content of a modified transudate. Hepatic lymph is protein-rich and, when the lymphatics are obstructed by intra- or posthepatic causes, it accumulates as protein-rich ascitic fluid. Only prehepatic portal hypertension (e.g. portal vein thrombosis, over-zealous PSS ligation), as well as simple hypoalbuminaemia, will cause a typical low-protein transudate. A modified transudate may indicate either primary hepatic disease or a 'post-hepatic' problem such as cardiac tamponade or congestive heart failure causing hepatic venous congestion.

Coagulation times

The liver plays a central role in the coagulation and fibrinolytic systems, and subtle abnormalities may be detected by assay of individual factor activities. However, overall coagulation ability assessed by whole blood clotting time, one-stage prothrombin time (OSPT) and activated partial thromboplastin time (aPTT) (see Chapter 3), is usually only abnormal in severe disease. Whilst this will be expected if there is a history of generalised bleeding, an occult bleeding tendency should always be suspected, and a clotting profile is mandatory before a liver biopsy is performed.

Coagulation factor proteins, synthesized in the liver, are activated by carboxylation of a glutamate residue through a vitamin K-dependent process. Indirect measurement of inactive vitamin K-dependent coagulation factors, so-called 'proteins invoked by vitamin K absence or antagonism' (PIVKAs), assayed by their inhibition of the OSPT, detects subtle changes in production of active coagulation factors (Mount, 1986). PIVKAs are a more sensitive test than coagulation times but have only recently become available as a commercial assay. In their absence, some workers have advocated the routine administration of parenteral vitamin K 12 hours before liver biopsy.

As well as deficiencies of clotting factors and failure of vitamin K-dependent activation, bleeding tendencies in liver disease may reflect increased fibrinolysis, demonstrable as increased fibrin degradation products (FDPs), and platelet dysfunction, which is most easily assessed by determining the buccal bleeding time.

Occasionally bleeding occurs because of acquired vitamin K deficiency in complete bile duct obstruction, as lack of bile salts precludes intestinal absorption of this fat-soluble vitamin, particularly following antibiotic therapy. Both OSPT and aPTT are abnormal, reminiscent of coumarin toxicity. This problem has been reported most frequently in cats with biliary disease and in feline exocrine pancreatic insufficiency; it appears to be less characteristic of biliary disease in dogs.

Bilirubin

Serum bilirubin concentration in dogs and cats should not normally exceed 7 µmol/l; hyperbilirubinaemia results in jaundice (icterus), the yellow discoloration of tissues by bile pigments. Jaundice may be indicative of liver disease, but it can be caused by other conditions (Table 9.5). It should also be remembered that it is not invariably present in liver disease; for example, it is *not* seen in congenital PSS, steroid hepatopathy and rarely in metastatic disease.

Jaundice is best detected clinically in the sclera when concentrations exceed 25 µmol/l, as the human eye can usually only detect the yellow colour against pink mucous membranes at about 35 µmol/l. However, hyperbilirubinaemia can be seen in separated serum at about 17 µmol/l and thus will be detected sooner by blood testing. Also, because of the low renal threshold, bilirubinuria usually precedes jaundice in dogs.

In order to understand jaundice it is necessary to understand the physiology of bilirubin metabolism (Figure 9.7). Bilirubin is the major bile pigment and is a product of haemoprotein catabolism. The phago-cytic cells of the mononuclear phagocytic system (MPS), particularly in the liver, spleen and bone marrow, engulf free haemoglobin and senescent and abnormal RBCs, and convert haemoglobin to bi-lirubin via biliverdin. Free bilirubin is insoluble and is carried in the plasma to hepatocytes reversibly bound to albumin. Here it is taken up and, along with bilirubin produced within the hepatocytes from haemoproteins such as cytochromes, it is conjugated to bilirubin diglucuronide. Conjugation of bilirubin aids solubilization and excretion via the biliary canaliculi.

After gall bladder storage and biliary excretion, bile pigment is converted by intestinal bacteria to a number of faecal pigments including stercobilin which produce normal faecal colour (Figure 9.7). The pigment urobilinogen is also produced and some of it is reabsorbed. Most undergoes enterohepatic

recycling and re-excretion in bile, but about 20% passes through the glomerulus. Thus the presence of urobilinogen in urine is normal and indicative of functional bile excretion.

Hyperbilirubinaemia can be caused by three basic mechanisms:

- Prehepatic causes: increased production of bilirubin exceeding the liver's ability for excretion
- Hepatic causes: abnormal uptake, conjugation or secretion by hepatocytes
- Posthepatic causes: obstruction of either intra- or extrahepatic biliary excretion.

Increased production of bilirubin is invariably associated with haemolytic anaemia. Genetic defects of bilirubin uptake and excretion, as seen in Southdown and Corriedale sheep, respectively, have not been described in dogs and cats. In primary liver disease hepatocyte abnormalities and intrahepatic cholestasis usually coexist. Posthepatic obstruction occurs with bile duct and pancreatic disease.

The van den Bergh test has been advocated for differentiation of the three major types of icterus by measuring the relative proportions of unconjugated and conjugated bilirubin. However, the results are very unreliable and the test is *not* recommended. Nevertheless, the types of hyperbilirubinaemia can often be distinguished by combination with other laboratory tests such as haematocrit and hepatocellular and cholestatic marker enzymes.

Haemolysis: Jaundice in the presence of a low PCV is suggestive of haemolysis. Initially the accumulated bilirubin is predominantly unconjugated, but gradually conjugated bilirubin accumulates as well. Spherocytosis and a positive Coombs' test support a diagnosis of immune-mediated haemolytic anaemia (see Chapters 3 and 6). Faeces are likely to be orange and there will be significant bilirubinuria. Hypoxia may cause some increase in liver-specific enzymes that may be misleading, but if the haematocrit is normal or there is only mild anaemia, any jaundice present is not of haemolytic origin.

Liver disease: Increased liver enzymes associated with jaundice are suggestive of primary hepatic disease, but it should be remembered that enzymes may not be increased in terminal cirrhosis. Jaundice is usually the result of a combination of hepatocyte dysfunction and intrahepatic cholestasis, and thus both unconjugated and conjugated bilirubin may appear in the blood, and both ALT and ALP are usually increased. Bilirubinuria and urobilinogen are expected on urinalysis.

Extrahepatic cholestasis: The expected rise in conjugated bilirubin alone, as predicted by the van den Bergh test, is not always found because by the time clinical signs occur there is significant dysfunction of the conjugation mechanism in hepatocytes as well. Increased cholestatic markers (ALP, GGT) and hypercholesterolaemia are found. Faeces are grey (acholic) and urine urobilinogen is absent if obstruction is complete. Ultrasound examination of the biliary tree can be helpful in locating the site of obstruction.

One reason why the van den Bergh test is unreliable is because of the variable presence of bilirubin bound irreversibly to serum albumin. Covalently bound δ-bilirubin (biliprotein) cannot be taken up by hepatocytes and adds to icterus, but it is found in very variable amounts (2–96% of circulating bilirubin). The clearance of δ-bilirubin is as slow as the turnover of albumin (i.e. half-life up to 3 weeks), and therefore jaundice occasionally persists well beyond the time of clinical and other laboratory evidence of resolution because of the existence of δ-bilirubin. The author has seen persistent jaundice after clinical recovery most frequently in dogs with obstructive jaundice associated with acute pancreatitis. Persistent jaundice should not be mistaken for persistent disease and in such cases laboratory abnormalities (hyperbilirubinaemia) must be interpreted in light of other clinical features.

Dynamic liver function tests

These tests rely on analysis of paired blood samples to assess the liver's capacity to clear endogenous (bile acids, ammonia) or exogenous (bromosulphthalein, indocyanine green) substances from the circulation. Impaired clearance is taken as evidence of hepatocellular dysfunction and/or portosystemic shunting, and is used as justification for performing further tests, including portography and biopsy, to differentiate the type of disease. Dynamic tests are redundant if the patient is icteric. Scintigraphy is also a dynamic test that can be used to assess both hepatic macrophage phagocytic function and shunting, but the need for radioisotopes and expensive equipment precludes its use in general practice.

Exogenous excretion tests

These tests are of historical interest only, being redundant now the serum bile acid assay is readily available.

Bromosulphthalein (BSP) retention test: Intravenous administration of the organic dye BSP (5mg/kg in a 50mg/ml aqueous solution) was followed by blood sampling at 30 minutes and measurement of the percentage retention of the dye. In normal cats and dogs, <3% and <5%, respectively was retained. As BSP follows the same excretory pathway as bilirubin (except for conjugation with glutathione not glucuronic acid) abnormal retention is suggestive of abnormal hepatic perfusion, hepatocellular function, or bile flow.

The method was prone to numerous problems and errors. The dye was irritant if accidentally given perivascularly, and there was a potential for contamination of the 30-minute sample. Decreased hepatic perfusion for non-hepatic reasons prolonged retention and hypoalbuminaemia enhanced clearance as less dye was bound. Presence of ascites also produced false results and lipaemia and haemolysis interfered with assay of BSP. However, the major reasons the test is no longer used are: concerns over carcinogenicity; BSP is no longer commercially available; and bile acid assay became widely available.

Indocyanine green (ICG) retention test: The ICG test was developed to replace the BSP test. ICG is handled by the liver the same way as bilirubin and BSP, except that it is not conjugated, and the test was thus prone to similar errors. The test did not find favour because experimentally it was not as sensitive as the BSP test, and offered no advantage over bile acid measurement. Normal dogs and cats retained <15% and <10% ICG, respectively, at 30 minutes.

Endogenous metabolic tests

These tests assess the liver's metabolic capacity; unlike BSP and ICG tests, they are not 'flow-limited'.

Plasma ammonia and ammonia tolerance test: Fasting blood ammonia concentration provides a relatively insensitive measure of hepatic function, and is only meaningful if increased. Ammonia is produced by intestinal bacteria and should be effectively cleared from the portal blood by the liver. Normal portal blood contains up to 350 μmol/l ammonia, but <60 μmol/l enters the systemic circulation from the liver. Increased resting ammonia concentration is evidence of hepatic dysfunction and/or portosystemic shunting (Figure 9.13). Very rarely, hyperammonaemia is caused by a genetic defect in the urea cycle, and in this situation only will serum bile acids (see below) be normal. The degree of hyperammonaemia correlates very roughly with the severity of hepatoencephalopathy; it is a marker for the condition, but other toxic metabolites are also involved in the causation of clinical signs.

Fasting blood ammonia concentration is only meaningful if increased, as resting concentrations are frequently normal in liver disease and in some patients with PSS. The sensitivity of the test can be improved by administering exogenous ammonia to the gastrointestinal tract to determine whether ammonia intolerance exists. The ammonia tolerance test, when ammonium chloride is administered (100 mg/kg to a maximum of 3 g) by stomach tube or enema, has been described. After peroral administration, a blood sample is taken at 30 minutes. Plasma ammonia concentration does not increase significantly in normal patients; marked elevations (>80 μmol/l) are seen in PSS.

The peroral test is quite sensitive but can cause vomiting, and is dangerous in patients, especially cats, that are already encephalopathic. The rectal ammonia tolerance test has the advantage of not provoking immediate vomiting but the absorption of ammonia is more variable and samples must be taken at 20 and 40 minutes. The test will detect PSS but not more subtle dysfunction. The colon also has to be prepared by enema, and since the results are less sensitive this method is rarely used.

Whilst the ammonia tolerance test is a sensitive test, particularly for PSS, it is not the preferred test of hepatic function because of methodological difficulties. Plasma needs to be harvested on ice and ammonia assayed within 30 minutes to produce meaningful results, as storage increases the ammonia content of blood. Thus the test is limited to institutions and practices with immediate access to a human laboratory. Dry chemistry ammonia tests are available in veterinary practice but the results are frequently unreliable.

P-450 cytochrome oxidase activity: Hepatic metabolic degradative capacity can be assessed by measuring clearance of substances such as antipyrine and caffeine by the hepatic P-450 cytochrome oxidase system and conversion of lignocaine to monoethylglyexylidide (MEGX). These tests have not yet been used in veterinary medicine.

Serum bile acids (SBA): Bile acids are a major constituent of bile, but are *not* the same as bile pigments. Fasting serum total bile acid concentration (FSBA) is a reflection of the enterohepatic circulation of bile acids (Figure 9.14). Bile acids are synthesized in the liver at

a rate to compensate for small faecal losses, but the enterohepatic circulation maintains a larger pool of bile acids that is recycled several times a day. Hepatic dysfunction and/or portosystemic shunting releases bile acids into the systemic circulation.

Bile acids (cholic and chenodeoxycholic acid) are synthesized in the liver from cholesterol, and are conjugated predominantly with taurine and some glycine before biliary excretion. Conjugation of bile acids causes ionization at intestinal luminal pH and lipid insolubility, preventing absorption through the gut wall. Only when fat absorption through micellarization has been completed are bile acids reabsorbed on specific ileal receptors. Some of the primary bile acids are metabolized by intestinal bacteria to deoxycholic and lithocholic acids before reabsorption. Only about 5% escape recycling and are lost in faeces. On return to the liver, bile acids are efficiently removed from the portal blood by hepatocytes and re-excreted.

The rate of synthesis and the bile acid pool size and distribution can be abnormal in liver disease if there is reduction in hepatocellular mass, impaired hepatocyte function or disturbed enterohepatic circulation. Thus FSBA will be abnormal if hepatic function is suboptimal or if there is a portosystemic shunting. It must be stressed that increased SBA concentrations merely indicate liver dysfunction and are not indicative of specific disease types.

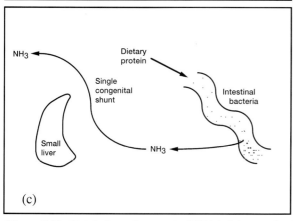
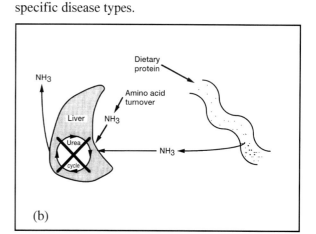
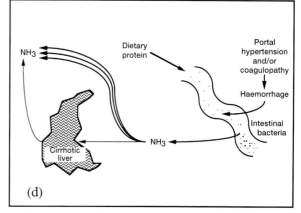

Figure 9.13: Metabolism of ammonia (NH3) in (a) normal animals, and animals with (b) urea cycle enzyme defect (rare), (c) congenital portosystemic shunting and (d) cirrhosis with multiple secondary acquired shunts.

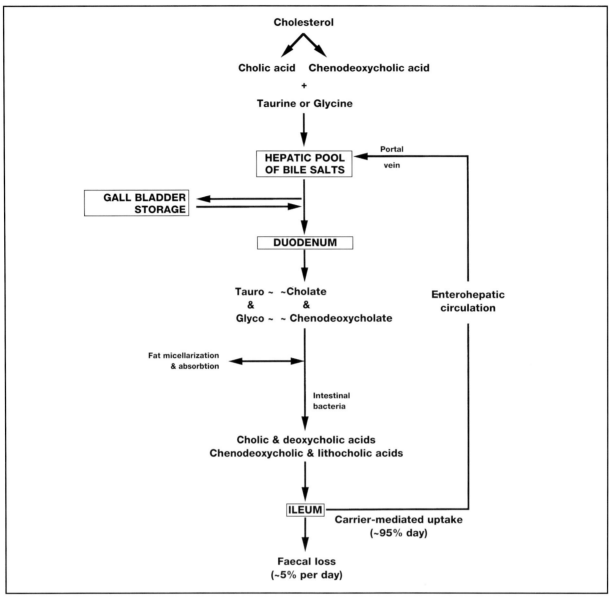

Figure 9.14: *Schematic representation of the normal enterohepatic circulation of bile salts.*

The value of measuring FSBA is in the detection of PSS and chronic hepatitis/cirrhosis before the development of jaundice. Hopes that the test would be highly sensitive and specific have been tempered with the evidence of mild increases in FSBA in non-hepatic diseases. The test is simple and sensitive and is readily available to veterinary practitioners. However, bile acids probably should not be measured as part of a routine biochemical screen, but only when there is a suspicion of liver disease.

Sensitivity of the test is reported to be improved by measurement of a 2-hour postprandial serum bile acid concentration (PPSBA). The principle of the dynamic test is that eating stimulates release of bile by gall bladder contraction, providing an endogenous tolerance test of the enterohepatic recycling ability of the liver.

Bile acids can be measured accurately by radioimmunoassay but in most veterinary laboratories enzymatic fluorimetric or spectrophotometric methods are used; inadequate laboratory technique as well as haemolysis can unfortunately produce spurious results. Reference ranges for bile acids are somewhat controversial, not only because of methodological problems in some laboratories, but because of the effect of secondary hepatic disease. Initially established criteria of <5 μmol/l FSBA and <10 μmol/l PPSBA are probably too strict, and double these values can be normal. A higher cut-off increases the specificity of the test but at the expense of sensitivity. Concentrations above 25 μmol/l for both FSBA and PPSBA have been shown to correlate with histological lesions, but these may still be caused by secondary disease.

The value of PPSBA measurement is still controversial, although undoubtedly some patients with PSS do have normal FSBA and wildly abnormal PPSBA concentrations. However, the efficiency of the two tests is approximately the same, and confusing decreases in the postprandial sample are sometimes

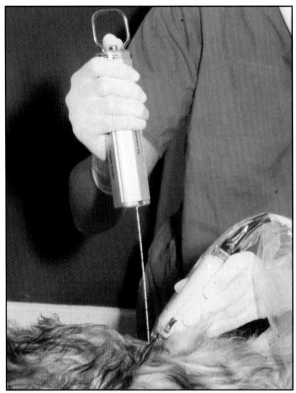

Figure 9.15: Ultrasound-guided percutaneous needle biopsy of the liver using a needle and automated gun to fire the biopsy needle. The ultrasound probe is covered in a sterile sleeve.

found. The reason for this is not clear but may be a result of inherent variability, failure to store all new bile in the gall bladder, incomplete gall bladder contraction, and intestinal bacterial metabolism.

A FSBA concentration of >30 µmol/l is usually taken as conclusive evidence of hepatic dysfunction and a need to perform further tests such as a biopsy unless an underlying disease can be identified. The magnitude of

the FSBA over ~100 µmol/l apparently has little predictive value for the severity of any particular hepatopathy, and some cases of PSS have normal FSBA and massively raised (up to 800 µmol/l) PPSBA. FSBA concentrations between 20 and 30 µmol/l are in a grey area, and recommendations for these patients are:

- Look for extrahepatic disease
- Repeat FSBA with a PPSBA and look for at least a 2-fold increase
- Repeat FSBA in 2-4 weeks

or

- If clinical signs and other results suggest liver disease, pursue the diagnosis by other tests, including biopsy.

In the future, fractionation of serum bile acids into specific acids such as cholic and chenodeoxycholic acids may have diagnostic utility in the identification of specific hepatopathies.

LIVER BIOPSY

Indications and techniques

As has been stressed earlier, identification of specific hepatopathies usually requires liver biopsy. Indications for liver biopsy include:

- Persistent elevations of liver enzymes
- Increased FSBA with no apparent underlying disease
- Altered liver size or ultrasonographic architecture
- Progressive signs of liver disease
- Monitoring response to therapy.

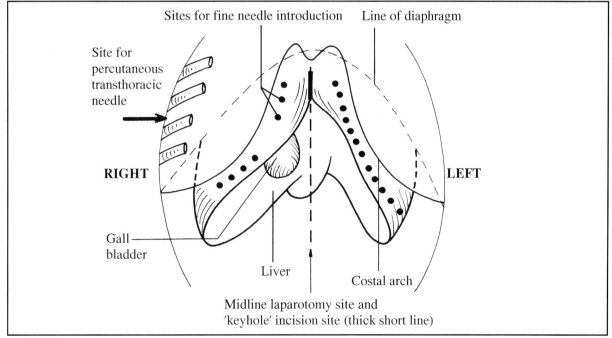

Figure 9.16: Sites for hepatic biopsy.

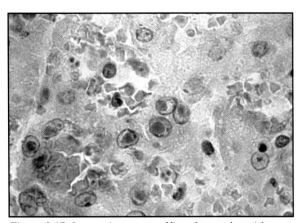

Figure 9.17: Impression smear of liver from a dog with infectious canine hepatitis showing characteristic intranuclear inclusions.

Liver biopsies can be collected by a number of methods, but it is mandatory that a coagulation profile is performed before biopsy because of the dangers of potential haemorrhage. In practice, liver biopsy is often limited to wedge biopsy at exploratory laparotomy. However, percutaneous biopsy techniques have been devised and have become increasingly safer with the advent of ultrasound-guided needle biopsy (Figure 9.15).

General anaesthesia is not usually required. However, percutaneous liver biopsy under sedation and local analgesia is contraindicated if there is:

- Lack of operator confidence
- An uncooperative patient
- A small liver or focal disease, unless ultrasound guidance is available
- Hepatic cysts, abscess or vascular tumour
- A bleeding disorder or severe anaemia
- Extrahepatic cholestasis
- Peracute hepatitis and jaundice associated with sepsis.

| Chronic infections and inflammation: |
| Severe dental disease |
| Pyelonephritis |
| Diabetes mellitus |
| Hyperadrenocortisolism |
| Hyperlipidaemia |
| Hypothyroidism |
| Inflammatory bowel disease |
| Neoplasia |
| Pancreatitis |
| Treatment with glucocorticoids |

Figure 9.18: Causes of vacuolar hepatopathies.

The sites for liver biopsy are shown in Figure 9.16, and the techniques used are described in detail in the *BSAVA Manual of Canine and Feline Gastroenterology* (Else, 1996).

Cytology

It is also possible to perform cytological examination of liver cells collected either by fine needle aspiration or by a touch preparation of a liver biopsy specimen. This may enable a tentative diagnosis and initiation of appropriate immediate treatment before confirmation by histopathological examination. The presence of intranuclear inclusion bodies is considered diagnostic of infectious canine hepatitis (Figure 9.17) but this examination is usually only performed post mortem.

Staining fine needle aspirates for copper granules with rubeanic acid has been used to identify copper hepatotoxicosis in Bedlington Terriers and other canine breeds, but histopathological staining and biochemical quantitation of copper content are necessary to avoid false negatives. Infiltration with neoplastic cells, including lymphocytes or mast cells, may be detected in primary and metastatic liver disease and in hepatic lymphosarcoma and mastocytoma, respectively.

Feature	Special stain
Amyloid	Congo red
Bacteria	Gram, Ziehl–Neelsen
Bile	Fouchet's, van Gieson
Collagen	Masson's trichrome, van Gieson
Copper	Rhodamine, rubeanic acid
Copper-associated protein	Orcein
Elastin	Elastic van Gieson, Weigert's
Fibrin, fibrinoid	Martius scarlet blue (MSB)
Glycogen	Periodic acid–Schiff (PAS) (diastase-positive), Best's carmine, Bauer–Feulgen (frozen)
α_1-Antitrypsin	PAS (unreliable), immunostaining
Iron (ferric)	Perl's Prussian blue
Lipid	Oil-red-O (frozen)
Lipofuscin	Schmorl, Ziehl–Neelsen
Reticulin	Reticulin stain

Table 9.16: Some of the special stains available for characterization of hepatic pathological changes.

Chronic hepatopathies can be subdivided into vacuolar hepatopathies and inflammatory hepatopathies (infectious hepatitis, chronic hepatitis) by cytological examination. Classification of chronic hepatitis can only be achieved by histological examination. Many causes of vacuolar hepatopathies are listed in Figure 9.18; the cytological finding of enlarged cells with vacuolated cytoplasm is not very helpful diagnostically.

Histopathology

A number of stains, in addition to routine haematoxylin and eosin, are available to facilitate characterization of hepatic pathology (Table 9.16). However, the clinician needs to work with the pathologist, providing all the relevant historical, clinical and clinicopathological information, in order that appropriate stains are used and an appropriate diagnosis reached. Liver biopsy specimens can also be investigated by electron microscopy after appropriate fixation and processing, but this technique is costly and is not done as a routine procedure.

Pieces of hepatic tissue about the size of 1 cm cubes are required for accurate determination of hepatic copper content by atomic absorption spectrophotometry. Formalin-fixed tissue can be used.

PROGNOSTIC INDICES

As well as identifying and helping characterize hepatopathies, laboratory testing can provide some prognostic information.

Good prognostic signs are:

- Decreasing hyperbilirubinaemia

- Decreasing liver enzymes. With resolution of an acute hepatic insult, ALT should fall approximately 50% every 3-4 days. Initially increasing ALT may indicate regeneration rather than continued hepatocyte damage. ALP may continue to rise after the injury and take several weeks to normalize (see Figure 9.9)

- Normoglycaemia

- Normal coagulation times

- Increasing serum albumin, not due to dehydration. In inflammatory disease albumin is frequently subnormal as a negative acute phase response, but serum protein electrophoresis at that time will show normal to elevated haptoglobin and α_1-antitrypsin. This is a good prognostic sign (Figure 9.9)

- Increasing cholesterol concentration (if previously low).

Bad prognostic signs are:

- Increases in AST and arginase as well as ALT, suggesting more severe hepatocellular damage

- Persistent elevation of liver marker enzymes indicative of continuing damage

- Hypoglycaemia and prolonged prothrombin time in chronic hepatitis. In Dobermanns with copper-associated chronic hepatitis, they were shown to be portents of imminent death

- Hypoalbuminaemia, if it is due to failure of synthesis. A decrease in albumin and other acute phase proteins on serum protein electrophoresis is indicative of end-stage disease and carries a poor prognosis (Figure 9.19).

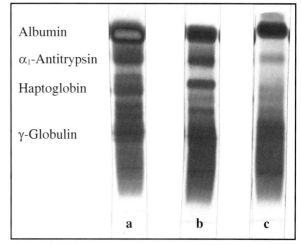

Figure 9.19: Serum protein electrophoresis from one healthy dog (a), one dog with chronic progressive hepatitis and good prognosis (b) (note the weak staining of albumin and the distinct α_1-antitrypsin and haptoglobin fractions), and one dog with late stage cirrhosis and poor prognosis (c) (note the weak staining of albumin and the almost abolished α_1-antitrypsin and haptoglobin fractions).

INTERPRETATION OF LIVER TEST PATTERNS

Apart from liver biopsy, there is rarely any one test that provides a definitive diagnosis. It must also be remembered that laboratory artefacts may produce abnormal results and that laboratory errors may occur. The bile acid assay is quite problematical in some laboratories and some dry chemistry analysers are inaccurate, especially when measuring ammonia. Results must always be interpreted in light of the whole clinical picture, because if poor-quality or unsuitable samples are presented to the laboratory, results may be inaccurate and misleading. Some of the common artefacts are listed in Table 9.7.

The author does not believe that a diagnosis should be reached by trying to match laboratory test results to a

Analyte	False increase	False decrease
Bilirubin	Severe haemolysis Lipaemia	UV light Viscous serum (dry chemistry)
Bile acids	Hypertriglyceridaemia Increased serum dehydrogenases	Severe chylomicronaemia Haemolysis
Ammonia	Delayed assay Strenuous exercise Dry chemistry analyser	
BSP retention	Haemolysis Hypoalbuminaemia Jaundice Lipaemia	Faulty collection
ALT	Severe haemolysis Lipaemia	
AST	Severe haemolysis Lipaemia Ketoacidosis	
ALP	Jaundice Lipaemia Storage (haemolysis)	Fluoride Oxalate Citrate EDTA
GGT	Lipaemia Fluoride and oxalate	

***Table 9.7:** Potential laboratory artefacts affecting liver test results.*

table of expected results, and such a table is not included here. Laboratory tests are used to identify suspected liver disease, but particular patterns of clinicopathological abnormalities, when interpreted in light of the clinical findings, can often provide a high index of suspicion of certain diseases. The characteristic clinicopathological features of certain conditions are described below.

Acute hepatitis and hepatic necrosis
Acute inflammatory conditions, whether due to toxic or infectious causes, usually cause rapid, moderate to marked increases in ALT. Other hepatocellular enzymes are likely to be increased, but rises in AST and arginase activity are indicative of more severe damage. Intrahepatic cholestasis, caused by hepatocyte swelling, induces a slower rise in ALP and GGT. Depending on the severity of the hepatic damage there will be varying impairment of bile acid circulation, and in severe cases hyperbilirubinaemia will ensue. Hypoalbuminaemia is not a feature because of the acuteness of the condition.

Chronic hepatitis
Isoelectric focusing can be used to characterize α_1-antitrypsin-associated chronic hepatitis (Figure 9.12). However, in general the specific type of chronic hepatitis can only be determined by liver biopsy; laboratory testing merely provides evidence of persistent damage and dysfunction, identifying the need for biopsy. Moderate to severe increases in ALT/AST and ALP/GGT are typical,

but persistence of the elevations is most characteristic (Figure 9.9). The absolute activities can fluctuate spontaneously and the clinician should not assume that a decrease in enzyme activity at one time point is necessarily indicative of remission.

Persistent elevation in enzyme activity or increased FSBA are indications for liver biopsy. Jaundice suggests significant hepatic impairment and may herald the development of cirrhosis. Late in the disease, serum albumin is likely to be decreased and may be a poor prognostic sign (see above).

Cirrhosis
Hepatic fibrosis and nodular regeneration in cirrhosis, the end result of various forms of chronic hepatitis, is associated with significant hepatic dysfunction, demonstrated by increased serum bile acids and eventually jaundice. Hypoalbuminaemia, low blood urea and ultimately coagulopathies, hypoglycaemia and ascites may develop. Serum protein electrophoresis may show hypoalbuminaemia and decreases in acute phase proteins. Serum enzyme activities may be elevated, but can be normal if there is no active inflammation or only minimal hepatocellular tissue left.

Congenital portosystemic shunts
The absence of hepatic inflammation and cholestasis in most cases of congenital PSS is reflected in the absence of, or only minimal increases in, liver en-

zymes. Shunting and hepatic bypass is characterized by increased FSBA and/or PPSBA, and hyperammonaemia and/or ammonia intolerance. Serum urea, albumin, cholesterol and occasionally glucose may all be decreased. Haematology quite frequently shows microcytic anaemia and poikilocytosis (Figure 9.6), and urate crystalluria (Figure 9.8) may be found.

Glucocorticoids

Both endogenous and exogenous glucocorticoids typically induce an increase in ALP/GGT with minimal increases in ALT/AST in dogs; cats appear resistant to these changes. The response in dogs is quite variable but can persist for at least 6 weeks after the administration of even a single dose of steroid in some individuals. When severe steroid hepatopathy is present, moderate increases in ALT may develop but the increase is generally disproportionate to the magnitude of the increase in ALP. There may be mild hepatic impairment and slight increases in FSBA, but jaundice is exceptionally rare. There may be some increase in serum albumin, hyperglycaemia and hypercholesterolaemia. If there is no history of exogenous steroid administration then dynamic hormone tests for Cushing's disease (see Chapter 17) should be considered if there are signs compatible with the diagnosis.

Benign nodular hyperplasia

A common incidental finding in older dogs, nodular hyperplasia is usually considered to produce no significant laboratory test abnormalities and overall liver function is apparently unaffected. However, there can be a marked rise in serum ALP with minimal changes in ALT (Meyer, 1996b). In this situation the major differential diagnosis would be hyperadrenocortisolism as there should be no signs of liver disease. Nodular hyperplasia may thus explain occasional cases where Cushing's disease is suspected because of increased ALP but where the endocrine status is normal by dynamic hormone testing.

Primary hepatic neoplasia

Primary hepatocellular tumours may be associated with increases in ALT and/or ALP, dependent on the presence of associated inflammation and/or intrahepatic cholestasis. Biliary carcinomas may cause increases in ALP and obstructive jaundice; other tumours cause jaundice infrequently. Hypoglycaemia may be noted with large hepatomas, but many are functionally 'silent'.

Mctastatic liver disease

Primary hepatic or metastatic haemangiosarcoma is frequently identified by the regenerative anaemia that occurs because of intraperitoneal haemorrhage and microangiopathic haemolysis. However, it is not unusual for there to be minimal increases in enzyme

| Azathioprine |
| Barbiturates (including phenobarbital, primidone) |
| Glucocorticoids (dogs) |
| Griseofulvin |
| Halothane |
| Ketoconazole |
| Mebendazole |
| Paracetamol (acetaminophen) |
| Sulphonamides |

Figure 9.20: *Important hepatotoxic drugs known or suspected to cause increases in ALT.*

activity despite extensive infiltration with any metastatic disease. This is particularly true for hepatic lymphosarcoma, but increases in FSBA, hepatomegaly and, sometimes, hypercalcaemia are usually enough to indicate the need for biopsy. Other metastatic disease is best detected ultrasonographically or by biopsy.

Feline idiopathic hepatic lipidosis

Massive fatty infiltration of the liver is associated with marked hepatic dysfunction with increased FSBA and often jaundice. Cholestatic markers would be expected to be increased, but interestingly there is often an increase in ALP but no significant rise in GGT. The mechanism of the discrepancy between ALP and GGT is not understood.

Cholangiohepatitis

In dogs, cholangiohepatitis and associated cholecystitis appear to be most commonly associated with ascending infection, and an inflammatory leucogram may be seen. Increases in ALT as well as ALP suggest extension of the inflammation into the hepatic parenchyma in addition to intrahepatic cholestasis. The diagnosis may be suspected by ultrasound scan changes in the gall bladder wall, but diagnosis is usually made on histological examination of biopsy tissue, supported by bacteriological culture of bile and/or liver tissue.

Lymphocytic cholangiohepatitis in cats is not uncommon and increases in liver enzymes, hyperglobulinaemia and liver dysfunction are expected; occasionally lymphocytosis is seen. Sometimes protein-rich ascitic fluid is present, and the major differential diagnosis would be feline infectious peritonitis.

Bile duct obstruction

Bile duct obstruction is classically associated with jaundice, increased ALP and hypercholesterolaemia; increases in hepatocellular marker enzymes are often smaller in magnitude. Initially obstruction is associated with increased ALP, but if it persists bilirubinuria and then hyperbilirubinaemia develop. Obstruction by biliary and pancreatic tumours or by chronic inflammatory lesions is usually gradual in onset. Acute pancreatitis can also cause temporary bile duct obstruction, but the onset of jaundice is often acute and may be preceded by the more typical signs of acute pancreatitis. Laboratory tests will reflect not only bile duct obstruction but also changes due to pancreatic inflammation and secondary toxic hepatic changes (see Chapter 8). Ultrasound examinations in cases of biliary obstruction can be very helpful in determining a cause before exploratory surgery.

Drugs

Toxic hepatopathies may be associated with increases in hepatocellular enzyme markers if there is hepatocellular damage. Certain drugs such as glucocorticoids and anticonvulsants induce production of ALP/GGT, and anticonvulsants, to a lesser extent, can induce synthesis of ALT. Figure 9.20 lists some of the more important known or suspected hepatotoxic drugs that can cause increases in ALT in dogs and cats.

Metabolic disease

Various hormonal and metabolic diseases cause secondary hepatopathies. Vacuolar hepatopathies with accumulation of lipid (diabetes mellitus, feline idiopathic hepatic lipidosis) or glycogen (hyperadrenocortisolism) can cause increases in liver enzymes, but usually overall hepatic function is minimally impaired. Identification of the primary disorder usually precludes the need to investigate the liver beyond measuring SBA.

REFERENCES AND FURTHER READING

Bunch SE (1993) Hepatotoxicity associated with pharmacologic agents in dogs and cats. *Veterinary Clinics of North America - Small Animal Practice* **23**, 659–670

Bunch SE, Jordan HL, Sellon RK, Cullen J and Smith JE (1995) Characterisation of iron status in young dogs with portosystemic shunt. *American Journal of Veterinary Research* **56**, 853–858

Center SA (1990) Liver function tests in the diagnosis of portosystemic vascular anomalies. *Seminars in Veterinary Medicine and Surgery - Small Animal* **5**, 94–99

Center SA (1993) Serum bile acids in companion animal medicine. *Veterinary Clinics of North America - Small Animal Practice* **23**, 625–657

Center SA (1995) Pathophysiology, laboratory diagnosis, and liver diseases of the liver. In: *Textbook of Internal Veterinary Medicine, 4th edn*, ed. SJ Ettinger and EC Feldman, pp. 1261–1357. WB Saunders, Philadelphia

Center SA (1996) Liver: normal structure and function; Pathophysiology of liver disease: normal and abnormal function; Acute hepatic injury: hepatic necrosis and fulminant hepatic failure; Chronic hepatitis, cirrhosis, breed-specific hepatopathies, copper storage hepatopathy, suppurative hepatitis, and idiopathic hepatic fibrosis; Hepatic lipidosis, glucocorticoid hepatopathy, vacuolar hepatopathy, storage diseases, amyloidosis, and iron toxicity. In: *Strombeck's Small Animal Gastroenterology*, ed. WG Guilford et al., pp 540–632; 654–802. WB Saunders, Philadelphia

Center SA, Baldwin BH, Dillingham S, Erb HN and Tennant BC (1986) Diagnostic value of serum γ-glutamyl transferase and alkaline phosphatase activities in hepatobiliary disease in the cat. *Journal of the American Veterinary Medical Association* **188**, 507–510

Center SA, Baldwin BH, Erb HN and Tennant BC (1985) Bile acid concentrations in the diagnosis of hepatobiliary disease in the dog. *Journal of the American Veterinary Medical Association* **187**, 935–940

Center SA, Baldwin BH, Erb H and Tennant BC (1986) Bile acid concentrations in the diagnosis of hepatobiliary disease in the cat. *Journal of the American Veterinary Medical Association* **189**, 891–896

Center SA, Baldwin BH, King JM and Tennant BC (1983) Hematologic and biochemical abnormalities associated with induced extrahepatic bile duct obstruction in the cat. *American Journal of Veterinary Research* **44**, 1822–1829

Center SA, Erb HN and Joseph SA (1995) Measurement of serum bile acid concentrations for diagnosis of hepatobiliary disease in cats. *Journal of the American Veterinary Medical Association* **207**, 1048–1054

Center SA, Leveille CR, Baldwin BH and Tennant BC (1984) Direct spectrometric determination of serum bile acids in the dog and cat. *American Journal of Veterinary Research* **45**, 2043–2050

Center SA, Manwarren T, Slater MR and Wilentz E (1991) Evaluation of twelve-hour preprandial and two-hour postprandial serum bile acid concentration for diagnosis of hepatobiliary disease in dogs. *Journal of the American Veterinary Medical Association* **199**, 217–226

Center SA, Randolph JF, Manwarren T and Slater M (1991) Effect of colostrum ingestion on γ-glutamyl transferase and alkaline phosphatase activities in neonatal pups. *American Journal of Veterinary Research* **52**, 499–504

Center SA, Slater MR, Manwarren T and Prymak K (1992) Diagnostic efficacy of serum alkaline phosphatase and γ-glutamyltransferase in dogs with histologically confirmed hepatobiliary disease: 270 cases (1980–1990). *Journal of the American Veterinary Medical Association* **201**, 1258–1264

Center SA, Thompson M and Guida L (1993) 3-α-Hydroxylated bile acid profiles in clinically normal cats, cats with severe hepatic lipidosis, and cats with complete extrahepatic bile duct occlusion. *American Journal of Veterinary Research* **54**, 681–688

Cornelius CE (1989) Liver function. In: *Clinical Biochemistry of Domestic Animals, 4th edn*, ed. JJ Kaneko, pp. 364–397. Academic Press, New York

Dillon R (1985) The liver in systemic disease - an innocent bystander. *Veterinary Clinics of North America - Small Animal Practice* **15**, 97–117

Else R W (1996) Biopsy collection, processing and interpretation. In: *BSAVA Manual of Canine and Feline Gastroenterology*, ed. D.A. Thomas et al., pp. 37–66. BSAVA, Cheltenham

Engelking LR (1988) Disorders of bilirubin metabolism in small animal species. *Compendium of Continuing Education for the Practicing Veterinarian* **10**, 712–722

McConnell MF and Lumsden JH (1983) Biochemical evaluation of metastatic liver disease in the dog. *Journal of the American Animal Hospital Association* **19**, 173–178

Meyer DJ (1983) Serum γ-glutamyl transferase as a liver test in cats with toxic and obstructive hepatic disease. *Journal of the American Animal Hospital Association* **19**, 1023–1026

Meyer DJ (1986) Liver function tests in dogs with portosystemic shunts: measurement of serum bile acid concentration. *Journal of the American Veterinary Medical Association* **188**, 168–169

Meyer DJ (1996a) Hepatic tests: reflections of hepatobiliary pathophysiology. *Waltham Symposium: Liver Disease: Practical Perspectives*, 8–11

Meyer DJ (1996b) Hepatic pathology. In: *Strombeck's Small Animal Gastroenterology*, ed. WG Guilford et al., pp. 633–653. WB Saunders, Philadelphia

Meyer DJ and Center SA (1986) Approach to the diagnosis of liver disorders in dogs and cats. *Compendium of Continuing Education for the Practicing Veterinarian* **8**, 880–888

Meyer DJ and Chiapella AM (1985) Cholestasis. *Veterinary Clinics of North America - Small Animal Practice* **15**, 215–227

Meyer DJ and Harvey JW (1994) Hematologic changes associated with serum and hepatic iron alterations in dogs with congenital portosystemic vascular anomalies. *Journal of Veterinary Internal Medicine* **8**, 55–56

Mount ME (1986) Proteins induced by vitamin K absence or antagonists ("PIVKA"). In: *Current Veterinary Therapy IX*, ed. RW Kirk, pp. 513–515. WB Saunders, Philadelphia

Roth L and Meyer DJ. (1995) Interpretation of liver biopsies. *Veterinary Clinics of North America - Small Animal Practice* **25**, 293–303

Rothuizen J and van den Ingh TSGAM (1982) Rectal ammonia tolerance test in the evaluation of portal circulation in dogs with liver disease. *Research in Veterinary Science* **33**, 22–25

Sevelius E and Jönsson L (1996) Liver diseases. In: *BSAVA Manual of Canine and Feline Gastroenterology*, ed. DA Thomas et al., pp. 191–220. BSAVA, Cheltenham

Taboada J and Meyer DJ (1989) Cholestasis associated with extrahepatic bacterial infection in five dogs. *Journal of Veterinary Internal Medicine* **3**, 216–221

Twedt DC (1985) Cirrhosis: a consequence of chronic liver disease. *Veterinary Clinics of North America – Small Animal Practice* **15**, 151–176

CHAPTER TEN

Respiratory Tract and Cardiovascular System

Malcolm Cobb

INTRODUCTION

Clinical signs resulting from diseases of the cardiovascular system and/or the respiratory tract are commonly seen in small animal practice and the signs associated with diseases of the two systems are frequently very similar. Thoracic radiography is one of the most useful diagnostic aids in these patients, but a number of other procedures such as endoscopic examination of the respiratory tract and ultrasound examination are becoming available in many practices, significantly improving the clinician's ability to diagnose cardiorespiratory disease accurately. This chapter will review the methods available to help establish a diagnosis in patients with a variety of presenting clinical signs referable to the cardiac and respiratory systems.

SNEEZING AND NASAL DISCHARGE

Diagnosis
This is a common clinical presentation, especially in cats, in which viral infection is the most frequent cause. Diagnosis of feline viral upper respiratory tract disease

is generally based on clinical signs, and treatment is supportive.

Additional investigations are generally pursued: in canine and feline patients in which the clinical signs persist despite treatment; in patients in which clinical signs recur following treatment; and in patients in which epistaxis is a presenting clinical sign. Common causes of epistaxis in dogs and cats include foreign bodies, tumours, clotting defects, and fungal infections, in particular aspergillosis.

Additional investigations
Ancillary diagnostic aids that are frequently employed include radiography of the skull, nasal chambers and frontal sinuses, and rhinoscopy.

Haematology
Routine haematology may show results suggestive of inflammatory disease but inflammation is likely to accompany most conditions causing sneezing or nasal discharge. In patients with epistaxis, haematology will allow assessment of the severity of any anaemia resulting from the blood loss and a platelet count is indicated to rule out thrombocytopenia as a cause of epistaxis

(some patients suffer from both immune-mediated thrombocytopenia and haemolytic anaemia).

Clinical biochemistry

Although not usually helpful in making a diagnosis of the cause of the upper respiratory tract disease, a biochemical profile may be helpful in identifying co-existing and concurrent diseases, allowing a more accurate prognosis to be given.

Clotting function

Tests of clotting function, plus a platelet count, may be indicated in patients with epistaxis where thrombocytopenia or a coagulopathy may be a primary cause of the condition (or possibly a complicating factor).

FIV and FeLV

In cats with chronic or recurrent upper respiratory tract disease, testing for feline immunodeficiency virus (FIV) and feline leukaemia virus (FeLV) is indicated. The immunosuppressive effects of infection with FIV and FeLV predispose the infected animal to a number of opportunistic infections, including chronic upper respiratory tract infections.

Serology

Serology may be helpful in the diagnosis of nasal aspergillosis. This condition can be difficult to diagnose and a combination of diagnostic procedures is frequently required. These include culture of the nasal discharge, radiological examination of the nasal chambers and direct visualization of *Aspergillus* colonies through rhinoscopy or on exploratory rhinotomy. Detection of circulating antibodies to *Aspergillus*, with ELISA or agar gel immunodiffusion, usually gives reliable results in that these tests generally only give a positive result in the presence of clinical infection. A positive result in combination with appropriate clinical signs and characteristic radiological findings is usually enough to allow a confident diagnosis to be made.

Outbreaks of viral respiratory tract disease may occur in some cat populations, and serological tests to assess the involvement of feline herpesvirus or feline calicivirus are often complicated by prior vaccination. Serum samples are best obtained in the acute phase of the disease and taken again 2 weeks later in an effort to identify a rising antibody titre. Cats recovering from acute calicivirus infection develop high serum levels of neutralizing antibodies, whereas antibody levels tend to rise more slowly and to lower levels in cats infected with feline herpesvirus.

Cytology, histopathology and microbiology

Specimens for cytological and microbiological examination can be obtained by direct swabbing or by lavage of the nasal chambers. These result in the collection of material from the surface of the mucosa only. In some cases cells infected with viruses, for example feline

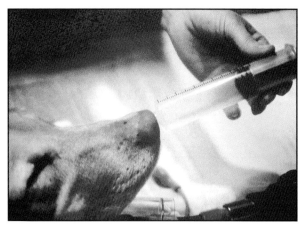

Figure 10.1: *Nasal flush biopsy. The flush is delivered by syringe which fits snugly into the nostril.*
Courtesy of Dr J.V. Davies.

herpesvirus, may be demonstrated in smears by immunofluorescence.

Often more effective is the performance of a nasal flush. This dislodges material in a retrograde manner and is often effective in collecting tissue for cytology, histology and microbiology, as well as occasionally dislodging foreign material. The animal is anaesthetized, a cuffed endotracheal tube is placed in the trachea, and the pharynx is packed with moist gauze swabs. The flush is delivered by syringe (luer fitting or catheter tip depending on the size of the animal) into the nostril (Figure 10.1). A bolus of saline is delivered at a dose of 0.5–1.0 ml/kg in an attempt to dislodge material which is collected from the back of the pharynx in a previously placed collection device (a uropipette or custom-made device fashioned from a plastic 5 ml, 10 ml or 20 ml syringe case; Figure 10.2) or on gauze swabs (use sterile swabs if the samples are required for microbiology). The collection system must fit snugly into the patient's pharynx (Figure 10.3). Some bleeding may occur but this ceases rapidly. In cases with nasal neoplasia, tissue samples rather than cytological samples will frequently be delivered (Figure 10.4).

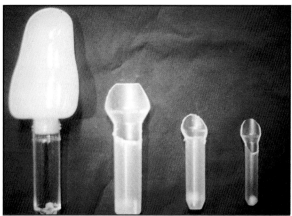

Figure 10.2: *Collection devices suitable for collecting material dislodged by nasal flush biopsy. A uropipette can be used or custom-made devices can be fashioned from plastic syringe cases.*
Courtesy of Dr J.V. Davies.

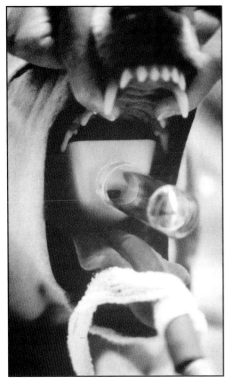

Figure 10.3:
The collection
system shown
fitting snugly
into the
patient's
pharynx.
Courtesy of Dr J.V.
Davies.

Tissue samples for cytology, histology and microbiology can sometimes be obtained from intranasal mass lesions by aspirating tissue from a lesion with a blunt cannula. A rigid plastic tube is measured against the length from the external nares to the medial canthus of the eye and cut; this avoids the tube reaching the cribriform plate. The tube is inserted into the lesion, vigorous aspiration is performed, and cores of tissue are frequently obtained (Clercx *et al.*, 1996).

Samples for cytology, histology and/or microbiology can be obtained by taking fine needle aspirates, using biopsy forceps or a cytology brush, or by using a biopsy needle. However, safe and accurate tissue sampling using these methods can usually only be achieved with endoscopic or rhinoscopic guidance or at exploratory rhinotomy.

Conjunctival biopsy specimens stained with haematoxylin and eosin may show intranuclear inclusion bodies in cats infected with feline herpesvirus.

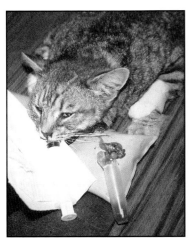

Figure 10.4:
A tissue sample
delivered by nasal
flush biopsy of
a cat.
Courtesy of Dr J.V. Davies.

Conjunctival scrapings from cats with *Chlamydia* infections may show intracytoplasmic inclusions within 2 weeks of infection.

COUGHING AND PULMONARY PARENCHYMAL DISEASE

Diagnosis

The clinical history and physical examination will often localize a disease to the lower respiratory tract. Further diagnostic tests are usually required in order to define more clearly the disease responsible and to assess the severity. Thoracic radiography is probably the single most useful diagnostic aid in patients with coughing and pulmonary parenchymal disease. Tracheal and bronchoalveolar lavage are minimally invasive procedures that may assist in the establishment of a definitive diagnosis and the institution of appropriate treatment. They are also useful procedures for the identification of complicating or coexisting problems in patients with structural diseases of the respiratory tract, such as tracheal collapse.

Cytological examination of cells and culture of swab material from the oropharynx is of very limited value in the coughing patient.

Additional investigations

Tracheal lavage

Tracheal lavage, or a 'tracheal wash', is a procedure whereby a representative sample of cells, mucus and microorganisms is obtained from the trachea and large airways. It is particularly useful for patients with evidence of airway disease, or diseases of the pulmonary parenchyma that also involve the airways, such as bronchopneumonia. A tracheal wash can be performed in an anaesthetized patient via the endotracheal tube (endotracheal lavage) or in a conscious or sedated patient using a catheter inserted through the skin into the trachea (transtracheal lavage). The advantage of the transtracheal technique is that the patient does not require general anaesthesia and this is preferred in patients considered to be at high risk from anaesthesia. With either technique, contamination with cells and bacteria from the oropharynx is minimized (Hawkins, 1992). Tracheal lavage does have limitations and the results must be carefully related to clinical signs and results of other ancillary diagnostic aids. It is usually indicated when bronchoalveolar lavage cannot be performed, either because the patient is compromised or as a result of a lack of facilities or equipment.

Transtracheal lavage: The animal is restrained in a sitting position or in sternal recumbency; sedation is rarely necessary but may be required in difficult patients. The head is lifted and the neck extended.

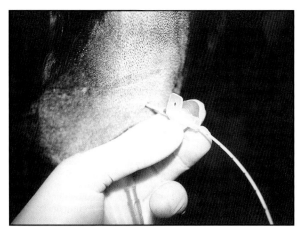

Figure 10.5: An over-the-needle catheter inserted through the cricothyroid ligament through which a sterile tube has been advanced to the level of the bronchial bifurcation.

The skin over the larynx is clipped and prepared as it would be for surgery.

Local anaesthetic is instilled into the subcutaneous tissue in the midline over the cricothyroid ligament, which can be palpated as a depression just cranial to the cricoid cartilage. A small incision is made in the skin at this site with a scalpel blade.

A 4 cm long, over-the-needle catheter is used; 14 or 16 gauge is suitable for most large or medium-sized dogs, 18 gauge for small dogs. The catheter is inserted through the cricothyroid ligament (the catheter can be felt to puncture the ligament easily) into the lumen of the larynx. The stylet is then removed and a sterile tube of an appropriate size, pre-loaded with warm sterile saline, is advanced through the catheter to the level of the bronchial bifurcation (Figure 10.5); the catheter from a through-the-needle jugular catheter or the suction catheter from an endoscope (Figure 10.6) is frequently used. At this point the patient usually coughs. The advantage of this system is that the stylet can be completely removed, minimizing the risk of cutting off the catheter during the procedure. An alternative method involves the use of a 25 or 30 cm long, through-the-needle jugular catheter (14 or 16 gauge for most large or medium-sized dogs). The needle is inserted as

described above and the catheter advanced through the needle down the trachea. Once the catheter is placed the needle is withdrawn.

In larger dogs, the catheter can be placed between the tracheal rings halfway down the cervical trachea (Figure 10.7).

Once the catheter is placed in the lumen of the trachea, approximately 0.25–0.5 ml/kg of warm sterile saline is instilled gently. It is important to ensure that the saline used does not contain a bacteriostatic agent. At the end of the instillation, the saline is re-aspirated immediately. A small quantity of fluid (usually 10–40% of the volume initially instilled) is usually recovered with floating material visible. It may be necessary to repeat the procedure before a satisfactory sample is recovered. The catheter is then gently removed.

Samples are collected into EDTA for cytology and into plain tubes for bacteriological culture. If possible, smears of the aspirated material should be made at once. In the presence of excessive mucus it is often worth making a 'squash' preparation to reduce cell clumping on the slide (see Chapter 7). If only very small volumes of material are recovered, examination of centrifuged samples ('cytospin' preparations) may be required. Unfortunately the equipment required to produce these preparations is generally only available in referral centres with their own laboratories.

Although complications associated with the procedure are rare, patients should be observed carefully after transtracheal lavage for problems such as pneumomediastinum or airway obstruction.

Transtracheal lavage is difficult in cats.

Endotracheal aspiration: A soft catheter (e.g. an endobronchial suction catheter that has had the proximal attachment replaced by a three-way tap; Figure 10.8) is passed down the lumen of the endotracheal tube (ideally a sterile endotracheal tube is used if the sample is required for bacteriological culture) in an anaesthetized patient (Figure 10.9).

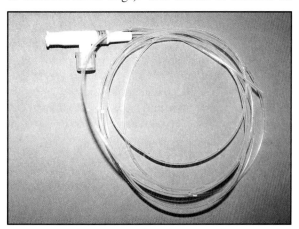

Figure 10.6: The suction catheter from an endoscope used to aspirate material from the trachea in a transtracheal lavage.

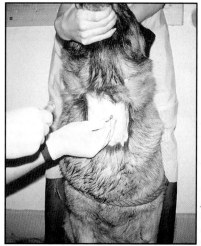

Figure 10.7: A transtracheal wash being performed in a large-breed dog in which the catheter has been placed between the tracheal rings halfway down the cervical trachea.

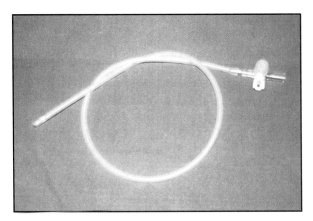

Figure 10.8: A modified endobronchial suction catheter that has had the proximal attachment replaced with a three-way tap; this is often used for endobronchial aspiration from the respiratory tract.

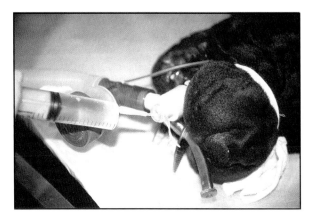

Figure 10.9: Endobronchial aspiration from the respiratory tract performed by passing the suction catheter down the lumen of the endotracheal tube (ideally through an adaptor as shown) in an anaesthetized patient.

Alternatively, endobronchial aspiration is performed under endoscopic guidance. This allows the catheter to be guided into areas of interest and visible material can be selected and sampled. Warm sterile saline (0.25–0.5 ml/kg) is infused into the airway and immediately re-aspirated as described above.

Bronchoalveolar lavage

This technique is particularly useful in patients with pulmonary parenchymal disease in which the examination of a tracheal wash may not be helpful. It can only be performed in anaesthetized patients.

The procedure is often performed using a suction catheter passed down the biopsy channel of an endoscope or a suction catheter that can be guided endoscopically; in both cases the procedure can provide material from specific sites. Sites within the respiratory tract to be sampled are selected for lavage on the basis of radiographic and endoscopic findings. In the presence of diffuse pulmonary parenchymal disease, an endobronchial suction catheter can be carefully passed blindly down the endotracheal tube until resistance is met as the catheter lodges in an airway. The suction catheter or the endoscope is introduced into the airway until a tight fit is achieved; enough warmed, sterile saline is infused into a small airway to flood the dependent alveoli and immediately re-aspirated. The volume of saline required will vary with the size of the patient and the diameter of the endoscope/catheter and therefore the volume of lung being sampled. Generally, between 1 and 3 ml/kg will be required. Lavage can be repeated for several lung lobes if diffuse parenchymal disease is suspected.

The patient is allowed to breathe 100% oxygen until extubated and the lungs are gently inflated several times before extubation. Hypoxaemia is rare and usually responds to oxygen supplementation.

Typical findings of bronchoalveolar and tracheal lavage

In normal animals a tracheal wash normally contains predominantly ciliated, columnar respiratory epithelial cells, a few macrophages and occasional neutrophils and/or eosinophils. Bronchoalveolar lavage typically results in the aspiration of saline containing more than 70% macrophages and a small number of ciliated, columnar respiratory epithelial cells. Very few lymphocytes, neutrophils or eosinophils are found in normal animals, although significant numbers of eosinophils are occasionally seen in washes from clinically healthy cats.

Excessive amounts of mucus and large numbers of non-degenerate polymorphs, particularly neutrophils, as well as increased numbers of goblet cells are often seen in washes from patients with chronic inflammatory airway disease such as bronchitis. In patients with bacterial bronchitis or bronchopneumonia, the neutrophils tend to have a degenerate appearance and may contain intracellular bacteria. This latter feature is helpful in differentiating active airway infection from oropharyngeal contamination that may result in extracellular bacteria in the preparation. Occasionally foreign material or a causative organism is evident, either free in the wash fluid or contained within phagocytes.

Eosinophilic polymorphs are the predominant cell type in patients with eosinophilic conditions, such as pulmonary infiltrates with eosinophilia (Corcoran *et al.*, 1991). Samples obtained by airway lavage from cats with feline 'asthma' frequently contain excessive numbers of polymorphonuclear leucocytes. Non-degenerate neutrophils are often the predominant cell type, though in some cases eosinophils will predominate, and variable numbers of macrophages are frequently seen (Corcoran *et al.*, 1995). Excessive numbers of eosinophils are also seen in washes from patients with infestations of parasites, such as *Oslerus osleri*, and worm larvae may be evident in the wash.

Neoplastic cells may be seen in patients with pulmonary neoplasia, but their absence does not rule out neoplasia as a cause of the clinical signs. Frequently the material recovered from patients with pulmonary or airway neoplasia is normal or suggests chronic inflammation only.

Haematology

Some conditions, particularly acute conditions such as bronchopneumonia, may be associated with an inflammatory haemogram. More chronic conditions may have a normal haemogram, or there may be evidence of chronic inflammation. A peripheral eosinophilia may be a feature of conditions such as pulmonary infiltrates with eosinophilia (PIE), feline 'asthma' or *Oslerus* infestation, but its absence does not rule out these conditions. Anaemia or polycythaemia may be associated with some primary pulmonary conditions and may contribute to the clinical signs. Anaemia may develop as a result of a coagulopathy which, again, can result in respiratory signs in patients that develop pulmonary haemorrhage.

Clinical biochemistry

Biochemistry may identify complicating or coexisting problems and may also assist diagnosis. For example, hyperglobulinaemia may be evident in inflammatory conditions; hypercalcaemia may occur in some patients with pulmonary neoplasia.

Testing for FeLV and FIV

In cats, examination of serum samples for evidence of FIV, FeLV and perhaps *Toxoplasma* infection may be indicated, since all these can be associated with various forms of intrathoracic disease. For example, FeLV infection may be associated with anterior mediastinal lymphoma.

Clotting function

An assessment of clotting function and a platelet count may be indicated in patients with pulmonary haemorrhage.

Airway and lung biopsy

Biopsy of the lining of the airways or lesions within the airways can be performed under endoscopic guidance.

Fine needle aspiration or tissue core biopsies (using a biopsy needle) can be performed for pulmonary mass

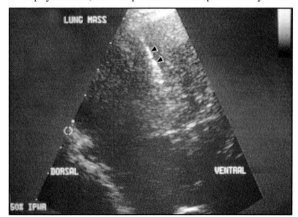

Figure 10.10: *Ultrasound image of a biopsy needle within a pulmonary mass lesion. Arrowheads mark the position of the needle within the mass.*
Courtesy of C.R. Lamb.

lesions under the guidance of ultrasound (Figure 10.10) or fluoroscopy, particularly if the lesion is adjacent to the body wall (Teske, 1995). This should be attempted only by experienced operators, great care should be taken and the patient monitored carefully for the development of pneumothorax or haemorrhage following any pulmonary biopsy procedure. Such procedures are contraindicated in patients with coagulopathy, pulmonary emphysema or bullous lung disease.

Similar methods can be used to obtain samples from other intrathoracic mass lesions, such as cranial mediastinal masses.

Fine needle aspiration samples can often be obtained from larger intrathoracic mass lesions without ultrasound or fluoroscopic guidance by 'blind' percutaneous aspiration. The site for aspiration is chosen based on the results of plain radiography and is clipped and prepared for surgery, and infiltrated with local anaesthetic. This is not a benign procedure, however; strict asepsis is required and the patient should be carefully monitored for the development of pneumothorax or haemorrhage in particular after the aspirate has been obtained.

Aspirated material can be submitted for cytological and microbiological examination, while tissue biopsies are submitted for histopathology and microbiological examination.

Techniques for obtaining blind percutaneous biopsy samples of lung parenchyma have been described (Teske, 1995) but these are associated with a significant degree of risk, particularly of pneumothorax and pulmonary haemorrhage. They may be useful in patients with diffuse pulmonary parenchymal disease, such as chronic inflammatory disease, and metastatic lung disease. The biopsy site is clipped and prepared for surgery, and infiltrated with local anaesthetic, taking care to ensure that the parietal pleura are infiltrated with anaesthetic. In patients with diffuse pulmonary disease, the diaphragmatic lung lobe is biopsied through the dorsal third of the seventh, eighth or ninth intercostal space. A 20 gauge disposable needle of an appropriate length, with a stylet (such as a spinal needle), is advanced into the lung parenchyma. The stylet is quickly removed and a gloved finger placed over the needle hub to prevent air being aspirated into the chest. Cells and fluid are then aspirated from the lung using a 10 or 20 ml syringe and submitted for cytological examination.

Tissue biopsies of the lung may also be obtained at exploratory thoracotomy, but this represents a significant surgical procedure.

Serology

While aspergillosis, usually the nasal form, is the only fungal infection commonly seen in patients in the United Kingdom, infections with other fungal agents, including *Histoplasma capsulatum*, *Coccidioides immitis* and *Blastomyces dermatitidis*, occur elsewhere. Following inhalation of these agents a variety of clinical syndromes can develop, although pulmonary parenchymal disease is a common consequence of infection. These conditions are usually diagnosed on the basis of the clinical signs seen in a patient from an area where the diseases are enzootic, the appearance of thoracic radiographs and direct visualization of the organism within, or the isolation of the organism from, material collected from the lower respiratory tract through tracheal or bronchoalveolar lavage. In addition, a variety of serological tests is available, being used most commonly to help diagnose blastomycosis and coccidioidomycosis.

BLOOD GAS ANALYSIS

Evaluation of blood pH and blood gases is not widely available in general practice because of the high cost of buying and maintaining the equipment required to perform the assays; local hospitals and referral practices may be able to offer the service. Lower-cost equipment and methods of assessing indirect indicators of some parameters, such as using the total CO_2 content to reflect the plasma bicarbonate level, may make some assessment of acid–base status more readily available in the near future.

Venous blood taken from the jugular vein is most useful for the evaluation of the whole body acid–base status.

Arterial samples (obtained from the femoral or the dorsal metatarsal artery) allow the oxygenation of the blood to be evaluated and are most useful for evaluation of respiratory function.

It must be remembered that the partial pressure of oxygen in the arterial blood (PaO_2) and the partial pressure of carbon dioxide in the arterial blood ($PaCO_2$) must be interpreted in relation to the clinical state of the patient and the indicators of acid–base balance, particularly the pH and the bicarbonate level.

Arterial carbon dioxide

Under normal circumstances, metabolic production of CO_2 is constant and the arterial CO_2 level ($PaCO_2$) is determined by the rate of elimination of CO_2 from the lungs. CO_2 diffuses readily from the capillary venous blood into the alveoli down the gradient of partial pressure that exists between these two areas. If lung function is normal and the patient is breathing room air, an elevated arterial CO_2 level is probably due to decreased elimination through hypoventilation and respiratory acidosis is the result. The normal $PaCO_2$ in dogs and cats is 35–45 mm Hg.

Hyperventilation results in a fall in arterial $PaCO_2$, and the development of a respiratory alkalosis.

Arterial oxygen

Arterial PaO_2 is a useful indicator of pulmonary function. The normal PaO_2 in a dog or cat breathing room air (which contains 20% oxygen) is 85–100 mm Hg. As a general rule, PaO_2 is usually 5 times the fraction of the inspired gas that is oxygen (FiO_2). In a patient receiving nasal oxygen, FiO_2 will be approximately 40% and PaO_2 should therefore be about 200 mm Hg; when breathing 100% oxygen, the PaO_2 should be 500 mm Hg.

There are two major situations in which a low PaO_2 can occur in patients breathing room air at sea level: hypoventilation — usually accompanied by a high $PaCO_2$ (see above); and poor oxygenation of the arterial blood.

Venous blood can reach the left ventricle without being adequately oxygenated in three ways:

- In patients with right-to-left shunting, blood passes from the systemic venous circulation through an anatomical venous-arterial shunt directly into the systemic arterial circulation and never passes through a ventilated area of the lung. Shunts can be generated by intrapulmonary disease, e.g. if blood is delivered to areas of the lung that are consolidated or atelectatic and consequently not functioning. Alternatively, the shunt may be extrapulmonary, e.g. in congenital cardiac diseases such as tetralogy of Fallot.

- There may be uneven blood flow and ventilation throughout the lung (ventilation-perfusion mismatching). This is common in patients with pulmonary parenchymal disease, and occurs as a result of uneven pulmonary ventilation and inefficient gas exchange. It can also occur as a result of normally ventilated lung being inadequately perfused with blood, e.g. in cases of pulmonary thromboembolism.

- Damage to, or thickening of, the capillary endothelium or the alveolar wall results in diffusion impairment, which prevents normal gas exchange and results in poor oxygenation of arterial blood and a low PaO_2.

In many patients with chronic pulmonary disease more than one mechanism frequently contributes to the development of hypoxia.

The alveolar–arterial oxygen difference

Calculation of the alveolar-arterial oxygen difference $(A–a)PO_2$ is a useful way of determining whether a patient with hypoxaemia has intrinsic pulmonary disease or whether some extrapulmonary disorder is responsible for the changes seen. The alveolar-arterial oxygen difference is calculated as follows:

$$(A{-}a)PO_2 = (150 - PaCO_2) - PaO_2$$

The normal value is 10–25 mm Hg.

In cats and dogs with hypoxaemia, as determined by arterial blood gas analysis, calculation of $(A-a)PO_2$ and the response to increased oxygenation can help determine the likely cause of the hypoxaemia. For example, the PaO_2 of patients with right-to-left shunting fails to increase to normal, even when breathing 100% oxygen, whereas arterial oxygenation in patients with a ventilation–perfusion mismatch can be improved by administering 100% oxygen (DiBartola and de Morais, 1992).

Pulse oximetry

PaO_2 is a measure of the amount of oxygen in arterial blood. Pulse oximetry allows the immediate determination of arterial haemoglobin saturation (SaO_2). Pulse oximeters transmit light through the skin or mucous membrane and sense the difference between the light absorbed during arterial pulsations and the background absorption resulting from venous blood and surrounding tissues. From these measurements values for haemoglobin saturation and pulse rate are calculated (Hendricks, 1995).

Pulse oximetry is a non-invasive method of obtaining information on the delivery of oxygen to the tissues (assuming the patient has adequate peripheral perfusion) and correlates with the PaO_2, although it must be remembered that the two are not related linearly (the relation between SaO_2 and PaO_2 is represented by the oxygen–haemoglobin dissociation curve).

PLEURAL EFFUSIONS

Diagnosis

A diagnosis of the presence of a pleural effusion is often made based on the clinical history and the results of physical examination. Thoracic radiography may be necessary to confirm the presence of a pleural effusion. In a dyspnoeic animal in which pleural effusion is suspected, thoracocentesis should be performed before thoracic radiography is attempted

in order to improve the animal's ability to oxygenate and thereby reduce the risk of worsening respiratory function developing as a result of any stress associated with radiography.

Thoracocentesis

The thorax can either be drained intermittently or an indwelling drain can be placed. The latter is useful where further production of fluid is anticipated or where there is persistent production of fluid.

Following thoracocentesis, additional diagnostic tests might include repeating thoracic radiography and thoracic ultrasound examination. However, the latter is often best performed before thoracocentesis because the thoracic fluid makes visualization of intrathoracic structures much easier.

Intermittent drainage

The procedure is usually performed in conscious patients. The hair coat must be clipped from a suitable site on the thoracic wall and the site prepared as it would be for surgery. Local anaesthetic is instilled into the subcutaneous tissue, the body wall and the pleura lining the thorax, which are very sensitive; animals often show discomfort as the needle or catheter is introduced. A common site used is the seventh or eighth intercostal space, at or just below the level of the costochondral junction. An appropriate site for drainage can also be identified from thoracic radiographs, if available. It may be necessary to drain both sides of the chest, although often aspiration from one side will adequately drain the contralateral hemithorax. Rarely, an effusion is unilateral. The patient is allowed to adopt the most comfortable position, usually sternal recumbency, and minimal manual restraint is applied.

A small incision is made in the skin with a scalpel blade. A 2–7 cm (0.8–2.8 inches) long, over-the-needle catheter of appropriate size (21–23 gauge in cats and small dogs, up to 16 or even 14 gauge in larger dogs) attached to extension tubing, is connected via a three-way tap to a 20 or 60 ml syringe (Figure 10.11).

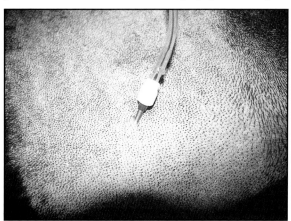

Figure 10.11: A catheter placed in the pleural cavity and attached to extension tubing for aspirating pleural fluid.

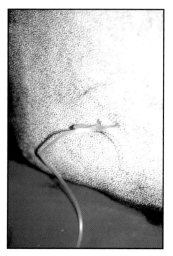

Figure 10.12:
A butterfly catheter placed in the pleural space is sometimes useful for aspirating pleural fluid in cats and smaller dogs. The needle or catheter is advanced perpendicular to the chest wall, as shown; once the pleural space has been entered, the needle or catheter is directed ventrally to minimize the risk of lung damage, as shown in Figure 10.11.

A butterfly catheter is sometimes useful in cats and smaller dogs (Figure 10.12). The needle or catheter is advanced perpendicular to the chest wall into the pleural space in the centre of the costochondral junction. Once the pleural space has been entered, the needle or catheter is directed ventrally to minimize the risk of lung damage. Gentle negative pressure is then applied via the syringe and fluid is aspirated from the thorax.

Thoracocentesis helps to relieve respiratory distress and provides samples of fluid that can be submitted for cytology (collected into a tube with EDTA), aerobic and anaerobic culture (plain tube) and biochemical analysis (plain tube). Several direct smears should be made for cytology, or unfixed material can be submitted for cytocentrifuge preparation if available at a nearby laboratory. Care should be taken when handling the fluid since it may be infectious.

Types of effusion

The nature of the pleural fluid present can usually be established on the basis of the gross appearance, protein content, specific gravity (SG), total nucleated cell count and cytological characteristics of any cells, as well as biochemical parameters such as the levels of triglyceride, cholesterol and glucose. These are used to characterize certain types of effusion, as summarized in Table 10.1 (Relford *et al.*, 1996). The characteristics of the fluid may change, depending on how long the fluid has been present in the pleural space and on attempts made to drain the fluid.

Pure transudates (hydrothorax), usually only occur where there is a low protein level in the plasma (hypoproteinaemia); they occasionally occur in congestive cardiac failure. In these cases there is often concurrent anasarca and/or ascites.

A modified transudate will typically accumulate in conditions where there is a high venous and capillary hydrostatic pressure, such as congestive heart failure or obstruction of veins and/or lymphatics by intrathoracic mass lesions, and can also develop in patients with diaphragmatic rupture or a lung lobe torsion, or if a pure transudate has been present in the pleural space for some time.

Chylous effusions typically occur if lymph drains into the thoracic cavity as a result of a rupture of the thoracic duct in the thorax. This may be the result of intrathoracic lymphangiectasia secondary to functional or structural obstruction or trauma, although in many cases the effusions are idiopathic. Chylothorax may also occasionally develop in cats with cardiac failure and pseudochylous effusions in patients with intrathoracic neoplasia. The triglyceride content of a chylous effusion is greater than the plasma level while the cholesterol level in a chylous effusion is usually less than the plasma cholesterol level (in pseudochylous effusions the cholesterol level in the effusion is greater

than plasma cholesterol).

Haemorrhagic exudates are usually obvious in gross appearance, and often very dark. They are highly cellular and usually have a PCV approaching that of circulating blood. Haemorrhagic exudates usually will not clot because they become defibrinated within the body cavity. This failure to clot does not mean that the haemothorax is a consequence of a coagulopathy. Haemorrhagic effusions typically accumulate in the pleural space as a result of a coagulopathy, thoracic trauma or, most commonly, in the presence of a bleeding intrathoracic tumour.

Exudates are differentiated into septic and nonseptic exudates. Culture of a septic exudate may isolate a pathogen if prior antibiotic therapy has not been administered. Septic exudates occur: in inflammatory conditions such as intrathoracic sepsis associated with the presence of a foreign body; following thoracic surgery; in association with penetrating wounds of the thorax, oesophagus or airway; or through the extension of an infectious process involving the lungs or mediastinum. However, the cause of a septic exudate is often not identified.

Non-septic exudates are negative on culture. They may occur as a result of an immune-mediated process (testing the fluid for antinuclear antibodies may be indicated; see Chapter 6), or as a result of parasitic or neoplastic processes. Some remain idiopathic. In cats, feline infectious peritonitis (FIP) results in a non-septic exudate that is clear or slightly opaque, yellow, viscous and has an SG greater than 1.030 and a protein level greater than 30 g/l.

Neoplastic cells may be identified in neoplastic effusions. They may be difficult to differentiate from reactive mesothelial cells, although the identification of clumps of cells with a large nuclear to cytoplasm ratio is significant (see Chapter 7). The absence of tumour cells does *not* rule out intrathoracic neoplasia as a cause of the effusion.

Additional investigations

Haematology
Routine haematology may be helpful in identifying changes associated with intrathoracic disease, e.g. anaemia associated with intrathoracic tumours such as haemangiosarcoma or lymphoma, or a degenerative left shift associated with a septic exudate.

Serology
In cats, particularly those with recurrent or chronic disease, testing for FeLV, FIV and FIP is often indicated, since these can be primary (FIP) or predisposing (FeLV infection) causes of pleural effusion.

Clotting function
An assessment of clotting function may be indicated in patients with haemothorax.

Effusion type	Appearance	Protein content (g/l)	Total nucleated cell count (x10⁹/l)	Cell types typically present	Useful biochemical parameters
Transudate	Clear, maybe yellow or colourless	5–10	0.5–1.0	Mesothelial cells, some WBC	
Modified transudate	Clear or slightly turbid; usually red/orange or yellow	15–30	1–5	Mesothelial cells, macrophages, PMN, some RBC	
Chylous	Milky white or pink	30–85	Variable: 2–60	Small lymphocytes	Triglyceride, cholesterol
Haemorrhagic	Dark red, sanguinous	40–80		RBC, variable WBC content	
Septic exudate	Variable: cloudy, turbid, maybe granular; often coloured	>25	50+	PMN (usually degenerate) ±organisms, macrophages, mesothelial cells	
Non-septic exudate	Clear or turbid; maybe coloured yellow/ orange	>30	25+	Variable, mesothelial cells, macrophages, PMN, lymphocytes	
Neoplastic	Variable: clear or red/orange; maybe slightly turbid; maybe sanguinous	30–80	Variable	Mesothelial cells, macrophages, PMN, maybe neoplastic cells	

Table 10.1: *Characteristics of different types of pleural fluid.*
WBC: white blood cells; RBC: red blood cells; PMN: polymorphonuclear neutrophils

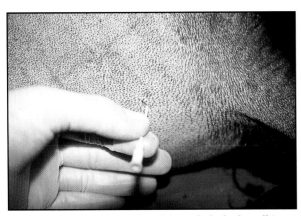

Figure 10.13: A catheter placed through the body wall into the pericardial sac to drain a pericardial effusion. The stylet has already been removed.

Clinical biochemistry

Tests may help to identify complicating or coexisting abnormalities and assist diagnosis. For example, hypoproteinaemia may be identified as a cause of a thoracic transudate; hyperglobulinaemia may be seen in inflammatory conditions and in cats with FIP; and hypercalcaemia may occur in some cases of thymic lymphoma, particularly in dogs.

PERICARDIAL DISEASE

Pericardial disease is usually characterized by an accumulation of fluid within the pericardial sac known as a pericardial effusion. The effusion is categorized on the basis of the type of fluid present (Jones, 1979; Lombard, 1983; Berg and Wingfield, 1984).

Diagnosis

A tentative diagnosis can often be made based on the clinical history and the results of physical examination, which usually indicate right-sided congestive cardiac failure. Ancillary diagnostic aids, particularly thoracic radiography and two-dimensional echocardiography, are commonly used to confirm the presence of pericardial disease and cardiac tamponade (compromised ventricular filling resulting from the elevated intrapericardial pressure; Miller and Fossum, 1992).

Pericardiocentesis

Pericardiocentesis relieves cardiac tamponade and provides fluid for analysis. Cytological examination of

pericardial fluid is, however, an unreliable method of distinguishing neoplastic from non-neoplastic pericardial disorders (Sisson *et al.*, 1984). The measurement of glucose level and pH, to assist the differentiation of various types of effusion, is currently being investigated (Edwards, 1996; Relford *et al.*, 1996). Drainage of the effusion usually results in resolution of the clinical signs within 2–3 days.

The patient is allowed to adopt the most comfortable position, usually sternal recumbency, and minimal manual restraint is applied. A common site for pericardiocentesis is the fifth intercostal space on the right side, at the level of the costochondral junction. The skin over the pericardiocentesis site is clipped and prepared as it would be for surgery. Local anaesthetic is instilled into the subcutaneous tissue, the body wall and the pleura lining the thorax. The procedure is usually performed in conscious patients, although light sedation may be necessary. Continuous ECG monitoring is also advisable in order to identify any sustained dysrhythmias that may develop during the procedure.

A small incision is made in the skin with a scalpel blade and an over-the-needle catheter is advanced through the body wall (Figure 10.13); the stylet can usually be felt to puncture the tense pericardial sac. A 14 or 16 gauge catheter, at least 7–15 cm long is suitable for most large or medium-sized dogs, whilst an 18 or 20 gauge catheter, 5–8 cm long is suitable for most small dogs and cats. A commercially available catheter, specifically designed for the purpose, is also available (Figure 10.14). At this point the effusion will usually appear in the hub of the stylet. The catheter is advanced into the pericardium and the stylet is withdrawn. The catheter is then connected to the extension set of an intravenous fluid administration set and this is connected, via a three-way tap, to a 60 ml syringe. Gentle negative pressure is then applied via the syringe and fluid is aspirated from the pericardium (Figure 10.15).

Figure 10.16 lists the common types of pericardial effusion found in dogs and cats, along with the most common underlying causes of the effusions. Blood is the most common fluid type identified in dogs with pericardial disease, due either to bleeding from tumours within the pericardium (commonly from heart base tumours, such as chemodectomas, or right atrial haemangiosarcomas, especially in the German Shepherd Dog) or as a result of bleeding from the

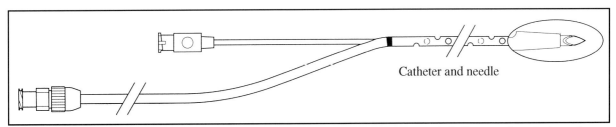

Catheter and needle

Figure 10.14: A commercially available catheter specifically designed for draining pericardial effusion in dogs. Redrawn by kind permission of Cooks Veterinary Products.

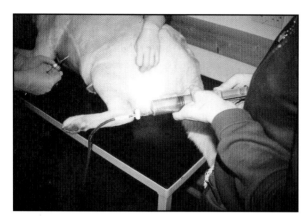

Figure 10.15: *Sanguinous effusion being aspirated from the pericardium of a dog with idiopathic pericardial haemorrhage.*

pericardial vessels themselves (Figure 10.17). The cause of this latter problem, idiopathic pericardial haemorrhage, is unknown. Sanguinous effusion aspirated from the pericardium can be differentiated from blood tapped from the heart by accidental cardiac puncture (Figure 10.17) by the fact that the former will contain no fibrin as a result of having been in the pericardium for some time and consequently will not clot; sanguinous effusion from the pericardium will usually have a lower PCV than peripheral blood.

Thoracotomy and subtotal pericardectomy are indicated in patients with evidence of intrapericardial neoplasia and are often effective for treatment of recurrent idiopathic haemorrhagic effusions. A sample of the pericardium can be submitted for histopathology.

Transudate / Modified transudate
Congenital pericardio-peritoneal hernia
Right-sided congestive heart failure
   (usually with ascites and/or anasarca)
Hypoalbuminaemia
   (usually with ascites and/or anasarca)
Idiopathic

Haemorrhage
Left atrial rupture
Intra-pericardial neoplasia*
Trauma
Coagulopathy
Idiopathic benign pericardial haemorrhage*

Exudate
Infection

Figure 10.16: *Common causes of pericardial effusion.*
* most common

HEART DISEASE AND HEART FAILURE

Congestive cardiac failure

Diagnosis
A tentative diagnosis can often be made based on the patient's details, the clinical history and the results of physical examination. Ancillary diagnostic aids, particularly thoracic radiography, are commonly used to confirm the presence of cardiac failure and to assess the severity.

Routine tests, in particular clinical biochemistry, may reflect the haemodynamic effects of cardiac failure, the effects of any therapeutic agents used, or the presence of concurrent extracardiac disease. Careful monitoring of the patient's metabolic condition is essential, particularly when agents such as diuretics and angiotensin-converting enzyme (ACE) inhibitors are part of the management regimen.

Additional investigations

Haematology: Many patients in heart failure have a neutrophilia, sometimes a mild left shift, and sometimes an eosinopenia and lymphopenia associated with the stress of the disease. Anaemia, particularly chronic anaemia, may precipitate cardiac failure. Neutrophilia and monocytosis can indicate inflammation, e.g. in cases of infective endocarditis.

Clinical biochemistry: In severe cardiac failure there is commonly evidence of prerenal azotaemia. Total protein and serum albumin values may be slightly low; this may be a dilutional effect as water is retained or may be due to reduced protein synthesis or absorption. Elevated globulin levels may reflect an underlying infectious or inflammatory disease.

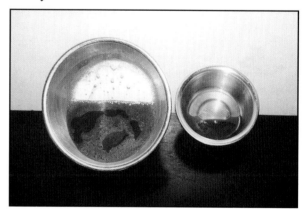

Figure 10.17: *A non-clotting sanguinous effusion is the most common fluid type identified in dogs with pericardial disease, due either to bleeding from tumours within the pericardium or as a result of idiopathic pericardial haemorrhage. Sanguinous effusion aspirated from the pericardium (left) can be differentiated from blood tapped from the heart by accidental cardiac puncture (right) by the fact that the effusion will not clot and will usually have a lower PCV than peripheral blood.*

Elevations of the activities of serum alanine aminotransferase (SALT) and serum alkaline phosphatase (SALP) are common in animals with cardiac failure, particularly right-sided congestive cardiac failure. However, there is usually minimal compromise of hepatic function and serum bile acid levels are usually within normal limits.

Changes in electrolyte level can occur as a result of treatment of cardiac failure. In severe cardiac failure high aldosterone levels may result in marginal hypokalaemia and excessive antidiuretic hormone secretion may result in hypochloraemia and hyponatraemia.

Some assessment of thyroid function may be indicated in individuals in which hypo- or hyperthyroidism might be considered to be contributing to the disease state.

Circulating markers of neurohumoral activation: Congestive heart failure is a clinical syndrome in which there are substantial data to indicate that activation of a number of neurendocrine mechanisms contributes to the overall clinical syndrome. There have been a number of studies in the last decade, in both human and veterinary patients with naturally occurring cardiac failure, designed to assess the prognostic importance of measurement of various neurohumoral factors in the circulation. Factors assessed include plasma noradrenaline and adrenaline, renin activity, angiotensin II, aldosterone, atrial natriuretic peptide, metabolites of vasodilator prostaglandins, antidiuretic hormone and endothelins. Although measurement of these factors is not yet routinely available, their use may be validated and become more routine in veterinary patients in the future.

Myocardial disease

Circulating markers of myocardial damage

For many years, circulating biochemical markers of myocardial damage have been used in human medicine to assess the severity of any myocardial damage and to monitor the response to treatment, particularly following myocardial infarction. Traditionally markers such as total creatine kinase, creatine kinase-2 and lactate dehydrogenase have been used, though these are now being replaced by more cardiac-specific markers such as myoglobin, myosin light chains, troponins and isoforms of the various creatine kinase isoenzymes (Bhayana and Henderson, 1995).

The use of these circulating markers in veterinary patients with heart disease has not become routine. This is probably because of the nature of the myocardial diseases seen in veterinary patients, being principally degenerative rather than the result of an acute ischaemic episode.

Specific heart muscle diseases

A number of specific heart muscle diseases have been described that may present as cardiomyopathy.

In these cases the cause of the myocardial disorder is known or the myocardial damage is the result of an identifiable primary systemic or metabolic disorder (e.g. the development of dilated cardiomyopathy in cats with taurine deficiency; Pion *et al.*, 1992). As our understanding of the aetiology of myocardial disease improves, evaluation of these patients for various deficiencies or other primary causes may be indicated.

Endomyocardial biopsy

Diagnosis of a specific myocardial disorder may require endomyocardial biopsy. Myocardial biopsy has been in routine use for several decades in human patients suspected of having myocardial disease, and in transplant patients to assess the degree of rejection postoperatively. Typically, the procedure is performed by the transvenous introduction of a biopsy catheter or 'bioptome' into the right ventricle, usually to obtain samples of the interventricular septum. Techniques for endomyocardial biopsy have been described in the dog and cat, but they are not in routine use (Burk *et al.*, 1983).

INFECTIVE ENDOCARDITIS

Diagnosis

Definitive diagnosis of infective endocarditis is difficult. The occurrence of fever, a murmur (especially a murmur not previously identified in an individual or a murmur with variable characteristics) and evidence of embolic disease in an individual is, however, suggestive of infective endocarditis. The clinical history, findings on physical examination and the results of routine investigations may alert the clinician to the possibility of the disease (Thomas, 1992). Two-dimensional echocardiography is particularly useful for the demonstration of vegetations and the secondary effects of valvular damage, such as chamber dilation as a result of volume overload due to valvular incompetence (Elwood *et al.*, 1993).

Additional investigations

Haematology

There may be evidence of acute inflammation — a leucocytosis as a result of neutrophilia accompanied by a left shift with toxic change evident in the neutrophils — in cases of acute, ulcerative infective endocarditis but such findings are rare. Evidence of chronic inflammatory disease — leucocytosis as a result of a mature neutrophilia often accompanied by a monocytosis — is more common. There is often evidence of a mild nonregenerative anaemia of chronic disease; and occasionally a secondary autoimmune haemolytic anaemia develops. Thrombocytopenia may be evident in cases that develop disseminated intravascular coagulation or secondary immune-mediated thrombocytopenia.

Clinical biochemistry

Chronic inflammation may result in an elevation of total protein due to an elevation of serum globulin, but albumin levels may be low if there is significant renal protein loss. There may be biochemical evidence of dysfunction in organs affected by embolization or multifocal infection, e.g. renal insufficiency, elevated muscle enzyme levels.

Urinalysis

Bacterial infections of the urinary tract may be primary or secondary. Renal infarction is common, and there may be pyuria, haematuria and evidence of casts in the urine sediment. Significant proteinuria may accompany a glomerulonephropathy that may develop in some patients secondary to the endocarditis as a result of deposition of amyloid or immune complexes.

Joint fluid and cerebrospinal fluid analysis

If indicated by the clinical findings, these investigations may demonstrate septic or aseptic inflammation of joints or meninges.

Tests for immune-mediated disease

Tests for antinuclear antibodies and the Coombs' test, for example, are sometimes positive if patients develop secondary immune-mediated disease (see Chapter 6).

Blood culture

Culture of blood samples is indicated in order to detect the presence of bacteraemia and to identify the organism(s) involved, together with their sensitivity to antibacterial agents. The more samples that are taken, the greater the likelihood of identifying the organism involved, and at least three samples should ideally be taken. Recommendations concerning the timing of the sampling vary but sampling every 3 hours for 12 hours is suggested as a reasonable protocol. Skin preparation at the venepuncture site is as for surgery. Samples should be incubated aerobically and anaerobically; growth of the same organism from two or more samples is strongly suggestive of significant bacteraemia.

Any site suspected of being the primary source of a significant bacteraemia, e.g. the urinary tract, should also be submitted to culture.

Necropsy

In some cases, definitive diagnosis is only obtained at postmortem examination (Figure 10.18).

PARASITES OF THE HEART AND RESPIRATORY TRACT

Angiostrongylus vasorum

Angiostrongylus vasorum is an intravascular parasite that is found in the UK. The adult worms live in the pulmonary arteries and the presenting clinical features can be very variable, although evidence of respiratory distress, tachypnoea, haemorrhage or peripheral oedema are fairly common (Martin *et al.*, 1993).

Angiostrongylus is diagnosed by detecting larvae in the faeces.

Lungworm in the dog: *Oslerus osleri*

Oslerus osleri infection is an uncommon cause of a chronic, dry cough.

Radiography shows nodules in the trachea if large; bronchoscopy is usually diagnostic. The larvae are frequently evident in a tracheal wash and may be evident in a faecal sample (Baermann method; this requires an experienced parasitologist and false-negative results are common).

Lungworm in the cat: *Aleurostrongylus abstrusus*

Aleurostrongylus abstrusus is a self-limiting infestation in young cats, and there are usually no clinical signs. Occasionally it may cause coughing in young cats, and rarely secondary infection and bronchopneumonia.

Radiography may show a diffuse interstitial pattern, sometimes with associated nodules. Larvae may be evident in a tracheal wash or in a faecal sample.

Heartworm: *Dirofilaria immitis*

Heartworm disease due to *Dirofilaria immitis* is enzootic in many tropical and subtropical areas of the world, but is only seen in the United Kingdom in dogs (it is only occasionally reported in cats) imported from these regions.

The adult worms live primarily in the pulmonary artery and also the right ventricle and the females produce first-stage larvae (microfilariae). These are ingested by feeding mosquitoes in which they develop into infective third-stage larvae. A mosquito injects the infective larvae into a susceptible host; the larvae then migrate through the body tissues until the fifth-stage larvae of young adults enter the vascular system and travel to the pulmonary artery.

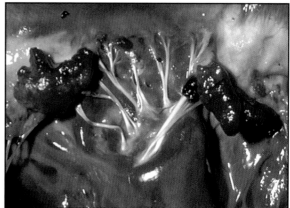

Figure 10.18: Postmortem specimen showing severe vegetative endocarditis lesions affecting the leaflets of an atrioventricular valve.

Infestation can result in a number of clinical syndromes in affected individuals depending on the number of parasites present and the duration of the infestation, including pulmonary hypertension and right-sided heart failure, and caval syndrome which can develop if large numbers of worms are present, resulting in their presence in the caudal vena cava and subsequent hepatic damage. Glomerulonephritis or pneumonitis can develop as a result of the presence of the microfilariae produced by the adult worms.

Diagnosis is based upon the clinical history and the clinical, radiographical and echocardiographical findings. It is confirmed by identifying microfilariae in the circulating peripheral blood, ideally using a method such as the modified Knott technique which concentrates the microfilariae. However, a significant number (approximately 20%) of patients will have an 'occult' infestation, with adult parasites present in the absence of a circulating microfilaraemia. Consequently, serological tests, in particular commercially available ELISA tests which detect circulating heartworm antigen, are now commonly used to confirm the diagnosis in affected individuals. For a detailed discussion of the diagnosis and treatment of heartworm disease the reader is referred to Knight (1995).

REFERENCES AND FURTHER READING

Berg JR and Wingfield W (1984) Pericardial effusion in the dog: a review of 42 cases. *Journal of the American Veterinary Medical Association* **20**, 721-730

Bhayana V and Henderson R (1995) Biochemical markers of myocardial damage. *Clinical Biochemistry* **28**, 1-29

Burk RL, Tilley LP, Henderson M and James VC (1983) Endomyocardial biopsy in the dog. *Veterinary Clinics of North America* **13**(2), 355-363

Clercx C, Wallon J, Gilbert S, Snaps F and Coignoul F (1996) Imprint and brush cytology in the diagnosis of canine intranasal tumours. *Journal of Small Animal Pracitice* **37**, 423-427

Corcoran BM, Foster DJ and Luis Fuentes V (1995) Feline asthma syndrome: a retrospective study of the clinical presentation in 29 cats. *Journal of Small Animal Practice* **36**, 481-488

Corcoran BM, Thoday KL, Henfrey JI, Simpson JW, Burnie AG and Mooney CT (1991) Pulmonary infiltration with eosinophils in 14 dogs. *Journal of Small Animal Practice* **32**, 494-502

DiBartola SP and de Morais HS (1992) Respiratory acid-base disorders. In: *Fluid Therapy in Small Animal Practice, e*d. SP DiBartola, pp. 258-276. WB Saunders, Philadelphia

Edwards NJ (1996) The diagnostic value of pericardial fluid pH determination. *Journal of the American Animal Hospital Association* **32**, 63-67

Elwood CM, Cobb MA and Stepien RL (1993) Clinical and echocardiographic findings in 10 dogs with vegetative bacterial endocarditis. *Journal of Small Animal Practice* **34**, 420-427

Hawkins EC (1992) Tracheal wash and bronchoalveolar lavage in the management of respiratory disease. In: *Current Veterinary Therapy, XI*, ed. RW Kirk and JD Bonagura, pp.795-800. WB Saunders, Philadelphia

Hendricks JC (1995) Pulse oximetry. In: *Current Veterinary Therapy, XII*, ed. JD Bonagura and RW Kirk, pp.117-119. WB Saunders, Philadelphia

Jones CL (1979) Pericardial effusion in the dog. *Compendium of Continuing Education for the Practising Veterinarian* **1**(9), 680-685

Knight DH (1995) Guidelines for the diagnosis and management of heartworm *(Dirofilaria immitis)* infection. In: *Current Veterinary Therapy XII*, ed. JD Bonagura and RW Kirk, pp.879-887. WB Saunders, Philadelphia

Lombard CW (1983) Pericardial disease. *Veterinary Clinics of North America* **13**, 337-353

Martin MWS, Ashton G, Simpson VR and Neal C (1993) Angiostrongylosis in Cornwall: clinical presentations of eight cases. *Journal of Small Animal Practice* **34**, 20-25

Miller MW and Fossum TW (1992) Pericardial disease. In: *Current Veterinary Therapy, XI*, ed. RW Kirk and JD Bonagura, pp.725-731. WB Saunders, Philadelphia

Pion PD, Kittleson MD, Thomas WP, Delellis LA and Rogers QR (1992) Response of cats with dilated cardiomyopathy to taurine supplementation. *Journal of the American Veterinary Medical Association* **201**, 275-284

Ramsey IK, Foster A, McKay J and Herrtage ME (1997) *Pneumocystis carinii* pneumonia in two Cavalier King Charles Spaniels. *Veterinary Record* **140**, 372-373

Relford RL, Thomas JS, Thompson JA and Whitney MS (1996) Effusions and neoplasia. In: *Proceedings of the 14th Forum of the American College of Veterinary Internal Medicine, San Antonio, Texas, USA, May 1996*. pp.14-16

Sisson D, Thomas WP, Ruehl WW and Zinkl JG (1984) Diagnostic value of pericardial fluid analysis in the dog. *Journal of the American Veterinary Medical Association* **184**(1), 51-55

Teske E (1995) Cytological evaluation of bronchoalveolar lavage and fine needle aspiration biopsies of the lung. In: *Proceedings of the 5th Annual Congress of the European Society of Veterinary Internal Medicine, Cambridge, England, September 1995*. pp.44-45

Thomas WP (1992) Update: infective endocarditis. In: *Current Veterinary Therapy, XI*, ed. RW Kirk and JD Bonagura, pp.752-755. WB Saunders, Philadelphia

Locomotor System

Roderick W. Else

INTRODUCTION

The locomotor system comprises an interrelated group of body organs – bones, joints, skeletal muscles, and the nervous system (central and peripheral). Diagnosis of disease conditions therefore requires a consideration of the relative involvement of one or more of these systems. This can be a clinically technically difficult, time-consuming and financially expensive undertaking and may only be realistic in a well equipped referral centre or specialist unit.

Conditions involving these tissues are truly unusual in the overall pattern of disease prevalence. The increasingly sophisticated nature of canine and feline clinical work, coupled with greater owner awareness and demand, however, has resulted in an increased need for more accurate diagnosis. For example, whilst joint disease has always been recognized as a common feature of the wider spectrum of canine disease, the advent of new techniques and more accurate assays has meant that the rather vague general diagnosis of 'arthritis' can now be further delineated and more accurate prognoses made using newer and less invasive, yet accurate, techniques such as arthroscopy and serological analysis.

In human beings the diagnosis of skeletal muscle disease is a well practised and sophisticated exercise, involving ancillary clinical diagnostic aids, such as electromyography, in combination with muscle biopsy examination and histochemistry. In contrast, muscle disease in all the domestic species, with a few notable exceptions such as nutritional myopathy ('white muscle disease'), is poorly recognized, not understood and rarely fully investigated. A major stumbling block has been the fact that many diseases of the locomotor system of the veterinary species have similar clinical symptoms, and special expertise with extended clinical examination is required to differentiate the neurological or primarily myogenic nature of some diseases. This is not made any easier in acquired conditions, i.e. in adult animals, which are usually presented as individual cases in the dog and cat. There is, however, a growing demand to investigate myogenic diseases in particular. Refinements in technique, and new assays and investigatory methods are becoming more readily available to veterinary surgeons and it is to be expected that identification of locomotor diseases will progress beyond simple delineation of origin as neurogenic, myogenic, arthrogenic or a combination of these, to more precise diagnosis and prognosis. In addition, such improvements should assist in elucidating the aetiology of some conditions beyond the broad categories of congenital or acquired disease.

In this chapter the main emphasis is on the techniques currently available for assisting the identification and diagnosis of skeletal muscle, with reference also to bone and joint disease. Because nerve abnormalities are responsible for, or sometimes part of, a locomotor syndrome there is brief comment on peripheral nerve sampling. This topic is also discussed in Chapter 13.

INVESTIGATION OF SKELETAL MUSCLE DISORDERS

The principal sign of muscular or neuromuscular disorders is muscular weakness. This may be manifested as functional weakness (gait abnormalities, paresis, paralysis, exercise intolerance, dysphagia or regurgitation phenomena) and/or as physical deficits (muscle deformity or atrophy/hypoplasia, apparent skeletal deformity), or compensatory hypertrophy.

It is important to differentiate between primary muscle disease (myopathy) and secondary myogenic disease resulting from a neuromuscular disorder (Table 11.1). The latter usually involves the motor nerve unit and may be a primary neural deficit (i.e. neuropathy involving the spinal cord, brain or peripheral nerves) or a disorder of neuromuscular transmission.

The clinical presentation (Figure 11.1) may be that of muscle disease but thorough examination, with coordination of clinical and special examinations (neurological 'work-up', radiography and electrodiagnostic tests such as electromyography and motor/sensory nerve conduction velocity), together with selected laboratory assays should reveal the true level of involvement of the nervous and muscular systems. As mentioned above, sophisticated examinations can usually only be effected in a specialist referral centre.

Disease of the skeletal musculature in the dog and cat can be recognized clinically as being of either congenital (Table 11.2) or acquired type. In many instances, even where a familial or sibling distribution of congenital abnormalities is identified, it is not possible to deduce the exact aetiology of the condition or to predict its occurrence. An exception to this is Duchenne-type muscular dystrophy which has been reported in dogs (Kornegay *et al.*, 1988) and cats (Carpenter *et al.*, 1989; Gaschen *et al.*, 1992). In infant male human beings the disease is an X-linked recessive disorder characterized by a deficiency of the

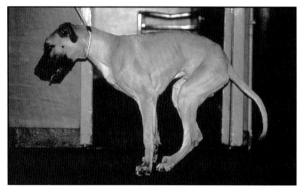

Figure 11.1: *A Great Dane with abnormal stance and muscle atrophy associated with myopathy.*

Courtesy of A.C. Stead.

Type of disorder	Examples
Neurogenic muscle disorders (secondary myopathies)	Motor neuron disease Spinal cord disorders (dysraphism, syringomyelia, tumours) Peripheral neuropathies (giant axonal neuropathy, diabetic neuropathy)
Disorders of neuromuscular transmission	Myasthenia gravis

Primary myopathies	Destructive:
	    Traumatic
	    Vascular disease
	    Toxin or drug-induced
	    Polymyositis/connective tissue disease
	    Dystrophy (Duchenne-type)
	Inflammatory (myositis):
	    Bacterial
	    Parasitic
	    Viral
	    Idiopathic (polymyositis)
	Congenital:
	    Fibre-type deficiency
	    Mitochondrial abnormality
	Metabolic:
	    Storage disease (glycogenosis, lipid storage)
	    Mitochondrial disease
	Selective Type II fibre atrophy:
	    Polymyositis (idiopathic)
	    Endocrinopathy (hypothyroidism, hypoadrenocorticism)
	Tumours of muscle:
	    Rhabdomyosarcoma
	    Myoblastoma

Table 11.1: *Classification of neuromuscular disorders.*

Disorder	Features
Hereditary canine myopathy	Labrador Retrievers over 6 months Abnormal head and neck and posture; stiff, hopping gait; muscle hypoplasia, myotonia Progressive loss of myofibres
Progressive canine muscular dystrophy	Golden Retrievers, Irish Terriers Stiff gait; dysphagia; poor exercise tolerance; progressive muscle atrophy; cardiomyopathy Dystrophin deficiency
Feline dystrophy	Male DSH cats 'Bunny hopping'; myotonia with hypertrophy; muscle necrosis/fibrosis Systrophin deficiency
Myotonia	West Highland White and Fox Terriers, Chows, German Shepherd Dogs, Bull Terriers 'Bunny hopping' gait with muscle spasm
Muscular hyper-tonicity ('Scottie cramp')	Scottish Terriers Non-painful spasm of back, neck, forelimb muscles; precipitated by fright CNS or somatostatin defect?
Familial canine dermatomyositis	Collies, Shetland Sheepdogs Muscle atrophy and skin lesions Immune-mediated?
Glycogenosis	No specific breed Glycogen storage disease Phosphofructokinase deficiency
Myasthenia gravis (dog; ?cat)	Jack Russell Terriers Muscle weakness; exercise intolerance; megaoesophagus Acetylcholine receptor deficiency or autoimmunity to receptors

Table 11.2: Congenital muscle disorders.

cytoskeletal protein dystrophin. A similar mutation has been identified for the dog (Sharp *et al.*, 1992) but not the cat. Identification of genetic mutations is costly and time-consuming and so remains the province of research workers rather than diagnostic assay.

Diagnostic methods for evaluating muscle disease

Clinical and general laboratory assays

The most important clinical assessment is that of neurological examination, specifically noting the presence of neurological deficits and abnormal reflexes. Neurological clinical examination (see Chap-

ter 13) is well within the capabilities of the average practising veterinary surgeon and is an important step in establishing whether the muscle disorder is a primary myopathy or a secondary neuromuscular disease. This preliminary classification should be done before further specialized clinical diagnostic tests or laboratory-based assays are contemplated, and certainly before referral to a specialist centre.

General haematological and clinical chemistry screening should be carried out to identify possible infections, or immune or metabolic abnormalities.

Muscle-specific serum enzyme assays

An important step in distinguishing neuropathies from myopathies is the measurement of the activities of muscle-specific enzymes. In a healthy state the concentrations of these enzymes in serum and plasma are low because they are located within muscle fibres. Damage to muscle, or increased output of the enzymes to the peripheral circulation in muscle disease results in elevation of serum/plasma levels, roughly in proportion to the amount of muscle tissue involved.

The enzymes mainly evaluated are: creatine kinase (CK) and its isoenzymes (three), lactate dehydrogenase (LDH) and its isoenzymes (five), and aspartate aminotransferase (AST; formerly known as glutamine oxaloacetic transaminase, GOT). Both LDH and AST are found in a wide variety of tissues, and therefore are less specific for muscle than is CK. This is particularly true of AST, which is found in abundance in the liver and in red blood cells. (See also Chapter 4.)

Creatine kinase: CK makes ATP available for muscle contraction through the phosphorylation of ADP from creatine phosphate. The isoenzymes are made up of different combinations of subunits of CK of muscle type (M) or brain type (B): CK = BB; CK_2 = MB; CK_3 = MM. A fourth variant, CK-Mt, is found in mitochondrial membranes and seems to be important in cardiac CK activity. The importance of the different isoenzymes lies in the fact that they can be used to assist in determining which tissue or organ is involved in raised CK situations. Although raised levels of CK are seen in some purely nervous diseases (e.g. polioencephalomalacia) as well as in central nervous system diseases that involve motor function, elevations of CK are generally higher in myopathies than in neuropathies. This is because myonecrosis is more prevalent in primary myopathies (Figure 11.2) and CK is specific for muscle necrosis. Elevated CK activity in serum indicates that there is active or recent myonecrosis. Persistently elevated levels of serum CK indicate that the myonecrosis is continuing or still active. In chronic muscle damage, or where myonecrosis is no longer active, however, the circulating CK level may fall to normal or be only slightly elevated. This is because the rate of myofibre damage is comparatively slow.

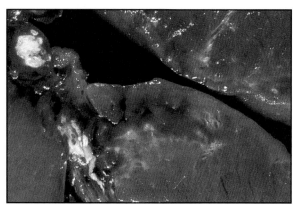

Figure 11.2: *Muscle necrosis in a dog, associated with trauma.*

In addition to pathological muscle or brain damage, CK levels may vary from normality with regard to age and sex (Table 11.3), degree of physical activity (raised in exercise), and whether the patient has had injections likely to cause local myonecrosis. Markedly raised CK levels are associated with crush injuries such as from road traffic accidents.

CK isoenzymes can be identified using electrophoresis, chromatography or immunological techniques.

Lactate dehydrogenase: LDH measurements are not organ-specific. Combinations of muscle (M) and heart (H) parent molecules result in five isoenzymes, usually identified by serum electrophoresis (Cardinet, 1997). LDH (M4) is predominantly found in skeletal muscle whilst LDH1 (M4) is a cardiac isoenzyme; this distribution reflects their relatively more anaerobic (M type) or aerobic (H type) metabolisms. There is marked species variation in absolute LDH levels and in isoenzyme pattern. In general, however, total LDH activity and muscle-specific LDH activity are higher in fast-twitch (type 2, see below) muscle fibres than in slow-twitch (type 1, see below) fibres (see Table 11.5).

Because of the wide tissue distribution of LDH (especially in liver and red cells where there are several isoenzymes) it is inadvisable to interpret total serum LDH levels in isolation. Isoenzyme analysis is helpful but only in association with CK and AST levels. In addition, the reference range for the laboratory carrying out the assay should be taken into account in reaching an interpretation of possible skeletal muscle damage.

Aspartate aminotransferase: Serum AST levels are useful as a diagnostic aid in muscular disease but only in parallel with simultaneous evaluation of CK and LDH. There are high concentrations of AST in liver, red cells and other organs, so it is not organ-specific for skeletal and cardiac muscle. Whilst CK levels rise rapidly with myonecrosis, LDH and AST levels rise less quickly. Thereafter, LDH elevation persists for a few days post-damage whilst AST levels usually remain raised for up to a week after a single damage episode. Where repeated waves of damage occur, the levels of both AST and LDH tend to remain elevated. Again it is important always to note the reference range of the laboratory carrying out assays.

In general, therefore, levels of the muscle-specific enzymes are useful aids to diagnosing muscle damage but the CK, LDH and AST levels should not be interpreted in isolation from each other.

Muscle-specific serum proteins and antibodies
Although enzyme markers of muscle damage have proved very useful, detection of muscle-specific proteins and serum antibodies associated with muscle disease or malfunction has always been an attractive proposition for more accurate and specific assessment of myoabnormality. The advent of sensitive assays with greatly enhanced specificity, such as enzyme-linked immunosorbent assay (ELISA), radioimmuno-

Enzyme	Age	Dog (IU/l)	Cat (IU/l)	Reference
Creatine kinase	Adult	48±18	69±31	Tasker (1978)*
	Adult	0–60	–	Greene et al. (1979)*
	Adult	–	48–177	Nilkumhang & Thornton (1979)*
	Adult	9.9±28.8	–	Heffron et al. (1976)†
	4–6 months	0.4–5.6	–	Cardinet (1969)
		0.0–7.5	–	Cardinet (1969)
	6–12 months	0.4–5.6	–	Cardinet (1969)
	4–6 months	0.0–7.5	–	Cardinet (1969)
	>12 months	0.2–2.6	0.4–3.4	Cardinet (1969)
		0.0–1.8	0.0–4.5	Cardinet (1969)
Lactate dehydrogenase	Adult	29±18	61±30	Tasker (1978)*
	Adult	0–100	–	Kornegay et al. (1980)*
	Adult	–	92–684	Nilkumhang & Thornton (1979)*

Table 11.3: *Normal levels of muscle-specific enzymes.*
* Quoted by Doxey (1983); † quoted by Cardinet (1997)

assay (RIA) and immunocytochemistry, is beginning to have beneficial effects on diagnosing neuromuscular disorders.

Myoglobin: Myoglobin is a heme-derived protein that transports and stores oxygen in muscle fibres. Myonecrosis and other more chronic muscle breakdown often result in raised levels of myoglobin in plasma and in renal clearance. The latter may become excessive, with resultant myoglobinuria and renal tubular destruction (myoglobin is accumulated in distal convoluted tubule cells). The level of plasma myoglobin as an indicator of exercise-associated myonecrosis has been validated in horses but there is no account of its significance in dogs and cats to date.

Anti-acetylcholine receptor antibodies: The detection of circulating autoantibodies to acetylcholine receptors in dogs with immune-mediated myasthenia gravis has been reported (Shelton *et al.,* 1988). The initial studies utilized an immunoprecipitation assay or RIA. Improvements in reagents and techniques have led to development of cheaper and more convenient immunohistological assays for circulating acetylcholine receptors (Cain *et al.,* 1986). This type of assay demonstrates localization of IgG at the neuromuscular junctions of affected dogs.

Myosin and troponin proteins: There is now considerable use of sensitive and specific ELISA and immunoelectrophoresis assays for myosin light chain proteins in the diagnosis of human myositis and myocardial infarctions. Similar assays are in vogue for troponin I in the diagnosis of human acute 'silent' myocardial infarction. There is every reason to expect that such protein assays will become available for aiding diagnosis of small animal muscle disease.

Assays for infectious agents and parasites

Bacterial and fungal infections: Bacterially induced myositis is not a common problem in dogs and cats in the northern hemisphere, although immunocompromised animals are at risk. Traumatic deep wounding, particu-

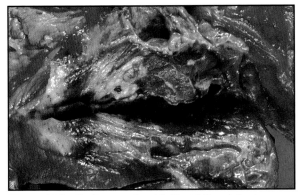

Figure 11.3: *Canine muscle with* Clostridium *infection following a puncture wound.*

larly puncturing, may lead to the introduction of unusual pathogens. Puncture wounds may, rarely, lead to gangrenous myositis in rural dogs as a result of *Clostridium* spp. infection (Figure 11.3). Staphylococcal infection may result in deep pyomyositis but in the author's experience this is a rare event.

Where lesions are suspected as being of bacterial origin, standard methodologies of swabbing or tissue sampling followed by culture (see Chapters 1 and 5) and antibiotic sensitivity assay are appropriate. If *Clostridium* infection is suspected, immunofluorescence tests (IFTs) using specific antisera may be appropriate.

Deep fungal infestations, usually in the wake of severe myonecrosis or persistent muscle damage, with degenerate tissue providing a suitable environment for fungal growth, are rare in dogs and cats in the UK. Similarly, infections by yeasts and related organisms are rare in the UK. Where such agents are suspected, isolation and identification by culture on suitable media such as Sabouraud's (see Chapters 1 and 5) should be attempted. Antibody assays (ELISA or IFT) may also be used.

Viral infections: Viral infections do not usually cause significant myopathies in the dog and cat, with the exception of distemper and parvovirus in the dog, and feline leukaemia virus (FeLV) and feline immunodeficiency virus (FIV)-related disease in the cat.

The most appropriate identification assays are ELISA and IFT, using paired serum samples (infection and post-infection) if possible for antibody detection. Viral isolation is costly and time-consuming and may not be cost-effective. The major problem with viral identification is knowing which virus to screen for.

Parasites: The most significant parasitic disease in dogs is polymyositis caused by *Toxoplasma gondii.* Muscle lesions are rarely associated with toxoplasmosis in cats, which are the definitive hosts. The lesions are necrotizing foci in muscles; chronic disease may lead to tissue cysts in the liver and brain. The infection can be detected using IFT or ELISA in both dogs and cats.

Neospora caninum infection may lead to peripheral or central neuropathy with secondary muscle effects. Again, IFT or ELISA of serum are useful in making a positive diagnosis.

Muscle biopsy
Although much circumstantial information can be derived from enzyme assays coupled with the clinical and electrophysiological evidence of muscle disease, a definitive evaluation of a myopathy can only be made by examination of a skeletal muscle biopsy sample. Not only does such a biopsy confirm the clinical and electrophysiological findings, it allows examination of myofibres, intramuscular nerves and, given the correct sample and technique, neuromuscular junctions, as well as associated connective tissue and blood vessels.

An important additional feature of an appropriately prepared muscle biopsy specimen is that histochemical assessment may provide information on the morphological and biochemical properties of myofibres in addition to the routine formalin-fixed samples. In addition, recent advances in immunocytochemical techniques and reagents (mainly antibodies to muscle proteins) has extended the possibilities of recognizing new lesions and defining changes in muscle more accurately.

Criteria for muscle biopsy

There are a number of criteria to be considered when choosing a muscle biopsy site:

- The chosen muscle must be affected by the disease being investigated. In acute disease, choose a severely affected muscle. In chronic disease, choose a moderately affected or normal-looking muscle (avoid scarred muscles)
- Accessibility
- Avoid adjacent vital structures (nerves, blood vessels, tendons, joints)
- Choose a muscle for which the normal distribution of histochemical fibre types and fibre size is known
- Use a standard technique
- Consider using a site that allows peripheral nerve biopsy also.

Biopsy samples should be taken from both forelimbs and hindlimbs. Samples of flexor and extensor muscles should be obtained. Suitable biopsy sites are listed in Table 11.4.

Technique

Muscle biopsy technique is described in standard surgical texts (e.g. Bojrab *et al.,* 1990) and specialist articles (Braund, 1991, 1994). Most canine and feline muscle biopsies are carried out as open sampling under general anaesthesia. In aged or high-risk patients, sedation and local anaesthesia may be employed. In open biopsy sampling a longitudinally oriented cylindrical segment of muscle approximately 1.5 cm long and 1 cm in diameter is excised with sharp scissors. Multiple samples may be obtained. Muscle clamping, using special apparatus such as a Price clamp, is not advocated unless samples are being obtained for electron microscopy (see below).

In human patients single or multiple samples are commonly obtained using wide-bore cutting needles such as 'Tru-cut' (see Chapter 1) or modified Bergström needles. Such needles, with the exception of the 'Tru-cut', are not commonly used in veterinary work and in the current state of experience open biopsy sampling remains the method of choice.

Sample processing

On removal from the main muscle mass the biopsy should ideally be placed on a piece of physiological saline-moistened gauze sponge to prevent dehydration. If the sampling is done at a referral centre or within easy reach of the laboratory then subsequent handling options are relatively easy.

Samples for transmission electron microscopy (TEM):
Although this is an expensive and specialist requirement it may be contemplated in special cases. If TEM is to be undertaken it is important that the biopsy sample is not allowed to contract. Some authorities believe that this is best achieved by the use of a special clamp apparatus (e.g. Price clamp) at the time of excision. The reasoning behind this is to have a compromise between the rapid fixation required for preservation for electron microscopy, and the contraction effect in residually excitable muscle when placed immediately into aldehyde fixatives. A good compromise seems to be that advocated by other authorities (Loughlin, 1993) where the muscle is allowed to 'bench rest' and adhere to a piece of card or wooden spatula for 4–5 minutes post-excision prior to small segments being subjected to immersion in 4% glutaraldehyde fixative. The fixative is diluted to 4% in 0.1M cacodylate buffer at pH7.2. Samples are fixed for 2

Location	Muscle	Function	Comments
Forelimb	Triceps brachii: distal third of long or medial heads	Extensor	
	Superficial digital flexor: proximal third	Flexor	Can sample ulnar nerve here
Hindlimb	Biceps femoris: distal third	Extensor	Can sample peroneal nerve here
	Vastus lateralis: distal third	Extensor	
	Gastrocnemius: lateral head, proximal third	Flexor (stifle)	
	Cranial tibial: proximal third	Flexor (hock)	

Table 11.4: Muscle sampling sites.

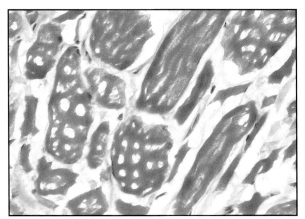

Figure 11.4: Freezing artefact in a cryostat section of canine muscle. H&E.

hours at 4°C and then transferred to cacodylate buffer prior to being post-fixed with osmium tetroxide and finally embedded in resin for ultrathin sectioning. These procedures are not normally carried out in veterinary practice situations although the sampling and fixation stages up to the transfer into cacodylate buffer can be undertaken if the referring veterinary surgeon has the correct reagents and the inclination to carry out the task. Samples in cacodylate can then be posted to a laboratory. Glutaraldehyde should be handled with care; it is extremely irritant to oral and ocular mucosae and should only be handled under a fume hood. These are specialist techniques and are probably best carried out in referral centres.

Samples for histochemistry: Histochemical analysis is probably the most important type of examination performed on muscle biopsy specimens. Most diagnoses of myopathy are made after histochemical examination. Success depends on producing a correctly frozen sample. If the freezing can be done in-house and the sample transferred easily to the laboratory then good tissue sections should be possible and accurate diagnosis guaranteed, given expertise in examining the sample. Where samples have to be transported to a receiving laboratory the procedure becomes more fraught. It is best if the biopsy specimen, or part of it, is frozen by the sampling surgeon and transferred, still frozen, to the laboratory. It is important that the sample does not thaw out in transit or undergo a freeze–thaw–freeze cycle which causes artefactual change. At worst, the sample of muscle can be sent to the laboratory in an air-tight bottle surrounded by frozen ice-packs in an insulated container, using a rapid delivery system.

The biopsy sample should be handled gently and the ends of the specimen, which may have been gripped during excision, should be trimmed with a clean sharp razor blade. This procedure allows enough 'bench rest' time for the sample, and samples should be frozen within 1 hour of removal in-house to prevent loss of enzymes. The sample to be frozen should be trimmed to approximately 1 cm length and 0.5 cm diameter. It is then placed on a cork disk (1.5 cm across) and adhered to the disc with optimum cutting temperature medium (OCT) or 10% gum tragacanth. It is usual to position halves of the specimen, or duplicate specimens, so that muscle bundles are cut both longitudinally and transversely.

The cork and specimen are then snap-frozen by immersion in isopentane (2-methylbutane) penetrant cooled in liquid nitrogen. A freeze bath of dry ice in methanol can be used as an alternative to liquid nitrogen, which is expensive and dangerous to handle. The tissue should be immersed in isopentane for 10 seconds; shorter periods of immersion result in artefacts in muscle bundles and too lengthy an immersion causes fissuring of the block. If the specimen is cooled too slowly or is subjected to thawing–refreezing cycles, ice crystals form in the myofibres and these appear as holes in the muscle bundle sections (Figure 11.4).

Samples are stored at –40 to –70°C prior to being cut as histological sections (5–8 μm thick) at –20°C on a cryostat and then stained for histochemical examination (see below). Frozen sections can also be stained with 'routine' stains such as H&E (Figure 11.5), Mallory trichrome and Van Giesson.

Samples for routine histology: Parallel muscle samples or part of the same biopsy taken for histochemistry may be fixed in 10% buffered formalin after 'bench rest' or adherence to card or a wooden spatula. The

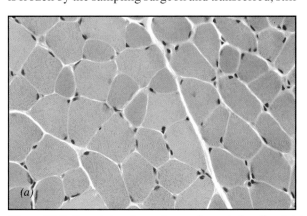

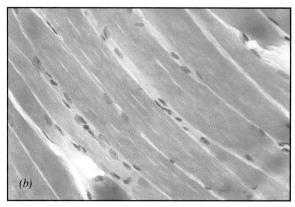

Figure 11.5: Cryostat sections of normal muscle bundles: (a) transverse; (b) longitudinal. H&E.

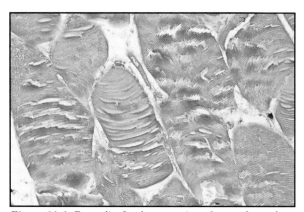

Figure 11.6: Formalin-fixed wax section of normal muscle, with artefactual changes masquerading as pathological change. H&E.

sample can then be processed to paraffin wax for routine histological sections (4-6 μm thick) stained with H&E or other selected tissue stains. An alternative option is to embed the tissue in plastic or in epoxy or hydroscopic resin.

It is often stated that formalin-fixed muscle is of limited diagnostic value but it is the most suitable tissue for the identification of inflammatory reactions (cells and infectious agents). In addition, many veterinary pathologists feel more 'morphologically comfortable' with a routine section in addition to the histochemical preparations. It is important, however, that sections for routine histology are of good quality,

as artefacts can lead to difficulty in interpretation (Figure 11.6).

Histochemical analysis
The objectives of histochemical examination of a biopsy specimen are:

- Recognition of distribution of muscle fibre types compared with normal muscles
- Recognition of fibre-type deficiencies or deletion diseases
- Recognition of abnormal myofibres which appear normal with routine stains (H&E)
- Diagnosis of specific enzyme deficiencies or abnormalities.

Muscle fibre typing is based on the reactivity of muscle adenosine triphosphatase (ATPase) with ATPase substrate under acidic and alkaline pre-incubation conditions (Figure 11.7). The different pH conditions are used to inactivate the different ATPase systems that exist in skeletal muscle.

There are three different types of fibre identified in mature canine muscle, dependent on the pre-incubation pH value (Table 11.5). The fibre types are essentially similar to the human muscle classification, with the exception that a human Type II B analogue does not occur in the dog, although Type II B has been reported in cats (Braund, 1991).

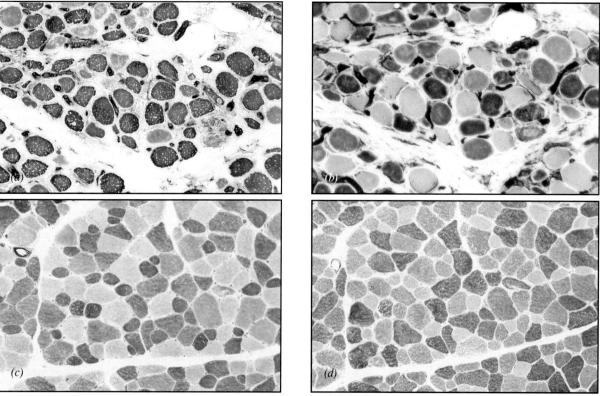

Figure 11.7: ATPase staining of normal canine muscle. (a) Triceps stained at pH 9.4, showing light-staining type I fibres. (b) Triceps after preincubation at pH 4.3, showing dark-staining type I fibres. (a) and (b) are serial sections. (c) Biceps femoris after preincubation at pH 4.3. Type I fibres are dark; type II fibres are light. (d) Biceps femoris after preincubation at pH 4.6. Type I fibres are dark; type IIA are light; type IIC are intermediate in colour. (c) and (d) are serial sections.

Feature	Fibre types		
	Type I	**Type IIA**	**Type IIC**
Staining properties:			
ATPase pH9.4	Light	Dark	Dark
ATPase preincubation*at pH4.5	Dark	Light	Dark
ATPase preincubation* at pH4.3	Dark	Light	Light/Intermediate
NADH–TR	Dark/Intermediate	Light	Intermediate/Dark
Physiological properties:			
Colour	Intermediate	Pale/White	Red
Twitch contraction	Slow	Fast	Fast
Fatiguability	Resistant	Fatiguable	Resistant

*Table 11.5: Physiological and histochemical profile of muscle fibre types. (*Incubation times are critical.)*

In muscle samples from normal dogs there are recognizable distributions of different fibre types. Broadly, muscles of positive or constant vital activity, such as the diaphragm, have a high content of Type I fibres, while the muscle groups associated with 'quick burst' activity have a predominance of Type II fibres. In myopathies, these distributions change, staining affinity is lost, or fibre groupings become more apparent.

ATPase staining in dogs is most useful for identifying: muscular dystrophies (specific loss of Type II fibres); hypothyroid-associated myopathy (atrophy of Type II fibres); idiopathic myopathies (atrophy of Type I fibres); or denervation–reinnervation (normal mosaic of staining replaced by groupings of Type I or II fibres).

Other histochemical stains are also useful (see Figure 11.8), particularly nicotinamide adenine dinucleotide–tetrazolium reductase (NADH–TR), which exhibits a reciprocal pattern to alkaline ATPase activity. This oxidative enzyme is useful as an index of mitochondrial presence and function. Periodic acid–

Schiff (PAS) staining demonstrates the presence of glycogen and in dogs is useful for demonstrating Type II fibres.

There is less information on muscle histochemistry in the cat; according to Braund (1991), feline muscle has similar fibre types to the dog but with the additional presence of Type II B fibres, similar to human muscle. Most diagnostic assessment of muscle biopsies should therefore utilize a standard battery of histochemical and routine stains on both frozen and formalin-fixed muscle, as shown in Figure 11.9.

The histomorphological appearance of muscle tissue is the basis of biopsy diagnosis; it requires expert appraisal and a description of the features is outwith the remit of this text.

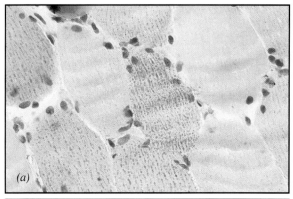

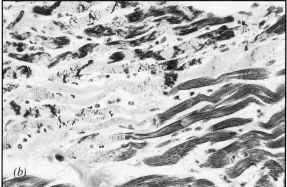

Figure 11.9: (a) Cryostat section of muscle with fatty change, seen as orange globules. Oil red O. (b) Routine muscle section, showing degenerate muscle stained pale brown with phosphotungstic acid–haematoxylin (PTAH).

Routine 'battery'
Haematoxylin and eosin (H&E)
Periodic acid–Schiff (PAS)
Oil red O (ORO)
Modified Gomori trichrome
*ATPase at pH 9.4
*ATPase at pH 4.5 and 4.2
*NADH–TR

Additional
Phosphotungstic acid haematoxylin (PTAH)
Heidenhain's haematoxylin
Martius scarlet blue (MSB)
Sudan black
*Succinate dehydrogenase (SDH)
*Phosphorylase
*Acid/alkaline phosphatases

*Figure 11.8: Stains used in muscle diagnosis. *These histochemical stains require frozen sections; other stains can be done on frozen or formalin-fixed tissue.*

A number of myopathies are idiopathic; they present a histopathological appearance of random muscle fibre degeneration (Figure 11.10) or bizarre bundle configurations, with or without atrophy (Figure 11.11). True myositis (acute or chronic) can usually be diagnosed from the presence of muscle bundle abnormality associated with inflammatory cells (Figure 11.12).

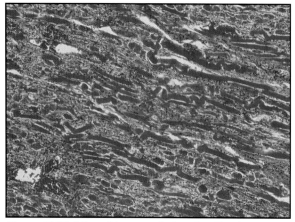

Figure 11.10: Idiopathic myopathy in a dog. Random degeneration of muscle fibre bundles shows as bright red staining. H&E.

MISCELLANEOUS MUSCLE CONDITIONS

Myasthenia gravis

Myasthenia gravis is recognized mainly in dogs but has also been reported in cats (Indrieri *et al.*, 1983). Two forms exist: the congenital form, and acquired autoimmune disease.

In the congenital condition there is reduced acetyl-choline receptor (AChR) density in the postsynaptic sarcolemmal membrane of the affected muscles. There are no specific assays for the condition; diagnosis is made on the basis of clinical features and positive responses (increased strength) to anti-acetyl cholin-esterase drugs (edrophonium).

The acquired disease is immune-mediated, involving the generation of autoantibodies against AChRs. Dogs may be affected at an early age (3–5 years) or when old (10+ years). They exhibit variable muscular weakness or ataxia, with or without dysphagia or megaoesophagus. The condition can be diagnosed by a combination of clinical and pharmacological investigations. In addition, however, definitive diagnosis can be made using immunocytochemical examination, either by demonstrating IgG bound to the sarcolemmal

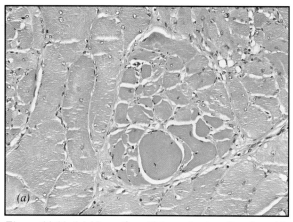
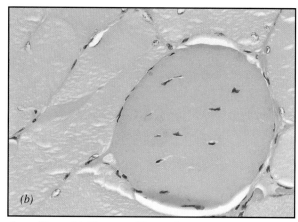

Figure 11.11: (a) Myopathy with irregular bundles alongside normal myofibres. (b) Giant myofibre with multiple centralized nuclei reflecting the abnormal nature of the bundle. Routine sections; H&E.

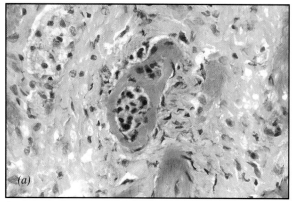
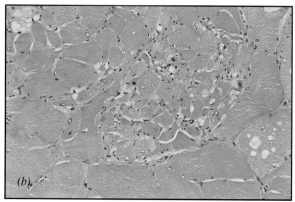

Figure 11.12: Myositis. (a) Cryostat section from a dog, showing disintegration of the muscle bundle and inflammatory cells. H&E. (b) Chronic myositis with irregular muscle bundles and a sparse infiltration of polymorphonuclear neutrophils. Routine section; H&E.

membrane using an immunoperoxidase method, or by the detection of circulating antibodies to the post-synaptic sarcolemmal membrane (Cardinet, 1997).

Myotonia

Myotonia is characterized by uncontrolled prolonged but painless contraction of skeletal muscles. In man myotonia is recognized as a congenital, non-progressive condition or, in adults, as a progressive dystrophy of unknown aetiology. In human infants myotonia is associated with diminished conductance of chloride ions across the sarcolemmal membrane. A congenital myotonia in dogs has been recognized (see Table 11.2) but whether this condition is related to chloride ion conductance has not been determined.

Canine masticatory myositis

This canine condition, also known as eosinophilic or atrophic masticatory myositis, affects only the masseter and temporal muscles. Type II fibres, which comprise the bulk of the masticatory muscles, are preferentially affected. The changes in the muscle are thought to be the result of autoantibodies directed against the Type II myofibres. Diagnosis can be made by examination of biopsy samples which show acute inflammation, often with eosinophils present, or more chronic changes (Figure 11.13); IgG may be demonstrated on the biopsied myofibres or circulating antibodies to Type II fibres detected using immunoperoxidase techniques.

Disorders of glycogen metabolism

Disorders of glycogen metabolism usually result in generalized excess storage of glycogen, with deposition of glycogen-containing vacuoles in muscle fibres. Such disorders are congenital in dogs and there are a

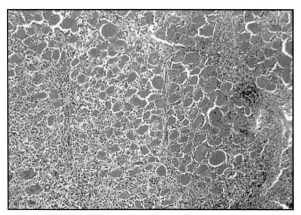

Figure 11.13: Chronic myositis in a German Shepherd Dog with masseter and temporal muscle atrophy. Routine section; H&E.

few reports of cats affected by similar enzyme deficiencies. The most frequent enzyme deficiencies are those of α-glucosidase and phosphofructokinase (PFK). Deficiency of PFK has been recorded in Springer Spaniels as an autosomal recessive trait characterized by intermittent severe haemolytic episodes rather than myopathy. There is reduced PFK activity in red blood cells, with reduced glycolysis in muscles on biochemical analysis. Muscle biopsies reveal PAS-positive vacuoles containing polysaccharide.

Endocrine myopathies

Muscle weakness is often part of an endocrinopathy syndrome in dogs.

Hyperadrenocorticism

Dogs with chronic natural or iatrogenic Cushingoid syndromes often develop muscle weakness and atrophy. The atrophy is predominantly of Type II

Nature of change	Agent involved
Necrosis/degeneration	Ionophores (monensin); oxytetracycline, corticosteroids; antimalarials (chloroquine); snake venoms; bacterial toxins (*Clostridium*); mycotoxins (aflatoxin)
Immune modulation	D-Penicillamine; procainamide
Altered neurogenic function	Neuromuscular blockage: aminoglycoside antibiotics Denervation: sulphonamides; nitrofurantoin; metronidazole; amphotericin B; antineoplastics (vincristine); chlorambucil; anti-rheumatics; phenytoin; ergotamine
Altered cell membrane and cytoskeletal structure	Bacterial toxins (*Clostridium*); ionophores; doxorubicin; vincristine; colchicine
Neuromuscular blockage (without morphological change)	Aminoglycoside antibiotics (neomycin, streptomycin, gentamycin, kanamycin); polypeptide antibiotics (polymyxin B); other antibiotics (oxytetracycline, lincomycin, clindamycin); cardiovascular drugs (quinidine, procainamide, propanolol); phenytoin; ketamine
Myotonia (without morphological change)	Propanolol; suxamethonium

Table 11.6: Agents causing toxic myopathy (Adapted from Van Vleet, 1997).

fibres but Type I fibres are also affected on histochemical examination. The changes are thought to be the result of decreased protein synthesis and increased protein catabolism following raised corticoid levels.

Hypothyroidism
Canine hypothyroidism is associated with Type II myofibre atrophy or deletion and Type I predominance. There is some indication that these changes may be mediated neurally since denervation abolishes the Type II atrophy generated by thyroidectomy in experimental studies.

Toxic myopathies
Many agents are potentially capable of causing myopathy through a number of different mechanisms, as shown in Table 11.6.

INVESTIGATION OF BONE DISEASES

Because bone is hard tissue it has frequently been regarded as a relatively static and unreactive organ system. This is untrue; normal bone matrix continually undergoes metabolic and microanatomical turnover and remodelling. It may also react dramatically in pathological states.

The range of bone diseases
The wide range of bone diseases is described in most pathology and clinical textbooks and the reader is referred to these standard accounts for detail. The major categories of inherited/congenital and acquired diseases occurring in the dog and cat are summarized in Table 11.7.

Many of the dysplasias and inherited conditions are detected in juveniles as a result of skeletal deformity, stunted growth, or syndromes of organ malfunction arising from deformities.

Nutritional or metabolic diseases tend to be manifested in young but still growing animals. In affluent societies these tend to be uncommon, with isolated cases arising either from misguided feeding regimens or maliciousness. Similarly, the idiopathic disorders or diseases of uncertain aetiology tend to occur in individual dogs and cats. Some (e.g. hypertrophic pulmonary osteoarthropathy) have been recognized for many years but remain unexplained aetiologically.

Increasingly sophisticated clinical care and preventive medicine, together with higher levels of owner education, have resulted in increased presentation of geriatric conditions. This implies that a greater number of skeletal neoplasms might be expected. In fact, bone neoplasia still affects relatively young dogs and cats as well as geriatrics; the reasons for this remain unknown.

Diagnostic methods

Clinically related investigations
In addition to clinical examination, techniques such as radiography and linear or computed tomography (CT) are of major assistance in diagnosis. Whilst tomography techniques are best accomplished in referral centres, most practising small animal veterinarians have access to good quality radiographic facilities. A good series of radiographs can go a long way towards making an accurate diagnosis.

More advanced techniques such as scintigraphy and magnetic resonance imaging (MRI) are usually prohibitively expensive or require special precautions for radioisotope handling and tend to be found only in a few specialist units.

Biochemical assays
Theoretically, the assay of serum calcium inorganic phosphate, alkaline phosphatase (ALP) activity and magnesium levels should be of assistance in diagnosing and monitoring bone disease. Although demineralization may be occurring, serum mineral levels usually remain within the reference range until the condition is advanced. ALP levels are raised with increased osteoblast activity but often rise non-specifically (e.g. in liver disease, see Chapter 9).

Biochemical assays are therefore advised only as secondary confirmation, in concert with clinical and radiological assessments, or where radiological changes are not diagnostic.

Routine haematological screening is helpful in inflammatory or necrotic disease; non-specific leucocytosis and neutrophilia are detected.

Bone biopsy
Bone biopsy is useful in the diagnosis of proliferative or lytic bone lesions and mandatory for the diagnosis and staging of neoplasia. If radiographical and clinical examination indicate the presence of an overt suspect neoplasm or a lesion that could be either neoplastic or lytic/necrotic (i.e. rarefaction and proliferative response in the same bone), then biopsy of the lesion provides a sample for definitive diagnosis (Figure 11.14).

Technique
A bone trephine (e.g. Michelle) or wide bore specialist needle such as a Jamshidi-type needle (see Chapter 1) should be used. Bone marrow biopsy needles have been advocated for this type of sampling but the author's experience is that they yield inferior small or fragmented samples.

It is important to remember that the Jamshidi-type needle is less robust (8–11 guage) than the Michelle trephine (3–5mm diameter) and is not suitable for sampling very dense bony lesions nor normal cortical bone.

Disease type	Examples	Features
Developmental dysplasias (inherited connective tissue disorders): juveniles affected, causing dwarfism	Chondrodysplasia Osteogenesis imperfecta Pituitary dwarfism	Hypo-/dys-chrondroplasia Multiple cartilaginous exostosis Fibrous dysplasia Bone fragility due to thin cortices Cystic or aplastic pituitary (German Shepherd Dogs)
Metabolic diseases (differences in juvenile and adult)	Rickets Osteomalacia Osteogenesis imperfecta (juvenile osteoporosis) Osteoporosis Osteodystrophia fibrosa Hypertrophic osteodystrophy (skeletal scurvy; Barlow's disease) Hypervitaminosis A	Abnormal endochondral ossification due to calcium/vitamin D (±phosphorus) deficiency or imbalance; juvenile Bone rarefaction due to calcium/vitamin D imbalance; adult Bone fragility due to calcium/phosphorus imbalance; juvenile Excessive bone resorption due to disuse, senility, malnutrition, endocrinopathy; adult Bone resorption with fibrous replacement (primary/secondary hyperparathyroidism); adult Failure of osteoid production due to vitamin C deficiency/imbalance; juvenile Cervical vertebral and joint fusion/exostosis due to excess dietary liver; adult cats
Inflammatory/necrotic states	Osteitis (+periostitis/osteomyelitis) Spondylitis/discospondylitis Spondylosis deformans Legg–Perthes disease	Infections or traumatic; juvenile and adult Vertebral disc infection; juvenile and adult Chronic/ageing change; adult Aseptic necrosis of femoral head; juvenile (small breeds)
Idiopathic/uncertain aetiology	Craniomandibular osteopathy ('Lion jaw') Hypertrophic pulmonary osteoarthropathy (Marie's disease) Canine hypertrophic osteodystrophy Osteochondrosis (+ osteochondrosis dessicans) Panosteitis 'Wobbler' syndrome	Multiple exostoses of the head; juvenile (Scottish, West Highland White and Cairn Terriers) Periosteal osteophytic proliferation of limb bones; adults (+chronic lung lesion) Metaphyseal inflammation/ossification; juvenile and young adults (large breeds) Disordered endochondral ossification; juvenile and young adults (large breeds) Osteomyelitis and endosteal ossification forelimbs; juvenile (large breeds) Cervical vertebral stenotic myelopathy; juvenile and young adults (Great Dane, Dobermann)
Neoplasia: usually adults but some young adults affected	Primary tumours Secondary tumours Tumour-like lesions	Benign (uncommon); malignant (osteosarcoma, fibrosarcoma, chondrosarcoma, myeloma) Malignant (carcinomas, haemangiosarcoma) Bone cysts (rare)

Table 11.7: Skeletal diseases in dogs and cats.

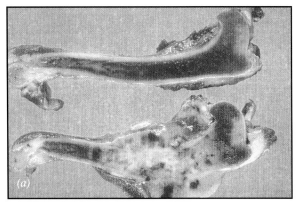
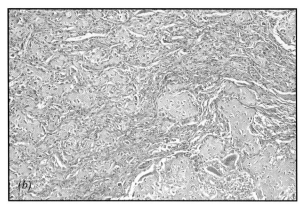

Figure 11.14: *(a) Osteosarcoma in the humerus of a dog. (b) Histopathological section of the tumour. H&E.*

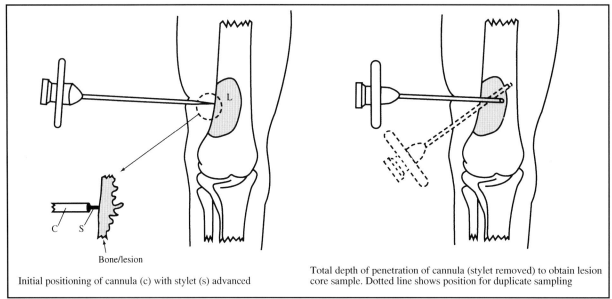

Initial positioning of cannula (c) with stylet (s) advanced

Total depth of penetration of cannula (stylet removed) to obtain lesion core sample. Dotted line shows position for duplicate sampling

Figure 11.15: *The technique of bone biopsy with a Jamshidi needle.*

Before attempting biopsy of the lesion, good quality lateral and dorsoventral radiographs of the bone and lesion should be obtained. It is important to use the radiographs to obtain representative samples. Ideally, at least one sample from the viable centre of the lesion (avoiding central lytic or necrotic regions in fast-growing tumours), and another at the junction of lesion and normal bone should be examined. The latter site may present problems. Sampling from too peripheral a site from a neoplasm or infective lesion may yield a 'false negative' of reactive bone or periosteal proliferation. Radiographs are important in delineating sites for sampling.

The technique of using the Jasmshidi needle is described in standard surgery textbooks (e.g. Bojrab *et al.,* 1990). Briefly, the needle, with sharp-point stylet advanced through the tip of the cannula, is pushed through soft tissue structures via a stab incision (2–3 mm). Once the desired site for sampling is reached, the stylet is withdrawn and the needle cannula advanced into the lesion or bone cortex until the medullary cavity is reached. The needle is then withdrawn and the bone or lesion core collected in the cannula is expelled using the special blunt probe supplied (Figure 11.15).

Trephines are used in essentially the same way. The trephine, with its stylet in place, is introduced through a stab incision in the skin. Once the needle is against the bone shaft or lesion site, the stylet is withdrawn and the trephine driven into the bone using a firm rotary action. The depth of penetration can be gauged with the help of a scale marked on the trephine barrel. The plug of bone is excised from the cortical shaft by a gentle rocking action of the trephine. The trephine is then withdrawn and the stab incision closed. Haemorrhage is not usually a problem.

Sample processing
After collection the bone core should be gently removed from the needle or trephine cannula using the stylet. The core should not be allowed to dehydrate and is generally best expressed from the cannula directly into 10% buffered formalin to fix. Calcified or osseous samples must be decalcified in commercially available decalcification fluids before sectioning for histology. These agents are usually based on formic acid. Softer tissue samples may be obtained with the use of chelating agents such as EDTA. The types of core sample obtained by the apparatus described above will be

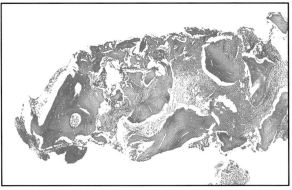

Figure 11.16: Typical bone core obtained with a Jamshidi needle. Decalcified section; H&E.

decalcified within 72–96 hours and are thereafter processed to paraffin wax sections (Figure 11.16) for routine or special staining. Frozen undecalcified bone biopsies for histochemistry or immunohistological assay require special cutting procedures; similarly, undecalcified bone cores (which do yield better histomorphometry) can only be cut as resin-embedded tissue using heavy duty microtome equipment.

Biochemical and hormone markers of bone metabolism and neoplasia

Bone turnover
Interest has focussed on examination of bone turnover (remodelling by new formation and osteoclastic resorption), by measurement of circulating biochemical and hormonal markers.

Bone resorption can be assessed by measuring the serum or urinary concentrations of osteoclast-derived enzymes or collagen breakdown products. Bone formation can be indirectly assessed by evaluating serum levels of osteoblast-associated proteins, enzymes or precursor peptides associated with collagen synthesis.

Because of natural circadian rhythms of bone turn-

over and wide normal variation, lack of bone specificity and higher levels in immature animals compared with adults, serial samples over a period of time need to be taken and each sample should be collected at the same time of day. Some of the markers are indicated in Table 11.8, together with the techniques used for their assay.

Although pituitary dwarfism is not a common condition, it has familial occurrence in German Shepherd puppies. The assessment of growth hormone levels using RIA is relevant for diagnosis.

Humoral hypercalcaemia of malignancy
Three mechanisms of increased serum calcium induced by neoplasms have been recognized: humoral hypercalcaemia of malignancy (HHM); haematological malignancies (multiple myeloma and lymphoid neoplasia); and hypercalcaemia induced by bone metastases. The last of these is uncommonly encountered in dogs and cats.

The characteristic features of HHM include hypercalcaemia, hypophosphataemia, hypercalciuria, increased excretion of phosphorus, and increased osteoclastic bone resorption. The latter feature is associated with increased release of calcium from bone. The tumours associated with HHM therefore induce a syndrome that mimics primary hyperparathyroidism. It is now known that these tumours secrete a factor with parathormone (PTH)-like activity but which is antigenically unrelated to PTH; this factor is parathyroid hormone-related protein (PTHrP). In bone PTHrP stimulates osteoclastic bone resorption. In addition, cytokines such as interleukin-1 (IL-1), tumour necrosis factor-α (TNF-α) and transforming growth factors (TGFs) are thought to have a synergistic role with PTHrP. This synergism is seen in anal sac gland adenocarcinoma in the bitch, where high levels of PTHrP have been identified, together with IL-1 and TGFs in serum.

Similar enhanced osteoclastic activity is seen in some canine lymphosarcomas where there is hypercalcaemia

Marker	Method of assay

Bone resorption markers:
    Serum:
        Tartrate-resistant acid phosphatase
    Urine markers:
        Collagen cross-link proteins
        (pyridinoline; deoxypyridinoline)
        Hydroxyproline
        Hydroxylysine glycosides
        (collagen breakdown product)
	Immunoassay
	
	Immunoassay
	
	Colorimetric
	Chromatography

Bone formation markers:
    Alkaline phosphatase
    (total or bone-specific isoenzyme)
    Osteocalcin
    (non-collagenous bone protein)
    Procollagen I carboxy terminal peptide
    (synthesized by osteoblasts)
	Immunoassay
	
	Radioimmunoassay
	
	Radioimmunoassay

Table 11.8: Biochemical markers of bone metabolism.

(20–40% of cases). The increased osteoclastic resorption seen is thought to be caused by PTHrP stimulation. Bone resorption may be generalized in these cases. In dogs with haematological malignancy affecting the bone marrow only (lymphosarcoma or myeloma), bone resorption may remain localized. Cytokines (such as IL-1, TNF-α, TGFs) and PTHrP have been implicated but there is some evidence that prostaglandin E_2 is important in this localized phenomenon.

INVESTIGATION OF JOINT DISEASES

The range of joint diseases

The reader is referred to the BSAVA *Manual of Small Animal Arthrology* (Houlton, 1994) for a full treatise on the clinical and surgical assessment, treatment and prognosis of arthrodial diseases. In addition, Table 11.9 gives an indication of the broad categories of joint abnormality that may require further specialized investigation and therapy.

Diagnostic methods

Clinically related investigations

Clinical investigation of joint disease involves detailed physical examination, with the use of diagnostic imaging techniques such as plain and contrast radiography, linear tomography or CT, and ultrasonography. Tomography is most likely to be in use in referral centres, though ultrasound scanning instrumentation is now more widely available. The more sophisticated

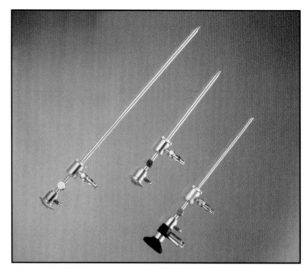

Figure 11.17: *Apparatus used for arthroscopy.*
Courtesy of G. Munroe.

and expensive techniques of MRI and scintigraphy are prohibitively expensive and require specialist units.

Arthroscopy: The technique of arthroscopy, which involves endoscopic examination of the synovial cavity (Figure 11.17), has recently achieved a higher profile in the range of diagnostic techniques available. The advent of smaller-bore flexible fibreoptic endoscopes with video recording facilities, in addition to direct visualization, has considerably enhanced the level of diagnosis of joint disease. Whilst this apparatus is currently largely the province of specialists in referral centres, there is no reason, other than financial,

Disease type	Examples
Dysplasias	Hip dysplasia Arthrogryposis syndromes (scoliosis, dysraphism) Congenital subluxations (toy breeds)
Inflammatory diseases	Infectious: 　　Acute suppurative or fibrinous; trauma-associated 　　Chronic non-suppurative (? possibly immune-mediated) Non-infectious: 　　Canine rheumatoid arthritis (erosive) 　　Polyarthritis 　　Non-erosive, immune-mediated 　　Progressive feline (FeLV-related)
Degenerative diseases	Osteoarthritis/osteoarthrosis: 　　Idiopathic, primary 　　Secondary Spondylosis deformans Degenerative intervertebral disc disease
Neoplasia	Primary: 　　Benign (chondroma, osteochondroma) 　　Malignant (chondrosarcoma, fibrosarcoma, haemangiosarcoma, synovial sarcoma) Secondary: 　　Metastases from carcinomas/sarcomas

Table 11.9: Joint diseases occurring in dogs and cats.

why many practising veterinary surgeons cannot undertake this technique.

The advantages of arthroscopy are: direct visualization of intra-articular structure in a minimally invasive manner; collection of synovial fluids and tissue biopsies without major arthrotomy; repeated investigations to monitor progress of disease or efficacy of therapy can be made. It is also possible to perform surgical procedures using this technique.

The procedure for arthroscopy does usually require general anaesthesia and thorough aseptic precautions.

Laboratory assays

The sampling and assessment of synovial fluid and synovial or other joint tissues are most useful. Routine haematological and biochemical screening assays are of assistance in the general assessment of a patient, particularly where systemic involvement is a clinical feature. In polyarthritides and syndromes involving joints with other organ systems, immunological assays are often appropriate; the indications and application of such tests are described in Chapter 6.

Synovial biopsy

Samples of synovial membrane can be obtained by wide-bore needle biopsy (e.g. 'Tru-cut'), arthrotomy or arthroscopy. The techniques of arthrotomy and arthroscopy are described in specialist texts devoted to joint disease. Arthroscopy is rapidly finding favour over arthrotomy for the reasons stated above, but yields relatively small samples. Where samples are obtained by opening the joint they are usually of sufficient size to be air-dried or pinned on to a piece of card or wooden spatula prior to fixation in 10% formalin for histopathological examination. Placing a biopsy wider than 2 mm directly into formalin fixative without support leads to distortion and this compromises interpretation (see Chapter 1). Duplicate samples (if the joint is large enough) or a portion of the biopsy may be used unfixed for microbiological culture or snap-frozen for immunohistological examination.

Biopsy findings are important in differentiating infectious inflammatory changes (acute, chronic) from degenerative, immune-mediated and neoplastic diseases (Figure 11.18). The morphology of a biopsy specimen should not, however, be viewed in isolation from other assays, such as serum analysis or clinical features, since degenerative and immune-mediated arthropathies may show similar histopathological changes.

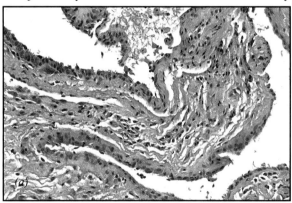

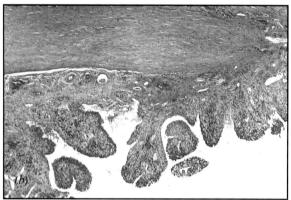

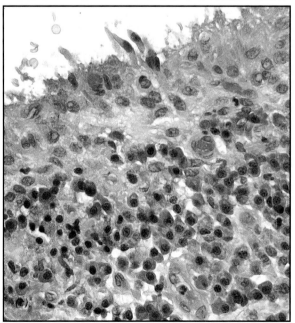

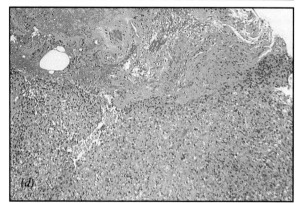

Figure 11.18: (a) *Chronic low-grade synovitis with mild synovial hyperplasia and sparse mononuclear inflammatory reaction.* (b) *Marked synovial villous hypertrophy associated with chronic synovitis.* (c) *Subacute inflammation with plasmacytes and neutrophils below the hyperplastic synovial lining.* (d) *Section of a biopsy specimen from a dog with synovial sarcoma in the stifle, showing a small layer of congested synovium above the sarcoma. H&E.*

Synovial fluid

One of the most useful examinations following the specialist clinical tests is that of sampling and analysis of synovial fluid. The technique can be applied where only one joint is apparently affected but is particularly useful for examination of polyarthropathies associated with joint effusions.

Collection

Collection of synovial fluid is by arthrocentesis using fine hypodermic needles (20–25 gauge, 10–35 mm long, depending on the joint involved). The surgical aspects of arthrocentesis are well described by Houlton (1994).

The sample should be correctly handled as soon as possible after removal. Normal synovial fluid does not coagulate but abnormal synovial fluid usually contains some fibrinogen, fibrin or other clotting factors. If a small amount of fluid is collected smears should be prepared immediately (see Chapters 3 and 7). Larger volumes should be expressed into anticoagulant; the author's preference is for EDTA but if measurement of viscosity or a mucin precipitation test (see below) is contemplated, heparin is preferred. Synovial samples in anticoagulant may gel on standing but can be reconstituted if gently shaken (important not to damage any cells present).

Analysis

A wide range of assessments can be applied to aspirated synovial fluid:

- Physical features: volume (relative increases); appearance (colour, turbidity, viscosity)
- Cell content: numbers and type
- Protein content and comparison with serum levels
- Glucose content and comparison with serum levels
- Mucin clot test: qualitative (firm, weak, none)
- Bacteriological/mycological examination/culture
- Crystal content and type

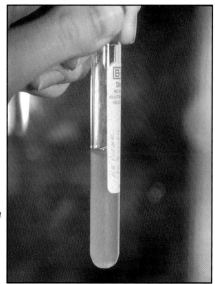

Figure 11.19: *Discoloured synovial fluid from a dog with immune-mediated arthritis.*

Courtesy of Dr A. Anderson.

- Immunological analyses: immunoglobulins; complement; antinuclear antibody; rheumatoid factor.

Volume and appearance: The volume of fluid obtained depends on the size of the joint and the degree of abnormality. Smaller volumes than anticipated are often collected, probably due to the presence of fibrin or exudate. The colour of synovial fluid can range from pale yellow, through orange, to overtly red and haemorrhagic, depending on the cell count, fibrin or other protein content, and the presence of pathological or iatrogenic haemorrhage (Figure 11.19). Similarly, viscosity will be influenced by cell content and protein, especially coagulable protein such as fibrin. The viscosity of synovial fluid is also affected by the amount of synovial mucin derived from polymerized hyaluronate within the joint. This change can be assessed using the mucin clot test which depends on the effect of 2% glacial acetic acid on synovial fluid. Addition of the acid to normal synovial fluid produces a firm clot. The test is usually performed by adding synovial fluid to acetic acid in a vial. In inflammatory states the clot quality or strength decreases, ranging from poor or weak to non-formed.

Cellular content and type: Normal synovial fluid should be virtually acellular, with a median nucleated cell count of <1000 cells/µl (upper limit 3000/µl in large breed dogs). Cell counts may be performed using automated counters or a manual haemocytometer (white blood cell diluting pipette with saline as diluent). Most

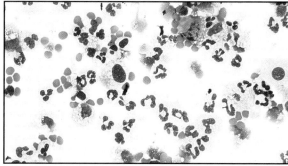

Figure 11.20: *Synovial fluid from a case of acute synovitis, showing red blood cells, PMNs and a few synovial lining cells. Leishman.*

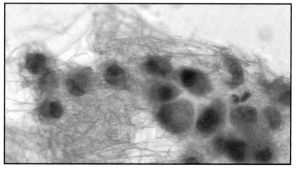

Figure 11.21: *Bizarre and degenerate tumour cells enmeshed in fibrin (same case as Figure 11.18d). H&E.*

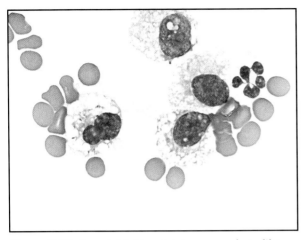

Figure 11.22: Synovial fluid containing macrophage-like cells of synovial origin. A PMN and several red blood cells are also present. Leishman.

pathologists will count cells from a Romanowsky-stained haematological-type smear (see Chapter 3) or a cytocentrifuge preparation.

The type of cells present is important. Normal synovial fluid should contain only sparse numbers of lymphocytes, neutrophils and mononuclear cells; the latter are probably derived from synovial lining, particularly if arthrocentesis has not been performed gently. In acute inflammation there is usually a dramatic increase in polymorphonuclear neutrophils (PMNs) (Figure 11.20); if there is an active bacterial infection many of these neutrophils will be degenerate or pyknotic. Large simple-lobed PMNs are indicative of possible toxin-associated inflammation with relative PMN immaturity. Bizarre cells may indicate neoplasia or degeneration (Figure 11.21) but care should be taken not to confuse significant cells of

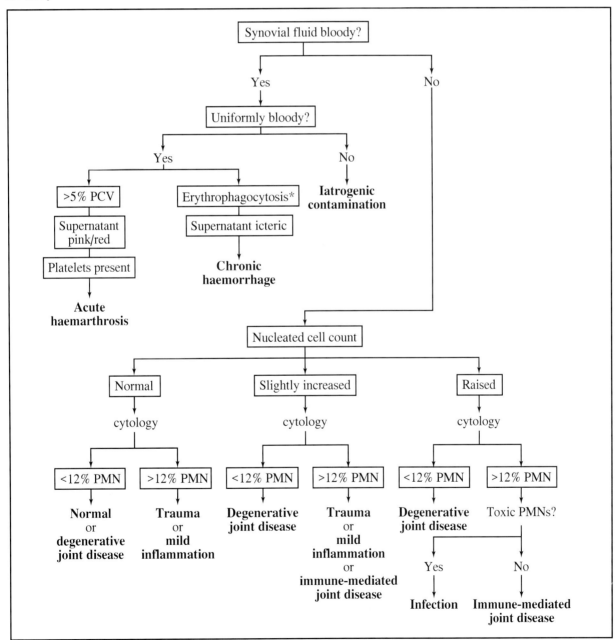

Figure 11.23: Approach to assessing the relative cell content of synovial fluid.

this type with transformed or so-called 'activated' synoviocytes, which may be sloughed from the synovial lining and assume macrophage-like morphology (Figure 11.22). The presence of bacteria in PMNs or macrophagic cells can be checked. A scheme for assessing the relative cell content of synovial samples, as suggested by Houlton and Collinson (1994) is shown in Figure 11.23.

Protein and glucose levels: Protein levels (total, globulin or albumin) should normally be minimal (<2.5 g/l). The presence of plasma-derived proteins is associated with inflammation and is usually paralleled by changes in serum levels. The content in synovial fluid can be measured biochemically or using a refractometer. Fibrin (see Figure 11.21) is the most commonly encountered protein precipitate in actively inflamed joints.

Fasting glucose levels in synovial fluid and serum are said to be helpful in indicating glycolytic activity induced by bacterial respiration in infected joints. The test, however, is not specific and active neutrophils in the absence of bacteria may induce rises in intra-articular glycolysis.

Other assays: Bacteriological examination (using Gram staining on smears and other stains where appropriate) is useful, followed by aerobic and anaerobic differentiation. Screening for viruses and mycoplasms is possible but is not often undertaken, on the grounds of cost and 'targetting' for viral specificity.

Immunological assays can be carried out on synovial fluid but are more easily assessed on serum samples (see Chapter 6).

Synovial fluid profiles in specific conditions

A suggested broad approach, relating characteristic changes in synovial fluid to disease conditions, is shown in Figure 11.24.

Infective arthritis:

- Increased synovial volume
- Usually yellow or orange
- Turbid
- Poor/non-formed mucin clot
- Raised protein (>25 g/l)
- Raised glucose (50–75% of serum level); may be misleading
- Raised cell count (100,000 per mm^3), mainly PMNs (Figure 11.25b), may be degenerate if infection is acute
- Common bacteria: *Streptococcus (?), Staphylococcus, Proteus*
- Occasionally, Lyme disease (*Borrelia burgdorferi*) or leishmaniasis in dogs (use ELISA?).

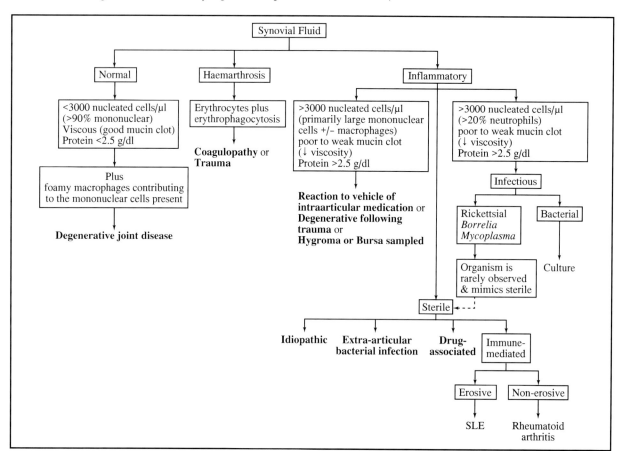

Figure 11.24: *Approach to the analysis of synovial fluid characteristics in disease states.*

Non-infective osteoarthritis: Osteoarthrosis or degenerative disease may be primary/idiopathic or secondary to non-infectious joint damage. Synovial fluid characteristics are:

- Increased volume
- Clear or pale yellow
- Reduced viscosity
- Normal mucin clot
- Slightly raised cell content (2000–4000 per mm³), mainly mononuclear cells (?synoviocytes) with up to 5% neutrophils (Figure 11.26)
- Articular cartilage fragments may be present.

Immune-mediated arthropathy: May be erosive (canine rheumatoid arthritis, CRA) or non-erosive (idiopathic or secondary). In CRA, the synovial fluid characteristics are:

- Serous, turbid or bloody
- Increased volume
- Raised cell count (>5000 per mm³), mainly neutrophils (see Figure 11.19)
- Rheumatoid factor-positive
- Anti-nuclear antibody (ANA)-positive (also serum).

In non-erosive idiopathic immune-mediate arthropathy, the synovial fluid characteristics are:

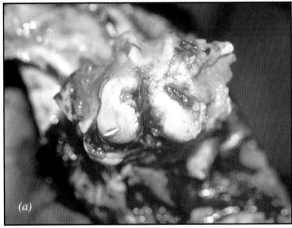

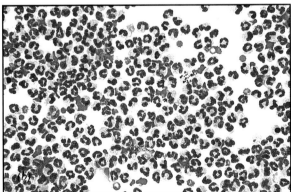

Figure 11.25: *Infective arthritis. (a) The stifle joint. (b) Synovial fluid sample showing acute inflammation with many PMNs. Leishman.*
(a) Courtesy of Dr A. Anderson.

- Serous, turbid or bloody
- Increased volume
- Raised cell count (>5000 per mm³), mainly neutrophils
- Rheumatoid factor-negative
- Anti-nuclear antibody (ANA)-negative
- Raised liver enzymes.

In addition, serum globulin concentrations are raised and there may be anaemia, leucocytosis or leucopenia.

Non-erosive secondary immune-mediated arthropathy may be of several types:

- Reactive, neoplastic and enteropathic-associated types: sterile chronic inflammation of joints with a primary inflammation elsewhere; probably related to immune complex deposition in the synovial membrane
- Systemic lupus erythematosus (SLE): polyarthritis associated with skin, renal, nervous, respiratory and haematological abnormalities; ANA-positive; synovial fluid profile similar to CRA but may have lupus cells present. A variant condition is polyarthritis–polymyositis syndrome of spaniels (Bennett and Kelly, 1987).
- Other conditions include: polyarteritis nodosa; Akita polyarthritis (with meningitis?); familial renal amyloidosis of Shar-Peis; post-vaccine reactive arthropathy; drug-induced arthropathy (e.g. lincomycin, some penicillins, sulphadiazine in Dobermanns and Golden Retrievers). These conditions are all probably mediated through immune complex deposition in the synovium.

PERIPHERAL NERVE BIOPSY

Sampling of peripheral nerve tissue is useful for assessing and diagnosing peripheral neuropathies that may lead to motor problems. The procedure involves sampling bundles (fascicles) of suitable nerves rather than transection and excision of a whole nerve segment (i.e. the majority of the nerve trunk is left intact).

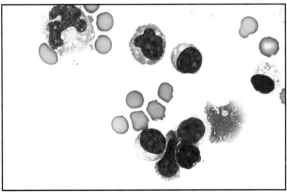

Figure 11.26: *Osteoarthrosis. Synovial fluid sample showing chronic inflammation with mononuclear cells and synovial cells. Leishman.*

There are several important criteria to be noted in undertaking nerve biopsy:

- The nerve selected should be affected by the suspected abnormality – determined by clinical neurological examination and, if possible, myographical assessment
- The nerve selected should have a constant anatomical location and should be readily identifiable
- The nerve selected should be located away from vital structures such as blood vessels, tendons and joints
- There must be no possibility of post-biopsy neurological deficit
- The nerve selected should be in a site protected from trauma
- Normal physiological and morphometric data for the selected nerve should be available.

Clearly, the aim of the biopsy is to obtain maximum morphological information on a nerve without creating any significant neurological deficit. The nerves that can be sampled without causing deficit are listed in Table 11.10. The majority are mixed, but purely sensory or motor nerves may be sampled. The most commonly used nerves are the common peroneal nerve (passing over the lateral head of the gastrocnemius muscle near the stifle joint) in the hindlimb, and the ulnar nerve in the forelimb (where it passes parallel to the medial head of the triceps brachii).

Technique

The aim of the peripheral nerve biopsy is to excise a fascicular sample no greater than 30% of the diameter of the whole nerve, except in the case of the plantar branches of the tibial nerve (see Table 11.10) where it is normal to resect a whole nerve sample. No sensory or motor deficits have been reported for the latter.

The excision sample should be no longer than 4 cm. After excision of the initial end of the selected fascicles the promixal end should be ligated with a fine 5-0 silk suture and the rest of the fascicles separated from the nerve using sharp, fine-pointed ophthalmic or similar surgical scissors.

Sample processing

The excised nerve sample should be pinned on to a wooden spatula or thick card in a slightly extended state. Clamping with special clamps or excision are not recommended. The tissue should be immediately fixed in 10% buffered formalin. If ultrastructural examination only is required, the nerve sample can be fixed in 2.5% glutaraldehyde and processed for transmission electron microscopy (TEM) thin sections as described above for muscle samples. It is usual, however, to fix in formalin and submit to the examining laboratory in this form.

The formalin-fixed nerve biopsy sample can be divided into several pieces for further processing, depending on which examinations are required.

For routine histopathology, the sample is processed through to paraffin wax sections and stained with H&E

Nerve	Type	Major functions	Comments
Common peroneal (hindlimb)	Mixed: Motor Sensory	Hock flexion; digital extension Skin of craniodorsal surface of paw, hock, stifle	Flat nerve Can combine nerve biopsy with muscle biopsy of lateral gastrocnemius and distal biceps femoris
Ulnar (forelimb)	Mixed: Motor Sensory	Carpal flexion; digital flexion Skin of caudal antebrachium	Biopsy can be difficult, as nerve runs near blood vessels and flexor tendons Difficult to separate fascicles Can combine nerve biopsy with muscle biopsy of medial triceps and superficial digital flexor
Tibial ± plantar branches (hindlimb)	Mixed: Motor Sensory	Hock extension; digital flexion Skin of plantar paw and metatarsus	Plantar branches are too small for fascicle resection; sample whole nerve
Caudal cutaneous antebrachial (foreleg)	Sensory only	Two-thirds caudolateral antebrachium	Subcutaneous from caudal part of ulnar nerve Passes over medial olecranon process

Table 11.10: Peripheral nerves recommended for biopsy.

and possibly special stains (Gomori trichrome, luxol-fast blue, silver impregnation). For TEM, small cubes (3-4 mm) of nerve are post-fixed in 1% osmium tetroxide and processed through resin to be cut as semithin (1-2 μm) and ultrathin sections.

The myelin sheath and any axonal changes can be studied by examining nerve fibres that have been teased out of their fascicular arrangement. Samples of the original formalin-fixed nerve are post-fixed in 1% osmium tetroxide then passed through 66% glycerin and finally stored and teased out in 100% glycerin. Individual fibres can be mounted on a microscope slide in glycerin and examined under a dissecting or high-power microscope.

Sample processing for TEM and teased nerve examination is best carried out in referral centres; submissions from veterinary surgeons in practice are best presented as fascicular nerve samples, correctly fixed in formalin. Where biochemical studies are contemplated (e.g. assessment of myelin content or storage disease enzyme assays), samples should be snap-frozen in liquid nitrogen.

REFERENCES AND FURTHER READING

Armstrong RB (1982) Distribution of muscle fiber types in the dog. *American Journal of Anatomy* **163**, 87-98

Bennett D and Kelly DF (1987) **Article title?** *Journal of Small Animal Practice* **28**, 891-908

Bojrab MJ, Birchard SJ and Tomlinson JL (1990) *Current Techniques in Small Animal Surgery, 3ʳᵈ edn.* Lea & Febiger, Philadelphia

Braund KG (1991) Nerve and muscle biopsy techniques. *Progress in Veterinary Neurology* **2**, 35-56

Braund KG (1994) Pediatric myopathies. *Seminars in Veterinary Medicine and Surgery (Small Animal)* **9**, 99-107

Cain GR, Cardinet GH III, Cuddon PA, Gale RP and Champlin R (1986) Myasthenia gravis and polymyositis in a dog following fetal haematopoietic cell transplantation. *Transplantation* **41**, 21-25

Cardinet GH III (1997) Skeletal muscle function. In: *Clinical Biochemistry of Domestic Animals, 5th edn*, ed. JJ Kaneko *et al.*, pp. 407-440. Academic Press, San Diego

Carpenter JL, Hoffman EP, Romanul, FC, Kunkel LM *et al.* (1989) Feline muscular dystrophy with dystrophin deficiency. *American Journal of Pathology* **135**, 909-919

Doxey DL (1983) The locomotor system. II. Muscles. In: *Clinical Pathology and Diagnostic Procedures, 2ⁿᵈ edn,* ed. DL Doxey, pp.229-240. Baillière Tindall, London

Gaschen FP, Hoffman EP, Gorospe JR, Uhl EW *et al.* (1992) Dystrophin deficiency causes lethal muscle hypertrophy in cats. *Journal of Neurological Science* **110**, 149-159

Houlton JEF and Collinson RW (1994) *Manual of Small Animal Arthrology.* BSAVA, Cheltenham

Indrieri RJ, Creighton SR, Lambert EH and Lennon VA (1983) Myasthenia gravis in two cats. *Journal of the American Veterinary Medical Association* **182**, 57-60

Jones TC, Hunt RD and King NW (1996) *Veterinary Pathology, 6ᵗʰ edn.* Williams & Wilkins, Baltimore

Kornegay JN, Tuler SM, Miller DS and Levesque DC (1988) Muscular dystrophy in a litter of golden retriever dogs. *Muscle and Nerve* **11**, 1056-1064

Loughlin M (1993) *Muscle Biopsy: A Laboratory Investigation.* Butterworth-Heinemann, Oxford

Meyer DJ and Harvey JW (1998) *Veterinary Laboratory Medicine: Interpretation and Diagnosis, 2ⁿᵈ edn.* WB Saunders, Philadelphia

Sharp NJ, Kornegay JN, Van Camp SD, Herbstreith MH *et al.* (1992) An error in dystrophin mRNA processing in golden retriever muscular dystrophy, an animal homologue of Duchenne muscular dystrophy. *Genomics* **13**, 115-121

Shelton GD, Cardinet GH III and Lindstrom JM (1988) Canine and human myasthenia gravis autoantibodies recognize similar regions on the acetylcholine receptor. *Neurology* **38**, 1417-1423

Van Vleet JF (1996) Skeletal muscle. In: *Veterinary Pathology, 6th edn,* ed. TC Jones *et al.*, pp. 873-897. Williams and Wilkins, Baltimore

CHAPTER TWELVE

Lymphoreticular System

Christopher J. Clarke

CHAPTER PLAN
Introduction
Lymph nodes
        Sampling
Spleen
        Sampling
Thymus
References and further reading

INTRODUCTION

The lymphoreticular system comprises the lymph nodes, spleen and thymus plus a considerable amount of organized lymphoid tissue scattered throughout the mucosal surfaces of the body systems (e.g. gut, respiratory tract). Collectively the tissues have a major role in host defence and act as filters for the lymph and blood.

LYMPH NODES

Lymph nodes filter lymph delivered by afferent lymphatics and may therefore reflect pathological changes that occur at distant tissue sites. Nodes act as sites for concentrating antigen and immune cells in one place and are involved in antigen recognition and the generation of cell-mediated and humoral immunity.

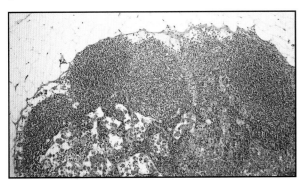

Figure 12.1: Low-power view of a normal canine lymph node showing the capsule and subcapsular sinus, and cortical and medullary areas. Surgical haemorrhage related to sampling has allowed some erythrocytes to drain into the medullary sinuses. H&E.

The node contains several cell types that are distributed in specific areas, including macrophages that act as phagocytes, dendritic cells (antigen-presenting cells) and lymphocytes of T and B lineages (Figure 12.1). The paracortex contains predominantly T cells (Figure 12.2) that are involved in immunoregulatory, proinflammatory and cytotoxic activities whilst cortical follicles contain B cells (Figure 12.3) that can differentiate to antibody-secreting plasma cells that populate the medullary cords (Figure12.4). Nodes may be affected singly or in regional groups indicating a local process, or more generally, reflecting a systemic condition.

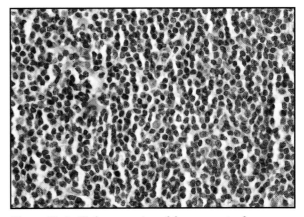

Figure 12. 2: High-power view of the paracortex from a normal canine lymph node. Small, round lymphocytes (mostly T cells) populate the area. H&E.

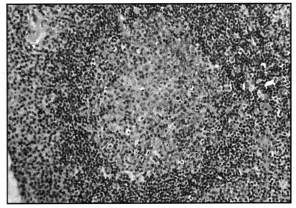

Figure 12. 3: Section of canine lymph node cortex showing a secondary lymphoid follicle with a pale germinal centre, indicating reactivity of the B cell area. H&E.

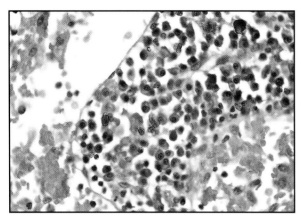

Figure 12.4: High-power view of canine lymph node medulla showing cords containing plasma cells mostly, plus some haemosiderin-laden macrophages. H&E.

Assessment of the size of lymph nodes by observation and palpation is an important clinical indicator of disease but is of limited diagnostic value without further clinicopathological information.

Lymph node enlargement is a common clinical sign and there are three basic causes:

- Reactive hyperplasia that reflects the response of the node to antigenic stimulation, with an increase in cellularity with or without oedema

- Inflammation directly involving the node (lymphadenitis) usually involving infection by bacteria, parasites or fungi

- Neoplasia arising from cells resident in or circulating through the node, or from metastatic lymphatic spread from malignant tumours.

Atrophy and involution of lymph nodes is less commonly detected than enlargement but may occur with senility, cachexia or radiation damage and following infections with lymphotrophic viruses such as the parvoviruses. Examination of good cytological or histological preparations can give a strong indication of the type of pathological process affecting the node.

Sampling

Lymph nodes may be sampled by fine needle aspiration (FNA), wide-bore needle biopsy, and excision or incisional biopsy, followed by smear, impression smear or routine section examination, respectively.

Fine needle aspiration

Fine needle aspiration of superficial lymph nodes is an increasingly popular, rapid and convenient technique of providing cells for cytological examination. Sedation and local anaesthesia are usually recommended.

Cytological examination of smears should identify cell types and their frequencies in the sample but it will rarely give any useful information on tissue architecture as this will have been disrupted in the preparation. Full interpretation of smear cytology usually requires

a veterinary pathologist but some broad indication of diagnosis may be possible with experience. A representative sample from a normal node contains about 85–95% small lymphocytes, each about 7–10 µm in diameter, with a typical round, densely basophilic nucleus and a very thin rim of pale cytoplasm (Figures 12. 5 and 12.6). Medium and large lymphocytes (up to 25 µm in diameter) represent lymphoblasts with larger, paler nuclei, possibly with recognizable nucleoli and more cytoplasm. In a normal node lymphoblasts constitute only a small percentage of total cells. Plasma cells (0–5% of the node) are 'egg-shaped' with small, eccentric, 'clock-face' nuclei with condensed chromatin aggregates and basophilic cytoplasm.

Macrophages are large cells with abundant pale, sometimes vacuolated and granular, cytoplasm and large, oval to indented, open nuclei. Occasional stromal cells (connective tissue and vascular), polymorphonuclear neutrophils, eosinophils and mast cells are seen in preparations from normal nodes. Erythrocytes, platelets and other blood-derived cells may also be present, originating from vessels within the node or from sampling haemorrhage.

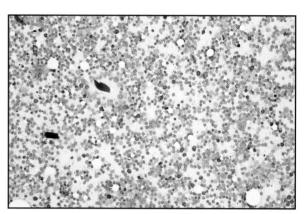

Figure 12.5: FNA smear from a slightly reactive canine lymph node, showing predominantly small, round lymphocytes and some larger, paler lymphoblasts.
Two 'squames' of epithelial origin have been introduced into the sample by the transcutaneous sampling procedure. Leishman.

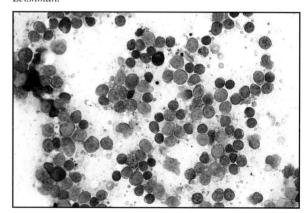

Figure 12.6: Higher-power view of an FNA smear from a moderately reactive canine lymph node showing small lymphocytes and larger lymphocytes, as well as a few macrophages. Leishman.

Skin and subcutaneous cells may also be introduced into the sample during the FNA procedure. Sampling and smearing will damage a proportion of cells, generating cytoplasmic and nuclear fragments that may form homogeneous basophilic and eosinophilic blobs or streaks, sometimes known as 'smear cells'. Air-dried smears cause cells to flatten, making nuclei and cells larger than in fixed sections. In smears wet-fixed with alcohol, nuclear shape may be better preserved.

Reactive hyperplasia in a node is indicated by an increased proportion of lymphoblasts (up to 15%), and if the reaction is of long standing plasma cells may be strongly represented. Sinus hyperplasia is indicated by a high proportion of macrophages.

Inflammatory cells may indicate drainage of inflamed tissues or lymphadenitis. The presence of many neutrophils (>5%) suggests a bacterial infection (Figure 12.7). Eosinophils (>3%) suggest drainage of an area affected by a hypersensitivity reaction or the presence of parasites. Granulomatous inflammation is indicated by many macrophages and possibly even multinucleate giant cells and may be associated with chronic persistent inflammation seen in infections

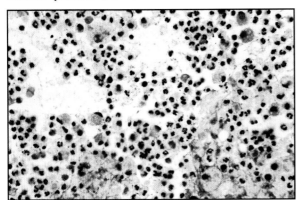

Figure 12.7: *FNA smear from an acutely inflamed (bacterial infection) canine lymph node, showing predominantly neutrophil polymorphs plus some macrophages (purulent lymphadenitis). H&E.*

with agents such as mycobacteria, *Leishmania, Toxoplasma*, and other protozoal and fungal infections. Foreign bodies such as plant awns and other material may also provoke strong pyogranulomatous inflammatory responses. Special stains for bacterial (Gram, Ziehl–Neelsen), fungal (Grocott's, periodic acid–Schiff) and parasitic agents (Leishman's) can be useful when inflammatory lesions are present.

Neoplasia of lymphocytes (lymphoma, malignant lymphoma, lymphosarcoma) may be difficult to diagnose but is usually indicated by an increased proportion of immature lymphocytes, often in excess of 50% of the population. Lymphomas can be classified in various ways including by anatomical distribution, tissue architecture (diffuse or follicular), cellular morphology and immunostaining pattern. Morphological classification is made according to the state of

differentiation of the lymphocyte and varies along a spectrum from well differentiated lymphocytic cells with a low mitotic rate, through cells with an intermediate differentiation state, to poorly differentiated, lymphoblastic cells with a high mitotic rate (based on the World Health Organization system). 'Histiocytic' or large cell lymphomas are recognized as a separate category. As many as 18 distinct types of lymphoma have been described, but some useful, general cytological indicators can be mentioned.

On cytology, lymphosarcoma may show either an unexpected increase in immature lymphocytes or a very monomorphic lymphocyte population. Diagnosis is easy and usually reliable with the former but much more difficult with the latter presentation.

Neoplastic cells are usually larger than the normal, small lymphocyte with a larger nucleus, often with an irregular and sometimes cleaved outline, and prominent and sometimes multiple nucleoli. Chromatin is granular and dispersed and the cytoplasm tends to be basophilic. Mitotic figures, represented by intensely condensed basophilic chromatin structures, may also be seen (Figures 12.8 and 12.9). The immaturity of the cell often confers an excessive fragility leading to an

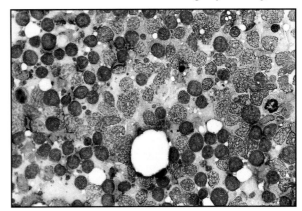

Figure 12.8: *FNA smear from a canine lymph node affected by lymphoma. Neoplastic cells have large, pale, pleomorphic nuclei and indistinct cytoplasm and cell borders compared to the normal lymphocytes with round, basophilic nuclei. A mitotic figure is present at the right edge of the field. Leishman.*

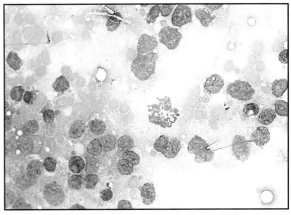

Figure 12.9: *FNA smear from a canine lymph node affected by lymphoma. Virtually all lymphocytes here are neoplastic with pale, irregular nuclei. Leishman.*

increased amount of cell debris in these preparations. Poorly differentiated lymphoid cells are often difficult to categorize definitively and it is impossible to assign cells to the B cell or T cell series on appearance in routinely stained smear preparations. Enzyme histochemical stains such as non-specific esterases have been used occasionally to detect T cells, but this is open to confusion as cells of the mononuclear phagocyte series are also stained. The continued development of monoclonal antibodies to lymphoid cell markers of the dog and cat will clarify this area considerably, as it has done in human pathology.

In human lymphomas morphological features can be correlated with a prognosis and have allowed a useful grading system (National Cancer Institute Working Formulation) to be developed. These features are less well investigated in domestic animals, although some authorities have assigned the equivalent tumours in animals to the same low-, intermediate-, and high-grade groups, with the latter having the most rapid development and poorest prognosis if left untreated. Paradoxically, the tumours with highest mitotic rates are the most amenable to chemotherapy.

Metastatic neoplasia in a node should be suspected if there are cell types not normally present (e.g. epithelial cells) or an increase in numbers of a resident cell type (e.g. mast cells, spindle cells). Searching for metastasized cells in lymph node samples is useful for staging tumours by the 'TNM' system, that defines the potential progress of neoplastic cells from the area of the primary tumour, to local and distant lymph nodes, and via metastatic spread to other organs, respectively.

Wide-bore needle aspiration
Wide-bore needle or core biopsy sampling may be performed using local anaesthesia and sedation. Samples may be taken using cutting needles of different gauges (14–18) but 14/15 gauge needles are usually adequate. The sampled tissue plug may be fixed in formol saline for histological examination or used to prepare smears for cytological staining. Unlike FNA samples, fixed sections of a core biopsy will provide some information on the tissue architecture as well as cell types and proportions. Core sample interpretation, however, will require time for fixation, transport and processing to routine sections for interpretation.

Incision biopsies
Incision biopsies are not usually indicated for lymph nodes because it is almost always easier to excise the whole node. Occasionally nodes may be closely adhered to, or infiltrated by, adjacent tissues making complete excision difficult. Core biopsies and FNA techniques should be considered before incisional biopsies in these circumstances, as healing in such areas is often poor.

Impression smears may be made directly from the cut surfaces of nodes and treated as smear preparations.

Surfaces should be blotted with absorbent paper before touching them gently on to a glass slide.

Excision biopsies
Excision biopsy of nodes using standard surgical procedures and general anaesthesia provides the most complete information on pathology and may be necessary if FNA or core biopsy techniques are inconclusive. Many pathologists are happier with a node excision sample. Freshly removed nodes may be transected and used for touch impressions that are then treated as smears for a rapid result, or may be fixed in 10% buffered formol saline and processed to routine sections for histological examination. The standard rules for tissue fixation of using a 1:10 ratio of tissue to fixative volume, and a maximum tissue diameter of 1 cm should be followed. Excised tissues should be kept in a clean, sterile dish or on moist polyester foam matting to avoid desiccation if there is any delay in their handling. If the node is large then it should be cut cleanly into slices parallel to the long or short axis so the cortical and medullary areas are obvious to the receiving pathologist.

The gross appearance of the cut surface of the node is often a useful indicator of the disease. Reactive nodes are large with discernible white, nodular, outer cortical areas (representing cortical hyperplasia) and an inner tan- to cream-coloured medulla. Acutely inflamed nodes are large, red and wet in the early stages, possibly with purulent lesions. More chronically inflamed tissues may appear as reactive hyperplasia grossly.

Nodes affected by lymphoid neoplasia are classically enlarged with a homogeneous cream-coloured tissue replacing the usual cortical and medullary zones and bulging from the surface. Red and black foci and streaks throughout the tissue may be present, representing areas of haemorrhage and necrosis. In cases of secondary neoplasia lesions in the node may be confined to one portion or may be more generalized.

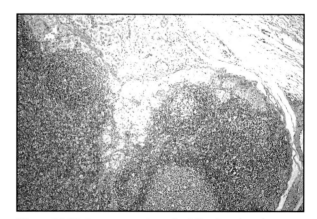

Figure 12.10: *Low-power view of a feline lymph node showing metastasized adenocarcinoma tumour cells occupying the subcapsular sinus and sinus channels leading into the node. Note the relative lack of hyperplastic or inflammatory reaction in the node. H&E.*

Metastatic tissue in a node may have the texture and appearance of the mature tissue of origin, even bone.

Pigment of endogenous origin (e.g. melanin, haemosiderin) or exogenous origin (e.g. soot, tattoo ink) may darken the medullary areas of some lymph nodes. Fixation of the excised node tissue usually takes about 24 hours.

Histological examination of sections often provides a definitive diagnosis because the microarchitecture of all areas of the node can be seen. Particular areas of interest include the cortex, which may show evidence of follicular or paracortical hyperplasia in reactive hyperplasia or a prolonged inflammatory reaction. Very marked follicular hyperplasia is sometimes seen in feline immunodeficiency virus (FIV) infection. Medullary areas exhibiting sinus hyperplasia or medullary cord hyperplasia also may indicate antigenic or inflammatory reactions. The subcapsular sinus contains the cell types draining into the node and can be a useful indicator of inflammatory or neoplastic conditions (Figure 12.10). The well recognized 'sinus histiocytosis' response of human lymph nodes to neoplastic cells within the sinus channels is not

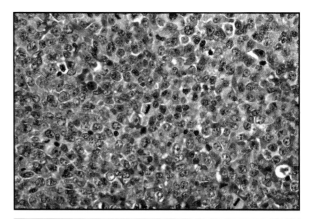

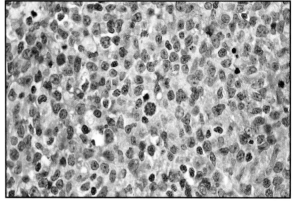

Figure 12.13: High-power views of sections from two cases of lymphoma in canine lymph nodes. Note the pleomorphic, pale nuclei, the mitotic figures and the loss of architecture. H&E.

very obvious in animals, supporting the concept of tumour-related immunosuppression. Indeed, resident tissue areas in nodes infiltrated by metastatic cells are usually poorly reactive. Subcapsular and medullary areas are usually most affected by oedema. With severe inflammatory and neoplastic changes the node architecture can be markedly disrupted and even obliterated (Figures 12.11–12.13).

Sampling of nodes at necropsy may be indicated sometimes. These should be treated as surgically-removed tissues with particular attention paid to labelling samples if multiple nodes are taken.

Figure 12.11: Low-power view of a canine lymph node affected by lymphoma. The typical 'flat field' of closely packed, neoplastic lymphocytes obliterates the node architecture. A few focal areas of haemorrhage are also present. H&E.

SPLEEN

The spleen is a highly vascular organ that filters blood and has no afferent lymphatic supply. It comprises red pulp areas containing vascular channels and cords of phagocytes and plasma cells, and white pulp areas of lymphoid tissue (Figure 12.14).

Splenomegaly may be detected by palpation, radiography or ultrasonography and may be due to reactive hyperplasia, immune-mediated disease, 'splenitis', circulatory changes (e.g. engorgement) or neoplasia. Barbiturate anaesthetics cause circulatory changes resulting in splenomegaly; this is to be expected as a 'normal' postmortem change therefore (especially in dogs) when euthanasia has been performed.

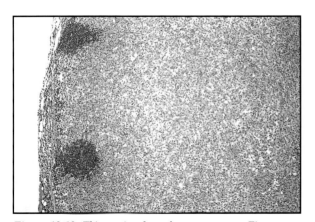

Figure 12.12: This section from the same case as Figure 12.11 shows the two small foci of normal basophilic lymphocytes that are the only surviving areas of normal cortical tissue. The remainder of the field is filled with neoplastic lymphocytes. H&E.

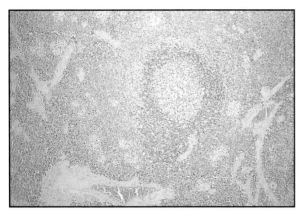

Figure 12.14: *Low-power view of normal canine spleen, showing the white pulp area (periarteriolar lymphatic sheath and B cell follicle) and red pulp area (cords and sinuses). H&E.*

Splenomegaly may be diffuse as in generalized hyperplastic conditions, hyperaemia, congestion, extramedullary haematopoiesis and neoplasia of lymphoid or myeloid origin. Nodular lesions are relatively common and may be due to haematomas, nodular hyperplasia or neoplasia. Diagnosis of splenomegaly may be assisted by haematology, bone marrow examination and tests for autoimmunity (Coombs' test, antinuclear antibody, rheumatoid factor; see Chapter 6).

Sampling

Sampling of splenic tissue by FNA or core biopsy should not be attempted lightly. The spleen is highly vascular and in many conditions of enlargement the tissue is very friable and needle trauma may cause significant haemorrhage. This is particularly so for conditions such as circulatory disturbances, haematoma, haemangioma and haemangiosarcoma. Furthermore, the large amount of blood present in many of these lesions often precludes a specific diagnosis being made. Aspiration techniques may be safer and more useful in cases of suspected lymphoid or myeloid neoplasia where the spleen is usually firmer.

FNA sampling of the spleen may be performed on sedated animals with a surgically prepared abdominal skin site over the position of the spleen. Local anaesthesia of the abdominal wall may be indicated. During the procedure the spleen is immobilized gently against the abdominal wall. The technique is similar to that described earlier for the lymph node but a longer needle may be required. If the sampled tissue has the consistency of blood then smears should be prepared as for blood, using glass slides. Those samples with apparent tissue fragments should be squashed gently between two glass slides before being smeared across the surface. A thin, even smear is the ideal preparation.

Because of the potential risk of haemorrhage from aspiration or incisional techniques, in many instances pathological examination of splenic tissue is concerned with entire spleens removed at surgery or necropsy. Gross examination of the spleen including

tissue consistency and nodular size may be very helpful in suggesting a diagnosis. Diffuse enlargement with marked congestion may occur with splenic torsion whilst firmer, cream-coloured parenchyma could be consistent with lymphoid neoplasia. Nodular hyperplasia is rather common in older dogs and lesions are often multiple and usually small (<2 cm diameter) with parenchymal-type tissue, i.e. both red and white pulp elements present (Figure 12.15). Haematomas may be large but will contain fresh or coagulated blood. Haemangiomas are firm to soft and ooze blood if cut open.

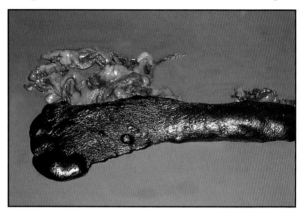

Figure 12.15: *Canine spleen showing a few, focal, firm areas of nodular hyperplasia.*

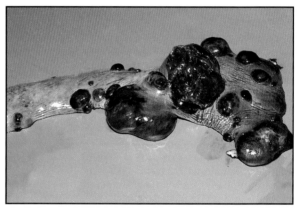

Figure 12.16: *Canine spleen with multifocal, soft, haemorrhagic, large nodular lesions of haemangiosarcoma.*

Haemangiosarcoma is a common neoplasm and may attain a very large size (>15 cm diameter) with areas of ulceration and haemorrhage in very friable tissue (Figure 12.16).

Fresh spleen tissue may be used to make impression smears. A fresh, clean cut is made across the spleen and the parenchymal surface is gently blotted with absorbent paper to remove excess blood and tissue fluid. Failure to observe the blotting step may result in lesions being obscured by normal blood components. Immediately after blotting, a glass slide is gently touched on to the cut surface to transfer exfoliated cells. If smears are thin enough they may be fixed and stained without further interference; very thick smears may require further spreading with another glass slide. It is sensible to make multiple smears to allow for special stains if required.

For FNA and impression smear preparations the principles of air-drying, wet fixation and staining outlined for cytology apply (see Chapter 7).

Normal splenic cytology is rich in leucocytes and red blood cells with additional lymphocytes, lymphoblasts, plasma cells, macrophages and platelets plus a few mast cells and stromal cells. Contamination by blood may be greater or less in impression smears or FNA samples depending upon the case and the technique used. Splenic conditions of hyperplasia may be indicated by an increase in numbers of macrophages, lymphoblasts and plasma cells. The phagocytic macrophages are an important cellular component of the spleen and examination of the cytoplasm is always indicated. Excessive levels of phagocytosed red blood cells or haemosiderin may indicate a haemolytic condition. Also, pathogens such as bacteria and blood protozoans (e.g. *Leishmania*) may be seen. Red blood cells may also be examined for evidence of shape and size changes, parasites (e.g. *Haemobartonella felis*) and Heinz bodies indicating damage.

Neoplasia of lymphoid and myeloid lines affecting the spleen is usually indicated by smears dominated by a monotonous population of the transformed cells. Lymphoid tumours are often represented by large, immature, lymphoblastoid cells; neoplasms of the erythroid, granulocytic, megakaryocytic and other series may also occur. Bone marrow and blood investigations are often useful adjuncts in these cases. Neoplasia of other tissue types is also relatively common in the spleen. Haemangiosarcoma smears often show numerous large, plump, pleomorphic endothelial cells, sometimes clumped into vascular-type structures (Figure 12.17). Other tumours seen in the spleen include mast cell tumour, fibrosarcoma, leiomyosarcoma, plasmacytoma and others, but definitive diagnosis often needs histopathological examination.

Extramedullary haematopoiesis may occur in the spleen in cases of chronic haemolytic and hypoplastic anaemia. Compensatory haematopoiesis in the spleen is indicated by increased numbers of erythroid cells plus megakaryocytes and granulocyte precursors.

Splenic tissue from splenectomy or necropsy can also be fixed in formalin and processed routinely to sections for examination. This is a sensible back-up for impression smears as lesions may be missed on small samples. The rules about 1cm-thick tissue and a 1:10 ratio of tissue to fixative apply for optimal results. It may be impractical to submit the entire spleen because of its large size. If so, a selection of carefully chosen blocks including both normal and abnormal tissue may suffice. Care should be taken to select areas of spleen that are not just zones of blood as the diagnostic value of these is usually limited. A diagram of the spleen and lesions and selected areas is often helpful to the pathologist.

THYMUS

The thymus is part of the primary lymphoid system concerned with lymphopoiesis of T cells, and contains cortical and medullary areas (Figure 12.18). It does not react to antigen as the lymph nodes and splenic tissue do but it may be affected by involution and by inflammatory and neoplastic changes. The thymus is small and involuted in normal adult animals. Probably the most common grossly obvious thymic abnormality in

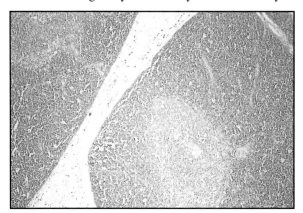

Figure 12.18: Low power view of normal canine thymus (puppy) showing cortical and medullary areas and lobules. H&E.

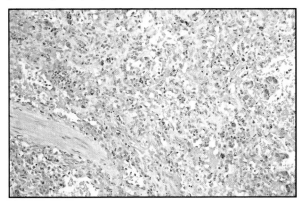

Figure 12.17: Low-power view of canine splenic haemangiosarcoma showing proliferating, pleomorphic endothelial cells forming irregular clefts. Such clefts are usually filled with red blood cells. H&E.

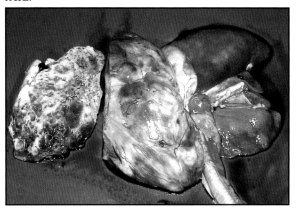

Figure 12.19: A large thymic lymphoma cranial to the thoracic viscera, from an adult cat. The cut surface of the tumour shows cystic and haemorrhagic areas.

small animals is thymic neoplasia. This may present as a large mass within the cranial thorax associated with dyspnoea and a pleural effusion (Figure 12.19). Diagnosis may be assisted by radiography, ultrasonography and thoracocentesis. Aspiration techniques may be helpful and can be applied as described above, with the cautionary reminder of the presence of vital structures locally.

Lymphoid neoplasia is seen often in cats with and without feline leukaemia virus infection; it is less common in dogs. Cytological preparations in such cases usually show large numbers of medium to large lymphocytes with neoplastic features, including mitotic figures. Grossly, tumour tissue is often firm, cream-coloured and structureless, possibly with some cystic, haemorrhagic and necrotic areas. Routine sections usually reveal a typical flat field of lymphoid cells. Lymphoepithelial tumours with lymphoid and epithelial elements are rare.

REFERENCES AND FURTHER READING

Else RW (1986) Biopsy - principles and specimen management. *In Practice* **8**, 112–116

Else RW (1989) Biopsy - special techniques and tissues. *In Practice* **11**, 27–34

Duncan JR (1993) The lymph nodes. In: *Diagnostic Cytology of the Dog and Cat*, ed. RL Cowell and RD Tyler, pp. 93–98. American Veterinary Publications Inc., Goleta, California

Jarrett WF and Mackey LJ (1974) Neoplastic diseases of the haematopoietic and lymphoid tissues. In: *International Histological Classification of Tumours of Domestic Animals. Bulletin of the World Health Organization* **50** (1-2), 21–34

MacWilliams PS (1993) The splenic parenchyma. In: *Diagnostic Cytology of the Dog and Cat*, ed. RL Cowell and RD Tyler, pp, 199–206 American Veterinary Publications Inc., Goleta, California

Moulton JE and Harvey JW (1990) Tumors of the lymphoid and hematopoietic tissues. In: *Tumors in Domestic Animals*. ed. JE Moulton, pp. 231–307. University of California Press, Berkeley.

Morris JS and Dobson JM (1992) Solid neoplasms. *In Practice* **14**, 18–24

Valli VEO (1993) The haemopoietic system. In: *Pathology of Domestic Animals, 4th edn*, ed. KVF Jubb, volume 3, pp. 209–251. Academic Press, San Diego

Nervous System

Nick Carmichael

INTRODUCTION

Clinical investigation of the nervous system is a challenging area of small animal practice. Routine diagnostic procedures that are applicable to other body systems, such as biopsy, are both technically demanding and potentially damaging to the patient and access to appropriate imaging modalities such as computed tomography and magnetic resonance imaging is relatively limited. Many cases, however, can be satisfactorily investigated in practice using relatively simple procedures coupled with some basic knowledge of clinical neurology. Laboratory tests can be a useful part of investigation both to exclude possible systemic causes of neurological signs and (in the case of analysis of cerebrospinal fluid (CSF)) to assist in characterizing the type of disease process present. As with all laboratory tests, however, the diagnostic yield is dependent on careful test selection and on obtaining the best quality samples for analysis.

This chapter discusses the clinical approach to investigation, currently available laboratory tests and the routine diagnostic procedures undertaken in the investigation of neurological disease.

INITIAL DIAGNOSTIC EVALUATION

In cases of suspected neurological disease the initial diagnostic plan comprises taking a full history, plus physical and neurological examinations. Using the information gained it should be possible to: localize the problem within the nervous system; formulate a list of differential diagnoses and select appropriate further tests to help establish a definitive diagnosis.

Lesions at different sites within the nervous system produce consistent patterns of clinical signs and deficits on neurological examination. By comparing the findings from an individual case with these recognized clinical syndromes it is often possible to localize lesions without a detailed knowledge of neuroanatomy (Braund, 1994).

Persistent, assymetrical changes on neurological examination usually reflect structural disease. Investigative procedures in such cases are therefore targeted at neural tissue and the adjacent supporting structures (e.g. examination of cerebrospinal fluid (CSF), myelography, intracranial imaging).

Neurological signs can also reflect dysfunction arising as a consequence of a systemic metabolic disturbance. Such secondary neurological signs are often transient or episodic and persistent deficits on neurological examination are rare. Common manifestations include altered consciousness or seizures and may be accompanied by other systemic signs (Cuddon, 1996). Where secondary disease is a possibility, a clinical screening profile should be performed before more invasive testing is undertaken. An example of an appropriate profile is given in Chapter 4. Such a profile can also provide useful baseline data before initiating therapy or considering general anaesthesia.

It is important to recognize, however, that secondary neurological disease is comparatively rare and that most cases presenting with neurological signs will have primary or idiopathic disease.

Feline infectious peritonitis (FIP), feline leukaemia virus (FeLV) infection, feline immunodeficiency virus (FIV) infection and toxoplasmosis have all been reported to produce a variety of neurological signs in cats. Differentiating between these conditions on clinical signs alone can be difficult and, as a result, routine screening of all cats presenting with obscure neurological signs has been recommended (Evans, 1995). Interpretation of test results can be difficult, however. Low titres of coronavirus need not rule out FIP involving the CNS, while a high titre may reflect exposure rather than active disease. The tests currently available in the UK do not allow differentiation of active toxoplasmosis from prior exposure without the use of paired samples. The presence of anti-FIV antibodies or FeLV antigen may on occasion be an incidental finding in the context of the presenting neurological signs.

CEREBROSPINAL FLUID EXAMINATION

Indications and contraindications

Examination of cerebrospinal fluid (CSF) is indicated where structural disease of the brain and spinal cord is suspected. It is of greater diagnostic value in inflammatory disease, as the changes in degenerative, neoplastic and granulomatous conditions are often mild and non-specific.

Clinical indications for CSF examination include: the presence of persistent deficits on neurological examination; cervical pain; refractory seizures, and investigation of focal spinal cord disease in conjunction with myelography. Contraindications include: poor anaesthetic risk; instability or suspected fractures of the cervical spine; and suspected raised intracranial pressure. Removal of CSF in cases of the latter can precipitate or exacerbate brain herniation. Clinically, raised intracranial pressure should be suspected in animals with a rapidly deteriorating level of consciousness, head pressing and aniscorea.

Sampling procedure

CSF is routinely collected from the cerebellomedullary cistern (CMC) but may also be obtained from the lumbar subarachnoid space. Samples from the lumbar site are often small and have a greater level of blood contamination but they may be useful in cases of focal spinal cord disease (Thompson *et al.*, 1990).

For collection from the CMC, the animal is anaesthetized, intubated and positioned in right lateral recumbency (assuming a right-handed operator). The atlanto-occipital area is clipped and surgically prepared. An assistant holds the patient's neck flexed, with the nose perpendicular to the upper cervical vertebrae and parallel to the table surface. Care should be taken to ensure that the endotracheal tube does not kink or obstruct in this position.

Collection is made using a 20–22 gauge 3.8 cm spinal needle in all but very large dogs where an 8.9 cm needle is required. The needle is inserted in the dorsal midline at the level of the anterior border of the wings of the atlas vertebra (Figure 13.1) and is slowly advanced ventrally. The stylet is removed frequently to check for the presence of CSF as the needle is advanced towards the atlanto-occipital membrane. When the membrane is penetrated and the subarachnoid space is entered a sudden decrease in resistance is often felt and CSF wells up at the needle hub.

CSF is allowed to drip freely into collection pots. The first few drops often contain mild blood contamination and are discarded. Plain samples and samples collected into EDTA are then obtained. One millilitre of CSF per 5 kg body weight can be collected safely.

Complications of collection

While excessive advancement of the spinal needle can result in trauma to the spinal cord or brainstem, the risks of iatrogenic damage are slight where due care is

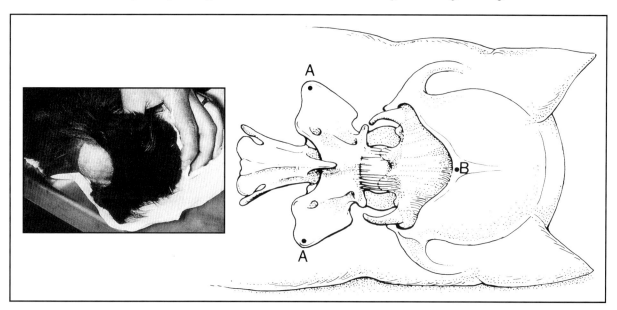

Figure 13.1: *The correct site for collection of CSF from the cisterna magna is shown in the photograph. The drawing shows the important landmarks of the atlas vertebra (A) and the occipital protuberance (B).*

1. Ensure the counting chamber is clean. Place a clean coverslip over the central area. Refraction spectra will be seen if this is placed correctly.

2. Fill the chamber with well mixed CSF, using a glass capillary tube. Touching the edge of the coverslip with the tube will cause the chamber beneath to fill by capillary action. Be careful not to overfill the chamber. Fill the other side of the chamber to allow duplicate counts to be performed.

3. Allow cells to settle for 5–10 minutes.

4. Count all cells seen in the nine large squares. By lowering the microscope condenser and examining cell size, outline and granularity it should be possible to determine which are red blood cells and which are nucleated cells without special staining. The total number of each kind of cell divided by 9 and multiplied by 10 gives the cell count per ml.

5. Repeat the cell counts on the other side of the chamber to ensure results are consistent. Record the presence of any artefacts that may affect cell counts (e.g. clumped cells, presence of debris).

Figure 13.2: Technique for CSF cell counts using the improved Neubauer haemocytometer.

taken during the procedure. It is advisable to practise CSF collection on a number of fresh cadavers before undertaking the procedure in live clinical cases.

Where orientation of the needle deviates from the midline the dorsal vertebral sinuses may be entered, resulting in venous blood appearing at the needle hub. Penetration of these vessels is not harmful to the patient and does not usually result in contamination of the CSF. The needle should be removed and a fresh needle inserted in the correct position.

Where the spinal cord is correctly positioned, mild blood contamination arising from penetration of small vessels within the meninges is common, particularly in samples collected from the lumbar subarachnoid space.

Sample handling

While the protein content and enzyme concentrations of CSF are relatively stable, cells lyse rapidly, necessitating processing or fixation of samples within 30 minutes of collection. Approaches to this problem include: performing manual cell counts in practice (Figure 13.2); using of sedimentation techniques to concentrate cells (Figure 13.3); and cytofixation using formalin or methanol.

In the author's laboratory, addition of one drop of 10% neutral buffered formal saline to 1 ml of fresh CSF

1. Prepare a 1–2 cm diameter cylinder and attach this to a microscope slide using a thin smear of paraffin jelly. A suitable cylinder can be made from the barrel of a 5 ml syringe.

2. 1 ml of well mixed CSF is placed in the cylinder and cells are allowed to sediment on to the slide for 30 minutes.

3. The cylinder is removed and any remaining jelly is scraped off. The slide is rapidly air-dried and submitted to the laboratory.

Figure 13.3: Technique for sedimentation preparations of CSF.

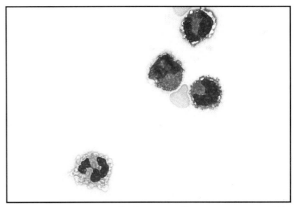

Figure 13.4: CSF sample showing inflammatory neutrophils.
Courtesy of Dr R.W. Else.

1. To prepare the Pandy reagent take 10 mg of carbolic acid and make up to 100 ml with distilled water. Alternatively, this reagent can be purchased ready prepared.

2. Place 1 ml of Pandy reagent in a clear test tube. Add a few drops of CSF.

3. Agitate the tube thoroughly.

4. Increased globulin presence within the sample will result in the development of white turbidity, the extent of which is proportional to the globulin increase.

Figure 13.5: Technique for the Pandy test. Normal CSF produces undetectable or very slight turbidity only.

has been shown to be helpful if preserving cell numbers and morphology during transit. Cells are subsequently concentrated using a cytocentrifuge following postal submission of a preserved sample.

Sample analysis

Routine analysis comprises physical evaluation (colour, turbidity), counts of red blood cells and nucleated cells, measurement of protein concentration and cytological examination. Accurate determination of CSF protein and detailed assessment of cell morphology usually require the use of an external laboratory familiar with CSF analysis.

Cytology is indicated on all samples, including those in which cellularity is within normal limits. Significant cytological abnormalities (Figure 13.4) have been reported to be present not infrequently in such samples (Christopher *et al.,* 1988).

Use of urine dipsticks to check for increased protein content and the Pandy test (Figure 13.5) for increased globulins can be useful while awaiting results from external laboratories. The finding of 2+ protein or greater in CSF reliably predicts an increased CSF protein concentration (Jacobs *et al.,* 1990)

Depending upon the clinical and routine analysis findings more specialized tests may be undertaken.

Where the protein content of CSF is increased, electrophoresis can be useful to assess if this change reflects altered blood–brain barrier permeability, production of antibody locally within the CNS, or a combination of both processes.

Changes in permeability are reflected in alteration of the ratio of albumin in CSF to that in serum (the albumin quota). Calculation of this ratio requires submission of a serum sample together with sufficient CSF for electrophoresis (2–3 ml). Changes in other protein fractions (alpha-, beta- and gamma-globulins) can be useful in identifying inflammatory, degenerative and neoplastic disease when combined with the clinical signs (Sorjonen, 1987).

Demonstration of specific antibody production within the CNS can be used to confirm the diagnosis of a variety of protozoal, viral and fungal diseases and is likely to be used increasingly in future (Munana, 1996). Increased creatine kinase (CK) can be associated with CNS parenchymal damage in the dog; however, this finding need not be associated with a poor prognosis and results can be affected by blood contamination of the sample.

Culture of CSF for microorganisms is rarely positive, given the low incidence of bacterial meningitis in the dog and cat, but it should be undertaken where cellularity is increased.

Effects of blood contamination
The low protein and cellular content of CSF means that even mild blood contamination can affect sample analysis. Red blood cells (RBCs) are not normally present in CSF and the RBC count can be used to give a guide to the extent of contamination. In studies in normal cats RBC counts as low as 500 per microlitre can be associated with spuriously increase nucleated cell counts (Rand *et al.,* 1990).

A number of different formulae have been applied in an attempt to compensate for the effects of blood contamination of CSF. Based on studies in normal dogs and cats a reduction of one nucleated cell per 500 RBCs in the dog and one nucleated cell per 100 RBCs in the cat has been recommended to give a corrected whire blood cell (WBC) count in mildly contaminated samples (<5000 RBCs/µl)(Chrisman, 1992). A factor of 1 mg/dl total protein for each 1000 RBCs/µl has also been recommended in the dog (Bailey and Higgins,1985). These factors may overestimate the changes associated with contamination and may not be reliable in more severely contaminated samples.

Interpretation of CSF results
CSF changes are often non-specific and can only usefully be interpreted in the light of the clinical signs and other tests. For example, mild to moderate increases in protein without any change in cells (albuminocytological dissociation) is a common finding and can reflect inflammatory, degenerative, compressive or neoplastic disease. Differentiation may require consideration of the history, neurological localization and possibly further diagnostic tests (CSF protein electrophoresis, albumin quota, myelography). Detailed discussion of CSF interpretation is beyond the scope of this chapter; however, a number of recent reviews are available (Chrisman, 1992; Parent, 1994; Evans, 1995).

EXAMINATION OF THE PERIPHERAL NERVOUS SYSTEM

Diseases of individual nerves (mononeuropathy) or multiple nerves (polyneuropathy) are being recognized with increasing frequency in small animal practice. Clinical signs can include reduced or absent limb reflexes and muscle tone, weakness and paralysis. Sensory abnormalities and self-mutilation may be evident.

In a similar manner to the investigation of CNS problems, the initial diagnostic evaluation comprises taking a complete history, plus physical and neurological evaluation. The latter may be extended to allow more precise localization of the nerve(s) involved. Polyneuropathies can arise secondary to a variety of systemic diseases, including hypothyroidism, hypoglycaemia, diabetes mellitus and hyperchylomicronaemia, and a screening metabolic profile should be performed. Infections with *Toxoplasma, Neospora,* FeLV and FIV can all be associated with peripheral neuropathies and should be excluded where necessary, using commercially available serum assay kits.

In localized peripheral neuropathies it can be difficult to determine clinically whether signs reflect disease of the appropriate spinal cord segment, the nerve roots or the peripheral nerve trunk. In such cases myelography and CSF examination may be useful to help exclude involvement of the CNS.

Further diagnostic evaluation includes electrodiagnostic studies (e.g. electromyography (EMG), nerve conduction and nerve biopsy). While nerve biopsy techniques are well described (Braund, 1994) and not technically difficult in most cases, the procedure is most appropriately performed at referral centres. Difficulties relate to selecting appropriate nerves in the absence of electrodiagnostic data and appropriate processing of the material collected. This can include preparation of teased nerve fibres and fixation for electron microscopy and immuno-cytochemical staining. Routine examination of for-malin-fixed nerve samples is unlikely to provide diagnostic information.

Inflammation or, less commonly, neoplasia of the inner ear can be associated with signs of periph-eral vestibular disease characterized by head tilt, horizontal or rotary nystagmus and asymetrical ataxia. Otitis externa usually reflects extension from the middle ear cavity which itself may become involved secondary to otitis externa. Both the facial nerve and sympathetic trunk supplying the head pass through the middle ear and their function can be affected by the presence of the disease. As a result otitis media/externa can be associated with ipsilateral facial nerve paralysis and Horner's syndrome, in addition to signs of peripheral vestibular disease.

The relative inaccessibility of the inner ear makes it difficult to assess and in cases with peripheral vestibular signs the middle ear cavity and tympanic membrane are routinely examined rather than the inner ear itself. Routine diagnostic testing includes examination of the tympanic membrane otoscopically and radiographical examination of the bullae on lateral and open-mouth views. Where the tympanic membrane appears inflamed, myringotomy and cytological evaluation of aspirated material from the middle ear have been recommended (Rosychuk and Luttgen, 1995). However, these pro-cedures are not without risk in terms of iatrogenic damage to the ossicles and introduction of further infection from the external ear canal. In contrast, bulla osteotomy has the advantage of creating im-proved drainage of the middle ear cavity and allows collection of biopsy material for histopathology and culture.

Bulla osteotomy has the advantage of creating improved drainage of the middle ear cavity and allows collection of biopsy material for histo-pathology and culture (CJ Little, personal comm-unication, 1996).

MONITORING ANTICONVULSANT THERAPY

Phenobarbitone and primidone (which is predomi-nantly metabolized to phenobarbitone) remain the mainstay of anticonvulsant therapy in the dog and cat. Serum concentrations are affected by a number of variables, including extent of gastrointestinal absorp-tion, duration of therapy, induction of drug-metabo-lizing hepatic enzymes and the effects of concurrent drug therapy. As a result there is a poor correlation between oral dosage and serum levels, and individual patient monitoring is indicated in all cases. Stable serum concentrations are not achieved for the first 10–14 days of therapy and in routine cases samples are taken at this time, 3 months into therapy and 6-monthly thereafter. The serum therapeutic range is 20–40 µg/ml for the dog and 10–30 µg/ml for the cat (Schwarz Porsche, 1994). Additional sampling may be indicated if there is an increasing frequency of seizures or signs associated with overdosage (in-creasing somnolence, ataxia, polydipsia, polyphagia) are noted.

Ideally two samples are taken: a peak sample obtained 4–6 hours 'post-pill' and a trough sample immediately prior to the next dose (usually 12 hours 'post pill' if on twice-daily therapy). Where only a single sample can be obtained, trough values are usually of greater use, particularly if seizures are continuing. Recent work has shown that significant reductions in drug concentration can result from the collection or submission of samples in some serum separation tubes (Boothe *et al.*, 1996), but tubes produced by other manufacturers do not appear to produce these effects; if in doubt, it is best to contact the laboratory for advice.

Use of bromide salts as a secondary anticonvulsant in the dog has led to increased monitoring of serum bromide concentrations. These may take up to 3 months to stabilize after initiating therapy. The timing of sampling in relation to the last dosage is less critical with these salts. The therapeutic range is 0.7–2.0 mg/ml (Schwarz Porsche, 1994).

Barbiturate-induced changes in liver enzymes are common on routine profiles and can be difficult to differentiate from emerging drug-associated toxic changes or underlying primary hepatopathies (Forrester *et al.*, 1989). Increases in alkaline phos-phatase up to a level of 2000–3000 IU/l, with lesser increases in alanine aminotransferase (ALT) and gamma-glutamyl transferase (GGT), are not un-common and need not be associated with hepatic functional impairment or morphological change in biopsy samples (Bunch, 1992). The presence of increased bilirubin and particularly a decline in albumin are changes suggestive of hepatoxicity and serum phenobarbitone levels should be checked when these changes are quoted.

Persistently elevated levels of phenobarbitone above the therapeutic range are associated with an increased risk of hepatoxicity, particularly if accompanied by concurrent phenytoin therapy. The long-term use of primidone rather than phenobarbitone has also been associated with increased risk of hepatoxicity.

Monitoring of serum bile acids in addition to liver enzymes can provide useful further information with regard to hepatic function ahead of the emergence of overt hepatic failure. These can be included with a liver profile when sampling for anticonvulsant monitoring.

Where clinical signs could reflect drug-induced hepatoxicity it is advisable to perform a bile acid stimulation test (see Chapter 9) to improve the sensitivity of detection of impaired hepatic function.

REFERENCES AND FURTHER READING

Bailey C S and Higgins R J (1985) Comparison of total white blood cell count and total protein content of lumbar and cisternal cerebrospinal fluid of healthy dogs. *American Journal of Veterinary Research*

Boothe D M, Simpson G and Foster T (1996) Effects of serum separation tubes on serum benzodiazepine and phenobarbital concentrations in clinically normal and epileptic dogs. *American Journal of Veterinary Research* **57**, 1299-1303

Braund K G (1994) *Clinical Syndromes in Veterinary Neurology, 2nd edition.* Mosby, St Louis

Bunch S E (1992) Hepatobiliary diseases of the dog. In: *Essentials of Small Animal Internal Medicine,* ed. RW Nelson and CG Couto, p.416. Mosby Year Book, St. Louis

Chrisman C L (1992) Cerebrospinal fluid analysis. *Veterinary Clinics of North America: Small Animal Practice* **22**, 781–808

Christopher MM, Perman V and Hardy ,R M (1988) Reassessment of cytological values in canine cerebrospinal fluid by use of cytocentrifugation. *Journal of the American Veterinary Medicine Association* **192**, 1726-1729

Cuddon P A (1996) Metabolic encephalopathies. *Veterinary Clinics of North America: Small Animal Practice* **26**, 893-924

Evans R H (1995) Haematology, biochemistry, cerebrospinal fluid analysis and other clinicopathological investigations. In: *Manual of Small Animal Neurology, 2nd edition,* ed. S J Wheeler, pp 38-49. BSAVA, Cheltenham

Forrester S D, Boothe D M and Troy G C (1989) Current concepts on the management of canine epilepsy. *Compendium of Continuing Education (Small Animal)* **11,** 811-819

Jacobs R M, Cochrane S M, Lumsden J H and Norris A M (1990) Relationship of cerebrospinal fluid protein concentration determined by dye-binding and urinary dipstick methodologies. *Canadian Veterinary Journal* **31,** 587-588

Munana K R (1996) Encephalitis and meningitis. *Veterinary Clinics of North America: Small Animal Practice* **26,** 857-874

Parent J (1994) Neurological disorders. In: *Small Animal Clinical Diagnosis by Laboratory Methods, 2nd edition,* ed. MD Willard *et al.,* pp.287-295. W B Saunders, Philadelphia

Rand JS, Parent J, Jacobs R and Percy D (1990) Reference intervals for feline cerebrospinal fluid: cell counts and cytological features. *American Journal of Veterinary Research* **51,** 1044-1048

Schwarz Porsche D (1994) Seizures. In: *Clinical Syndromes in Veterinary Neurology, 2nd edition,* pp.244-245. Mosby Year Book, St Louis

Sorjonen D C (1987) Total protein, albumin quota and electrophoretic patterns in cerebrospinal fluid of dogs with central nervous system disorders. *American Journal of Veterinary Research* **48,** 301-305

Thompson C E, Kornegay J N and Stevens J B (1990) Analysis of cerebrospinal fluid from the cerebellomedullary and lumbar cisterns of dogs with focal neurological disease: 145 cases (1985-1987). *Journal of the American Veterinary Medical Association* **196**, 1841-1844

CHAPTER FOURTEEN

The Eye

Brian Wilcock

CHAPTER PLAN
Introduction
Investigation of conjunctivitis and/or keratitis
Investigation of proliferative extraocular lesions
 Neoplasms and proliferative
   lesions of the eyelid margin
 Enlargement of the third eyelid
 Proliferative lesions involving the
   bulbar conjunctiva, sclera or
   peripheral cornea
Investigation of intraocular disease
 Cytology
 Serology
References and further reading

INTRODUCTION

With the possible exception of the skin, the eye is unique in its accessibility to direct clinical examination by the unaided eye, or with magnification in the form of a head loop or an ophthalmoscope. Since the interior of the eye is filled with optically clear media, most intraocular lesions can be detected and characterized without the need for any kind of tissue sampling. This is fortunate, since the eye does not take kindly to the introduction of needles or other foreign objects for the purposes of microbiological, cytological, or histopathological sampling. For these reasons, the interior of the eye is not sampled very often, and then only by experienced veterinary surgeons who are well aware of its sensitivity to iatrogenic injury. On the other hand, tissues associated with the external aspect of the globe, including eyelids, conjunctiva, and cornea, can safely be sampled with relative ease when attempting to determine the aetiology of a suspected infectious disease, to characterize the nature of an inflammatory infiltrate when seeking therapeutic guidance, or to determine the nature of a proliferative lesion.

The discussion below focuses on those lesions or diseases most likely to require, at least occasionally, the use of ancillary laboratory aids when making the diagnosis. This means that some very prevalent or important diseases are not discussed at all, simply because their diagnosis does not usually involve any of these ancillary tests

INVESTIGATION OF CONJUNCTIVITIS AND/OR KERATITIS

The initial management of conjunctivitis and/or keratitis routinely involves a search for foreign bodies, examination of eyelid configuration to detect causes of irritation, measurement of tear production, and careful assessment of history to rule out environmental or traumatic causes. In many cases, these common inflammations are managed conservatively with topical broad-spectrum antibiotics or corticosteroids for a week or two without any more detailed laboratory investigation.

Indications for more detailed laboratory examination include cases in which: routine therapy has not had the desired effect; the initial lesion looks unusual or dangerous; the suspected clinical diagnosis carries important long-term implications for therapy or prognosis; or other animals are at risk.

Sampling methods

Culture
Samples for culture from the conjunctival sac or corneal ulcers may be obtained by gentle application of a moistened sterile swab. Although it has been suggested that prior use of topical anaesthetic be avoided because these agents may be bactericidal, recent work has demonstrated little effect of topical anaesthetics on the isolation of various conjunctival bacteria (Champagne and Pickett, 1995). There is no scientific basis for assuming that the organism that one recovers on culture is necessarily the cause for the inflammatory disease, because the organisms isolated are usually the same as those listed as normal conjunctival flora (Gerding *et al.*,1988). In dogs, these include *Staphylococcus* spp. in 40-90% of normal dogs, followed by *Corynebacterium* (20-75%), haemolytic *Streptococcus* spp. (10-55%) and *Bacillus* spp.(6-30%). Less frequent isolates include *Pseudomonas* and *Neisseria* spp. (Gaskin, 1980). In cats, the range of bacteria is very similar, but the overall prevalence of bacterial isolation from the conjunctival sac of healthy cats or from cats with conjunctivitis is low, reported at 4-12% in one study (Shewen *et al.*,1980). Nonetheless, if one is

going to use antibiotics to treat bacterial infection (even if it is only opportunistic), it seems logical to be guided by the sensitivity pattern of those organisms known to be present on the basis of culture, rather than being guided just by 'best guess'. A notable exception would be in the case of a rapidly 'melting' ulcer in which waiting for a culture result would be disastrous. In such cases, one must gamble that the organism is either a *Streptococcus* or *Pseudomonas*, and treat appropriately and vigorously.

Cytology

After topical anaesthesia, corneal or conjunctival scrapings are obtained with a stainless steel spatula or similar instrument, and should be deep enough to obtain basal cells but ordinarily not to induce haemorrhage. The cellular harvest can then be gently teased or brushed on to a glass slide and the cells stained with any of the routine stains used in haematology or cytology.

While textbooks list corneal scraping as a method for the detection of infectious agents, or to characterize the inflammatory infiltrate as a guide to therapy, the experience of the author with this technique has been most disappointing. Corneal or conjunctival cytology ordinarily is only used for those cases in which the initial course of therapy has not been successful. By this time, the inclusion bodies typical of viral or chlamydial disease have disappeared, and the leucocytes have usually shifted to a non-specific mixture of lymphocytes and plasma cells. Exceptions certainly exist, and scrapings are very useful in the diagnosis of eosinophilic keratitis in cats, suspected mycotic keratitis in any species, and in the investigation of enzootic or epizootic outbreaks of infectious feline keratoconjunctivitis in which one has the opportunity to sample acutely affected kittens for the inclusion bodies typical of herpesvirus or *Chlamydia psittaci*.

Serology

Measurement of serum antibodies is of very limited value in the diagnosis of corneal or conjunctival inflammatory disease because of the ubiquitous nature of the most prevalent causal agents. It is used most often in cases of feline conjunctivitis when attempting to distinguish cases of herpetic keratoconjunctivitis from those caused by *Chlamydia*, calicivirus, or *Mycoplasma*. In most instances, absence of antibody titre can be used to rule out infection, but the presence of a titre cannot be interpreted as proof of causation because the prevalence of antibodies to each of these agents is quite high, even within the healthy cat population.

Surgical biopsy

Corneal or conjunctival biopsy is not performed frequently except in cases of suspected neoplasia. In inflammatory disease, the pattern of inflammation will have shifted to a chronic, non-specific lymphocytic–plasmacytic infiltrate by the time the

veterinary surgeon and the owner are frustrated enough to consider surgical biopsy. There are instances in which biopsy is useful in confirming or refuting suspicions of a few very specific disease entities, particularly feline eosinophilic keratoconjunctivitis or canine nodular granulomatous episcleritis. Both of these conditions ordinarily present as proliferative lesions and thus fall under the investigative logic outlined below.

INVESTIGATION OF PROLIFERATIVE EXTRAOCULAR LESIONS

Proliferative lesions involving the exterior of the eye include the familiar neoplasms that involve the eyelid margin, as well as less common neoplasms and immune-driven proliferative lesions of the third eyelid or conjunctiva. In most instances, diagnosis is based upon the precise anatomical location and clinical appearance of the lesion. Lesions that are unusual, or that have responded poorly to appropriate therapy, will usually be biopsied in order to establish a definitive diagnosis.

Alternatively, fine needle aspiration (FNA) can be used to harvest cells from proliferative superficial lesions involving any of the extraocular tissues. FNA is most useful in distinguishing neoplastic from granulomatous proliferative lesions, but in most instances it will not result in diagnosis of a specific syndrome. This is because many of these lesions involve proliferation of various mononuclear leucocytes and fibroblasts, and distinguishing among them requires examination of the architectural relationship among these cells, and between the infiltrating cells and the normal tissue constituents.

Most of these proliferative lesions, whether neoplastic or not, are highly site-specific and are thus presented below by specific anatomical location.

Neoplasms and proliferative lesions of the eyelid margin

Small nodules involving the free margin of the eyelid are very common in dogs, but are rare in cats. In dogs, they are almost all benign. Approximately 60% of these are Meibomian adenomas, 20% are melanomas, and about 10% are papillomas (Krehbiel and Langham, 1975; Gwin *et al.*, 1982; Roberts *et al.*, 1986). The remainder include a wide range of benign skin tumours, such as histiocytomas, mast cell tumours, and schwannomas. Almost all can be adequately treated by minor surgical resection, and ordinarily one does not attempt any prior histological or cytological sampling.

Chalazion

Chalazion is sterile granulomatous inflammation within and around a ruptured Meibomian gland. Almost all chalazia in the author's collection are associated with Meibomian adenoma, and on a clinical basis there seems to be little relevance to worrying about whether the nodule is a Meibomian adenoma, a chalazion, or both. The surgical approach and prognosis do not change.

Granulomatous marginal blepharitis

This is an idiopathic, presumably immune-mediated condition in which suppurating granulomas form in the palpebral conjunctiva of the lid margin. In some dogs the lesion begins as one or more discrete nodules that coalesce over several months into a continuous nodular thickening of the lid margin, unilaterally or bilaterally. The cause is unknown, and no infectious agent has been demonstrated. Diagnosis is based on detecting the coalescing suppurating granulomas in surgical specimens.

Enlargement of the third eyelid

Swelling of the bulbar aspect of the third eyelid may represent: prolapse of the gland of the third eyelid ('cherry eye') that has become engorged with congestion and oedema; a manifestation of nodular granulomatous episcleritis (nodular fasciitis, ocular fibrous histiocytoma); or genuine adenocarcinoma of the gland of the third eyelid. Since therapy and prognosis for these various third-eyelid disorders differ greatly, some kind of biopsy is recommended to distinguish among them. Tissue biopsy offers much greater accuracy than cytology, and something as simple as a 3 mm skin punch can be used, under topical anaesthetic, to obtain an adequate sample for diagnostic purposes.

Nodular granulomatous episcleritis

This occasionally involves the third eyelid, creating the same smooth, pink nodule as is typical of this syndrome in any of its locations (sclera, bulbar conjunctiva, peripheral cornea, or third eyelid). Particularly in Collies, the third-eyelid manifestation of this syndrome may be bilateral. It is still not clear whether all of these manifestations are of one disease, or simply represent a broad histological umbrella under which are sheltered several different disease entities. Diagnosis is usually based upon clinical criteria, but cases that do not respond appropriately to immunosuppressive therapy can be biopsied to confirm the clinical diagnosis (Paulsen *et al.*, 1987). Cytology is not usually considered useful because the diagnosis is based on the *arrangement* of the infiltrating mononuclear leucocytes and fibroblasts, rather than merely on the *presence* of these cells.

Plasmoma

Plasmoma is a nodular plasmacytic proliferative lesion within the palpebral conjunctiva of the third eyelid, with a strong breed predilection for German Shepherd Dogs. Although it has been given the name 'plasmoma', there is no evidence that this proliferative lesion is truly a neoplasm. The histological lesion is an intense, band-like subepithelial infiltration of plasma cells, similar to what is seen in other idiopathic inflammatory lesions involving mucous membranes.

Adenocarcinoma

Adenocarcinoma of the gland of the third eyelid is a rare tumour of very old (over 10 years) dogs. Initially it may be mistaken for the much more prevalent syndrome of prolapse of the gland of the third eyelid, but eventually its invasive behaviour will trigger recognition that this is something different. Local excision will provide a sample for diagnosis, but cure will require excision of the entire third eyelid. Less extensive surgery is not usually curative. Perhaps because of the late onset of disease, and what seems to be a very slow progression, metastasis has not been recorded (Wilcock and Peiffer, 1988).

Proliferative lesions involving the bulbar conjunctiva, sclera, or peripheral cornea

Nodular proliferative lesions of the canine bulbar conjunctiva, the underlying sclera, or the adjacent cornea include the common syndrome of nodular granulomatous episcleritis, as well as less common lesions such as limbal melanoma, conjunctival melanoma, necrotic scleritis, and vascular tumours. In most cases, biopsy is a combination of sampling for diagnosis and excision for attempted cure. There are, however, substantial differences among these lesions that influence the aggressiveness of surgery, or indeed whether such cases are better candidates for referral.

Vascular tumours

Vascular tumours are relatively common in dogs, and almost all of them occur along the free margin of the third eyelid and in the bulbar conjunctiva at the lateral limbus. They represent a continuum from telangiectasia to haemangioma and eventual haemangiosarcoma, but thorough surgical excision is curative. To date, there are no reported cases of metastatic disease from conjunctival haemangiosarcoma.

Limbal melanoma

Limbal melanoma is a heavily pigmented, benign lesion that occurs in both dogs and cats. It is a deep-seated lesion that develops from the melanocytes at the corneoscleral junction. Successful removal is complex surgery because grafting is frequently required to repair the excision site.

Conjunctival melanoma

Conjunctival melanomas originate within the conjunctiva, and differ sharply from the very prevalent melanomas that arise from the haired skin of the eyelid margin. The latter are virtually always benign and are easily cured by excision. The rare conjunctival melano-

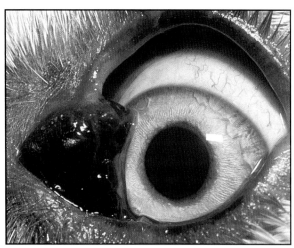

Figure 14.1: *Melanoma involving the medial canthus. In such instances, the single most important prognostic determinant is the exact site of origin: haired skin, conjunctiva, or the melanocytes resident at the corneoscleral junction.*

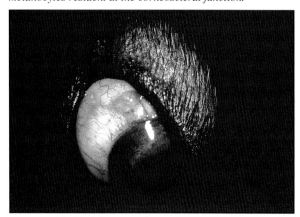

Figure 14.2: *Nodular granulomatous episcleritis, in its most classical appearance as a solitary, smooth grey–pink subconjunctival nodule a few millimetres caudal to the limbus.*

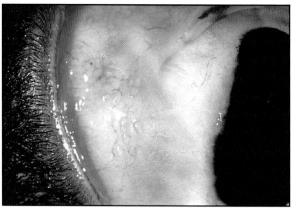

Figure 14.3: *Follicular conjunctivitis presenting with a collection of 1–2 mm glistening nodules just under the epithelium of the bulbar conjunctiva. This reflects chronic antigenic stimulation of resident lymphocytes and carries no aetiological specificity.*

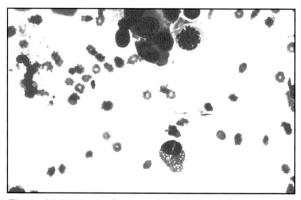

Figure 14.4: *A smear from a case of eosinophilic keratoconjunctivitis in a cat, stained with Diff Quik®. There are epithelial cells at the top of the picture, some red blood cells across the field and an eosinophil towards the bottom of the photo to the right of centre.*
Courtesy of S. Petersen-Jones

mas are both histologically and behaviourally more aggressive, with frequent recurrence after attempted local excision and a significant risk of metastatic disease (Collins *et al.*, 1994) (Figure 14.1).

Nodular granulomatous episcleritis
This occurs as a grey–pink, fleshy, raised, proliferative nodule protruding from the bulbar conjunctiva just caudal to the limbus (Figure 14.2). Almost all cases can be successfully treated with topical steroids or azathioprine, without the need for surgery (Paulsen *et al.*, 1987). Lesions that look atypical, or that have not responded well to immunosuppressive therapy, can be partially or completely excised and submitted for histological reassessment of the original clinical diagnosis.

Follicular conjunctivitis
This results from any type of chronic antigenic stimulation of the resident lymphoid tissue within the conjunctiva. The most frequent presentation is of numerous small (1mm) glistening nodules below the bulbar conjunctiva (Figure 14.3), although such nodules may occur under any conjunctival surface. Biopsy is occasionally necessary to distinguish this highly non-specific lesion from atypical presentations of other proliferative conjunctival diseases such as nodular granulomatous episcleritis, but the great majority of cases are recognized on purely clinical criteria.

Pannus keratitis
Pannus keratitis is a bilateral epithelial and superficial stromal keratitis that is seen most commonly in German Shepherd Dogs and in other sheep-herding breeds, although sporadic cases have been recorded in other types of dog. The proliferative clinical presentation is distinctive and is well recorded in clinical textbooks. Biopsy can be used to confirm the diagnosis in atypical cases but is rarely used. Cytology is not helpful since the diagnostic specificity lies in the histological detection of a lupus-like interface keratitis, not in any cytological features.

Feline eosinophilic keratitis
This uniquely feline lesion is seen clinically as a granular, raised, white-to-pink proliferative lesion af-

fecting the superficial corneal stroma near the limbus. Old lesions may cover almost the entire cornea. A shallow scraping will reveal huge numbers of eosinophils (Prasse and Winston, 1996) (Figure 14.4). In cases already treated with corticosteroids, plasma cells may predominate but a few eosinophils will persist and allow for a specific diagnosis.

LABORATORY INVESTIGATION OF INTRAOCULAR DISEASE

Cytology

There are only a few instances in which one would attempt to sample intraocular tissues, and even then many of these procedures should be left in the hands of experienced ophthalmologists. The only sampling that is commonly done in private practice is aspiration of the aqueous or vitreous humor in an attempt to confirm intraocular mycosis, particularly blastomycosis and cryptococcosis. In both of these diseases, organisms may be quite numerous, particularly within the vitreous and in the exudate that gathers below the detached retina. Most attempts at so-called vitreous aspiration are, in fact, unintended aspirations of the subretinal exudate. Because there is substantial risk of creating retinal holes and of intraocular heamorrhage, such aspirations are usually done only in those globes that are already irretrievably blind, and in animals in which the paramount need is for accurate diagnosis. In the absence of enlarged lymph nodes or draining skin lesions, the subretinal fluid may offer the best opportunity for such diagnosis. Preparing the slides is the same as would be done for any other cavity fluid, and the organisms can readily be identified with haematological stains.

Serology

Although serology has long been a standard part of the clinical investigation of uveitis in cats (and occasionally in dogs), objective assessment of the utility of such testing is hard to find. The great majority of cats with uveitis as the sole manifestation of disease are serologically negative for infections such as feline leukaemia virus (FeLV), infectious peritonitis, feline immunodeficiency virus (FIV), and toxoplasmosis (Davidson *et al.*, 1991). Indeed, the prevalence of seropositivity in cats with uveitis is the same as in the general cat population, making it impossible to evaluate the significance of the occasional case in which serology is positive. More reliable serology can certainly be obtained if one pursues paired serum samples, measures the more rapidly rising IgM antibodies, or obtains aqueous samples to measure aqueous:serum antibody ratios. Nonetheless, the expense of such pursuits should be weighed against the apparent rarity with which an otherwise healthy cat will yield any type of positive result. This it not to say that cats with feline infectious peritonitis, FeLV, FIV or systemic mycosis will not have uveitis, but that cats with uveitis alone are very unlikely candidates for any of these diseases.

REFERENCES AND FURTHER READING

Champagne ES and Pickett JP (1995) The effect of topical 0.5% proparacaine HCl on corneal and conjunctival culture results. *Proceedings of the Twenty-Sixth Annual Meeting, American College of Veterinary Ophthalmologists, Newport, Rhode Island*, p. 144

Collins BK, Collier LL, Miller MA and Linton LL (1994) Biologic behavior and histologic characteristics of canine conjunctival melanoma. *Progress in Veterinary and Comparative Ophthalmology* **3**, 135–140

Davidson MG, Nasisse MP, English RV, Wilcock BP and Jamieson VE (1991) Feline anterior uveitis: a study of 53 cases. *Journal of the American Animal Hospital Association* **27**, 77–83

Gaskin JM (1980) Microbiology of the canine and feline eye. *Veterinary Clinics of North America* **10(2)**, 303–316

Gerding PA, McLaughlin SA and Troop MW (1988) Pathogenic bacteria and fungi associated with external ocular disease in dogs: 131 cases (1981–1986). *Journal of the American Veterinary Medical Association* **193**, 242–244

Gwin RM, Gelatt KN and Williams LW (1982) Ophthalmic neoplasms in the dog. *Journal of the American Animal Hospital Association* **18**, 853–866

Krehbiel KP and Langham RF (1975) Eyelid neoplasms of dogs. *American Journal of Veterinary Research* **36**, 115

Paulsen ME, Lavach JD, Snyder SP, Severin GA and Eichenbaum JD (1987) Nodular granulomatous episclerokeratitis in dogs: 19 cases (1973–1985). *Journal of the American Veterinary Medical Association* **190**, 1581–1587

Prasse KW and Winston SM (1996) Cytology and histopathology of feline eosinophilic keratitis. *Progress in Veterinary and Comparative Ophthalmology* **6**, 74–81

Roberts SM, Severin GA and Lavach JD (1986) Prevalence and treatment of palpebral neoplasms in the dog: 200 cases (1975-1983). *Journal of the American Veterinary Medical Association* **189**, 1355–1359

Shewen PE, Povey RC and Wilson MR (1980) A survey of the conjunctival flora of clinically normal cats and cats with conjunctivitis. *Canadian Veterinary Journal* **21**, 231–233

Wilcock BP and Peiffer RL (1988) Adenocarcinoma of the gland of the third eyelid in seven dogs. *Journal of the American Veterinary Medical Association* **193**, 1549–1550

CHAPTER FIFTEEN

Skin and External Ear

Julie A. Yager and Ken Mason

INTRODUCTION

The skin is readily accessible to a wide range of diagnostic procedures. These procedures are, for the most part, easy to perform and the results may be interpreted by the clinician without involving laboratory assistance. Such tests include skin scrapings for parasites, bacteria and fungi, and the examination of plucked hairs.

More invasive techniques, such as skin biopsy, are also relatively simple to perform. They yield much diagnostic information, but do require specialized assistance in interpretation.

As with all diagnostic processes, data from several sources are pooled to reach a final and definitive diagnosis. This chapter will detail those procedures that are most commonly used in small animal veterinary practice in the elucidation of dermatological problems in dogs and cats. Skin cytology, a very important adjunct to dermatological diagnosis, is covered in Chapter 7. Immunological techniques, such as intradermal skin testing, are found in Chapter 6.

SKIN SCRAPING

Technique

Skin scraping is an easy technique, used routinely in the diagnosis of parasitic skin disease. The technique varies according to the habitat of the suspected parasite: scrapings may be superficial or deep and the techniques involved in each of these are quite different.

Superficial scraping

This technique samples loose and adherent surface scale. It is used to demonstrate the parasites that normally inhabit the stratum corneum – in particular the sarcoptid mites (*Sarcoptes scabiei, Notoedres cati, Trixacarus caviae*) and, rarely, short-bodied forms of *Demodex* spp. Superficial scraping may detect *Cheyletiella* spp., trombiculid mites and larval ticks. Superficial scraping is also used to collect scale or crust for the detection of *Malassezia* yeasts.

The area to be scraped should be selected carefully. When sarcoptid mites are suspected, erythematous papules or scaly plaques are best chosen, paying particular attention to the lateral aspects of the pinna, the elbow and the carpus, and avoiding excoriated or exudative lesions. Sampling as wide an area as possible and performing multiple skin scrapings increases the chance of recovering mites.

The equipment required includes clippers, scalpel blades (No. 10), medium, microscope slides and coverslips, and a microscope. Mineral oil such as liquid paraffin is most often used as the medium for collection. Propylene glycol, however, has the advantage of being miscible with water. Consequently, should air bubbles impede sample observation histologically, the addition of a drop of water or normal saline at the edge of the coverslip will clear the bubbles.

The hair is clipped, using a No. 40 blade, and the area is blown clear. This is an important step, as large amounts of contaminating hair can interfere with the collection of surface scale and can make the microscopic examination of the sample more difficult. The skin is steadied between the thumb and forefinger and several drops of medium, mineral oil or propylene glycol are spread over the area with a scalpel blade. The scalpel blade is then scraped across the skin to a point, so that a wide wedge-shaped area of skin is sampled. The material thus collected is transferred on to a glass slide and a coverslip is gently lowered on to the sample.

When checking for *Malassezia* oil or propylene glycol should not be used. The smear should be heat-fixed before staining.

Deep scraping

This technique is used to demonstrate follicular mites, in particular *Demodex canis* and *D. cati*. The mites reside deep within the follicles and may be difficult to dislodge. Animals with secondary bacterial folliculitis may have painful lesions, necessitating sedation, local or even general anaesthesia.

The selected area is clipped and free hair is removed. A drop of medium, either paraffin oil or propylene glycol, is applied to the skin or placed on a glass slide. A skinfold is picked up between the fingers and thumb and squeezed quite forcibly to extrude any parasites from the hair follicles. As this can cause some discom-

fort to the animal, adequate restraint is important and, in some cases, sedation may be required. A failure to apply sufficient deep pressure can lead to a false-negative result. It is also important to scrape the skin until true capillary bleeding is elicited (Figure 15.1).

The pustular lesions of demodicosis may be more easily sampled by simply expressing the contents of a pustule on to a glass slide.

Interpretation

It is important to be methodical and thorough in examining a slide for parasites. The entire slide should be scanned at low power (4X or 5X objective), checking for movements within the scale. Lowering the microscope condenser, which increases light diffraction, markedly enhances the visibility of adults, larvae and ova.

Observing the life-cycle stages present and performing an approximate count of live and dead mites may be useful, particularly when comparing sequential skin scrapings to monitor the success of treatment. Successful treatment is often reflected by a shift in population from immature to mature forms and from live to dead mites (Scott *et al.*, 1995).

The interpretation of skin scrapings is relatively easy as the morphology of the mites that cause the common parasitic infestations of companion animals is quite characteristic (Figure 15.2).

It is important to be aware that the mere presence of a parasite is not necessarily diagnostic of parasitic disease. *Demodex canis*, for example, is a commensal organism which may be sampled from the skin of normal dogs. The finding of a single mite from lesional skin is, however, suspicious and warrants further testing. Table 15.1 summarizes the techniques used in the laboratory diagnosis of parasitic disease and some of the factors to be considered in interpreting the significance of results.

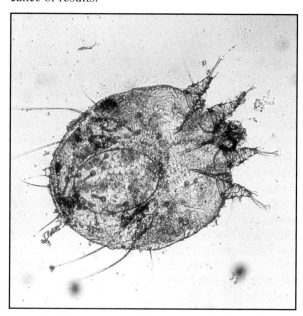

Figure 15.2: Sarcoptes scabiei. *Finding a single mite is diagnostic.*

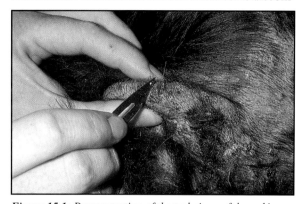

Figure 15.1: Demonstration of the technique of deep skin scraping. Note the capillary bleeding.

Parasitic disease	Appropriate diagnostic techniques	Interpretation
Canine demodicosis *Demodex canis*	Deep skin scraping Hair plucking (pododermatitis)	Simply finding a single follicular mite from a skin scraping in the area of the muzzle is not diagnostic. Diagnosis requires demonstration of several mites and preferably several life-cycle stages from multiple scrapings from clinical lesions.
Canine demodicosis Short-bodied species tentatively named *D. cornei*	Tape stripping Superficial skin scraping	Rare. Clinical significance unproven; may be a commensal or may be associated with pruritic dermatosis.
Feline demodicosis *Demodex cati*	Deep skin scraping	Any *Demodex* mite recovered from lesional skin in a cat is diagnostic.
Feline demodicosis Short-bodied form	Tape stripping Superficial skin scraping	The unnamed species is shorter and fatter than *D. cati*. It has been associated with a pruritic dermatosis.
Canine sarcoptic mange *Sarcoptes scabiei*	Superficial to deeper skin scraping (multiple)	A single sarcoptic mite is diagnostic. Repeated scrapings may be necessary to detect the parasite. A negative scraping does not rule out sarcoptic mange.
Feline notoedric mange *Notoedres cati*	Superficial skin scraping	Numerous mites are present, making diagnosis relatively easy. The mite is quite similar to *Sarcoptes* but has a dorsal rather than a terminal anus.
Canine otodectic mange *Otodectes cynotis*	Superficial skin scraping Tape stripping Cotton bud (ear sample)	Numerous mites are present, making diagnosis relatively easy.
Cheyletiellosis *C. yagsuri* (dogs) *C. blakei* (cats)	Direct examination with magnification Combing and brushing with KOH digestion & concentration techniques Tape stripping	Tiny white mites easily seen on a dark surface – 'walking dandruff' is diagnostic; characteristic, large palpal claws; non-operculated ova attached to hairs. Even the best technique (flea combing) is not sensitive – 15% false negatives in dogs, 58% in cats.
Cat fur mite *Lynxacarus radovsky*	Hair plucking	Differentiate from parasitic ova (lice or *Cheyletiella*). Only reported from tropical areas such as Florida, USA and northern Australia.
Lice *Trichodectes canis* *Heterodoxus spiniger* *Linognathus setosus* (dog) *Felicola subrostratus* (cat)	Visual examination Coat brushing Hair plucking Superficial scraping Tape stripping	The diagnosis is readily made by finding the adult lice on the body or the eggs attached to the hairs. Biting lice may be more difficult to find than less mobile sucking lice.

Table 15.1: *Techniques and interpretation in parasitic skin disease.*

TAPE IMPRESSION (Tape Stripping, Acetate Tape Preparation)

Tape impression is used to detect superficial parasites, surface bacteria and fungi. It is particularly useful for the identification of *Cheyletiella* spp. infestations in cats and dogs. In dogs, tape impressions are used also in the diagnosis of *Malassezia* yeast infection. They also may be used to detect the ear mite *Otodectes cynotis* and unusual mite infestations, such as the poultry mite *Dermanyssus gallinae* and the very rare short-bodied forms of *Demodex* (Chen, 1995). Tape

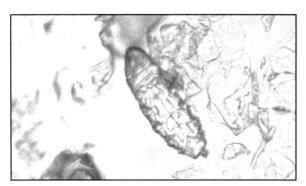

Figure 15.3: Superficial skin scraping from a dog reveals a rare infection caused by a short-bodied form of Demodex, *tentatively named* Demodex cornei.

stripping is also an effective method for sampling dermatophyte spores from the surface of fungal colonies, for the identification of dermatophyte species.

Parasitic infestation

A short strip of clear, not translucent, adhesive tape is used (Scott *et al.*, 1995). The hair is parted and the tape is pressed, adhesive side down, on to the skin surface so as to collect large amounts of scale. The process is repeated at different sites. The segment of tape is pressed, again with the adhesive side down, on to a glass slide and immediately scanned, in a methodical manner, for the presence of mites. Staining is not necessary to demonstrate mites, but lowering the microscope condenser is helpful. Using water as a mounting medium renders the short-bodied *Demodex* more visible (Figure 15.3). The presence of mites with the characteristic morphology is diagnostic.

Malassezia yeasts

The preferred sampling site is one that is inflamed and scaly. The area is prepared by clipping and blowing away the hair. A short length of clear tape is pressed firmly on to the skin surface, several times, until the tape is opaque from adherent material (Figure 15.4). One end of the tape (about 1 cm) is attached to a glass slide, leaving the remainder free but with the adhesive side facing the glass slide. The preparation is plunged into a Coplin jar (or some other dip-staining device) containing a basophilic dye. The slide is stained for 30 seconds, with no agitation. Irrigating the slide in tap water removes most, but not all of the stain. Leaving some residual stain and water on the slide, the tape is then pressed to the glass surface. Excess water is removed but the film of dye and water acts as a mounting medium. The preparation should be examined immediately as the tape may begin to wrinkle as it dries. In the absence of a staining jar, a drop of stain may be placed on to a glass slide before the tape is pressed to the surface .

The mere presence of the typical bottle-shaped yeasts (Figure 15.5) is not, in itself, diagnostic for *Malassezia* dermatitis. The presence of an occasional *Malassezia* (<1 per 40X high-power field) in scrapings

taken from lesions on the trunk may be suspicious, but this number would be insignificant in scrapings taken from perioral skin, the ear canal or the interdigital skin. More than three organisms per high-power field is suspicious of *Malassezia* dermatitis, irrespective of the sample site, and an average of five organisms per high-power field warrants a therapeutic trial.

Coccoid bacteria, usually *Staphylococcus intermedius*, are often present in conjunction with *Malassezia* yeasts (Figure 15.5). The conditions that predispose to overgrowth of one, often also apply to the other.

DETERGENT-SCRUB TECHNIQUE

This technique has been used to quantify *Malassezia* yeasts and bacterial flora on normal and diseased skin (Bond *et al.*, 1995 a,c) . The technique is of particular value for therapeutic trials, such as comparisons of the efficacy of shampoos (Bond *et al.*, 1995b). It is not in common usage in general practice.

The detergent solution used is 0.075M phosphate-buffered saline, pH 7.9, containing 0.1% Triton-X-100. Two millilitres of the wash fluid is poured into sterile, open-ended 22 mm-diameter cylinders of polytetrafluoroethylene. A sterile rod is used to rub the skin gently for 60 seconds. The wash fluid is transferred to a sterile container and aliquots are dispensed on to appropriate culture media for quantitation.

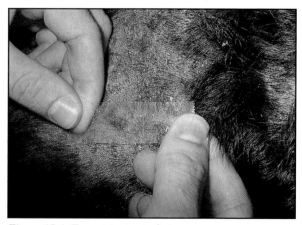

Figure 15.4: Tape stripping technique.

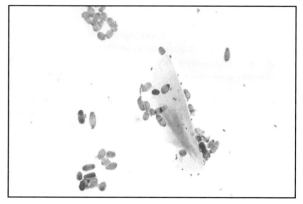

Figure 15.5: Bipolar Malassezia *yeasts, bacterial cocci and squames in a stained tape-strip preparation.*

COMBING AND BRUSHING TECHNIQUES

These techniques are used to detect flea and/or flea faeces and *Cheyletiella* mite infestation. The tooth-brush technique is the procedure chosen by most dermatologists to collect samples from cats suspected of having dermatophytosis (Moriello, 1990).

Flea infestation and cheyletiellosis

To detect fleas, the animal is positioned over a white surface – a white table top, a piece of white paper or material; a dark surface is preferable for *Cheyletiella*. The animal's coat is ruffled to loosen surface debris. A fine-toothed comb is run rapidly through the fur, paying particular attention to the tailbase, caudal aspects of the hindlegs and ventral neck when flea infestation is suspected and to the dorsal midline when cheyletiellosis is suspected.

In heavily flea-infested animals, the comb may become clogged with detritus (Figure 15.6). Adult fleas are readily visible and will leap off the comb's surface unless they are immobilized with alcohol. A hand lens or a dissecting microscope may be used for closer examination of the sample. The diagnosis of cheyletiellosis is markedly enhanced if digestion and concentration techniques are employed (see below).

Hair samples for dermatophyte culture

A new or sterilized toothbrush is used. The bristles may be shortened to facilitate transfer to the culture medium. The hair samples are placed in direct contact with the culture medium and are spread out to minimize overgrowth by saprophytes.

The technique is excellent for confirming dermatophyte infection in lesional cats and is also used to identify subclinically infected individuals. One disadvantage is that normal cats carrying *Microsporum canis* spores on their coats will also yield positive cultures with this technique. However, there are other clues that will help to distinguish truly asymptomatic infected cats from those acting simply as carriers (Moriello and De Boer, 1995).

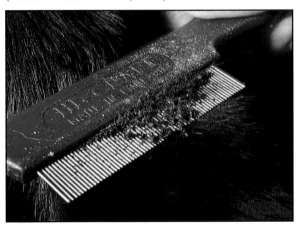

Figure 15.6: *The combing technique reveals a heavy flea infestation.*

HAIR PLUCKING (TRICHOGRAM, TRICHOGRAPHY)

Trichography refers to the microscopic examination of plucked hairs.

Technique

This is a simple technique requiring only a pair of forceps, adhesive tape, a glass slide and a microscope. A small tuft of hair is plucked from the skin and placed on the adhesive tape. This is inverted on to a microscope slide for examination.

When examining hairs for dermatophytes, the sample is mounted in paraffin oil or may be first subjected to 'clearing' by incubation with potassium hydroxide (KOH) or chlorophenolac (Scott *et al.*, 1995).

Ectoparasites

The technique will detect adherent parasites, such as fur mites (*Lynxacarus radovsky* on cats and *Lystrophorus gibbus* on rabbits) and adherent egg cases in lice infestations and cheyletiellosis. However, it is not the method of choice for diagnosing most parasitic skin disease.

Anagen:telogen ratios

Trichograms are used in human dermatology to determine anagen:telogen ratios in the evaluation of alopecic disorders. The ratio is determined by examining a large number of plucked hairs to assess the growth stage. Anagen hairs have a plump, smooth, shiny, rounded bulb whereas the base of the telogen hair is made up of the residual 'club' which is more spear-shaped and has an irregular contour. The technique has not found much favour in veterinary dermatology to date (Wilkinson and Harvey, 1994; Scott *et al.*, 1995). The normal range of anagen:telogen ratios has not been established for either dog or cat, a task made even more complicated by the cyclical nature of hair growth and the variations between breeds.

Hair abnormalities

The most useful application for trichography is to determine whether or not hair loss is associated with self-epilation. The tip of a normal hair is pointed; hairs with fractured or squared-off ends are indicative of coat barbering. Trichograms are also useful in the detection of dystrophic hairs, such as occur in canine colour dilution alopecia. Large clumps of melanin (aggregated macromelanosomes) (Figure 15.7) are irregularly dispersed along abnormal, often broken hair shafts (Miller, 1990).

Dermatophyte infection

Direct examination of hair is also used to detect dermatophyte infection although the procedure is time-consuming and tedious. Most dermatologists use the Wood's lamp to identify fluorescent hairs and pluck these for further examination. The most common in-

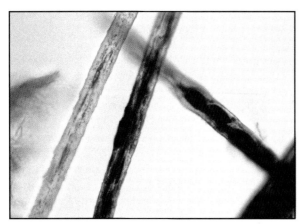

Figure 15.7: *Plucked hairs from a dog with colour dilution alopecia showing the characteristic pigment clumps.*

Courtesy of Dr Karen Beale and Dr Gail Kunkle.

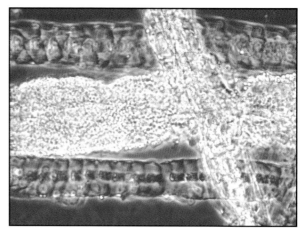

Figure 15.8: *A KOH-cleared preparation showing* Microsporum canis-*infected hairs flanked by normal hair shafts.*

fecting species of dermatophyte in both the dog and the cat, *Microsporum canis,* is usually fluorescent. It is important not only to warm up the Wood's lamp for at least 5 minutes, but to allow sufficient time for fluorescence to become apparent (Moriello and De Boer, 1995). Too hasty an examination can yield false negatives. False positives may be due to topical medications, keratin debris and some bacteria.

Interpretation of these preparations requires patience and some expertise in identifying infected hairs. Scott *et al.* (1995) recommend making test preparations from a known positive and heavily infected sample. Repeated examination of these samples, gradually increasing the number of non-infected hairs added to the preparation, allows one to become adept at picking out an infected hair from a mass of normal hairs (Scott *et al.,* 1995).

On microscopic examination the infected hairs appear damaged or broken. The cortex and cuticle are irregular and have a fuzzy outline because of the presence of ensheathing hyphae and arthroconidia. The hyphae of the common infecting species are branching and septate, approximately 2-3 µm in diameter. The arthroconidia of the most frequently isolated pathogenic species, *M. canis,* are small (2-3 µm), bead-like and coalesce to form a dense mosaic pattern on the outside of the hair shaft (ectothrix infection) (Figure 15.8). The arthroconidia of *Microsporum gypseum* are much larger (5-8 µm) and occur as sparse chains. Those of *Trichophyton mentagrophytes* and *T. verrucosum* are intermediate in size (3-7 µm). None of the pathogenic species produces macroconidia in tissue – thus the presence of macroconidia indicates a contaminating saphrophytic fungal species. Finally, it is important not to confuse melanin granules, normally present within the hair shaft, with fungal elements.

Some fungi, such as *Trichophyton terrestrae,* tend to associate with surface corneocytes. Culturing scale, as well as hair, improves the chance of fungal isolation.

Isolation and culture are necessary for fungal identification and all positive tests should be so confirmed.

DIGESTION TECHNIQUES

To aid in the microscopic visualization of dermatophytic fungi or parasites, it may be advantageous to 'clear' the keratin and debris from the sample by digestion with potassium hydroxide (KOH) or chlorophenolac alkaline solutions.

Dermatophyte infection

Since the common dermatophyte infections of the dog and cat are ectothrix in type, many veterinary dermatologists dispense with KOH techniques and simply suspend Wood's lamp-positive plucked hairs in mineral oil. However, clearing techniques will assist in the microscopic visualization of fungal hyphae and spores.

The few drops of a solution of 10-20% KOH are applied to hair, scale and/or claw samples placed on a glass slide. A coverslip is added and the slide is then heated to assist digestion. Placing the slide on the warm microscope lamp housing for 15-20 minutes is a recommended method for safely heating the slide (Scott *et al.,* 1995). Holding the slide high over a Bunsen burner flame for 15-20 seconds is a faster, but more risky technique. Alternatively, the preparation may be left at room temperature for 30 minutes.

Chlorophenolac, a mixture of chloral hydrate, liquid phenol and lactic acid (Scott *et al.,* 1995), is a somewhat simpler clearing agent to use, as there is no need to heat the suspension and the slide may be read almost immediately.

Stains, such as lactophenol cotton blue, may be added to enhance the visibility of the fungal elements. A new technique, which employs KOH as the clearing agent and the textile brightener, calcofluor white, to illuminate the fungal elements, is effective but has the disadvantage of requiring a fluorescent microscope to read the preparation (Sparkes *et al.,* 1994).

Ectoparasites

The digestion and concentration procedure is an adjunct to skin scraping, brushing and combing techniques. It increases the chance of detecting ectoparasites, particularly *Cheyletiella* spp. The KOH digestion is significantly more effective in the demonstration of *Cheyletiella* mites and ova than are skin scrapings or tape preparations (Noxon, 1995).

Accumulated scale and hair is placed in a test tube containing 10–20 ml 10% KOH and digested under gentle heat, such as provided by a 37°C water bath for about 30 minutes. When the debris is largely dissolved, the suspension is centrifuged at 1000 rpm for one minute and the supernatant decanted. The test tube is half-filled with water and topped up with a saturated sucrose solution. Sediment is collected by recentrifuging, or by allowing the suspension to sit for 15–20 minutes, then transferred to a glass slide. A coverslip is added and the slide is examined microscopically for the presence of mites or ova.

SAMPLING FOR FUNGAL CULTURE

Dermatophytes

The most reliable means of diagnosing a dermatophyte infection is by isolating the fungus by culture. The toothbrush technique is the preferred technique for sample collection in cats (Moriello and De Boer, 1995). If using plucked hairs, the chance of a positive culture is increased if the Wood's lamp is used as an aid to the selection of the sample. The collected hairs are placed directly on to the dermatophyte test medium (DTM), which contains an indicator system to detect dermatophyte species, or onto Sabaraud's dextrose agar plates. Dual culture systems, in which one plate contains an indicator and the other does not, are useful.

In a positive culture the DTM changes colour from yellow to red. The colour change should occur within 3–5 days and begin while the colony is still small. It is important to check the culture daily. Non-pathogenic fungi may cause a colour change if the culture period is prolonged (more than 10 days), yielding false-positive results. *Microsporum persicolor* may be wrongly discarded as a saprophyte because it causes a late colour change.

It is essential to confirm that a fungal colony isolated on DTM is truly a dermatophyte species, even if there has been an appropriate colour change. This is achieved by the microscopic demonstration of characteristic conidia produced by the sporulating fungus. Most dermatophytic fungi will sporulate on identification medium but some require subculturing upon non-indicator-containing medium (thus, the advantage of the dual culture system, which provides both types of media on one divided plate).

Tape impression is a simple way of transferring conidia to a glass slide for microscopic examination. A short length of tape is attached to the end of a spatula, forceps or the wooden stem of a swab – the so-called Roth's flag preparation. The adhesive side of the tape

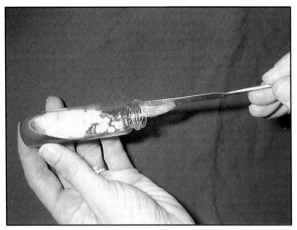

Figure 15.9: Using adhesive tape to collect a sample from the surface of fungal colonies growing on DTM (Roth's flag technique).

is on the outside. The tape is pressed against the surface of the fungal colony and then transferred to the glass slide, sticky side down (Figure 15.9). The slide is irrigated with stain, usually lactophenol blue, wiped free of excess stain and evaluated microscopically. The characteristic boat-shaped conidia are morphologically distinctive (Figure 15.10). Table 15.2 lists the chief cultural and anatomical features of the common dermatophyte species affecting the dog and cat.

Malassezia yeasts

This relatively simple method for the culture of *Malassezia* yeasts has been described recently by Bond *et al.*, 1994. The technique is readily performed in a clinical setting and provides valuable quantitative data with minimal expense and equipment. The technique can be used to monitor response to therapy.

The hair is removed with curved scissors and the culture dish containing a malt-extract agar-based medium (Bond *et al.*, 1994) is pressed on to the skin surface for 10 seconds. The plates are cultured at 32°C for 3 days under aerobic conditions. The white glistening colonies are enumerated and the colony counts per cm^2 of skin are calculated by dividing the colony count by the surface area of the plate.

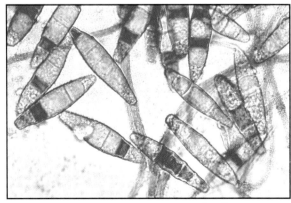

Figure 15.10: A tape preparation, prepared as shown in Figure 9, reveals macroconidia typical of dermatophyte infection.

Species	Colonial morphology	Anatomy of arthroconidia
Microsporum canis	White cotton-wool colonies with yellow to orange reverse pigment As colony ages, reverse pigment becomes brown, the centre is depressed and radial folds may develop	Thick-walled boat-shaped macroconidia Asymmetrical More than 6 cells Spines at the terminal end may cluster to form a knob
Microsporum gypseum	Cream to cinammon brown with yellow-tan reverse pigment Flat colony with a granular texture	Thin-walled Symmetrical Less than 6 cells No terminal knob
Trichophyton mentagrophytes	Cream with brown reverse pigment Powdery surface Flat colony	Cigar-shaped, thin-walled macroconidia Accompanying hyphae are often spiral Round microconidia along hyphae, sometimes in clusters

Table 15.2: The cultural and anatomical features of common dermatophytes infecting the dog and cat.
(Adapted from Wilkinson and Harvey, 1994, and Scott et al., 1995.)

Contact plate cultures collected from 8 of 10 normal dogs yielded no growth and the numbers of colonies collected from the two positive sites were low (Bond *et al.,* 1994). These results indicate that the technique does not pick up low concentrations of this commensal organism on normal skin. In lesional skin, the population is increased 100–100,000-fold.

SAMPLING FOR BACTERIA

Cytology

Cytology is the technique of choice in the evaluation of bacterial skin infections (see Chapter 7). Depending on the type of lesion to be sampled, material may be collected by: expressing the lesional content on to the end of a microscope slide, which is then used as a spreader to produce a direct smear; applying a microscope slide to the surface of the lesion to produce an impression smear; collecting exudates/secretions on a saline-moistened swab; superficial scrapings; or fine needle aspiration. Smears should be rapidly air-dried and stained with modified Wright's stain.

Staphylococcus intermedius is the most common pathogen causing pyoderma in dogs and it is readily visible cytologically. The presence of intracellular cocci in a properly collected sample is sufficient to warrant a therapeutic antibiotic trial (Scott *et al.,* 1995).

Bacterial culture

When bacterial culture is indicated, it is important to avoid surface contamination in the collection of samples and to submit them promptly to a laboratory well versed in veterinary microbiology.

The choice of sample is critical: if possible, culture from an intact pustule or papule. Moist erosions and crusts are heavily contaminated with bacterial and fungal opportunists. The surface of an intact pustule should be teased open with a sterile 25 gauge needle and the contents transferred to the tip of a sterile swab. Larger pustules may be penetrated with a 25 gauge needle and the contents aspirated. Papular lesions may be pierced, the fluid pus expressed and transferred to a sterile swab. The swabs are then placed in transport medium. Nodular lesions and fistulous tracts may be sampled by fine needle or by excisional biopsy.

Surface disinfection is not recommended in the culture of superficial lesions as it may lead to false-negative results. When deeper lesions are sampled, the surface is surgically prepared and the tissue biopsy is taken aseptically.

Knowledge of the resident and transient bacterial species found on the skin of the cat and dog is important in the interpretation of culture results (Table 15.3).

Communication between the laboratory and the clinician is critical when an unusual pathogen, such as atypical *Mycobacteria* spp. or *Nocardia*, is suspected. It is essential that the laboratory is aware of the differential diagnosis, so that appropriate cultural techniques are employed. Similarly, it is often necessary to request anaerobic cultures as many laboratories do not perform these routinely.

OTIC SAMPLING

The external ear canal is routinely sampled for cytology, detection of ear mites and/or *Malassezia* yeasts, and for bacterial culture.

The simple technique employs a cotton-bud swab, which is inserted deep into the vertical ear canal, and rotated against the walls of the canal until it is

Type	Bacterial species
Resident	**Dog and Cat:** *Micrococcus* spp.; *Staphylococcus epidermidis*; *S. simulans* (cat); other coagulase–negative staphylococci (*S. capitis, S. haemolyticus, S. hominis, S. sciuri, S. warneri*); *S. aureus* (transferred from humans); *Acetinobacter* spp.; α-haemolytic streptococci; *Streptococcus intermedius* (dog - resident status is controversial); *Clostridium* spp. (dog - abundant but not clear that these are true residents).
Transient	**Dog and Cat:** *Escherichia coli*; *Proteus mirabilis*; *Pseudomonas* spp.; *Bacillus* spp. **Cat:** *Alcaligenes* spp.; ß-haemolytic streptococci; *Staphylococcus* spp.
Pathogenic	*Staphylococcus intermedius* is the major pathogen in the dog and, most likely, of the cat. *S. aureus* is occasionally pathogenic. A variety of oral anaerobes are responsible for subcutaneous abscesses, particularly in cats.

Table 15.3: Transient, resident and pathogenic bacterial species on the skin of dogs and cats.

(Adapted from Scott et al., 1995 and Harvey and Lloyd, 1995.)

impregnated with aural wax and/or inflammatory exudates. If ear mites are suspected it may be advantageous to dampen the tip of the swab with a little liquid paraffin. A sterile plastic otic cone may be used to cut down contamination when culture samples are being collected.

The material may be smeared on to a glass slide for direct examination for mites, stained for cytological examination (see Chapter 7), or submitted for bacterial culture and antibiotic sensitivity testing.

SKIN BIOPSY

The taking of cutaneous punch biopsies for histopathological examination by a competent dermatohistopathologist is an extremely useful adjunct to dermatological diagnosis. However, the success of this diagnostic procedure depends upon several important points, some of which are under the control of the clinician and some of which are not (Dunstan, 1990).

Precautions

Select the biopsy sites carefully
Nothing is as important as the selection of the biopsy sites. The histological diagnosis of the lesions is highly dependent upon the selection of appropriate lesions, typically a primary lesion. If a secondary lesion is selected, such as a heavily ulcerated lesion, the diagnostic benefit from the histological examination of that tissue sample will be limited. A clinician must be able to identify primary lesions from which to select appropriate sites for biopsy (Figure 15.11).

Take multiple skin biopsies
Whenever possible, it is important to take several skin biopsies representing the range of clinical lesions present. Very often, only one of these several biopsies will demonstrate a diagnostic histological

lesion. It is important to take lesions at different stages of their evolution. It is also important, in the case of larger lesions to take biopsies from the centre as well as from the periphery.

Preserve the surface of the lesion
It is crucial that the biopsy site is not surgically prepared as this destroys much of the surface of the lesion, in which there may be important diagnostic clues for the pathologist. The presence of large numbers of acantholytic cells in surface crust, over a ruptured pemphigus foliaceus pustule, is just one example.

Be very careful not to crush or squeeze the biopsy
The technique described below is designed to minimize the chance of causing crush artefact. As Dunstan (1990) states, 'Diagnostic dermatopathology is as much an art as a science. To perform it well, the pathologist must collate a variety of patterns and colors into a diagnosis. Anything that causes artefactual alteration of these colours and patterns will greatly hinder histologic assessment.'

Do not let samples desiccate
For the same reason, it is important not to let samples dry out. Biopsy samples should be placed immediately into the formalin fixative. Surgery lights are extremely

Primary lesions		
Macule	Vesicle	Nodule
Papule	Wheal	Tumour
Pustule	Plaque	Cyst

Secondary lesions		
Scale	Erosion	Hyper/Hypopigmentation
Crust	Ulcer	Comedone
Scar	Excoriation	Lichenification

Figure 15.11: Primary and secondary lesions in dermatology.

dehydrating and samples left on gauze swabs will rapidly develop significant artefacts. This error is most likely to happen when taking multiple biopsies, and especially if samples are small punches.

Use generous volumes of buffered formalin and allow sufficient time for fixation

To avoid various artefactual changes (e.g. formalin pigment contamination, poor fixation) it is important to use fresh buffered formalin for sample submission. It is good practice to discard any unused formalin bottles that have been on the clinic shelf for more than 12 months. Artefact resulting from inadequate fixation due to insufficient fixative is seldom a problem with punch biopsies. It is easy to maintain the recommended ratio of fixative to sample volume of at least 10:1. Poor fixation may be a problem when large tumours are squeezed into small submission bottles (see Chapter 1).

Provide a summary of the clinical history, the clinical signs (including a diagram of the anatomic distribution of lesions), the treatments and response and a list of differential diagnoses or rule-outs

The pathologist requires, at the very least, a complete history and a list of rule-outs or differential diagnoses on the submission form. The clinician should indicate clearly the salient clinical findings associated with the biopsy and outline any treatments and their effect. Diagrams showing the location and extent of the lesions and the sites of the biopsies are very useful. Some clinicians simply submit a photocopy of the animal's entire case record – which in some instances may be pages long. While this can be helpful in some cases, most pathologists prefer to read the clinician's précis of the case.

Communication between the clinician and pathologist is the key

The importance of communication between the clinician and his or her routine pathologist cannot be overestimated. It has been said that if a clinician is not on a first name basis with his or her pathologist then they should consider changing to another pathologist.

If the pathologist's report does not fit well with the clinical signs, a telephone call to discuss the case will often yield further insights. A diligent pathologist will contact the submitting clinician when the histological findings appear to be at odds with the clinical history. A repeat biopsy at a later date may be recommended. It is only through this type of interchange that the maximum benefit from skin punch biopsy can be obtained.

Technique

Types of skin biopsy

There are two types of skin biopsy technique:

- Excisional or wedge biopsies
- Punch biopsies.

Excisional (or wedge) biopsies are indicated: for large solitary lesions, particularly if neoplasia is suspected; for lesions that may be destroyed by the shearing action of the biopsy punch, such as fragile vesicles or bullae; and in diseases of the panniculus, which are usually inadequately sampled by punch techniques.

The punch biopsy procedure is used more frequently, as it is simpler to perform and is ideal for multiple biopsies, and for biopsies from delicate sites, such as beside the eye.

Anaesthesia

Most punch biopsies are taken under local anaesthetic, unless the area is a particularly tender one, such as the nasal planum or footpad, or the animal is extremely fractious. The local anaesthetic, generally 2% lidocaine, is carefully injected into the subcutaneous tissue using a fine-gauge needle. Too shallow an administration of local anaesthetic can cause microscopic artefact in the dermis. The inclusion of adrenalin has been associated with histological artefact and is not recommended (Henfrey et al., 1991).

Surface preparation

The hair may be clipped away from the biopsy site carefully with scissors, but the site should not be shaved or surgically prepared. If antisepsis is required, 70% alcohol may be gently applied. Scrubbing is definitely contraindicated.

Skin punch biopsy technique

The instruments used for skin punch biopsy are illustrated in Figure 15.12. Skin punches are available in a range of sizes, from 3 mm to 8 mm in diameter. Most veterinary dermatologists prefer to use 6 mm punches. Exceptions are for areas in which the larger punch would be too destructive, such as nasal planum, ear margins or footpad. Here, a 3 mm punch is advisable. Very small primary lesions constitute another

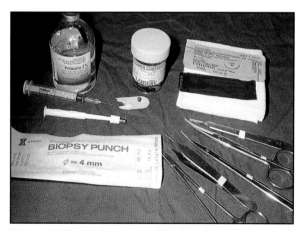

Figure 15.12: Equipment used in the taking of skin punch biopsies.

exception. Because the pathologist will automatically hemisection a punch biopsy, there is more chance that a small lesion may be missed in trimming. It is preferable to position a small vesicle, papule or pustule in the centre of a 3 or 4mm punch to ensure that it appears on the pathologist's slide.

The lesion should be centred in the punch field and the skin severed with a rotating movement. The punch is advanced, using gentle rotational force, into the subcutis. Some dermatologists choose a back-and-forth movement, others continue rotating in the same direction. It is important not to twist the punch too hard, as the shearing force on the tissues may cause tissue deformation and may lead to confusing artefact.

The small plug of loosened tissue is then gently removed. There are two methods, depending on the nature of the lesion sampled. In lesions that are not fixed to the subcutis, the biopsy can be popped up above the surface of the skin by applying gentle pressure to the panniculus beneath the punch (Figure 15.13). A needle point applied to the deep margin of the biopsy specimen will tease it from the attachments, which can be completely severed by sharp fine scissors. In lesions that are fixed to the subcutis, the biopsy sample is speared with a needle point just beneath the epidermis and lifted so that the attachments may be severed with sharp scissors . Mosquito haemostats or very fine forceps may be applied if necessary, but extreme care should be taken not to crush the tissue.

A single suture is usually sufficient to close the biopsy site created by a 6 mm punch. Larger incisions may be closed with simple interrupted sutures.

Sample submission
The biopsy samples should be immersed immediately in 10% neutral buffered formalin and submitted to the pathologist of choice with a form giving a detailed history and list of differential diagnoses or clinical rule-outs. Many pathologists suggest that punch biopsy samples are placed upon a piece of cardboard or a tongue depressor to stop the sample from curling and to prevent epidermal distortion. To be effective, the

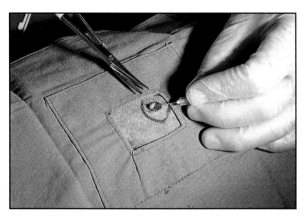

Figure 15.13: Using a needle, the skin sample is gently teased free of its attachments. The biopsy sample should never be grasped with forceps, as this leads to damaging artefact.

sample must be gently flattened so that it adheres to the cardboard or wooden surface before it is immersed in the formalin. Too often, the samples immediately separate from the cardboard surface, negating the value of the procedure. This procedure offers no advantage if samples are larger than 6 mm, as they do not usually curl.

A problem peculiar to cold climates such as in Canada and northern USA, is the freezing of samples during transit in the mail. This may be avoided by including 10% by volume 95% ethyl alcohol to the formalin.

It is usual to place multiple biopsies in a single container of formalin. In most laboratories, multiple skin biopsies are processed into one tissue block. If it is critical for individual biopsies to be identified with the location, it may be necessary to submit each biopsy in a separate bottle of formalin and to indicate clearly on the submission form that each tissue is to be processed into a separate block. This is particularly important when the clinical lesions are very different from biopsy site to biopsy site.

It is important that the clinician submits the punch biopsy sample in its entirety and does not attempt to section it prior to fixation. The only exception to this rule is when submitting very large samples (greater than 2–3 cm in any dimension) which will not fix properly. Large excisional biopsies should be incised deeply to facilitate the penetration of the formalin fixative.

The samples are trimmed after fixation is complete. Generally speaking, punch biopsy samples are hemisectioned in a sagittal plane. This allows full visualization of the hair follicles and enables accurate assessment of the hair growth cycle. In some instances it may be necessary to section the block horizontally, a process that is more commonly used in research, but which is used by some veterinary pathologists in the assessment of sebaceous adenitis.

Interpretation
The pathologist's report should include:

- A detailed histological description of the lesions in the biopsy submitted
- A morphological diagnosis, usually with a list of 'consistent' clinical diagnoses
- A definitive aetiological diagnosis (rare)
- Comment (the most useful part of the report).

Pattern analysis
Pattern analysis is the method by which dermato-histopathologists practise their art. Dermatological lesions have been mapped into nine pattern categories, which reflect basic pathological processes in the skin and subcutis (Table 15.4). Sometimes these patterns correlate with specific diseases: more often they

Pattern name	Diagnostic utility	Some associated diseases
Perivascular dermatitis	Low – poor discriminating power; often accompanies other more powerful patterns	Many and varied – this pattern reflects the 'dermatitis reaction'; it is therefore present to some extent in most skin biopsies. Eosinophilic perivascular dermatitis is the lesion of many allergic skin diseases
Interface dermatitis	High	Immune-mediated disorders including lupus erythematosus and drug eruptions, poorly understood 'lichenoid' diseases. Cell-poor interface dermatitis occurs in the genodermatosis of Collies and Shetland Sheepdogs known as dermatomyositis
Vasculitis	High	Immune-mediated diseases, drug eruptions and rare infectious diseases of blood vessels, e.g. Rocky Mountain spotted fever. Vasculitis of German Shepherd Dogs, Scottish Terriers, etc.
Intraepidermal vesiculopustular dermatitis	High	Bacterial skin disease; immune-mediated disorders such as pemphigus foliaceus; drug eruptions; some parasitic disease (here the pustules are eosinophilic); some fungal infections; idiopathic sterile eosinophilic diseases
Subepidermal vesiculopustular dermatitis	Intermediate – because the pattern can develop as a consequence of severe dermal oedema from many causes	Classic lesion of the rare immune-mediated disease bullous pemphigoid; epidermolysis bullosa-type genodermatoses; also seen secondary to vasculitis and following severe dermal oedema
Nodular to diffuse dermatitis	High – when an infectious agent or foreign body is demonstrated Intermediate in sterile diseases	The most common manifestation of this pattern is secondary to folliculitis and furunculosis in the dog. Infectious diseases of bacterial, mycotic and some protozoal aetiologies. Various poorly understood 'sterile' nodular diseases, such as sterile pyogranuloma syndrome
Folliculitis, furunculosis and sebaceous adenitis	High	Bacterial, fungal and parasitic diseases of the hair follicle. Some poorly understood sterile diseases such as eosinophilic furunculosis of the face (allergic reaction to insects?). Sebaceous adenitis is a genodermatosis of Standard Poodles
Panniculitis	High – if an infectious agent is present Intermediate in sterile forms	Many of the agents causing nodular to diffuse lesions also cause panniculitis. Some are more specifically targeted to the panniculus, e.g. nodular panniculitis; vaccine-associated lesions
Atrophic	Intermediate to low	Endocrinopathies, e.g. Cushing's disease (usually not hypothyroidism). Poorly understood follicular dystrophies. Metabolic disorders, e.g. cancer-associated alopecia in cats. Traction alopecia. Some genodermatoses – dermatomyositis

Table 15.4: Pattern analysis of inflammatory skin disease.

reflect the end stage of several pathogenic pathways. The patterns are not diagnoses *per se*, but they do narrow the diagnostic choices. Pattern analysis is not a perfect system but it is infinitely preferable to the alternative – 'non-specific dermatitis'. Learning the pattern classifications used routinely by dermatohistopathologists and understanding how they relate to clinical disease is now necessary for any veterinarian practicing dermatology. There are several recent textbooks published on this subject (e.g. Gross *et al.*, 1992; Yager and Wilcock, 1994).

Diagnosis

A definitive, aetiological diagnosis is seldom possible from skin biopsy alone when no aetiological agent is present or when the lesions are not pathognomonic for a particular disease. Exceptions, such as cases of demodectic pododermatitis, are always very welcome to dermatopathologists. The pathologist will indicate those diseases with which the biopsy lesions are compatible, often using the term 'consistent with'. Such diagnoses have been somewhat aptly named 'pathohedges' (Dunstan, 1990) and have been known to cause clinicians to gnash their teeth. As our knowledge of the pathogenesis and aetiology of veterinary skin diseases grows, the necessity for pathohedges will diminish but they are unlikely to disappear. The skin has only a limited repertoire of reactions to injury; different insults will produce morphologically similar lesions. Sorting out the pathogenesis and aetiology of these diseases awaits the application of modern molecular biological techniques, such as *in situ* hybridization and the polymerase chain reaction (PCR), to diagnostic biopsy samples.

Special stains may be very useful in the diagnosis of fungal infections, bacterial diseases and for the identification of abnormal products (such as amyloid) within the skin. Special stains such as periodic acid–Schiff or methenamine Gomori silver are used to diagnose fungal infections. In many instances, routine haematoxylin and eosin (H & E) staining will detect fungi but there are some infections, particularly those by *Trichophyton terrestrae* and *Microsporum persicolor*, in which the fungi are very difficult to see with H & E staining but can be detected by special stains. Special stains are also used to detect bacteria in granulomatous and pyogranulomatous diseases such as those caused by *Mycobacterium* spp. Most pathologists do not routinely perform special stains for *Staphylococcus intermedius* in cases of canine pyoderma. Special stains are not, however, a panacea. The majority of special stains produce no reaction, particularly those performed on cutaneous granulomatous lesions in the skin of dogs. Anticipation of a negative result should not, however, deter the pathologist from using these stains.

Comment

The most useful part of the pathology report is often the 'comment', which will discuss the list of differential diagnoses provided by the clinician and indicate in what ways the histological lesions may confirm or rule out these particular clinical conditions. In the comment, the pathologist may suggest additional tests to confirm a diagnosis suggested by the biopsy sample.

If the pathologist has any concerns about the case, he or she should contact the practitioner; conversely if the practitioner receives a biopsy report and diagnosis which does not fit with the clinical condition, it is generally very helpful to discuss the case further with the pathologist. Sometimes additional biopsies may be required; in other instances the pathologist may reassess the slides, take deeper sections, perform special stains or seek additional opinions. A good pathologist does not shy away from seeking second opinions. It is important to remember that the pathologist is working with 5–6 μm thin slices of tissue, representing only a merest glimpse of the disease process.

Ultimately, the diagnosis is made by the clinician and not by the pathologist.

To obtain the maximum benefit from skin biopsy remember that lesion selection is paramount and that communication between pathologist and clinician markedly increase the diagnostic benefit.

REFERENCES AND FURTHER READING

Bond R, Collin NS and Lloyd DH (1994) Use of contact plates for the quantitative culture of *Malassezia pachydermatis* from canine skin. *Journal of Small Animal Practice* **35**, 68–72

Bond R, Lloyd DH and Plummer JM (1995a) Evaluation of a detergent scrub technique for the quantitation of *M. pachydermatis* on canine skin. *Research in Veterinary Science* **58**, 133–137

Bond R, Rose JF, Ellis JW and Lloyd DH (1995b) Comparison of two shampoos for treatment of *Malassezia pachydermatis*-associated seborrhoeic dermatitis in basset hounds. *Journal of Small Animal Practice* **36**, 99–104

Bond R, Saijonmaa-Koulumies LEM and Lloyd DH (1995c) Population sizes and frequency of *Malassezia pachydermatis* at skin and mucosal sites on healthy dogs. *Journal of Small Animal Practice* **36**, 147–150

Chen C (1995) A short-tailed demodectic mite and *Demodex canis* infestation in a Chihuahua dog. *Veterinary Dermatology* **6**, 227–229

Dunstan RW (1990) A user's guide to veterinary surgical pathology laboratories. Or why do I still get a diagnosis of chronic dermatitis even when I take a perfect biopsy? *Veterinary Clinics of North America, Small Animal Practice* **20**, 1397–1417

Gross TL, Ihrke PJ and Walder EJ (1992) *Veterinary Dermatopathology. A Macroscopic and Microscopic Evaluation of Canine and Feline Skin Disease.* Mosby-Year Book, St Louis

Harvey RG and Lloyd DH (1995) The distribution of bacteria (other than staphylococci and *Proprionobacterium acnes*) on the hair and at the skin surface and within hair follicles of dogs. *Veterinary Dermatology* **6**, 79–84

Henfrey JI, Thoday KL and Head KW (1991) A comparison of three local anaesthetic techniques for skin biopsy in dogs. *Veterinary Dermatology* **2**, 21–27

Miller WH (1990) Color dilution alopecia in Doberman pinschers with blue or fawn coat colors: a study in the incidence and histopathology of this disorder. *Veterinary Dermatology* **1,** 113–122

Moriello KA (1990) Management of dermatophyte infections in catteries and multiple cat households. *Veterinary Clinics of North America, Small Animal Practice* **20,**1457–1474

Moriello KA and De Boer DJ (1995) Feline dermatophytosis. Recent advances and recommendations for therapy. *Veterinary Clinics of North America, Small Animal Practice* **25,** 901–921

Noxon JO (1995) Diagnostic procedures in feline dermatology. *Veterinary Clinics of North America, Small Animal Practice* **25,** 779–799

Scott DW, Miller WH and Griffin CE (1995) Laboratory procedures. In: *Small Animal Dermatology, 5th edn,* ed. DW Scott *et al.,* pp.94–118. WB Saunders, Philadelphia

Sparkes AH, Werrett G, Stokes CR and Gruffydd-Jones TJ (1994) Fluorescence microscopy with calcofluor white - improved sensitivity in the diagnosis of dermatophytosis. *Veterinary Record* **134,** 307–308

Wilkinson GT and Harvey RG (1994) Diagnostic tests and clinical pathology. In: *Color Atlas of Small Animal Dermatology. A Guide to Diagnosis, 2nd edn,* ed. GT Wilkinson and RG Harvey, pp. 33–52. Mosby-Wolfe, London

Yager JA and Wilcock BP (1994) *Color Atlas and Text of Surgical Pathology of the Dog and Cat. Volume 1. Skin and Skin Tumors.* Mosby-Wolfe, London

CHAPTER SIXTEEN

Thyroid Function

Carmel T. Mooney

CHAPTER PLAN

Introduction

Physiology of the thyroid gland

Basal thyroid hormone concentrations
   Total T4
   Total T3
   Free T4
   Free T3
   Reverse T3
   TSH

Tests of thyroid autoimmunity
   Antibodies to thyroglobulin
   Antibodies to T4 and T3

Dynamic thyroid function tests
   TSH stimulation test
   TRH stimulation test
   T3 suppression test

Summary

References and further reading

GLOSSARY

ALKP	Alkaline phosphatase
ALT	Alanine aminotransferase
AST	Aspartate aminotransferase
ELISA	Enzyme-linked immunosorbent assay
HDL	High-density lipoprotein
LDH	Lactate dehydrogenase
RIA	Radioimmunoassay
T3	L-Triiodothyronine
T4	L-Thyroxine
TBG	Thyroxine-binding globulin
TBPA	Thyroxine-binding prealbumin
TRH	Thyrotropin releasing hormone
TSH	Thyroid stimulating hormone (thyrotropin)

INTRODUCTION

Hypothyroidism and hyperthyroidism are the most common endocrine disorders of the dog and cat, respectively. In dogs, hypothyroidism is associated with vague and often non-specific clinical signs. Most cases exhibit some degree of mental dullness, lethargy and inactivity. Dermatological changes are common, including bilaterally symmetrical or asymmetrical alopecia and a dry brittle haircoat that is easily epilated (Figure 16.1). A variety of other clinical signs have been described and include bradycardia, peripheral neuropathies, reproductive abnormalities and constipation. Hyperthyroidism in cats is commonly associated with weight loss despite a normal or increased appetite, polyuria/polydipsia, hyperactivity and intermittent gastrointestinal signs of vomiting and/ or diarrhoea (Figure 16.2). Common findings on physical examination include cardiovascular abnormalities (tachycardia, murmurs) and palpable goitre.

Routine haematological and biochemical investigations are useful in providing both supportive evidence of hypo- or hyperthyroidism and eliminating other possible diagnoses in individual cases (Tables 16.1 and 16.2). Confirmation of the diagnosis requires

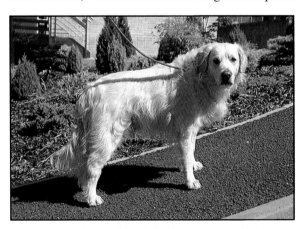

Figure 16.1: A 9-year-old male Golden Retriever exhibiting weight gain, poor haircoat and lethargy. Laboratory abnormalities included a mild anaemia, hypercholesterolaemia (11.4 mmol/l; reference range 2.0–7.0 mmol/l) and low serum total T4 (6.4 nmol/l; reference range 15–50 nmol/l). Serum total T4 concentrations did not respond to exogenous TSH administration, confirming a diagnosis of hypothyroidism.

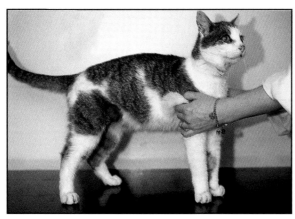

Figure 16.2: An 8-year-old female Domestic Shorthair cat with evidence of weight loss. A small goitre was palpable on physical examination. Serum total T4 concentration was elevated, at 74.2 nmol/l (reference range 8.5–46.2 nmol/l), confirming a diagnosis of hyperthyroidism. Serum total T3 concentration (0.72 nmol/l) remained within the reference range (0.13–1.27 nmol/l).

Abnormality	% of cases affected
Erythrocytosis	50
Macrocytosis	20
Increased ALT/ALKP/AST/LDH	90
Increased urea and creatinine	20–40
Hyperphosphataemia	10–20

Table 16.2. Haematological and biochemical abnormalities in feline hyperthyroidism.

Abnormality	% of cases affected
Mild normochromic/ normocytic anaemia	25–50
Hypercholesterolaemia	75
Hypertriglyceridaemia	30–50
Mild increase in creatine kinase	< 20
Mild increase in ALT/ALKP/LDH/AST	Occasional

Table 16.1: Haematological and biochemical abnormalities in canine hypothyroidism.

some evaluation of thyroid function, for which numerous tests have been recommended. Selection of the most appropriate test and subsequent interpretation depends on a knowledge of thyroid pathophysiology and the effects of non-thyroidal factors.

PHYSIOLOGY OF THE THYROID GLAND

Thyroxine (T4) is the main secretory product of the thyroid gland but 3,5,3'-triiodothyronine (T3), as well as small amounts of 3,3',5'-triiodothyronine (reverse T3 (rT3)), an inactive product, are also secreted. Approximately 60% of circulating T3 is produced by extrathyroidal enzymatic 5'-deiodination of T4. T3 is three to five times more potent than T4 and, although T4 possesses intrinsic metabolic activity it is considered a prohormone with activation to T3, a step which is autoregulated individually by peripheral tissues. Approximately 90% of circulating rT3 is produced by extrathyroidal 5-deiodination of T4.

In dogs, circulating T4 is bound to thyroxine-binding globulin (TBG) and to a lesser extent to thyroxine-binding prealbumin (TBPA), albumin, a high-density lipoprotein (HDL$_2$) and a very low-density lipoprotein. Cats depend on albumin and TBPA. Over 99% of circulating T4 is protein-bound in both species. The free fraction (approximately 0.1%) is metabolically active, while the bound fraction acts to buffer hormone delivery to target tissues. Most circulating T3 is also protein-bound while approximately 1% is free.

Overall control of thyroid function is mediated via negative feedback (Figure 16.3). The hypothalamus secretes thyrotropin releasing hormone (TRH) into the hypophyseal portal system and this acts on the anterior pituitary promoting the synthesis and secretion of thyrotropin (thyroid stimulating hormone, TSH). TSH acts on the thyroid cells, promoting iodide trapping and synthesis and release of thyroid hormone. The presence of excessive circulating free T4 and T3 produces a negative feedback on the anterior pituitary, which serves to decrease TSH synthesis and release and, subsequently, thyroid hormone production.

BASAL THYROID HORMONE CONCENTRATIONS

Total T4
Radioimmunoassay (RIA) is the preferred laboratory method for determining serum total T4 concentration but because of the radioisotope component RIAs are usually only used by commercial laboratories. Kits designed for use with human serum must be modified to allow for the measurement of the lower circulating total T4 concentrations in dogs and cats, and validated to compensate for differences in serum protein binding. Non-isotopic methods should be correlated with results of RIA before widespread use. Reference ranges for serum total T4 concentrations in dogs and cats vary between laboratories but generally fall between 10–15 (bottom) and 45–65 (top) nmol/l.

Sample collection
Plasma or serum can be used but serum decreases the risk of fibrin interference in the assay and is therefore

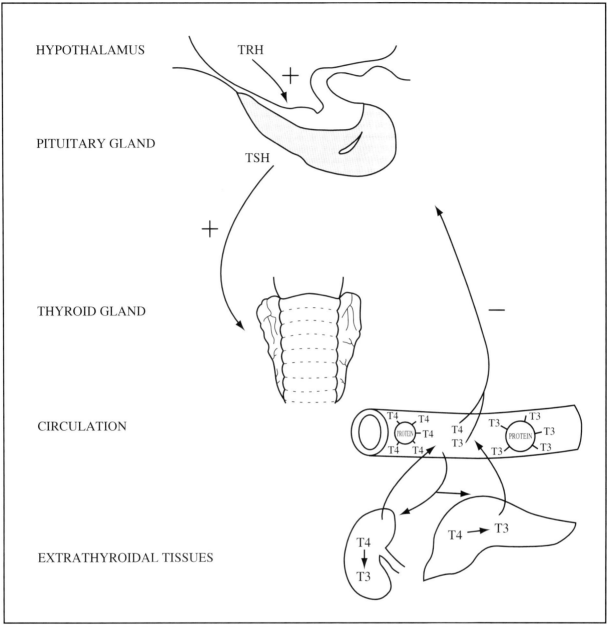

Figure 16.3: *The hypothalamic-pituitary-thyroid-extrathyroid axis, demonstrating the interaction between the various factors controlling thyroid function.*

+, stimulation; –, inhibition

preferred. Total T4 is stable in whole and clotted blood for up to 72 hours, or in serum for up to 8 days at room temperature and is unaffected by haemolysis, lipaemia, up to eight freeze–thaw cycles or fasting for 36 hours. There is no recommended time of day for sampling. A circadian rhythm does not occur but fluctuations in and out of the reference range have been reported (Miller *et al.*, 1992).

Effects of age, sex and breed
In the dog, normal serum total T4 concentrations are two to five times higher in the first 3 months of life and decrease significantly from adult values into old age (Reimers *et al.*, 1990; Casal *et al.*, 1994). In newborn kittens, serum total T4 concentrations are approxi-

mately half that of the mother, doubling within 2 weeks and reaching 62 ± 10 nmol/l by 4 weeks of age (Jones, 1997). In the adult cat, concentrations decrease in a non-linear manner until approximately 5 years of age and then increase again (Thoday *et al.*, 1984).

Male and female dogs have similar concentrations although with selection for specific reproductive states, serum total T4 concentrations are highest in dioestrus and in pregnant bitches (Reimers *et al.*, 1990). Female and neutered female cats have higher serum total T4 concentrations than males and neutered males (Thoday *et al.*, 1984).

Serum total T4 concentrations are higher in small than in medium and large-breed dogs, but breed has no

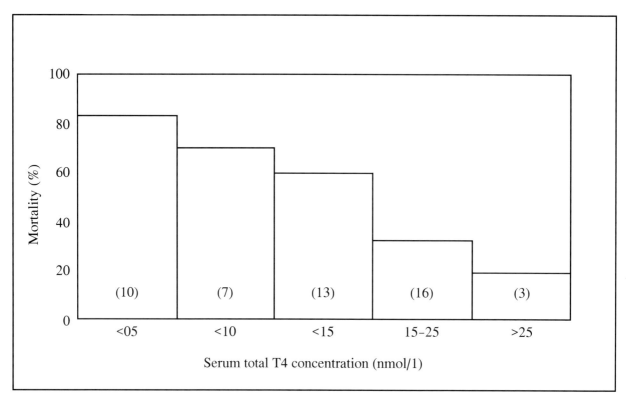

Figure 16.4: *The relationship of mortality to serum total T4 concentrations in 107 cats with a variety of non-thyroidal illnesses. The number of cats that died or were euthanased in each group is depicted in parentheses. Most cases died or were euthanased at initial presentation, on hospitalization or shortly afterwards.*

apparent effect in the cat (Thoday *et al.*, 1984; Reimers *et al.*, 1990). An increase in serum total T4 concentrations has been reported in obese dogs, presumably resulting from excessive caloric intake.

Effect of non-thyroidal illness

In human beings, a variety of acute and severe illnesses have a profound effect on circulating total T4 concentrations in the absence of intrinsic thyroid disease. This phenomenon appears to be a common response to illness in dogs and cats and is referred to as 'the euthyroid sick syndrome'. In the dog, hyperadrenocorticism, diabetes mellitus, hypoadrenocorticism, chronic renal failure, congestive cardiac disease, hepatic disease, diseases associated with cachexia, dermatological conditions and critical conditions requiring intensive care have all been implicated in the euthyroid sick syndrome (Peterson *et al.*, 1984; Peterson and Ferguson, 1989; Chastain and Panciera, 1995). In practice, any illness should be considered capable of such an effect. In cats, suppression of total T4 is related more to the severity of the illness than the disease process itself and T4 concentration is significantly inversely correlated with mortality, rendering its measurement useful as a prognostic indicator (Peterson and Gamble, 1990; Mooney *et al.*, 1996a) (Figure 16.4). Possible mechanisms involved include alterations in protein binding, hormone metabolism and, particularly in hyperadrenocorticism, inhibition of pituitary TSH

release. Affected animals are *not* hypothyroid; thyroxine therapy is not beneficial and may be detrimental for normalization of thyroid function during recovery.

Effect of drug therapy

A variety of drugs depress serum total T4 concentrations, including glucocorticoids, non-steroidal anti-inflammatory drugs (salicylates, flunixin and phenylbutazone), anticonvulsants (phenobarbital and phenytoin), anabolic steroids, sulphonamides and certain anaesthetic agents (Peterson and Ferguson, 1989; Chastain and Panciera, 1995). Other drugs increase or decrease serum total T4 concentrations in human beings, but many have not yet been evaluated in dogs or cats. The potential for interference should always be considered and, if possible, the drug should be withdrawn at least 6 weeks prior to testing.

Hypothyroidism

Serum total T4 concentrations are generally depressed in hypothyroid dogs. Unfortunately, because of the suppressive effects of non-thyroidal factors, a low serum total T4 concentration alone does not confirm a diagnosis (Figure 16.5). An extremely low value (<8 nmol/l), particularly in association with marked hypercholesterolaemia and a mild non-regenerative anaemia without evidence of non-thyroidal illness or a history of recent drug therapy, indicates a diagnosis of hypothyroidism (Panciera, 1994). Since such a combination of factors is rarely seen in practice, a serum total T4 estimation is more reliable in eliminating a diagnosis of hypothyroidism, because concentrations well within the reference range are rarely associated with this condition.

In congenitally hypothyroid cats, serum total T4 concentrations may be below or within the low end of the reference range. Depending on the underlying condition, concentrations may increase as the animal ages (Jones, 1997).

Hyperthyroidism

Serum total T4 concentrations are generally elevated in hyperthyroid cats and provide the most useful test for its diagnosis (Figure 16.5). A value that exceeds three standard deviations from the reference mean has been suggested to differentiate hyperthyroid cats from the small number of healthy individuals with values above the reference range (Thoday and Mooney, 1992). In a few hyperthyroid cats, serum total T4 concentrations may be in the mid-to-high end of the reference range because of early disease, hormone fluctuation or the suppressive effects of severe concurrent non-thyroidal disease (Peterson et al., 1987; Peterson and Gamble, 1990). In such cases, concentrations will increase into the diagnostic thyrotoxic range within 3-6 weeks or on recovery, or treatment of the concurrent disorder.

Serum total T4 concentrations will be elevated in rare cases of a hyperfunctioning thyroid tumour of the dog.

Monitoring thyroid hormone replacement therapy

Measurement of serum total T4 concentrations is valuable in ensuring adequate thyroid hormone replacement therapy. Samples should be evaluated 4-6 hours after tablet administration and concentrations should be within the higher end of the reference range at this time (Nachreiner and Refsal, 1992).

Monitoring treatment for hyperthyroidism

Serum total T4 concentrations may be below the reference range for weeks to months following treatment of hyperthyroid cats with radioactive iodine or by surgical thyroidectomy (Peterson et al., 1994b). Supplementation with thyroxine is unnecessary unless clinical signs of hypothyroidism are present. Values are also frequently low in hyperthyroid cats treated with carbimazole or methimazole (Mooney et al., 1992). Clinical signs of hypothyroidism do not occur, presumably because serum total T3 concentrations tend to remain within the reference range. Moderate to marked elevations in serum concentrations of the liver enzymes frequently occur in feline hyperthyroidism. Their progressive decline as euthyroidism is achieved provides a non-specific indicator of therapeutic efficacy.

Total T3

Circulating total T3 concentrations are often depressed in response to prolonged fasting, non-thyroidal illness or drug therapy and may fluctuate in and out of the reference range. Low serum total T3 concentrations are also frequently found in hypothyroid dogs but as for total T4, interpretation is complicated by the suppressive effects of the above factors. In addition, maintenance of reference range concentrations is a common response to early thyroid failure, presumably through increased T3 production and secretion by the thyroid gland and increased peripheral conversion from T4 (Panciera, 1994; Chastain and Panciera, 1995). Elevated serum total T3 concentrations are common in hyperthyroid cats but are more frequently within the reference range than serum total T4 concentrations (Thoday and Mooney, 1992). Thus, measurement of serum total T3 concentrations offers no advantages over serum total T4 estimations and is of limited value in investigating thyroid disease.

Free T4

Circulating free T4 concentrations are less affected by non-thyroidal illness and drug therapy and are therefore valuable in diagnosing hypothyroidism. Unfortunately, the validity of many free T4 assays, particularly analogue RIAs, has been seriously questioned and results probably reflect a proportion of the total hormone rather than a true free concentration (Ferguson, 1994). Reference ranges are often much lower than the constant average of 25 pmol/l reported for most vertebrate species. Where such assays have been used, serum free T4 concentrations have been found to be no better in assisting a diagnosis of hypothyroidism than a total T4

Decreased serum total T4
Hypothyroidism
Non-thyroidal illness
Drug therapy
Advanced age
Fluctuation
Anti-T4 antibodies
Treatment for hyperthyroidism (usually transient)

Increased serum total T4
Hyperthyroidism
Young age
Certain drugs
Anti-T4 antibodies

Figure 16.5: Factors associated with significantly decreased or increased serum total T4 concentrations in dogs and cats.

estimation (Nelson *et al.*, 1991). Equilibrium dialysis and ultrafiltration are the recommended standard techniques for measuring serum free T4 concentrations. Where such techniques have been used in dogs with non-thyroidal illness, serum free T4 concentrations tend to remain within the reference range when serum total T4 concentrations are depressed. Serum free T4 concentrations are, however, often depressed in dogs with hyperadrenocorticism and, therefore presumably those on long-term glucocorticoid therapy (Ferguson and Peterson, 1992).

There is a significant correlation between serum total and free T4 concentrations in hyperthyroid cats. However, in euthyroid cats with non-thyroidal illness, serum free T4 concentrations are occasionally elevated, particularly if serum total T4 concentrations remain within the reference range (Mooney *et al.*, 1996a). Thus, serum free T4 estimations are not recommended as the sole diagnostic test for confirmation of hyperthyroidism.

Free T3
Serum free T3 concentrations are depressed in non-thyroidal illness and are therefore unlikely to be helpful in the investigation of hypo- or hyperthyroidism.

Reverse T3
In human beings, serum concentrations of rT3 are increased in response to non-thyroidal illness but decreased in response to hypothyroidism. Unfortunately, in dogs non-thyroidal illness and fasting are associated with variable rT3 responses, including concentrations that are increased, decreased or unaffected (Ferguson and Peterson, 1992).

TSH
The potential value of serum TSH measurements for diagnosing hypothyroidism has long been speculated upon. A species-specific kit for measurement of canine TSH has recently become commercially available. In a study of 11 naturally occurring cases of hypothyroidism, 9 dogs had elevated serum TSH concentrations (> 0.6 ng/ml), while dogs with non-thyroidal illnesses had concentrations within the reported reference range (Dixon *et al.*, 1996). Unexpectedly lower values in hypothyroid dogs could result from secondary hypothyroidism, glucocorticoid excess, chronic stressful illnesses or non-specific hormone fluctuation. Inappropriately high TSH values can be found in euthyroid dogs, particularly if they are being treated with potentiated sulphonamide drugs or recovering from a non-thyroidal illness. A combination of serum total T4 and TSH measurements improves the sensitivity for diagnosing hypothyroidism. In human beings, the combination of TSH and free T4 measurements allows a diagnostic accuracy for

hypothyroidism of 100% and this may yet prove useful in the dog (Ferguson, 1994).

TESTS OF THYROID AUTOIMMUNITY

Primary hypothyroidism is the most common cause of naturally occurring thyroid failure in the dog, accounting for over 95% of cases. Immune-mediated destruction (lymphocytic thyroiditis) is considered to be an important mechanism and evidence for its presence may be obtained by measurement of circulating autoantibodies. (See also Chapter 6.)

Antibodies to thyroglobulin
Antibodies to thyroglobulin are often generated early in the course of lymphocytic thyroiditis and have been detected in approximately 50% of hypothyroid dogs using an ELISA. These antibodies should only be used as supportive evidence of hypothyroidism and its underlying cause. Antibody measurement may gain more widespread use as a possible predictor of impending hypothyroidism in susceptible breeds prior to embarking on a breeding programme (Chastain and Panciera, 1995).

Antibodies to T4 and T3
Anti-T4 and -T3 antibodies may also be produced during the course of lymphocytic thyroiditis. Interference with total T4 and T3 RIAs is possible with spuriously elevated or low concentrations, depending on the separation system used. Antibodies to T3 are more common but both occur most frequently in animals with circulating anti-thyroglobulin antibodies. Elevated serum total T4 or T3 concentrations should not be misinterpreted as hyperthyroidism in a dog suspected of hypothyroidism. The infrequent finding of a reference range serum total T4 concentration in a hypothyroid dog may result from anti-T4 antibodies (Chastain and Panciera, 1995). Extremely low or undetectable serum total T3 concentrations with reference range serum total T4 concentrations may also indicate the presence of anti-T3 antibodies (Ferguson, 1994). Antibodies to T3 and T4 can be measured directly by some laboratories or indirectly, by changing the assay system used.

DYNAMIC THYROID FUNCTION TESTS

Dynamic thyroid function tests confirm or refute a diagnosis of thyroid dysfunction. In cats they are only recommended for equivocal hyperthyroidism and are therefore rarely required, but they are frequently used to confirm hypothyroidism in dogs. If the endogenous canine TSH assay proves as valuable as suggested, it is likely that function tests will become obsolete. The most commonly used protocols are outlined in Table 16.3.

Test	Species	Dose	Route	Sampling times	Assay
TSH stimulation	Dog	0.1 iu/kg	Intravenous	0 and 6 hours	Total T4
	Cat	0.5 iu/kg	Intravenous	0 and 6 hours	Total T4
TRH stimulation	Dog	100 - 600 µg	Intravenous	0 and 4 hours	Total T4
	Cat	0.1 mg/kg	Intravenous	0 and 4 hours	Total T4
T3 suppression	Cat	20 µg 8-hourly for 7 doses	Oral	0 and 2–4 hours after last dose	Total T4, T3

Table 16.3: *Commonly used protocols for dynamic thyroid function tests.*

TSH stimulation test

Dogs

The administration of exogenous bovine TSH followed by measurement of serum total T4 concentrations is currently the definitive test for hypothyroidism. The total T3 response to TSH is of lower magnitude and greater variability and therefore of limited value (Sparkes *et al.*, 1995). Dogs with primary hypothyroidism show little or no response to TSH while in dogs with non-thyroidal illness or on drug therapy, the response parallels that in healthy dogs. Dogs with secondary hypothyroidism may respond to TSH administration (Feldman and Nelson, 1996). Interpretation should be based on the increment and absolute post-TSH total T4 concentration as supplied by each laboratory (e.g. a post-TSH concentration exceeding 23 nmol/l with an increment in excess of 1.5 x basal concentration). Calculation of formulae (e.g. $k = 0.5$ x pre-TSH + (difference in post-TSH and pre-TSH total T4 concentrations)) to confirm a diagnosis have not been found to improve diagnostic accuracy over the incremental and absolute response at 6 hours.

Bovine TSH is expensive, difficult to obtain, unlicensed and potentially antigenic, and therefore should be administered only once. If obtainable, reconstituted TSH can be stored at -20ºC for at least 200 days or at 4ºC for at least 3 weeks without loss of biological activity. The test can be performed concurrently with tests of adrenal function without significant effects on the results of either (Moriello *et al.*, 1987). For meaningful results, thyroxine therapy must be withheld for 4 weeks or longer before TSH stimulation testing is undertaken (Panciera *et al.*, 1989).

Cats

There is a lack of total T4 response after TSH administration in hyperthyroid cats. Recently, it has been shown that the response is negatively correlated with basal serum total T4 concentrations and as such is of limited diagnostic value (Mooney *et al.*, 1996b).

TRH stimulation test

Dogs

Given the problems with the TSH stimulation test, TRH has been recommended as a useful alternative. The higher doses of TRH are associated with frequent adverse reactions of salivation, elimination, miosis, tachycardia and tachypnoea (Ferguson, 1994). In addition, the serum total T4 response to TRH is of lower magnitude and greater variability than to TSH (Sparkes *et al.*, 1995). Thus, the test requires a T4 assay of high sensitivity and it is unclear if dogs with non-thyroidal illness or those on drug therapy can be adequately distinguished from hypothyroid dogs. A subnormal response to TRH stimulation in dogs with a normal response to TSH is indicative of secondary hypothyroidism (Feldman and Nelson, 1996).

Cats

There is a limited total T4 response to TRH in cats with hyperthyroidism compared to healthy cats and those with non-thyroidal illness (Peterson *et al.*, 1994a). Adverse reactions, including vomiting, salivation, tachypnoea and defecation are, however, common.

T3 suppression test

This test has been recommended to confirm a diagnosis of hyperthyroidism in equivocal cases (Peterson *et al.*, 1990; Refsal *et al.*, 1991). In euthyroid cats, there is marked suppression of T4 after T3 administration (usually to <20 nmol/l, representing a decrease of more than 50% from basal concentrations) while in hyperthyroid cats there is little or no suppression. Concomitant measurement of serum total T3 concentrations is recommended to ensure adequate administration and absorption of the drug, thereby increasing the expense of this test.

Summary

Figures 16.6 and 16.7 outline the procedures for using thyroid function tests in the diagnosis of canine hypothyroidism and feline hyperthyroidism.

REFERENCES AND FURTHER READING

Casal ML, Zerbe CA, Jezyk PF, Refsal KR and Nachreiner RF (1994) Thyroid profiles in healthy puppies from birth to 12 weeks of age. *Journal of Veterinary Internal Medicine* **8**, 158

Chastain CB and Panciera DL (1995) Hypothyroid diseases. In: *Textbook of Veterinary Internal Medicine, 4th edn*, ed. SJ Ettinger and EC Feldman, Vol 2. pp. 1487–1501. WB Saunders, Philadelphia

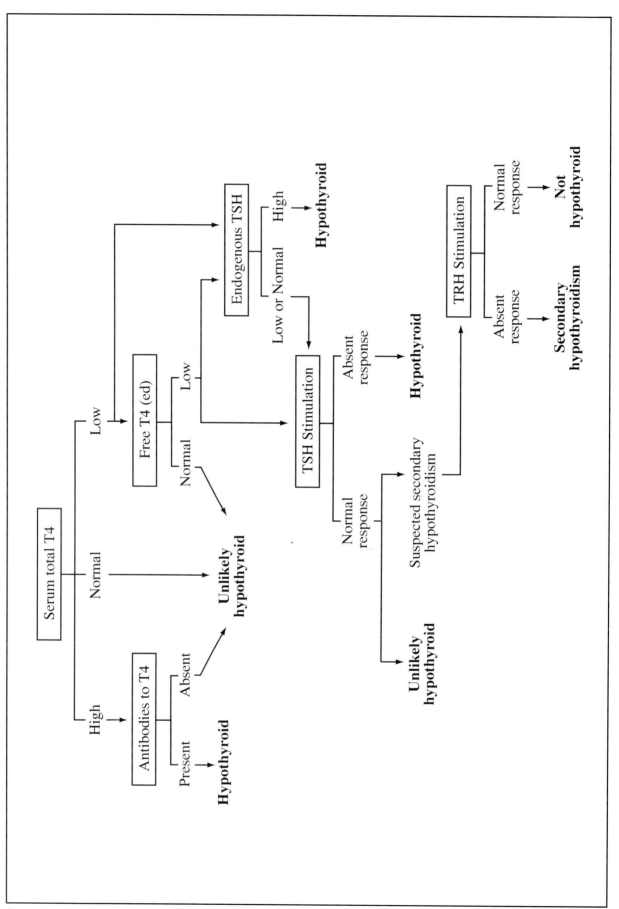

Figure 16.6: *Algorithm for using thyroid function tests in the diagnosis of canine hypothyroidism.*

T4, thyroxine; ed, equilibrium dialysis; TSH, thyroid stimulating hormone; TRH, thyrotropin releasing hormone

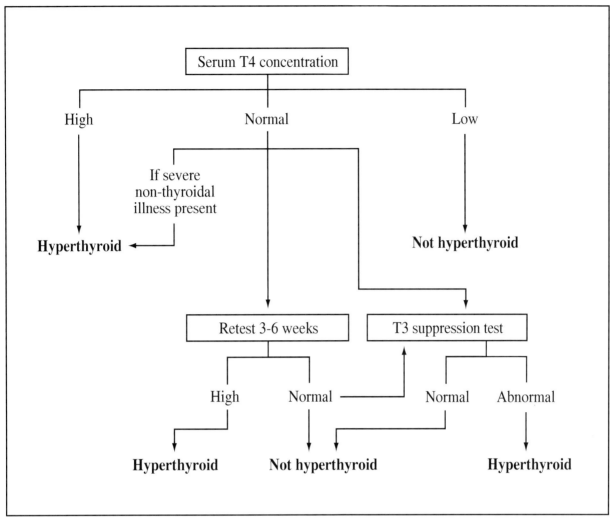

Figure 16.7: *Algorithm for using thyroid function tests in the diagnosis of feline hyperthyroidism.*

T4, thyroxine; T3, triiodothyronine

Dixon RM, Graham PA and Mooney CT (1996) Serum thyrotropin concentrations: a new diagnostic test for canine hypothyroidism. *Veterinary Record* **138,** 594-595

Feldman EC and Nelson RW (1996) The thyroid gland. In: *Canine and Feline Endocrinology and Reproduction, 2nd edn,* ed. EC Feldman and RW Nelson, pp 67-185 WB Saunders, Philadelphia

Ferguson DC (1994) Update on the diagnosis of canine hypothyroidism. *Veterinary Clinics of North America. Small Animal Practice* **24,** 515-539

Ferguson DC and Peterson ME (1992) Serum free and total iodothyronine concentrations in dogs with hyperadrenocorticism. *American Journal of Veterinary Research* **53,** 1636-1640

Jones BR (1998) Hypothyroidism in cats. In: *Manual of Small Animal Endocrinology, 2nd edn,* ed. A Torrance and CT Mooney. BSAVA Publications, Cheltenham (In preparation)

Miller AB, Nelson RW, Scott-Moncrieff JC, Neal L and Bottoms GD (1992) Serial thyroid hormone concentrations in healthy euthyroid dogs, dogs with hypothyroidism, and euthyroid dogs with atopic dermatitis. *British Veterinary Journal* **148,** 451-458

Mooney CT, Little CJL and Macrae AW (1996a) Effect of illness not associated with the thyroid gland on serum total and free T4 concentrations in cats. *Journal of the American Veterinary Medical Association* **208,** 2004-2008

Mooney CT, Thoday KL and Doxey DL (1992) Carbimazole therapy of feline hyperthyroidism. *Journal of Small Animal Practice* **33,** 228-235

Mooney CT, Thoday KL and Doxey DL (1996b) Serum thyroxine and triiodothyronine responses of hyperthyroid cats to thyrotropin. *American Journal of Veterinary Research* **57,** 987-991

Moriello KA, Halliwell REW and Oakes M (1987) Determination of thyroxine, triiodothyronine, and cortisol changes during simultaneous adrenal and thyroid function tests in healthy dogs. *American Journal of Veterinary Research* **48,** 458-462

Nachreiner RF and Refsal KR (1992) Radioimmunoassay monitoring of thyroid hormone concentrations in dogs on thyroid replacement therapy; 2,674 cases (1985-1987). *Journal of the American Veterinary Medical Association* **201,** 623-629

Nelson RW, Ihle SL, Feldman EC and Bottoms GD (1991) Serum free thyroxine concentration in healthy dogs, dogs with hypothyroidism, and euthyroid dogs with concurrent illness. *Journal of the American Veterinary Medical Association* **198,** 1401-1407

Panciera DL (1994) Hypothyroidism in dogs: 66 cases (1987-1992). *Journal of the American Veterinary Medical Association* **204,** 761-767

Panciera DL, MacEwan EG, Atkins CE, Bosu WTK, Refsal KR and Nachreiner RF (1989) Thyroid function tests in euthyroid dogs treated with L-thyroxine. *American Journal of Veterinary Research* **51,** 22-26

Peterson ME, Broussard JD and Gamble DA (1994a) Use of the thyrotropin releasing hormone stimulation test to diagnose mild hyperthyroidism in cats. *Journal of Veterinary Internal Medicine* **8,** 279-286

Peterson ME and Ferguson DC (1989) Thyroid diseases. In: *Textbook of Veterinary Internal Medicine: Diseases of the Dog and Cat, 3rd edn,* Vol 2. ed. SJ Ettinger, pp 1632-1675 WB Saunders, Philadelphia

Peterson ME, Ferguson DC, Kintzer PP and Drucker WD (1984) Effects of spontaneous hyperadrenocorticism on serum thyroid hormone concentrations in the dog. *American Journal of Veterinary Research* **45,** 2034-2038.

Peterson ME and Gamble DA (1990) Effect of nonthyroidal illness on serum thyroxine concentrations in cats: 494 cases (1988). *Journal of the American Veterinary Medical Association* **197,** 1203-1211.

Peterson ME, Graves TK and Cavanagh I (1987) Serum thyroid hormone concentrations fluctuate in cats with hyperthyroidism. *Journal of Veterinary Internal Medicine* **1,** 142-146.

Peterson ME, Graves TK and Gamble DA (1990) Triiodothyronine (T3) suppression test. An aid in the diagnosis of mild hyperthyroidism in cats. *Journal of Veterinary Internal Medicine* **4,** 233-238.

Peterson ME, Randolph JF and Mooney CT (1994b) Endocrine diseases. In: *The Cat. Diseases and Clinical Management, 2nd edn,* ed. RG Sherding, Vol. 2, pp 1403-1506 Churchill Livingstone, New York

Refsal KR, Nachreiner RF, Stein BE, Currigan CE, Zendel AN and Thacker EL (1991) Use of the triiodothyronine suppression test for diagnosis of hyperthyroidism in ill cats that have serum concentration of iodothyronines within normal range. *Journal of the American Veterinary Medical Association* **199,** 1594-1601

Reimers TJ, Lawler DF, Sutaria PM, Correa MT and Erb HN (1990) Effects of age, sex, and body size on serum concentrations of thyroid and adrenocortical hormones in dogs. *American Journal of Veterinary Research* **51,** 454-457

Sparkes AH, Gruffydd Jones TJ, Wotton PR, Gleadhill A, Evans H and Walker MJ (1995) Assessment of dose and time responses to TRH and thyrotropin in healthy dogs. *Journal of Small Animal Practice* **36,** 245-251

Thoday KL and Mooney CT (1992) Historical, clinical and laboratory features of 126 hyperthyroid cats. *Veterinary Record* **131,** 257-264

Thoday KL, Seth J and Elton RA (1984) Radioimmunoassay of serum total thyroxine and triiodothyronine in healthy cats: assay methodology and effects of age, sex, breed, heredity and environment. *Journal of Small Animal Practice* **25,** 457-472

CHAPTER SEVENTEEN

Pituitary and Adrenal Function

Michael E. Herrtage

PITUITARY FUNCTION TESTS

INTRODUCTION

The hypothalamus and pituitary form a complex functional unit that controls much of the endocrine system. The pituitary gland is a small ovoid structure that lies in a distinct fossa, the sella turcica, within the sphenoid bone just ventral to the hypothalamus. The pituitary consists of two functional and morphological parts which have separate origins: the anterior lobe of the pituitary, or adenohypophysis, develops from Rathke's pouch, which arises from the dorsal wall of the pharynx; the posterior lobe of the pituitary, or neurohypophysis, is a ventral extension of the hypothalamus.

The hypothalamus is important in the regulation of anterior and posterior pituitary function. The release of hormones from the anterior lobe of the pituitary is controlled by hypothalamic peptides which are transported to the anterior pituitary by the capillaries of the hypothalamic–hypophyseal portal circulation (Table 17.1). The hypothalamus contains a number of autonomic centres that control thirst, satiety, body temperature, emotional reactions and sympathetic nerve responses. It serves as an important link between the brain and the endocrine system.

The anterior lobe of the pituitary produces and releases a number of trophic hormones that control many of the endocrine glands (Figure 17.1) The anterior lobe consists of three components: the pars distalis, the pars intermedia and the pars tuberalis. Three cell types can be identified by special stains: acidophils, basophils and chromophobes. The acidophils include somatotrophs which secrete growth hormone (GH) and lactotrophs which secrete prolactin (PRL); basophils include gonadotrophs which secrete follicle-stimulating hormone (FSH) and luteinizing hormone (LH), and thyrotrophs which secrete thyroid-stimulating hormone (TSH); chromophobes include corticotrophs which secrete adrenocorticotrophic hormone (ACTH) and cells which secrete melanocyte-stimulating hormone (MSH). The actions of these hormones are summarized in Table 17.2.

In the case of those hormones that control a specific endocrine gland, for example the adrenal, there is a negative feedback mechanism whereby the hormone produced by the target gland affects the secretion of the relevant releasing factor from the hypothalamus and/or the trophic hormone from the anterior lobe of the pituitary (Figure 17.2).

In contrast, growth hormone, prolactin and MSH do not act through a target endocrine gland. Control of the release of these hormones is a balance of effects of

Anterior lobe hormone	Hypothalamic hormone (stimulatory)	Hypothalamic hormone (inhibitory)
TSH — thyroid-stimulating hormone	TRH — thyrotrophin releasing hormone	
ACTH — adrenocorticotrophic hormone	CRH — corticotrophin releasing hormone	
GH — growth hormone	GHRH — growth hormone releasing hormone (*somatocrinin*)	GHRIH — growth hormone release inhibitory hormone (*somatostatin*)
FSH — follicle-stimulating hormone	GnRH — gonadotrophin releasing hormone	
LH — luteinizing hormone	GnRH — gonadotrophin releasing hormone	
PRL — prolactin	PRH — prolactin releasing hormone	PRIH — prolactin release inhibitory hormone (*dopamine*)
MSH — melanocyte-stimulating hormone	MSHRH — MSH releasing hormone	MSH-RIH — MSH release inhibitory hormone

Table 17.1: *Hypothalamic control of hormone release from the anterior lobe of the pituitary.*

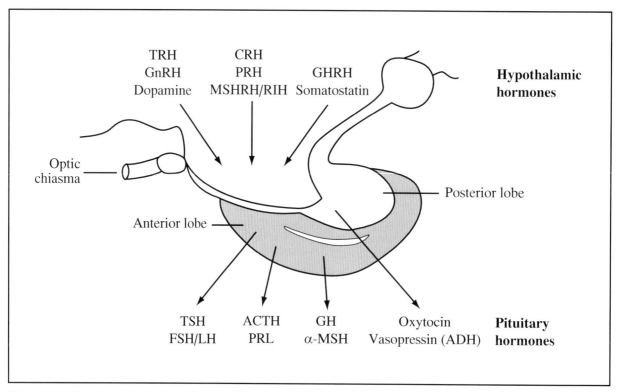

Figure 17.1: *Hypothalamic–pituitary physiology.*

Hormone	Action
TSH	Thyroid-stimulating hormone stimulates the biosynthesis of thyroid hormones and the release of thyroxine into the circulation
ACTH	Adrenocorticotrophic hormone maintains adrenocortical size and stimulates the adrenal to secrete glucocorticoids
GH	Growth hormone stimulates growth of the long bones provided the epiphyses are open. It also enhances protein anabolism and has marked anti-insulin activity. It is diabetogenic in adults
FSH	Follicle-stimulating hormone stimulates ovarian follicular growth and maturation in the female. In the male, it stimulates testicular growth and spermatogenesis along with testosterone
LH	Luteinizing hormone is required for ovulation and stimulates the formation of the corpus luteum. With FSH it stimulates maximum oestrogen secretion. In the male, LH (ICSH) stimulates the interstitial cells to produce testosterone
PRL	Prolactin, in conjunction with other hormones, induces mammary development and lactation. Prolactin also maintains lactation in the female. In the male it has a stimulatory effect on prostate growth
MSH	Melanocyte-stimulating hormone is produced primarily in the pars intermedia as part of the prohormone pro-opiomelanocortin (POMC). MSH controls melanin formation in the melanocytes of the epidermis

Table 17.2: *Actions of the hormones released from the anterior lobe of the pituitary.*

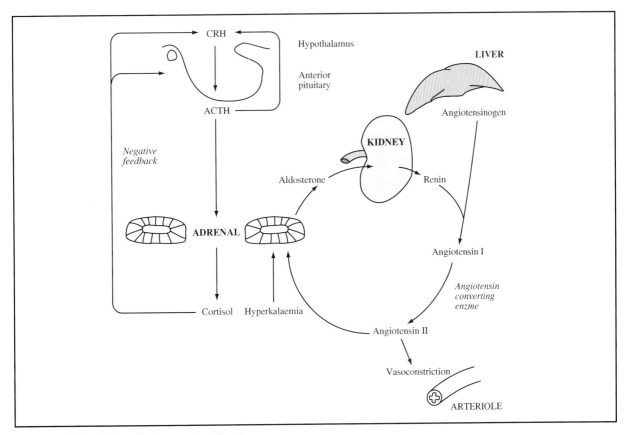

Figure 17.2: Regulation of adrenocortical function.

the relevant stimulatory and inhibitory factors produced by the hypothalamus on the anterior lobe of the pituitary (Figure 17.3).

ANTERIOR LOBE FUNCTION

Hypothalamic–pituitary–thyroid testing is dealt with in Chapter 16; hypothalamic–pituitary–adrenal testing is described below, under adrenocortical function tests. Gonadal function in small animals can be assessed by measuring progesterone, oestradiol and testosterone concentrations, although interpretation of the results can prove difficult (see Chapter 20). Assays for FSH and LH concentrations are not routinely available.

Conditions affecting growth hormone secretion are occasionally encountered in dogs and cats. Congenital hypopituitarism results in inadequate secretion of growth hormone with resultant retardation of growth (pituitary dwarfism) (Figure 17.4). This rare condition has been reported in a number of breeds of dog but is most commonly seen in German Shepherd Dogs, where it has been shown to be inherited as an autosomal recessive trait. Congenital hypopituitarism has also been reported in the cat.

Chronic hypersecretion of growth hormone in the adult results in acromegaly, an insidious condition associated with connective tissue and bone overgrowth. Acromegaly has been reported in the dog and cat, although the pathogenesis is different in the two spe-

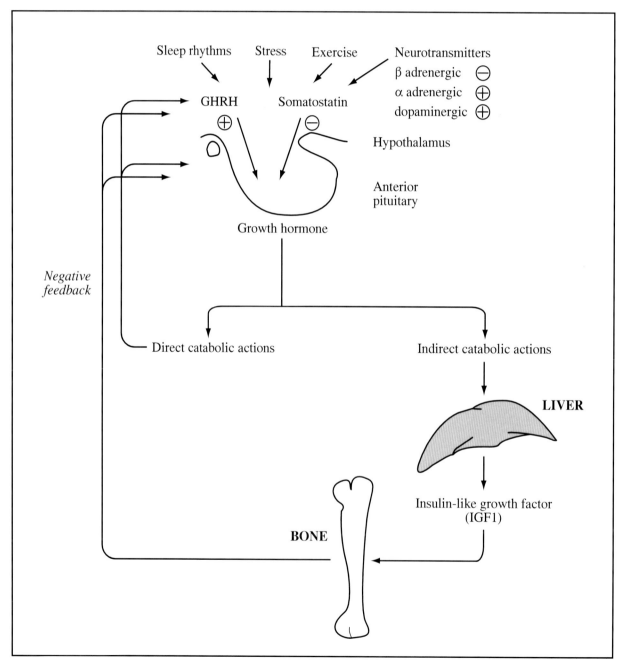

Figure 17.3: Regulation of growth hormone release.

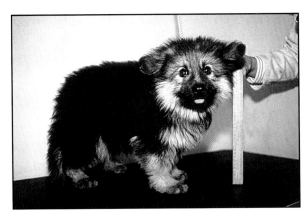

Figure 17.4: A 5-month old German Shepherd bitch with pituitary dwarfism.

cies. In the dog, acromegaly is caused by progestagen therapy or by endogenous progesterone produced during the metoestrus phase of the oestrous cycle. The progestin-induced growth hormone excess originates not from the pituitary, but from hyperplastic ductular epithelium in the mammary gland (Selman *et al.*, 1994). In the cat, acromegaly is caused by pituitary tumours that secrete excess growth hormone. This cause has not been reported in the dog.

Plasma growth hormone concentrations tend to fluctuate throughout the day and basal concentrations may be low even in healthy animals. For this reason a stimulation test should be performed to help distinguish hyposecretion or hypersecretion from normal.

Growth hormone stimulation test

Indication
The GH stimulation test is used to diagnose pituitary dwarfism (congenital panhypopituitarism) and acromegaly, and to evaluate patients with adult-onset growth hormone-responsive alopecia. Basal concentrations of growth hormone are often difficult to interpret due to the overlap between normal dogs and those with growth hormone deficiency. Therefore, provocative testing with an α_2-adrenergic agonist (such as clonidine or xylazine) is recommended.

Method
1. Collect 5 ml of blood into EDTA; centrifuge immediately and store plasma frozen (below -20°C) for measuring basal GH concentration.
2. Inject either: clonidine 10 µg/kg intravenously (maximum dose 300 µg) or xylazine 100 µg/kg intravenously.
3. Collect a second 5 ml blood sample into EDTA 20 minutes after injection; centrifuge immediately and store plasma frozen (below -20°C) for measuring GH concentration.

Samples should be sent for assay, frozen, to the Biochemical Laboratory, Department of Clinical Sciences of Companion Animals, Utrecht, The Netherlands.

Interpretation
The reference range in dogs for basal growth hormone concentration is 1-4 µg/l and peak post-stimulation value is 10-58 µg/l (Eigenmann and Eigenmann, 1981).[1]

GH concentrations are generally reduced in pituitary dwarfism (<1 µg/l) and show little or no response to stimulation with clonidine or xylazine.

Reduced GH concentrations, with little or no response to stimulation, may be found in adult-onset growth hormone-responsive alopecia. However, reduced responses may be found in dogs with hypothyroidism or hyperadrenocorticism and these more common disorders must first be excluded as possible diagnoses.

Basal GH concentrations are generally elevated in acromegaly (>100 µg/l) and are not usually further stimulated by clonidine or xylazine (Eigenmann *et al.*, 1984).

Basal serum insulin-like growth factor 1

Indication
This test is used in the diagnosis of pituitary dwarfism and acromegaly. Insulin-like growth factor 1 (IGF1) concentration is regulated by growth hormone and nutritional status and is less subject to fluctuation than is growth hormone. This makes a single determination more meaningful. The assay is readily available in the UK.

Interpretation
The reference range for IGF1 in normal adult dogs and cats is >200 ng/ml and for animals up to a year of age is >500 ng/ml (Evans and Walker, 1995).

Serum IGF1 concentrations are decreased in pituitary dwarfs (<50 ng/ml). The sensitivity can be increased by comparing IGF1 concentrations with those of normal littermates. IGF1 concentrations may be depressed in chronic debilitating disease.

Elevated IGF1 concentrations are seen in dogs and cats with acromegaly (>1000 ng/ml).

POSTERIOR LOBE FUNCTION

Vasopressin (ADH) concentrations are rarely measured in veterinary practice. Only indirect tests of vasopressin activity are used commonly in veterinary practice and these include the water deprivation test and the vasopressin response test.

Diabetes insipidus is characterized by severe polyuria, with the passage of large quantities of dilute urine and resultant polydipsia. It may be caused by either a partial or total failure to synthesize or release ADH (*central diabetes insipidus*) or a partial or total failure of the renal tubules to respond to ADH (*nephrogenic*

---

[1] The reference ranges given in this chapter should be used only as a guide. The actual values obtained from a laboratory should be compared with the reference range for that laboratory and the assay must have been validated in the species under investigation.

diabetes insipidus). Vasopressin excess (syndrome of inappropriate antidiuresis) results in hyponatraemia. It is a rare condition in dogs and cats and only a few cases have been reported.

Water deprivation test

Indication
The water deprivation test is used in the diagnosis of diabetes insipidus. It does not differentiate between the central and nephrogenic forms of the disease. The test should only be performed in animals with normal blood urea and creatinine concentrations.

Method
1. Collect 5 ml of urine and plasma if osmolality is being measured. If specific gravity is to be measured, only urine is required.
2. Weigh the patient.
3. Withhold all fluids and food.
4. Collect urine and plasma after 8 hours and then at 2-hour intervals until the test is complete. It is rarely safe, or necessary, to continue this test for 24 hours.
5. Weigh the patient each time urine and plasma is collected.

6. Stop the test if the patient demonstrates adequate concentrating ability (specific gravity >1.020) or becomes dehydrated and loses 5% of its body weight or more.

Interpretation
Cases of central or nephrogenic diabetes insipidus fail to concentrate urine (specific gravity <1.010) and urine osmolality remains low and does not exceed that of plasma (Table 17.3).

This test does not always give conclusive results, especially if plasma and urine osmolality are not measured.

Vasopressin (ADH) response test

Indication
The ADH response test is used to differentiate central diabetes insipidus from nephrogenic diabetes insipidus.

Method
1. Collect 5 ml of urine and plasma if osmolality is being measured. Only urine is required if specific gravity is to be measured.
2. Inject desmopressin intramuscularly. Use 2 μg for dogs less than 15 kg and 4 μg for dogs over 15 kg.
3. Collect urine and plasma samples every 2 hours.

Parameter	Before water deprivation	After water deprivation		
		CDI	**NDI**	**PP**
Urine				
Specific gravity	<1.010	<1.010	<1.010	<1.025
Osmolality	<300 mOsm/kg	<300 mOsm/kg	<300 mOsm/kg	<700 mOsm/kg
Plasma				
Osmolality	>300 mOsm/kg in CDI or NDI <295 mOsm/kg in PP	>310 mOsm/kg	>310 mOsm/kg	±310 mOsm/kg
Ratio of urine:plasma osmolality	<1.0	<1.0	<1.0	2–3
ADH response				
Urine specific gravity	<1.010	>1.015	<1.010	>1.015
Ratio of urine:plasma osmolality	<1.0	>1.0	<1.0	>1.0

Table 17.3: *Differentiation of central diabetes insipidus (CDI), nephrogenic diabetes insipidus (NDI) and psychogenic polydipsia (PP).*

Interpretation

Dogs with nephrogenic diabetes insipidus will show very little or no response to exogenous vasopressin and the urine specific gravity and osmolality will remain low.

Dogs with central diabetes insipidus will concentrate their urine usually within 6 hours (specific gravity >1.015); their urine osmolality will rise by 50% or more and the urine osmolality will exceed the plasma osmolality.

ADRENOCORTICAL FUNCTION TESTS

PHYSIOLOGY OF THE ADRENAL CORTEX

The adrenal cortex produces about 30 different hormones, many of which have little or no clinical significance. The hormones can be divided into three groups based on their predominant actions: mineralocorticoids, which are important in electrolyte and water homoeostasis; glucocorticoids, which promote gluconeogenesis; and small quantities of sex hormones, particularly male hormones that have weak androgenic activity.

Aldosterone is the most important mineralocorticoid and is produced by the zona glomerulosa. The principal glucocorticoid, cortisol, and the sex hormones are produced in the zona fasciculata and the zona reticularis. Glucocorticoid and mineralocorticoid release are controlled by different mechanisms.

Regulation of glucocorticoid release

Glucocorticoid release is controlled almost entirely by adrenocorticotrophic hormone (ACTH) secreted by the anterior pituitary, and this is in turn regulated by corticotrophin releasing hormone (CRH) from the hypothalamus (see Figure 17.2). CRH is secreted by the neurons in the anterior portion of the paraventricular nuclei within the hypothalamus and is transported by the portal circulation to the anterior pituitary, where it stimulates ACTH release. There is probably an internal or 'short loop' negative feedback control by ACTH on CRH. ACTH secreted into the systemic circulation causes cortisol release, with concentrations rising almost immediately. Cortisol has direct negative feedback effects on: (i) the hypothalamus, to decrease formation of CRH; and (ii) the anterior pituitary gland, to decrease the formation of ACTH. These feedback mechanisms help regulate the plasma concentration of cortisol.

Secretion of CRH and ACTH is normally episodic and pulsatile, which results in fluctuating cortisol levels during the day. Diurnal variation is superimposed on this type of release. It is usually stated that in the dog CRH, ACTH and thus cortisol levels are highest in the early hours of the morning and that in the cat, they are greatest in the evening. However, a true circadian rhythm of cortisol concentrations has been difficult to confirm in the dog and cat (Kemppainen and Sartin, 1984; Peterson et al., 1988). The episodic release of CRH and ACTH is perpetuated by the reciprocal effect of cortisol acting through negative feedback control. This reciprocal arrangement does not hold during periods of stress when both ACTH and cortisol are maintained at high levels, because the effects of stress tend to override the normal negative feedback control.

In summary, ACTH and CRH secretion are influenced by diurnal variation and stress as well as by negative feedback control.

Regulation of mineralocorticoid release

Aldosterone release is influenced primarily by the renin–angiotensin system and by plasma potassium levels (see Figure 17.2).

Renin is secreted into the blood by the cells of the juxtaglomerular apparatus, which consists of specialized cells in the wall of the afferent arteriole immediately proximal to the glomerulus and the specialized epithelial cells of the distal convoluted tubule adjacent to that arteriole, the macula densa. Renin release may be stimulated by stretch receptors in the juxtaglomerular apparatus in response to hypotension or reduced renal blood flow or by sodium and chloride receptors in the macula densa. Renin is also released by sympathetic nerve stimulation and is inhibited by angiotensin II, antidiuretic hormone, hypertension and increased reabsorption of sodium by the renal tubules.

Renin is an enzyme that splits circulating angiotensinogen, produced by the liver, into angiotensin I. Angiotensin I is converted to angiotensin II by angiotensin converting enzyme found almost entirely in the pulmonary capillary endothelium.

Angiotensin II is a powerful vasoconstrictor and stimulates aldosterone secretion from the zona glomerulosa. Through its action on the distal convoluted tubule, aldosterone has a negative feedback effect on the juxtaglomerular apparatus.

Potassium has a direct stimulatory effect on the zona glomerulosa cells to release aldosterone.

ACTH and sodium play a less significant role in aldosterone secretion. ACTH is necessary to maintain normal aldosterone output. In the absence of ACTH, the zona glomerulosa partially atrophies, causing mild to moderate aldosterone deficiency compared with almost total atrophy of the other zones.

TESTS FOR DISEASES OF THE ADRENAL CORTEX

The most common disorders affecting the adrenal cortex cause either hyperadrenocorticism (Cushing's disease) or hypoadrenocorticism (Addison's disease). Hyperadrenocorticism can be spontaneous or iatrogenic. Spontaneously occurring hyperadrenocorticism may be associated with inappropriate secretion of ACTH by the pituitary (*pituitary-dependent hyperadrenocorticism*) or associated with a primary adrenal disorder (*adrenal-dependent hyperadrenocorticism*). Pituitary-dependent hyperadrenocorticism accounts for over 80% of dogs with naturally occurring hyperadrenocorticism (Figure 17.5). Functional corticotrophic adenomas can be found in the majority of these cases. The remaining 15–20% of spontaneous cases of hyperadrenocorticism are caused by unilateral or bilateral adrenal tumours, which can be benign or malignant.

Feline hyperadrenocorticism is rare but resembles the canine disorder in many respects. The majority of cases are pituitary-dependent although adrenal-dependent cases have been reported.

Isolated increase in production of aldosterone by an abnormal zona glomerulosa appears to be very rare in dogs and cats.

Hypoadrenocorticism is a syndrome that results from a deficiency of both glucocorticoid and mineralocorticoid secretion from the adrenal cortices. Destruction of more than 95% of both adrenal cortices causes a clinical deficiency of all adrenocortical hormones and is termed *primary hypoadrenocorticism* (Addison's disease). *Secondary hypoadrenocorticism* is caused by a deficiency in ACTH which leads to atrophy of the adrenal cortices and impaired secretion of glucocorticoids. The production of mineralocorticoids, however, usually remains adequate.

Measurement of plasma, serum or urinary cortisol concentrations, particularly following dynamic manipulation, or the measurement of endogenous plasma ACTH concentrations can be used to assess the hypothalamic–pituitary–adrenal axis.

Basal plasma or serum cortisol

A single resting or basal plasma or serum cortisol determination is of very limited diagnostic value because of the overlap in cortisol concentrations ob-

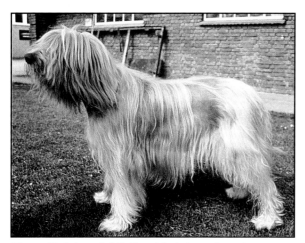

Figure 17.5: *Bearded Collie with pituitary-dependent hyperadrenocorticism, showing the pot-bellied appearance and bilaterally symmetrical alopecia.*

tained from normal and abnormal disease states. In particular:

* Stress associated with sample collection can result in higher than normal cortisol concentrations in samples from animals with normal hypothalamic–pituitary–adrenocortical axis (HPA) function

* Recent administration of glucocorticoids such as hydrocortisone, prednisolone or prednisone may result in elevated cortisol concentrations due to cross-reactivity in many cortisol assays. For this reason glucocorticoids should be withheld for at least 24 hours before testing. There is no cross-reactivity with dexamethasone, but dexamethasone will suppress cortisol concentrations in patients with an intact hypothalamic–pituitary–adrenal axis.

Plasma or serum cortisol values are only useful after dynamic manipulation with ACTH or dexamethasone.

ACTH stimulation test

Indication
The ACTH stimulation test is used: to screen for hyperadrenocorticism; to distinguish hyperadrenocorticism from iatrogenic Cushing's disease (secondary hypoadrenocorticism); to monitor the response to mitotane therapy; and to diagnose primary hypoadrenocorticism (Addison's disease).

Method
1. Collect 3 ml plasma or serum for measuring basal cortisol concentration (see note above about withholding glucocorticoids).
2. Inject 0.25 mg of synthetic ACTH intravenously to dogs 5 kg and over. Use only 0.125 mg in dogs under 5 kg.
3. Collect a second sample 30–60 minutes later for measuring cortisol concentration.

In cats, 0.125 mg of synthetic ACTH is administered intravenously and post-stimulation samples are collected after 60 and 90 minutes.

Interpretation
In normal dogs, pre-ACTH cortisol concentrations are usually between 20 and 250 nmol/l with post-ACTH cortisol concentrations between 200 and 450 nmol/l.

An exaggerated response (post-ACTH cortisol concentration >600 nmol/l) is expected in dogs and cats with hyperadrenocorticism (Figure 17.6). The ACTH stimulation test reliably identifies more than 50% of dogs with adrenal-dependent hyperadrenocorticism and about 85% of dogs with pituitary-dependent hyperadrenocorticism. Exaggerated responses to ACTH may also be seen in chronic illness, e.g. uncontrolled diabetes mellitus.

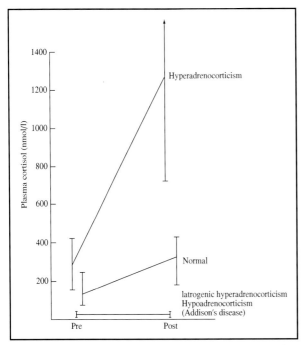

Figure 17.6: The ACTH stimulation test. Interpretation of plasma cortisol concentrations determined before and after administration of synthetic ACTH.

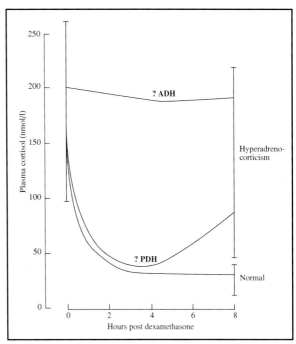

Figure 17.7: The low-dose dexamethasone test. Interpretation of plasma cortisol concentrations determined during low-dose dexamethasone screening.
?ADH represents the type of response seen in cases of adrenal-dependent hyperadrenocorticism. ?PDH represents a possible response in pituitary-dependent hyperadrenocorticism.

The ACTH stimulation test is the best screening test for distinguishing spontaneous hyperadrenocorticism from iatrogenic Cushing's disease, where reduced responses to ACTH are recorded due to adrenocortical suppression as a result of long-term or high-dose glucocorticoid administration.

Reduced responses to ACTH are also seen in primary hypoadrenocorticism (Addison's disease). Usually both pre- and post-ACTH cortisol concentrations are <15 nmol/l. Mineralocorticoid deficiency will usually result in hyponatraemia, hyperkalaemia and hypochloraemia. The ratio of sodium to potassium may be more reliable than the absolute values. The normal ratio of sodium to potassium varies between 27:1 and 40:1, whereas in patients with hypoadrenocorticism, the ratio is commonly less than 25:1 and may be below 20:1. However, 10% of cases of hypoadrenocorticism may have normal electrolyte levels at the time of presentation.

A flat response to ACTH is seen in mitotane-treated cases of hyperadrenocorticism. The post-ACTH cortisol concentration should not exceed 125 nmol/l if the disease is well controlled. At concentrations above 250 nmol/l clinical signs of hyperadrenocorticism are likely to be present.

Disadvantages of the ACTH stimulation test are that it does not reliably differentiate adrenal-dependent from pituitary-dependent hyperadrenocorticism and that a diagnosis of hyperadrenocorticism cannot be excluded on the basis of a normal ACTH response. If the clinical signs are compatible with hyperadrenocorticism, a low-dose dexamethasone suppression test would then be recommended.

Low-dose dexamethasone suppression test (LDDST)

Indication
The LDDST is used to screen for hyperadrenocorticism.

Method
1. Collect 3 ml plasma or serum for cortisol determination.
2. Inject 0.01 mg/kg of dexamethasone intravenously.
3. Collect a second sample for cortisol concentration 4 hours later, and a third sample 8 hours after dexamethasone administration.

Interpretation
A plasma or serum cortisol concentration >40 nmol/l at 8 hours is regarded as diagnostic for hyperadrenocorticism (Figure 17.7). The LDDST reliably identifies all dogs with adrenal-dependent hyperadrenocorticism and about 90% of dogs with pituitary-dependent hyperadrenocorticism. However stress during therapy may cause animals without hyperadrenocorticism to break the suppressive effect of dexamethasone.

The cortisol concentrations at 0 and 4 hours are not required for the diagnosis of hyperadrenocorticism but may be informative in the differential diagnosis. Suppression of the cortisol concentration to <30 nmol/l at 4 hours with a rebound escape of suppression at 8 hours would be suggestive of pituitary-dependent hyperadrenocorticism. Cases of adrenal-dependent hyperadrenocorticism do not show significant suppression of cortisol at 4 hours; however, up to 40% of dogs with pituitary-dependent hyperadrenocorticism will not show suppression at 4 hours either.

Urine corticoid:creatinine ratio

Indication
This test is used to screen for canine hyperadrenocorticism.

Cortisol and its metabolites are excreted in urine. By measuring urine cortisol in the morning sample, the concentration will reflect cortisol release over a period over several hours, thereby adjusting for fluctuations in plasma cortisol concentrations and the concentration in urine increases with increased plasma concentrations. Relating the urine cortisol concentration to urine creatinine concentration provides a correction for any differences in urine concentration.

Method
Urine (5 ml) is collected in the morning for cortisol and creatinine measurements. It is preferable for the dog to be at home for this test so that it is as little stressed as possible. The urine corticoid:creatinine ratio is determined by dividing the urine cortisol concentration (in μmol/l) by the urine creatinine concentration (in μmol/l).

Interpretation
The reference ratio for normal dogs is $<10 \times 10^{-6}$ (Stolp *et al.*, 1983).

The urine cortisol:creatinine ratio is increased above the normal ($> 10 \times 10^{-6}$) in dogs with hyperadrenocorticism. However the ratio is also increased in many dogs with non-adrenal illness (Smiley and Peterson, 1993). Therefore, while this simple test appears highly sensitive in detecting hyperadrenocorticism in dogs, it is not specific. The test does provide a good screening test for hyperadrenocorticism and values in the normal range make a diagnosis of hyperadrenocorticism highly unlikely.

High-dose dexamethasone suppression test (HDDST)

Indication
This test is used to differentiate pituitary-dependent hyperadrenocorticism from adrenal-dependent hyperadrenocorticism. It cannot be used as a screening test for hyperadrenocorticism.

Method
1. Collect 3 ml serum or plasma for cortisol determination.
2. Inject 0.1 mg/kg (although some authors recommend 1.0 mg/kg) of dexamethasone intravenously.

3. Collect two post-dexamethasone samples, one at 4 hours and a second at 8 hours after the dexamethasone.

Interpretation
A plasma cortisol concentration that declines by more than 50% from the pre-dexamethasone value at either 4 or 8 hours post-dexamethasone is consistent with pituitary-dependent hyperadrenocorticism. A decrease of less than 50% can be due to an adrenocortical tumour or to pituitary-dependent hyperadrenocorticism. About 20–30% of dogs with pituitary-dependent hyperadrenocorticism fail to suppress adequately to high doses of dexamethasone.

Endogenous plasma ACTH concentration

Indication
This test is used to differentiate pituitary-dependent hyperadrenocorticism from adrenal tumour in dogs with documented spontaneous hyperadrenocorticism and to distinguish primary from secondary hypoadrenocorticism.

Measurement of basal endogenous ACTH concentrations is of no value in the diagnosis of hyperadrenocorticism because of the episodic secretion of ACTH in the normal dog and the overlapping values with those dogs with hyperadrenocorticism.

Method
Blood (5 ml) is collected into a cooled plastic EDTA tube and centrifuged at 4°C immediately. The plasma should then be harvested and stored frozen (at less than –20°C) in a plastic tube. Samples must be transported to the laboratory frozen and must be kept frozen until assayed. Stringent and meticulous sample handling is crucial since hormone activity in the plasma will reduce rapidly, resulting in falsely low values and incorrect interpretation.

The endogenous ACTH assay must be validated for use in dogs, otherwise the test may provide spurious results that could be misleading to the clinician.

Interpretation
Endogenous ACTH concentrations in normal dogs range from 10 to 70 pg/ml. Dogs with adrenal tumours have very low endogenous ACTH concentrations (<20 pg/ml) whereas cases with pituitary-dependent hyperadrenocorticism tend to have high-normal to high concentrations (>40 pg/ml).

Dogs with primary hypoadrenocorticism have very high endogenous ACTH concentrations (>500 pg/ml).

Other tests
A CRH stimulation test has been described (Van Wijk *et al.*, 1994). Following the intravenous injection of ovine CRH, the ACTH concentrations usually peak at 5 minutes and the cortisol concentrations at 20 minutes

in normal dogs. In dogs with autonomously secreting adrenal tumours, CRH causes virtually no increase in release of endogenous ACTH or cortisol.

Plasma aldosterone concentrations may be measured in response to ACTH stimulation (as in the protocol above). Basal aldosterone concentrations are of little or no diagnostic value.

After stimulation with ACTH, plasma aldosterone concentrations should double, unless the basal concentration is already in the high-normal range (Golden and Lowthrop, 1988). In hypoaldosteronism, the basal aldosterone concentration is low, with minimal or no increase in the post-ACTH aldosterone concentration. Markedly increased basal and post-ACTH aldosterone concentrations would be suggestive of primary aldosteronism (Conn's disease). Aldosterone excess leads to increased sodium and water retention, potassium depletion and suppression of the renin–angiotensin system, but appears to be a rare condition in the dog and cat.

REFERENCES AND FURTHER READING

Eigenmann JE and Eigenmann RY (1981) Radioimmunoassay of canine growth hormone. *Acta Endocrinologica* **98**, 514–520

Eigenmann JE, Patterson DF, Zapf J and Froesch ER (1984) Insulin-like growth factor 1 in the dog: a study in different dog breeds and in dogs with growth hormone elevation. *Acta Endocrinologica* **105**, 294–301

Evans H and Walker M (1995) In: *SCL Veterinary Services Manual*, 6th edn, pp. 29–31. SCL Bioscience Services, Cambridge.

Golden DL and Lowthrop CD (1988) A retrospective study of aldosterone secretion in normal and adrenopathic dogs. *Journal of Veterinary Internal Medicine* **2**, 121–125

Kemppainen RJ and Sartin JL (1984) Evidence for episodic but not circadian activity in plasma concentrations of adrenocorticotropin, cortisol and thyroxine in dogs. *Journal of Endocrinology* **103**, 219–226

Peterson ME, Kemppainen RJ and Graves TK (1988) Episodic but not circadian activity in plasma concentrations of ACTH, cortisol and thyroxine in the normal cat. *American College of Veterinary Internal Medicine Scientific Proceedings, Washington, D.C.*, p. 721 (abstract)

Selman PJ, Mol JA, Rutteman GR, Van Garderen E and Rijnberk A (1994) Progestin-induced growth hormone excess in the dog originates in the mammary gland. *Endocrinology* **134**, 287–292

Smiley LE and Peterson ME (1993) Evaluation of a urine cortisol:creatinine ratio as a screening test for hyperadrenocorticism in dogs. *Journal of Veterinary Internal Medicine* **7**, 163–168

Stolp R, Rijnberk A, Meijer JC and Croughs RJM (1983) Urinary corticoids in the diagnosis of canine hyperadrenocorticism. *Research in Veterinary Science* **34**, 141–144

Van Wijk PA, Rijnberk A, Croughs RJM, Wolfswinkel J, Selman PJ and Mol JA (1994) Responsiveness to corticotropin releasing hormone and vasopressin in canine Cushing's syndrome. *European Journal of Endocrinology* **130**, 410–416

CHAPTER EIGHTEEN

Endocrine Pancreatic Function

Michael E. Herrtage

INTRODUCTION

Functionally the pancreas comprises two separate glands: an exocrine portion and an endocrine portion. Secretions from the exocrine pancreas contain digestive enzymes which are excreted into the intestinal lumen. The endocrine pancreas is composed of the islets of Langerhans, which secrete at least four hormones. Four cell types have been identified in the pancreatic islets with light microscopy on the basis of staining properties and histochemistry: alpha cells, which secrete glucagon; beta cells, which secrete insulin; delta cells, which secrete somatostatin; and F cells, which secrete pancreatic polypeptide. A number of other peptides, e.g. gastric inhibitory polypeptide (GIP) and cholecystokinin (CCK), are also found in the islet cells.

Insulin and glucagon are involved in the control of carbohydrate, lipid and protein metabolism and are particularly important in blood glucose homoeostasis. Glucose is the most potent stimulus for insulin secretion, although some other sugars and amino acids may also stimulate insulin release. The release of glucagon is inhibited by glucose, whereas the release of glucagon is stimulated by ingestion of protein, acute hypoglycaemia, catecholamines and glucocorticoids.

Diabetes mellitus is a heterogeneous condition characterized by a relative or absolute deficiency of insulin secretion by the beta cells of the islets of Langerhans in the pancreas. Carbohydrate metabolism and in particular blood glucose concentration is controlled by the balance between the actions of catabolic hormones, e.g. glucagon, cortisol, catecholamines and growth hormone, and of the principal anabolic hormone, insulin. A relative or absolute deficiency of insulin results in decreased utilization of glucose, amino acids and fatty acids by peripheral tissues, particularly liver, muscle and adipose tissue. Failure of glucose uptake by these cells leads to hyperglycaemia. Once the renal threshold for glucose reabsorption is exceeded, an osmotic diuresis ensues, with loss of glucose, electrolytes and water in the urine. A compensatory polydipsia prevents the animal becoming dehydrated. The loss of glucose leads to catabolism of the body's reserves, especially of fats. Excessive fat catabolism leads to the production and accumulation of ketone bodies and the onset of diabetic ketoacidosis. In diabetic ketoacidosis, the dog is unable to maintain an adequate fluid intake and becomes rapidly dehydrated due to the uncontrolled osmotic diuresis. The dehydration and acidosis requires emergency care if the animal is to survive.

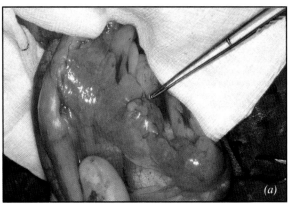

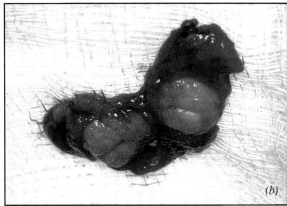

Figure 18.1: An insulinoma in the pancreas of a dog (a) and (b) its cut surface after surgical removal.

Functional islet cell tumours (insulinomas) are the most frequently occurring tumours of the endocrine pancreas in dogs (Figure 18.1). Most insulin-secreting tumours are malignant islet cell carcinomas which metastasize to regional lymph nodes and/or the liver. Early diagnosis is important as dogs with metastases have significantly reduced survival times. Insulin-secreting tumours are rare in cats.

ENDOCRINE PANCREATIC FUNCTION TESTS

Serum insulin

Indication
Measurement of serum insulin is used to diagnose insulin-secreting pancreatic tumours (insulinomas).

Insulin concentrations may be used to assess residual beta cell function in cases of diabetes mellitus, but such measurements have not been shown to be clinically useful.

Insulin measurements have also been used in diabetic dogs and cats to suggest the presence of insulin-binding antibodies in patients with insulin resistance.

Method
A serum sample (from 3–5 ml of whole blood) is collected from a fasted animal.

Serial serum insulin concentrations may be measured during an intravenous glucose tolerance test (see below).

Blood glucose concentration must be determined at the same time in order to evaluate the significance of the serum insulin concentration.

Interpretation
Serum insulin concentrations in normal fasting dogs are 5–20 mIU/l with a normal blood glucose (3.5–5.0 mmol/l).

A serum insulin concentration of >20 mIU/l with a low blood glucose (<3.0 mmol/l) is consistent with an insulinoma. If normal insulin concentrations are found in a hypoglycaemic dog then a insulinoma is still possible, but if the serum insulin is low, this diagnosis is unlikely.

The insulin:glucose ratio has proved useful in making a diagnosis of insulinoma in some cases. A ratio of more than 4.2 is consistent with an insulinoma.

Most dogs and cats with insulin-dependent diabetes mellitus have serum insulin concentrations of <10 mIU/l in the presence of hyperglycaemia, whereas insulin concentrations of >20 mIU/l in the presence of hyperglycaemia suggests some residual beta cell activity and the possibility of insulin antagonism (Nelson et al., 1994).

If a single antibody radioimmune assay is used to measure insulin, spuriously high concentrations of >400 mIU/l may be found 24 hours after exogenous insulin when significant insulin-binding antibodies are present. Serum insulin concentrations are typically <50 mIU/l 24 hours after the last insulin injection in diabetic dogs and cats without antibodies causing interference with the radioimmune assay (Nelson et al., 1994).

Serum fructosamine

Indication
Measurement of serum fructosamine is used to monitor glycaemic control in treated diabetic dogs and cats.

Measurement of glycated proteins such as fructosamine and glycosylated haemoglobin, are used increasingly in diabetic dogs and cats to monitor the response to treatment. The glycated protein is formed by an irreversible, non-enzymatic reaction between glucose and the protein, which in the case of fructosamine is mainly albumin. The serum fructosamine concentration therefore reflects the half-life of albumin and the time-averaged glucose concentration to which the albumin has been exposed. Thus the measurement of glycated proteins reflects the average blood glucose concentration over the preceding 1–2 weeks in the case of serum fructosamine and 2–3 months in the case of glycosylated haemoglobin (Jensen, 1995).

The assay can also be used as a screening test to identify diabetic dogs and cats and particularly to distinguish between transient hyperglycaemia (caused for example by stress, recent feeding, concurrent illness or medication) in non-diabetic patients and persistent hyperglycaemia in diabetic patients.

Serum fructosamine assay may be useful as a screening test for insulinoma.

Method
A serum sample (from 3–5 ml of whole blood) is collected from the patient.

Interpretation
The reference range for serum fructosamine in normal dogs is 250–350 μmol/l and in normal cats is 150–270 μmol/l.

Serum fructosamine concentrations of <400 mmol/l indicate good glycaemic control in dogs, whereas concentrations of >500 mmol/l are found in newly diagnosed or poorly controlled diabetic dogs (Reusch et al., 1993).

Serum fructosamine concentrations of >400 μmol/l in cats indicate insufficient glycaemic control or newly diagnosed diabetes (Thoresen and Bredal, 1996).

Low serum fructosamine concentrations may be found in dogs with insulinoma.

Glycosylated haemoglobin is less routinely available as an assay. Well controlled diabetic dogs have between 4 and 6 % glycosylated haemoglobin, whereas poorly controlled diabetics have more than 7% (Nelson, 1995).

Intravenous glucose tolerance test (IVGTT)

Indication
The IVGTT is used to evaluate glucose homoeostasis.

Serum insulin increases rapidly after intravenous administration of glucose in normal dogs and cats. Abnormal glucose tolerance may be identified in dogs and cats with suspected preclinical diabetes mellitus or in equivocal cases of insulinoma.

Method
Glucose 0.5g/kg body weight is injected slowly over 30 seconds into the cephalic vein using a 50% dextrose solution.

Blood samples (2 ml) are collected into fluoride anticoagulant from a different vein for glucose determinations at times zero (pre-injection), 5, 10, 15, 20, 25, 30, 45 and 60 minutes and, occasionally, at 75 and 90 minutes.

An intravenous catheter may be used, particularly in cats, where there may be difficulty in taking multiple blood samples. The first millilitre of each sample should be discarded to achieve accurate measurements.

Interpretation
In animals with normal glucose tolerance, the blood glucose concentration should return to normal by 60 minutes after intravenous administration of glucose.

Persistent hyperglycaemia (> 7 mmol/l) beyond 60 minutes would suggest carbohydrate intolerance and possible preclinical diabetes mellitus. With insulinoma, the blood glucose concentration may return to normal more quickly (< 30 minutes) and may fall further to hypoglycaemic levels (< 3 mmol/l).

The results of the IVGTT can be used to calculate the glucose half-life and the fractional clearance of glucose (*k* value) (Kaneko *et al.*, 1977; Dunn *et al.*, 1992).

There is considerable individual variation in the results of IVGTT from normal animals. In addition, the period of fasting, the carbohydrate content of the last feed, stress and drugs, such as sedatives or anaesthetic agents, will influence the result of the test. For optimal results, the test must be carried out using strict standard conditions that may be difficult to achieve in practice.

Other tests
An intravenous glucagon stimulation test (IVGST) has been described but offers no advantages over the IVGTT and is not recommended in cases of insulinoma because it may cause severe hypoglycaemia after the initial rise in blood glucose concentrations. Glucagon can also cause significant hypertension in animals with phaeochromocytoma.

REFERENCES AND FURTHER READING

Dunn JK, Heath MF, Herrtage ME, Jackson KF and Walker MJ (1992) Diagnosis of insulinoma in the dog: a study of 11 cases. *Journal of Small Animal Practice* **33**, 514–520
Jensen AL (1995) Glycated blood proteins in canine diabetes mellitus. *Veterinary Record* **137**, 401–405
Kaneko JJ, Mattheeuws D, Rottiers RP and Vermeulen A (1977) Glucose tolerance and insulin response in diabetes mellitus of dogs. *Journal of Small Animal Practice* **18**, 85–94
Nelson R W (1995) Diabetes mellitus. In: *Textbook of Veterinary Internal Medicine*, ed. SJ Ettinger and EC Feldman, pp. 1510–1537. WB Saunders, Philadelphia
Nelson RW, Turnwald GH and Willard MD (1994) Endocrine, metabolic and lipid disorders. In: *Small Animal Clinical Diagnosis by Laboratory Methods, 2nd edition*, ed. MD Willard *et al.*, p.159. WB Saunders, Philadelphia
Reusch CE, Liehs MR, Hoyer M and Vochezer R (1993) Fructosamine: a new parameter for diagnosis and metabolic control in diabetic dogs and cats. *Journal of Veterinary Internal Medicine* **7**, 177–182
Thoresen SI and Bredal WP (1996) Clinical usefulness of fructosamine measurements in diagnosing and monitoring feline diabetes mellitus. *Journal of Small Animal Practice* **37**, 64–68

Urinary System

Mike Davies

INTRODUCTION

The results of clinical pathology tests are often critical for the successful diagnosis, treatment and monitoring of a patient with urinary system disease. For example, an accurate diagnosis of the cause of polyuria cannot be made without laboratory investigations. Sometimes life and death decisions will be made based upon laboratory results and it is therefore essential that they are accurate and that the clinician interprets them correctly in the context of other clinical information about the patient.

This chapter reviews the clinical pathology tests that are used to assist in the diagnosis of renal and urinary tract diseases in the dog and cat, with the emphasis on assessment of system and organ function.

FUNCTIONAL ANATOMY AND PHYSIOLOGY

When collecting laboratory samples it is important to understand the anatomical relationships of organs from which the samples are being taken, as adjacent structures can affect the quality or quantity of sample taken. A good understanding of normal anatomy is also necessary for the correct interpretation of laboratory findings, for the proper application of other diagnostic aids such as imaging techniques (radiography and ultrasonography), for planning surgical approaches for sample collection, and for post-mortem examination.

Organs comprising the urinary system include the kidneys, ureters, bladder and urethra. Genital organs that share part of the urinary outflow tract are the prostate gland and testes in the male, and the uterus, vagina and vestibule in the female.

Kidneys

The kidneys lie in a retroperitoneal position, in the sublumbar region on either side of the aorta and posterior vena cava. The dorsal surface of each kidney is surrounded by fat which, in obese individuals, can make exposure and visualization difficult. The ventral surface is covered by peritoneum. The medial border is indented by the hilus from which the renal artery, vein, lymph vessels, nerves and ureter emerge. Great care must be taken to avoid trauma to this area during exploratory surgery or biopsy collection.

The kidneys are attached to local structures by fascia but they are not fixed in position and can move about naturally; hence they can be displaced by adjacent structures rather than be subjected to compression. This movement is useful for physical examination, as the kidneys can be palpated and, if necessary, manipulated for sample collection.

The surface of normal healthy kidneys should be smooth. Large kidneys with smooth soft fluid-filled protuberances may be cystic (Figure 19.1), although deep-seated or turgid cysts may feel hard on palpation. Large kidneys with hard, irregular swellings on the surface may be affected by neoplastic change (Figure 19.2), whereas small shrunken kidneys with a hard, irregular surface may be fibrosed due to chronic renal failure (CRF).

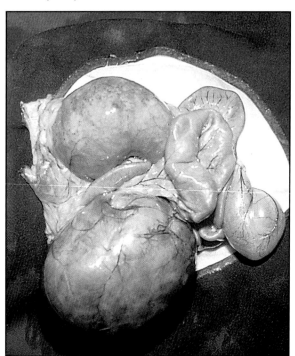

Figure 19.1: Polycystic kidneys from a cat.

Within the external fibrous capsule the kidney parenchyma consists of an outer cortex and an inner medulla. The functional unit of the kidney that produces urine is called the nephron and is comprised of a renal corpuscle and a portion of straight tubule. Renal corpuscles are only found in the cortex and not in the medulla. When assessing kidneys for renal disease,

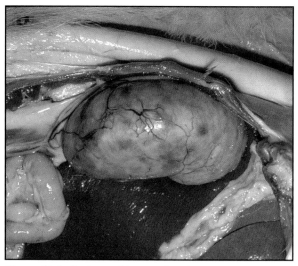

Figure 19.2: Canine multicentric lymphosarcoma.

good biopsies of the cortex are needed to evaluate the number and morphology of corpuscles.

Both absorption of substances from, and secretion of substances into, the urine take place along the excretory pathway after the initial glomerular filtration (Figure 19.3).

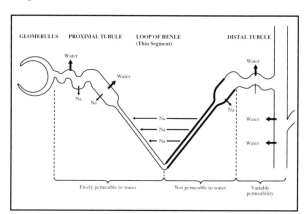

Figure: 19.3: The excretory pathway.

In normal kidneys substances passing through the capillary bed of a glomerulus can pass freely across the semipermeable membrane if they have a molecular weight of less than 68,000; this includes water, electrolytes and glucose. However, most of these substances are later conserved by the body through resorption from the tubules.

Albumin has a molecular weight of 66,000 and haemoglobin a molecular weight of 64,000 so these are on the borderline for filtration into the urine – but they do pass through. Other proteins are far too large to be filtered (molecular weight 160,000–900,000) and they also have a negative charge which is repelled by a negative charge in the glomerular membrane. The kidneys are therefore physiologically designed to conserve protein in the bloodstream. Also, any protein that does pass into the glomerular filtrate can later be resorbed very efficiently from the tubules.

Despite these mechanisms, small amounts of protein (up to 0.5 g/l) are found in normal urine from healthy individuals. This consists of Tamm–Horsfall protein, uromucoid, matrix substance A and polypeptides, along with other substances such as glycosaminoglycans (GAGs) and pyrophosphate. About half of the protein in normal urine is albumin that has come through the kidney, though over 90% of the albumin that passes through the glomeruli into the filtrate is reabsorbed in the proximal tubules. The rest of the protein is derived from the collecting tubules and lower urinary and genital tracts. The precise role of these proteins in the urine is not fully understood but it is believed that some are natural inhibitors to crystallization (e.g. GAGs, pyrophosphate and nephrocalcin).

Many substances have a renal threshold so that they only pass into the urine when the circulating blood concentration exceeds a certain level. In the case of glucose this is 10 mmol/l in dogs and 16 mmol/l in cats. The transient postprandial hyperglycaemia that occurs after a meal is unlikely to exceed the renal threshold, so glycosuria does not result. On the other hand, stress-related hyperglycaemia does give rise to glycosuria, particularly in fractious and excited or nervous cats.

Urine output (volume and rate of production) and urine content are determined by the net result of glomerular filtration, tubular secretion and tubular resorption. The control of these, and of water homeostasis in particular, is complex, involving both passive and active local mechanisms and several centrally mediated factors. For example, vasopressin (antidiuretic hormone, ADH), aldosterone, angiotensin, renin, adrenocorticotropic hormone (ACTH), atrial natriuretic hormone, sodium and potassium, parathyroid hormone (PTH) and vitamin D are all involved. (The role of vasopressin and adrenocortical function tests are discussed in Chapter 17.) It is important to remember that the glomerular filtration rate (GFR) is not necessarily the same as the urine output.

The ability of the kidneys to concentrate urine is dependent upon the number of functional nephrons. Like most major organs the kidneys have a huge functional reserve, and renal insufficiency (inability to concentrate urine) only occurs when 66% of nephrons have ceased to function. Clinical signs of renal failure will only be seen once 75% of nephrons have ceased to function. A diagnosis of renal failure is therefore extremely serious, as injured nephrons are irreversibly damaged and the patient will never regain full renal capacity.

The kidney should not be regarded solely as an excretory organ for waste products and toxins. Renal function is vitally important for the normal function of other body systems, including the cardiovascular system (blood volume, content and pressure) and the skeleton (bone homeostasis). Also, disorders in other systems can have a profound effect on renal function. This means that during the interpretation of clinical laboratory findings the possibility of primary and secondary disorders in other organ systems must always be considered.

Ureters

Numerous congenital anomalies of the ureters can occur, including duplication and ectopic locations whereby the ureters open in an abnormal site such as the bladder neck, urethra or vagina. Ectopic ureters are a commonly recognized cause of urinary incontinence in young dogs, often associated with secondary urinary tract infection due to impaired natural defence mechanisms against ascending infection.

Urinary bladder

The bladder stores urine, which is received passively from the kidneys through the ureters. An enlarged prostate (common in old male dogs) can displace the bladder into the abdomen and cause distension, and sometimes the bladder can be deflected back into the pelvic canal as part of a perineal rupture.

The cranial end of the bladder (fundus) usually lies in the midline in contact with the ventral wall of the abdomen just cranial to the pubic symphysis, extending to the umbilicus when full. This makes it easy to access for cystocentesis. The trigone is the area near the bladder neck where the ureters open into the lumen and where the urethral orifice is located; there are no mucosal folds in this area.

Blood supply is from the cranial and caudal vesicle arteries, which originate from the umbilical and urogenital arteries, respectively, and these should be avoided during biopsy or other surgery. Venous drainage is via the internal pudendal vein; the lymphatics drain into the internal iliac and lumbar lymph nodes.

The bladder is innervated by the pudendal nerve (somatic, originating from sacral nerves 1, 2 and 3) to the external sphincter and striated muscle of the urethra; stimulation causes voiding of urine. Stimulation of the hypogastric nerve (sympathetic) and the pelvic nerve (parasympathetic) causes contraction of the bladder and relaxation of the sphincter, resulting in urination.

Micturition is the expulsion of urine from the bladder down the urethra and is a complex process, involving both involuntary and voluntary control mechanisms. A failure to void urine regularly, or enforced urinary retention due to obstruction or a failure of the normal neurological control of micturition, such as frequently occurs following spinal trauma, can lead to stale urine, which can affect urinalysis findings and results in an increased risk for urinary tract infection. Prolonged urinary retention can lead to a retrograde build-up of pressure, resulting in hydronephrosis and irreparable renal damage (Figure 19.4).

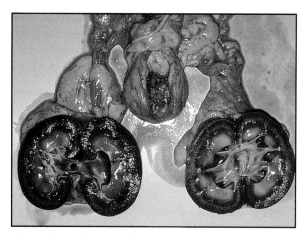

Figure 19.4: *Bilateral hydronephrosis secondary to a transition cell carcinoma in the bladder.*

Congenital anomalies of the bladder include diverticula, patent urachus and urachal cysts, and these can predispose a young dog to secondary diseases such as urinary tract infection and urolithiasis.

Urethra

Male
In the male dog the urethra extends from the bladder neck, passes caudally through the prostate gland, over the brim of the pelvis at the ischial arch, through the ventral groove of the os penis, and emerges at the tip of the glans penis. When attempting catheterization of the bladder via the urethra, natural resistance to passage of the catheter is frequently encountered when it reaches the os penis and at the ischial arch. These are also natural sites for obstruction of the urinary tract by uroliths and for trauma following repeated catheterization or clumsy attempts to free obstructions. Urethral fibrosis at the level of the os penis is a common complication following the relief of obstruction with uroliths.

When embarking upon catheterization, the approximate length of catheter required to reach the neck of the urinary bladder should be estimated prior to insertion. If too much catheter is inserted it can impinge on the wall of the bladder; if this is severely inflamed, ulcerated or neoplastic, there can be further damage or even perforation. Sometimes an excessively long catheter will deflect off the bladder wall and either kink (making collection of a urine sample difficult or impossible) or pass back in an arc through the neck of the bladder and emerge again at the urethral orifice.

Care is needed to avoid trauma to the lining of the urethra during catheterization or surgical procedures. Following injury the healing process often results in fibrosis, causing stenosis which can obstruct normal urine flow. Furthermore, injury to the distal urethra can lead to impaired natural defence mechanisms, leading to recurrent ascending urinary tract infection.

In males the urethra carries both urine and seminal secretions, so abnormal findings such as red blood cells, white blood cells, protein or cell debris in naturally voided urine could have originated from the kidneys, excretory urinary tract, prostate or testes.

Female
In bitches the distal urethral opening lies on the floor of the genital tract approximately 5 mm caudal to the vaginovestibular junction. A urinary catheter can usually be easily inserted into the urethra, though it is necessary to avoid the blind-ended folds of the vestibule on either side.

In the queen the distal urethral orifice lies along the ventral wall of the vagina; the common passage formed by the union of the urethra and vagina is called the urogenital sinus and opens at the urogenital aperture ventral to the anus.

The vagina lies ventral to the rectum, and faecal contamination of urine can occur if there is a connection between the two, as occurs with a rectovaginal fistula.

Prostate
The musculoglandular prostate gland of the male dog surrounds the neck of the bladder and the proximal part of the urethra. It can be spherical or ovoid, and weight and size vary with breed, age and body weight.

Prostatic enlargement is a common finding in old animals and is usually due to prostatic hypertrophy secondary to hormonal changes. The hypertrophy may be glandular, fibrous or both, and cysts may also be present. There may also be secondary infection and inflammation. It can be difficult to differentiate a large prostatic cyst from the urinary bladder by palpation alone, and contrast radiography may be needed prior to performing cystocentesis.

Prostatic hypertrophy can physically interfere with urination or defecation, causing straining and dysuria. It can also result in the urinary bladder being displaced cranially and ventrally. If the bladder is full, the prostate may get pulled cranially into the abdomen, so care is needed if urine is to be collected by cystocentesis.

In male cats the prostate is a small structure which lies near the union of the ductus deferens and the urethra.

Genital tract
The male and female genital tracts are discussed in Chapter 20.

THE ROLE OF CLINICAL PATHOLOGY

Clinical pathology tests in the evaluation of a patient for the presence of renal and/or urinary tract disease should be performed under the following circumstances:

Breed	Disorder
Abyssinian cat	Amyloidosis
Basenji	Fanconi syndrome
Beagle	Polycystic kidneys
Cairn Terrier	Polycystic kidneys
Cocker Spaniel	Cortical hypoplasia
Dobermann Pinscher	Progressive renal disease
Lhasa Apso	Progressive renal disease
Norwegian Elkhound	Progressive renal disease
Pembroke Welsh Corgi	Hydronephrosis and telangiectasia
Samoyed	Progressive renal disease
Shih-Tsu	Progressive renal disease
Soft-coated Wheaten Terrier	Renal dysplasia
Standard Poodle	Progressive renal disease

Table 19.1: Familial renal disorders that cause chronic renal failure.

- When primary or secondary urinary system disease is suspected from the presenting signs, clinical history or physical examination
- When a patient has a disease in another organ system that is known to be potentially associated with concurrent or secondary renal or urinary tract disease
- When screening 'at risk' patients as part of a general health check (e.g. as part of a geriatric screening programme, before general anaesthesia, or before administration of drugs that are known to be potentially nephrotoxic, such as non-steroidal anti-inflammatory drugs, aminoglycosides or oxytetracycline).

In the author's opinion a claim for negligence could be justified if a renal crisis such as acute renal failure (ARF) occurred in a patient that was in more than one 'at risk' group and which had not been screened prior to the administration of a general anaesthetic or a nephrotoxic therapeutic agent.

Examples of common groups 'at risk' for renal or urinary tract disease are :

- Animals with a familial predisposition
- Certain breeds (see Table 19.1)
- Old animals
- Animals with concurrent disease, e.g. diabetes mellitus, hepatic impairment.

The accurate diagnosis of renal and urinary tract diseases requires investigation by any or all of the following:

- Full history
- Full physical examination
- Imaging:
    Radiography – plain and contrast studies; sometimes dynamic studies
    Ultrasonography
- Urinalysis
- Blood chemistry
- Haematology
- Microbiological culture and sensitivity testing
- Tissue biopsy
- Surgical examination at laparoscopy or laparotomy
- Post-mortem examination.

Most commercially available clinical pathology diagnostic tests, particularly the newer dry chemistry tests, are easy to use and provide a high degree of accuracy. However, some do not, especially if they are tests designed and validated only for human use. Also, some veterinary practices may not always adopt good laboratory practice standards; regular quality control testing is of paramount importance if results obtained are to be relied upon.

In general, microbiological examinations, post-mortem examinations and infrequently performed tests are best conducted in a specialist laboratory environment rather than in general practice.

URINALYSIS

Urine is a complex substance which has evolved as an efficient medium for the excretion of waste products from the body. It is the main route by which metabolic products (e.g. creatinine and urea), minerals (e.g. calcium, magnesium and phosphorus), electrolytes (e.g. sodium, potassium and chloride) and water are eliminated from the body. The pH of the urine varies with its constituents and reflects the need for homeostatic maintenance of acid–base balance by the body.

Urine should be analysed when:

- There is a change in its physical appearance, e.g. discoloration
- An animal passes frank blood in its urine
- An animal exhibits polydipsia
- An animal exhibits polyuria
- An animal exhibits urinary tenesmus
- An animal licks its external genitalia excessively
- An animal exhibits increased urinary frequency
- An animal is dehydrated
- An animal is vomiting
- An animal has signs of fluid accumulation in the abdomen (i.e. ascites) or peripherally (subcutaneous oedema)
- Primary or secondary renal or urinary tract disease is suspected
- A urolith has been passed
- An animal exhibits pyrexia of unknown origin
- It is part of a routine screening test – juvenile, geriatric or before anaesthesia.

One of the main advantages of urinalysis is the wide range of information that it can provide for the clinician about systemic as well as local diseases. Urine collection is usually non-invasive and most tests can be carried out in the veterinary practice laboratory; with modern in-house laboratory equipment and commercial kits, reliably accurate results can be obtained very rapidly.

Urine should always be examined as soon as possible after it is collected. Samples will usually need to be transported to a commercial diagnostic laboratory for microbiological culture and sensitivity testing, for the quantitative analysis of sediment or uroliths, and for other non-routine chemical analyses. Transportation should be completed as soon as possible using, as appropriate, refrigerated samples, samples streaked by calibrated loop or pipette on to culture media such as blood agar and McConkey's agar, or samples with preservatives such as formaldehyde, thymol, toluene or boric acid.

Urinalysis includes one or more of the following :

- Physical examination
- Chemical examination
- Examination of sediment
- Bacterial culture
- Viral examination.

Methods of urine collection

Urine is a potentially hazardous substance because zoonotic organisms such as *Leptospira* may be present; hence, protective disposable gloves should be worn during the collection and handling of urine samples. Waste urine samples and soiled containers are classified as clinical waste and should be disposed of in accordance with the appropriate health and safety regulations (see Chapter 1).

There are three commonly used techniques for the collection of urine; each has its advantages and disadvantages.

Free flow

Urine is collected by free flow either during normal micturition, or during manual expression of urine from the bladder.

The timing of collection can be important. The first stream of urine flow is the best sample to collect for suspected lesions very low in the urinary tract, such as for the collection and identification of urethral plugs, crystals, uroliths, bacteria, viral infections, or haemorrhage. However, this sample is also the most likely to be contaminated with cells, bacteria and cell debris/sperm from the genital tract and surrounding skin and hair.

The mid-stream urine flow is the best sample to collect for most examinations. End-stream urine flow is the best sample to collect for examination for prostatic disease and, in some circumstances, for the collection of sediment or haemorrhage that may have collected on the floor of the bladder.

As much urine as possible should be collected in an inert, sterile, ceramic, steel or plastic container and then transferred to a commercial sterile container.

Urine collected by free flow is nearly always contaminated with bacteria. Nevertheless, it is an acceptable method for the collection of urine to be examined for physical appearance, pH, chemistry and microscopic appearance.

Manual expression of urine is convenient when the bladder contains sufficient urine to be isolated manually on palpation of the abdomen. In large dogs the urinary bladder can easily be expressed manually. If strong resistance is met, care needs to be taken so as not to rupture the bladder, especially if the bladder may have been subjected to trauma, if the outflow tract is obstructed or if there may be a destructive lesion (such as a neoplasm) which could have weakened the bladder or urethral wall. Care is needed especially when compressing the bladder of male cats with urethral obstruction. Pressure on the bladder can result in retrograde reflux of urine up the ureters from the bladder, which may be detected during dynamic retrograde contrast urography.

Cystocentesis

Cystocentesis involves the passage of a needle through the abdominal wall and into the urinary bladder. The urine-filled bladder is identified by palpation and held against the caudal ventral abdominal wall. The area of skin overlying the bladder is clipped and surgically prepared. A 50–75 mm 23 gauge hypodermic needle is inserted through the midline of the abdominal wall, at a 45° angle in a caudal and dorsal direction. Urine in the bladder is drained off into a suitable sterile syringe or collection vessel so that it can be used for analysis and/or microbiological culture and sensitivity.

Cystocentesis is well tolerated in most conscious animals, which is important for patients in which the administration of a general anaesthetic could be hazardous. Cystocentesis has been described (Elliott, 1996; Scott-Moncrieff, 1996) as the method of choice for the collection of urine because it provides a sample not contaminated by bacteria and cells from the distal urethra and so allows more accurate interpretation of culture and sensitivity results.

Haemorrhage into the urine is a common complication of cystocentesis and a recent report (Kruger *et al.*, 1991) claims that 46% of cats developed cystocentesis-induced microscopic haematuria. According to Chew and DiBartola (1986), urine obtained by cystocentesis should only contain up to three red blood cells per high-power microscope field, which is within the normal range of 0–8.

Cystocentesis is contraindicated or inappropriate if the urinary bladder cannot be isolated easily on abdominal palpation, or if the patient has ascites, thrombocytopenia or other clotting defects. Some authors (Macdougall and Curd, 1996) have recently suggested that cystocentesis is contraindicated if the bladder is severely overdistended, as it may be in cases of urinary tract obstruction. This author disagrees with this view. In such cases cystocentesis is a good procedure to use to collect urine and it has the advantage of providing a rapid reduction in intraluminal pressure in the bladder, which is an important clinical objective. It is also necessary to drain the bladder by cystocentesis before uroliths obstructing the lower urinary tract can be removed by retrograde flushing.

Catheterization

Catheterization involves the passage of a man-made tube into the urinary bladder via the urethra to collect urine. It is also a useful procedure for identifying the position of total or partial obstructions of the urethra, especially uroliths, stenosis or foreign bodies. Catheterization is also used in studies designed to monitor urine volume and rate of production, particularly in post-surgical cases, and it is essential when conducting dynamic tests of urine output in renal failure studies, for the administration of contrast media in radiography, and for the measurement of post-micturition urine volume in the bladder.

Catheterization is a minimally invasive procedure that is well tolerated by many male dogs but it frequently requires sedation or general anaesthesia in

bitches, queens and entire tom cats. Although a commonly performed procedure it has disadvantages. Organisms in the distal part of the genital tract and urethra can be transported up the urethra into the urinary bladder, leading to urinary tract infection (Biertuempfel *et al.*, 1981; Comer and Ling, 1981). Also, these organisms can complicate the interpretation of culture and sensitivity results. Also, the procedure can cause trauma to the urinary tract, leading to haemorrhage and later fibrosis and stenosis. According to Chew and DiBartola (1986), samples of urine collected by catheterization can contain up to five red blood cells per high-power microscope field (within the normal range of 0–8). Unnecessary catheterization should therefore be avoided.

Catheters are available in a range of different materials and sizes. The author prefers to use flexible polypropylene catheters, although these can sometimes be rough and cause minor trauma during passage – particularly to the male urethra. Metal catheters are too rigid. Catheters are sized according to the 'French' system in which 1 French = one third of a millimetre, so a 9F catheter has a diameter of 3 mm. Urinary catheters have a variable number (up to six) of holes in the end to facilitate fluid movement in both directions, but sometimes it is necessary to cut off the end if a high-pressure stream of fluid is needed, such as when performing retrograde flushing to free a calculus lodged in the urethra. Jackson catheters have been specifically designed to minimize trauma to the penile urethra during catheterization in cats with lower urinary tract obstruction.

Examination of urine

Physical examination

Visual appearance: Abnormalities in colour, smell, turbidity or content may be noticed on visual inspection (Table 19.2).

Urine volume: Total urine output should be collected over a 24-hour period, which requires that the animal is kept in a metabolism cage unless it has an indwelling catheter *in situ* and the urine is collected into a bag or other container.

According to Bush (1991) daily urine output is usually within the range of 20–40 ml/kg body weight for dogs and 18–25 ml/kg body weight for cats. An increase in urine output, though within the normal physiological range, occurs with increased intake of fluid, food, protein or salt.

Polyuria exists when urine output exceeds the normal range by more than 50 ml/kg per day and can be due to many causes, including renal and urinary tract disorders. The differential diagnosis of polyuria can be difficult, because of the number of possibilities (Table 19.3).

Test	Normal range	Abnormal increase	Abnormal decrease
Odour:	Pheromones (e.g. tom cats), diet-related (e.g. fish —volatile fatty acids)		
Ammonia		Due to urease-positive bacteria (e.g. *Proteus*) if a urinary tract infection; otherwise stale sample	
Acetone (sweet)		Ketoacidotic stage of diabetes mellitus	
Putrefaction		For example, bladder necrosis following strangulation in a perineal rupture	
Therapeutic agents		For example, penicillin	
Colour:	Clear to pale yellow (due to urochrome)		
Very pale			Due to dilution
Dark yellow		Due to concentration	
Red or pink		Due to haematuria, haemoglobinuria, myoglobinuria, porphyrins, phenytoin, bromsulphthalein, phenolsulphonphthalein	
Red to brown to black		Myoglobin or methaemoglobin	
Yellow to orange		Bilirubin, drugs (nitrofurantoin), riboflavin, phenolsulphonphthalein (in acid urine)	
Blue		Methylene blue	
Green		Biliverdin (old sample), myoglobin, *Pseudomonas* infection	
Turbidity: White	Transparent	Crystalluria	
Buff		Urate crystals Casts	
Cloudiness	Clear	Bacteria, secretions (e.g. semen, mucus, prostatic fluid)	
Cells	None	Blood, epithelial, other	

Table 19.2: Normal and abnormal urine odour and colour.

Oliguria (decreased urine output) occurs when urine output falls below 7 ml/kg per day. Although anuria literally means 'no urine production', according to Bush (1991) anuria occurs when urine output is below 2 ml/kg per day. Causes of oliguria are listed in Table 19.4.

In acute renal failure (ARF) there is reduced rate of urine formation, with oliguria or anuria, but sometimes urine output can be normal or even increased, particu-larly due to polyuria in the later stages (Bush, 1991). In chronic renal failure (CRF) the rate of urine production is usually increased (polyuria) but sometimes it is normal or decreased.

The volume of urine produced affects its density and thus its specific gravity (SG) which can affect the quantitative analysis of urine contents (e.g. concentration of protein).

Cause	Comments

Causes of impaired ADH secretion:
   Central diabetes insipidus
   Overhydration due to i.v. fluid therapy
   Therapeutic agents
   Psychogenic polydipsia
   Insulinoma
   Phaeochromocytoma
	Produces very high urine volumes
	
	Adrenaline, atropine, phenytoin, clonidine
	Uncommon. Very high urine volumes

ADH inhibition:
   Renal diabetes insipidus
   Hyperadrenocorticism (Cushing's syndrome)
   Toxaemia (eg pyometra)
   Hypercalcaemia
   Hyperthyroidism
   Liver disease
   Hypokalaemia
   Therapeutic agents
	
	e.g. Paraneoplastic syndrome
	Cats
	
	Methoxyfluorane, amphotericin B,
	glucocorticoids, prostaglandins, demeclocycline

Excess solute:
   Diabetes mellitus
   High-protein or high-salt diet
   Osmotic diuretics
   Chronic renal failure
   Acute renal failure
   Fanconi syndrome
   Primary renal glycosuria
   Nephrotic syndrome
   Hyperviscosity
   Acromegaly
	
	Mannitol, dextrose
	Common
	Including post-renal causes, e.g. obstruction
	Uncommon
	Uncommon
	Uncommon
	Uncommon
	Uncommon

Diuresis:
   Loop diuretics
   Thiazide derivatives
   Aldosterone antagonists
   Carbonic anhydrase inhibitors
	Frusemide, ethacrynic acid
	Hydrochlorthiazide
	Spironolactone
	Acetazolamide

Other:
   Hypoadrenocorticism
   Liver disease
   Low-protein diet
   Pyelonephritis
   Hypocalcaemia
   Lymphocytic thyroiditis
	
	Uncommon
	Uncommon
	Uncommon
	Uncommon

Table 19.3: *Differential diagnosis of polyuria. (Modified after Bush, 1991.)*

Specific gravity: On commercially available dipstick test strips, the SG results are unreliable for dogs and cats because they have been designed and validated for human urine (Bush, 1991). SG is best measured with a refractometer (Figure 19.5) which has a calibrated scale for SG based upon the refractive index, which is what it actually measures. Normal and abnormal SG measurements are summarized in Tables 19.5 and 19.6.

Urine SG measurement is one of the most important tests to include when screening old animals, as this will detect abnormalities in urine-concentrating ability, which can alert the clinician to the presence of subclinical chronic renal disease, which is very common in this population.

Cause	Comments
Pre-renal acute renal failure (ARF)	Specific gravity >1.030 (dogs) Specific gravity >1.035 (cats) Due to dehydration, shock, haemorrhage, hypoadrenocorticism, cardiac failure, hypoproteinaemia
Renal ARF	Specific gravity <1.030 (dogs) Specific gravity <1.035 (cats) Due to acute interstitial nephritis
Post-renal ARF	Specific gravity variable
Chronic renal failure (CRF)	Terminal stage only Specific gravity <1.030 (dogs) Specific gravity <1.035 (cats)

Table 19. 4: Causes of oliguria. (SG values from Bush, 1991.)

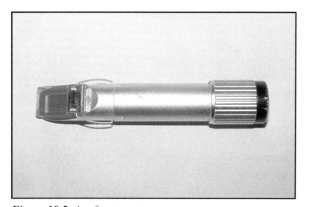

Figure 19.5: A refractometer.

Test	Range
Reference value for dogs	1.015–1.045
Reference value for cats	1.035–1.060
Maximum possible range in dogs	1.001–1.065
Maximum possible range in cats	1.001–1.080
Glomerular filtrate	1.008–1.012 290–300 mOsm/kg (same as plasma)

Table 19.5: Urine specific gravity. (Values from Bush, 1991.)

Cause	Comments
Increased water loss but no increased loss of solutes	Causes low or low normal SG See Table 19.2 – Causes of polyuria, due to ADH inhibition and diuresis
Increased water loss and increased loss of solutes	Normal or slightly increased SG See Table 19.2 – Causes of polyuria, due to excess solute loss, except ARF and CRF
Decreased loss of water and no decreased loss of solutes	High SG Severe shock, haemorrhage, cardiac failure, dehydration, renal infarction

Inability of kidneys to dilute or concentrate urine	Following loss of 66% of functional nephrons – results in a stable SG of:
	    dogs: 1.007–1.029
	    cats: 1.007–1.034
	Seen in renal and post-renal ARF and in CRF
	NB In early primary glomerular disease azotaemia may occur prior to the inability to concentrate urine
	A loss of 75% of functional nephrons leads to isosthenuria (same SG as glomerular filtrate)

Table 19.6: Causes of abnormal urine specific gravity (SG). (Values from Bush, 1991.)

Chemical examination

Many of the laboratory tests in common use in veterinary practice have been designed for use in human patients and they may give misleading results in dogs and cats. Common examples are:

- A dipstick 'positive' result for protein (equates to 0.5 g/l) is normal in dogs
- A dipstick 'positive' result for bilirubin may be normal in dogs
- A dipstick test for nitrite gives false-negative results
- A dipstick test for urobilinogen gives false-positive and false-negative results.

Many substances interfere with test results and can cause erroneous results. Drugs that can alter laboratory findings for tests of importance in relation to the renal and urinary systems are listed in Tables 19.7 and 19.8. It is important to be aware of the effects of drugs, particularly when laboratory tests are being used to monitor progress whilst an animal is on concurrent treatment. Drug interference may sometimes provide the explanation for an otherwise bizarre set of results.

Urine pH: pH is a measure of the hydrogen ion concentration. A pH of 7 is regarded as neutral, a higher pH (7–14) is alkaline, and a lower pH (0–7) is acidic. In the dog and cat the maximum feasible range is 4.5–8.5. Urine pH is usually measured using commercially available test strips but a pH meter or other indicator paper can also be used. The urine pH for normal dogs and cats is usually slightly acidic, within the range of pH 5.5–7.5. The causes of abnormal increases and decreases in urine pH are listed in Tables 19.9 and 19.10.

The pH of urine affects the solubility of urine constituents and so can affect their solubility products and can increase or decrease the likelihood of crystallization of solutes. Urine pH is extremely important in the aetiopathogenesis of some forms of urolith (see below).

A strongly alkaline urine is often the result of urease-producing urinary tract infections such as with *Staphylococcus* or *Proteus* spp. Renal tubular dys-

Urine parameter	Drugs and other substances that can affect laboratory estimations
Acetone	Acetaminophen, bromsulphthalein, phenylsulphonphthalein, salicylates
Albumin	Ampicillin, iodides, penicillin, salicylates, radiographic contrast media
Blood	Iodides, methenamine, vitamin C (–), radiographic contrast media
Calcium	Anabolic steroids, methenamine, sodium bicarbonate (–), thiazides (–), triamterene (–), viomycin (–), vitamin D
Colour	Anthraquinones, chloroquine, furazolidone, methocarbamol, methylene blue, phenazopyridine, PSP, phenothiazines, quinacrine, quinidine, sulphonamides
Creatinine	Anabolic steroids, corticosteroids, thiazides (–), triamterene (–)
Glucose	Bismuth salts, corticosteroids, epinephrine, intravenous glucose, isonazid, morphine, nicotinic acid, salicylates, tetracyclines, thiazides, vitamin C
Phenylsulphonphthalein	Acetazolamide (–), anthraquinones, cephaloridine, furazolidone, iodides (–), methenamine, penicillin (–), phenazopyridine, probenecid, salicylates (–), sodium bicarbonate (–), sulphonamides (–), thiazides (–), triamterene (–)
Total protein	Aminophylline, amphotericin B, ampicillin, arsenicals, dithiazanine, gentamicin, griseofulvin, isoniazid, kanamycin, methicillin, neomycin, oxacillin, penicillin, penicillamine, polymyxin B, salicylates, viomycin, vitamin D, radiographic contrast media
Specific gravity	Ampicillin, dextrans, dithiazanine, radiographic contrast media
Uric acid	Acetazolamide (–), corticosteroids , probenecid, salicylates, thiazides (–), triamterene, vitamin C
Urobilinogen	Ampicillin (–), BSP, cephaloridine (–), chloramphenicol (–), cloxacillin (–), erythromycin (–), gentamicin (–), kanamycin (–), methicillin (–), neomycin (–), oxacillin (–), phenazopyridine, phenothiazines, procaine, streptomycin (–), sulphonamides, tetracyclines (–)

Table 19.7: Agents that can influence urine tests. (–) indicates agent causes a false-negative depression of value.

Blood parameter	Drugs and other substances that can affect laboratory estimations
Alkaline phosphatase	Allopurinol, ampicillin, anabolic steroids, androgens, barbiturates, bromsulphthalein, cephaloridine, cephalothin, chloramphenicol, chlordiazepoxide, cloxacillin, colchicine, erythromycin, oestrogens, fluoride (–), frusemide, intravenous glucose, indomethacin, meperidine, morphine, oxacillin, penicillamine, phenothiazines, primidone, progesterones
Ammonia	Acetaminophen, chlorthalidone, heparin, isoniazid, lincomycin, methicillin, neomycin (–), sodium bicarbonate (–), sodium chloride (–), spironolactone
Blood urea nitrogen	Aluminium antacids, amphotericin B, arsenicals, bacitracin, calcium antacids, cephaloridine, chlorthalidone, colistin, dextrothyroxine, ethacrynic acid, frusemide, gentamicin, indomethacin, kanamycin, magnesium antacids, mercurials (–), methicillin, methocarbamol, neomycin, nicotinic acid, oxacillin, polymixin B, propranolol, spironolactone, stilbophen, streptokinase, sulphonamides, tetracyclines, triamterene, vancomycin, radiographic contrast media
Calcium	Anabolic steroids, androgens, bromsulphthalein, calcium antacids, oestrogens, EDTA (–), intravenous glucose (–), heparin (–), iodides (–), magnesium antacids (–), methicillin (–), progesterones, sodium bicarbonate , sodium chloride, viomycin (–)
Chloride	Acetazolamide, anthraquinones, corticosteroids (–), corticotrophin (–), ethacrynic acid (–), frusemide (–), kanamycin (–), mannitol (–), phenylbutazone , potassium chloride, thiazides (–) triamterene
Creatinine	Amphotericin B, barbiturates, bromsulphthalein, colistin, kanamycin, mannitol, methicillin, PSP, streptokinase, triamterene, viomycin (–)
Glucose	Acetaminophen (–), caffeine, chlorthalidone, corticosteroids, corticotropin, diphenylhydantoin, epinephrine, oestrogens, ethacrynic acid, fluoride (–), frusemide, intravenous glucose, heparin, indomethacin, iodides, isoniazid, nicotinic acid, phenacetin (–), phenothiazines, potassium chloride (–), propranolol (–), salicylates (–), tetracyclines (–), thiabendazole, thiazides, triamterene
Platelet count	Acetazolamide (–), amphotericin B (–), arsenicals (–), chloramphenical (–), chloroquine (–), chlorthalidone (–), colchicine (–), oestrogens (–), ethacrynic acid (–), methotrexate (–), penicillin (–) , phenylbutazone (–), quinidine (–), quinine (–), salicylates (–), sulphonamides (–), thiazides (–)
Phosphorus	Phosphate binders (–)
Potassium	Acetazolamide (–), amphotericin B (–), anthraquinones (–), chlorthalidone (–), corticosteroids (–), corticotropin (–), epinephrine, ethacrynic acid (–), frusemide (–), iodides (–), iron, isoniazid , mannitol (–), mercurials (–), penicillamine (–), penicillin, phenothiazines (–), potassium chloride, salicylates (–), spironolactone, tetracyclines (–), thiazides (–), triamterene, viomycin (–)
Sodium	Anabolic steroids, androgens, anthraquinones (–), calcium antacids (–), corticosteroids, corticotropin, ethacrynic acid (–), frusemide (–), heparin (–), iron, mercurials (–), methicillin, penicillin, phenylbutazone, potassium chloride, reserpine, salicylates, sodium chloride, spironolactone (–), triamterene (–)
Uric acid	Acetazolamide, allopurinol (–), cephaloridine, chlorthalidone, corticosteroids (+/–) , corticotropin (–), epinephrine , ethacrynic acid (+/–), frusemide, mercurials, methicillin, methotrexate (–), nicotinic acid, phenothiazines (–), phenylbutazone, piperazine, salicylates (–), spironolactone, thiazides, triamterene
White blood cell count	Acetaminophen (–), allopurinol , chloramphenicol (–), chlordiazepoxide (–), chloroquine (–), chlorthalidone (–), colistin (–), corticosteroids , corticotropin , diiodohydroxyquin (–), erythromycin, ethacrynic acid (–), frusemide (–), indomethacin (–), methicillin (–), methocarbamol (–), methotrexate (–), novobiocin (–), oxacillin (–), penicillamine (–), phenothiazines (–), phenylbutazone (–), primidone (–), propylthiouracil (–), quinine (–), sulphonamides (–), thiabendazole (–), vitamin A (–)

Table 19.8: Agents that can influence blood tests of relevance to the urinary system. (–) signifies agent reduces values.

Cause	Comments
Renal or urinary tract in origin:	
Urinary tract infection	Due to urease-producing bacteria (*Proteus, Staphylococcus*). Can reach pH of 8.5, and this cannot be corrected by the use of urinary acidifiers
Urinary retention	Obstruction leading to bacterial contamination and decomposition of urea
Proximal renal tubular acidosis (rare)	Causes excess loss of bicarbonate
Other causes:	
Diet	Low-protein diets During postprandial period — called postprandial alkaline tide. Caused by relative alkalosis due to secretion of gastric acids
Respiratory alkalosis	Due to losses of carbon dioxide through hyperventilation in respiratory disease
Vomiting	Due to loss of gastric acid. Usually indicates chronic vomiting or pyloric obstruction
Alkalinizing drugs	Sodium bicarbonate, chlorthiazides, acetazolamide, sodium lactate, potassium citrate
False results:	
Contamination	Ammonia products or detergents

Table 19.9: *Causes of alkaline urine (pH >7).*

Cause	Comments
Renal or urinary tract causes:	
Severe azotaemia	Acidosis in acute renal failure due to waste product accumulation from protein catabolism
Other causes:	
Severe vomiting	Lactic acidosis develops with dehydration, loss of duodenal contents (alkaline) and increased hydrogen and chloride resorption
Respiratory acidosis/ hypoxia	Pulmonary or cardiac disease resulting in respiratory depression and decreased carbon dioxide excretion Respiratory depression due to anaesthesia
Shock	Reduces oxygenation, leading to accumulation of acidic metabolites
Ketoacidosis	Common sequel to diabetes mellitus
Severe diarrhoea	Due to decreased resorption of bicarbonate ions
Acidifying diets	Used in the management of urolithiasis
Acidifying drugs	Ammonium chloride, methionine, frusemide, sodium chloride, sodium acid phosphate
Metaldehyde poisoning	Produces acidic metabolites
Ethylene glycol poisoning	Produces acidic metabolites
Increased protein catabolism	High-protein diets Catabolic disorders — major organ disease Glucocorticoids Hyperthyroidism Pyrexia Malignant neoplasia

Table 19.10: *Causes of acidic urine (pH<7).*

function (tubular acidosis) often leads to an inability to produce acidic urine due to excessive bicarbonate ion excretion in the urine and this can be checked using the ammonium chloride test (see below).

Proteinuria: A small amount of protein is found in normal urine (see above). The commercial strip tests in common use are most sensitive to albumin and may therefore underestimate the concentrations of other proteins that are found in urine. Sulphosalicylic acid (20%) can be used in an alternative test which is more sensitive to other proteins. Both types of test can produce false results (see Table 19.11). The commercial tests for protein in urine are not as sensitive as those for protein in blood, so a 'negative' result does not preclude the presence of haemoglobin or myoglobin in the sample. Unfortunately, commercial test strips can also miss Bence–Jones protein (immunoglobulins produced in great numbers, usually in multiple myeloma). This form of protein needs to be identified using 20% sulphosalicylic acid or electrophoresis. Both electrophoresis and paper chromatography are useful tests because they produce highly specific separation profiles for individual proteins or amino acids.

A trace reading for protein on dipstick test strips (equates to 0.3 g/l) is of no clinical significance. Very high readings are significant and usually signify glomerular disease or the presence of a urinary tract infection.

There are numerous causes of proteinuria (Tables 19.11 and 19.12) and interpretation can be misleading unless certain influencing factors are taken into consideration. For example, protein concentrations in urine must always be interpreted with a knowledge of the urine volume being produced. This is best done by :

- Examination of urine SG. Dilute urine will reduce the protein test result; concentrated urine will increase it
- Measurement of daily protein excretion in urine. This requires collection of all urine voided in a 24-hour period, which may present practical difficulties in a practice environment. Healthy dogs can lose up to 30 mg protein per kilogram of body weight (average 15 mg/kg) per day

Cause	Comments

RENAL IN ORIGIN
   Severe proteinuria (>10g/l):
      Advanced glomerulonephritis,
      advanced amyloidosis
	Part of the nephrotic syndrome

Proteinuria up to 10g/l :
   CRF, ARF, early amyloidosis, diabetic
   glomerulosclerosis, Fanconi syndrome,
   chronic passive cardiac congestion,
   infectious disease (leptospirosis, feline
   leukaemia, infectious canine hepatitis,
    feline infectious peritonitis), fever, primary
   renal glycosuria, physiological causes
   (extreme heat or cold, exercise or stress)
Specific proteinuria – abnormal trace
	One of the reasons why these disorders may result in only a low to moderate increase in proteinuria is because they may be associated with polyuria which effectively dilutes the quantity of protein in the urine
	In early glomerulonephritis or amyloidosis with only moderate proteinuria, may get nephrotic syndrome without oedema
	
	Enzyme gamma-glutamyltransferase in urine

NON-RENAL CAUSES
   Mild to moderate proteinuria:
      Urogenital tract inflammation, haematuria,
      haemoglobinuria, myoglobinuria,
      hyperproteinaemia, genital secretions	

FALSE-POSITIVE RESULTS Strip tests	Stale urine Sample contaminated with cetrimide, benzalkonium chloride, chlorhexidine, polyvinyl pyrrolidone Excessive soaking of strip with the urine sample
20% sulphosalicylic acid	Presence of thymol, tolbutamide, radiographic contrast media, penicillins, cephalosporins or sulphafurazole

Table 19.11: Causes of proteinuria.

Cause	Usual findings	Other tests	Dipsticks
PRERENAL CAUSES			
Haemolytic anaemia	Haemoglobinuria	Haematology	Easily detected
Azotaemia (rhabdomyolysis)	Myoglobinuria		Easily detected
Multiple myeloma	Bence–Jones immunoglobulins	Radiography	Not easily detected
Lymphoma	Immunoglobulins		Not easily detected
Leukaemia	Immunoglobulins	Haematology Serology	Not easily detected
Hyperproteinaemia due to parenteral plasma administration			Easily detected
RENAL CAUSES			
Glomerulopathy:			
Glomerulonephritis	Albumin: Usually large amounts present (>1g/l)	Biopsy	Easily detected
Renal amyloidosis			
Glomerulosclerosis (unusual complication of diabetes mellitus)			
Primary renal glycosuria (Cocker Spaniel and Elkhound)			
Tubular disorders:			
ARF (interstitial nephritis, acute tubular necrosis)	Enzymes Polypeptide hormones Immunoglobulins	Haematology Serology	Not easily detected
CRF (hydronephrosis, nephrolithiasis, polycystic kidney, end-stage renal disease)	Fibrin degradation Retinol-binding protein Microglobulins	Renal biopsy – as appropriate	
Fanconi syndrome			
Renal parenchymal disease:			
Pyelonephritis	Inflammatory exudate	Urine microscopy and culture Fine needle biopsy and culture Serology	Not easily detected
Neoplasia (e.g. lymphoma)	Neoplastic cells, cell debris and inflammatory exudate	Radiography Fine needle biopsy	
Passive venous congestion		Full clinical work-up for cardiac, hepatic disease or abdominal mass	
POSTRENAL CAUSES			
Urinary tract inflammation:			
Urinary tract infection (especially cystitis)	Inflammatory exudate	Urinalysis Culture	Not easily detected
Urolithiasis			
Trauma			
Prostatitis			
Vaginitis			
Neoplasia (lower urinary tract):			
Bladder and urethral neoplasia	Neoplastic cells and inflammatory exudate	Cytology Radiography	Not easily detected
Other:			
Any cause of haematuria, haemoglobinuria or myoglobinuria			Easily detected
Normal urogenital secretions (e.g. semen, prostatic secretions, oestrus-related secretions)			Not easily detected

Table 19.12: *Test results with different causes of proteinuria.*

- Determination of the ratio of urine creatinine to urine protein (best done in a commercial laboratory) in a random sample. This can allow an extrapolated value to be calculated for daily protein loss because the creatinine is excreted at a constant rate (Barsanti and Finco, 1979). Normal protein to creatinine ratio values in urine are 0.08-0.29 in dogs and 0.13-0.42 in cats (Barsanti and Finco, 1979). High ratios are caused by a protein meal, glomerulonephritis and amyloidosis. This technique cannot differentiate between the latter, so renal biopsy is still needed to differentiate these conditions.

The specific diagnosis of proteinuria can be complicated and requires a logical rule-in/rule-out approach (see Table 19.13). Blood components consist of protein; hence it is necessary to consider causes of haematuria and haemoglobinuria as well (Tables 19.14 and 19.15).

Increased protein concentrations in urine must always prompt an examination of urine sediment for cells and casts, which will help to determine whether the protein is of renal or of lower urinary tract origin.

Glycosuria: Glucose does not appear in the urine unless its blood concentration exceeds the renal threshold or there is renal damage that allows leakage into the glomerular filtrate. There are many causes of glycosuria and it is important to differentiate between those associated with hyperglycaemia and those which are *not*. Renal causes are *not* associated with hyperglycaemia.

Examination of sediment

For accurate interpretation of urine sediment a freshly collected sample of urine should be examined immediately by microscopy, or urine can be centrifuged and the sediment removed for examination. Delay in examination results in cell lysis and can cause a change in pH and precipitation of non-significant crystals.

The findings on examination of urine sediment that are of clinical significance are summarized in Table 19.16; crystals that are commonly found in the sediment of dog and cat urine, and their significance, are summarized in Table 19.17. Figure 19.6 illustrates some of the common crystals. The reader is also referred to a recent review of crystalluria (Osborne *et al.*, 1990).

Bacterial culture

Urinary tract infections (UTIs) are common in both cats and dogs but finding bacteria in the urine does not, in itself, confirm a diagnosis of UTI as the organisms found might be commensals or contaminants. Diagnosis is based upon identification and culture of a pathogenic organism which is present in large numbers in a fresh urine sample. Clinical signs need to be compat-

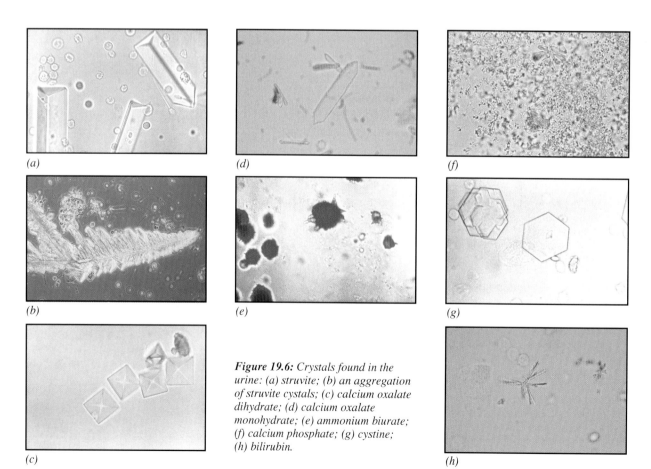

(a) *(d)* *(f)*

(b) *(e)* *(g)*

(c)

Figure 19.6: Crystals found in the urine: (a) struvite; (b) an aggregation of struvite cystals; (c) calcium oxalate dihydrate; (d) calcium oxalate monohydrate; (e) ammonium biurate; (f) calcium phosphate; (g) cystine; (h) bilirubin.

(h)

Stage	Test	Sample	Positive	Negative
1	Dipstick test	Voluntary or manually voided urine	Indicates presence of albumin (**Go to stage 2**)	Very low amounts of albumin present
2	Dipstick test	Urine collected by cystocentesis	Indicates urine in bladder contains albumin (**Go to stage 3**)	Recheck another sample of urine
3a	Centrifuge sample and examine any sediment under microscope	Examine sample for red and white blood cells, other cells (neoplastic, epithelial or inflammatory), crystals, casts, parasites and microorganisms (bacteria, yeast) Urine collected in different ways can be helpful in localizing a lesion (see section on methods of urine collection)	Sediment present (but no tubular casts): can be upper or lower urinary tract disorder Sediment present with casts: upper urinary tract disorder (**Go to stage 4**)	No sediment or haemoglobinuria found Quantify proteinuria: calculate protein to creatinine ratio (**Go to stage 5**)
3b	Visual inspection of urine for colour change. Dipstick test for haemoglobin	Any fresh sample	Haemoglobin: pink or red discoloration Myoglobin: brown discoloration (usually; can be red-brown to black) Positive dipstick result (**Go to stage 6**)	
4a	Perform full blood chemistry panel for renal and urinary tract disorders	Fresh blood sample	Pursue likely diagnosis: upper or lower urinary tract disorder (See individual disease panels)	
4b	Examine urine for presence of glucose	Fresh urine sample	**Tubular functional defect** if patient has normal blood glucose concentrations	
4c	Culture urine		**Urinary tract infection**	
4d	Imaging	Radiography/Ultrasonography	Urolithiasis, neoplasia, renal abnormalities in shape/size	
5a	Creatinine to urea ratio normal or slightly elevated (i.e. <0.5-1)	**Transient proteinuria:** repeat test in 2 weeks **Concentrated urine:** check urine SG and measure urine output. Perform haematology to see if animal has increased packed cell volume. **False-positive** dipstick test:repeat test in 2 weeks		
5b	Creatinine to urea ratio elevated (i.e. >1 to <13)	Check blood chemistry Check for urine glucose Check haematology	Elevated creatinine and urea: **Glomerular cause of proteinuria** Glycosuria (normal blood glucose): **Tubular functional defect** Hyperproteinaemia: **Pre-renal proteinuria**	
5c	Ceatinine to urea ratio very high (i.e. >13.0)		**Glomerular cause of proteinuria**	
6	Haematology	Red cell count and PCV	Anaemia: Look for causes of **Pre-renal (intravascular) haemolysis** No anaemia: Look for causes of **Post-renal or Renal causes of haemorrhage and subsequent haemolysis in the urinary tract**	

Table 19.13: Differential diagnosis of proteinuria. (Modified after Barber, 1996.)

Cause	Comments

Systemic causes:
    Disorders leading to defective
        haemostasis
	Warfarin poisoning
	Thrombocytopenia

Hepatic failure	Due to impaired prothrombin production by the liver, and consequential defective haemostasis
Septicaemia	Any
Toxaemia	Any
Viraemia	Any
Chronic passive venous congestion	Cardiac failure
Any part of the urinary tract: Inflammation	Bacteria: localized in the bladder is the most common cause of haematuria Cyclophosphamide: haematuria is a side effect of this widely used anti-cancer drug
Urolithiasis or nephrolithiasis	Particularly rough surfaced stones such as calcium oxalate
Neoplasia	Often malignant transition cell carcinomas located near the bladder neck, but can be caused by any neoplasm including benign polyps
Trauma	Catheterization Cystocentesis Road traffic accidents *Capillaria plica* infection (rare)
Renal in origin: Acute leptospirosis	Due to *Leptospira canicola*. Confirmed by urine examination for presence of leptospires
Acute tubular necrosis	Due to ischaemia or nephrotoxicity
Glomerulopathies	Due to glomerulonephritis or amyloidosis
Renal injury due to infarction	Primary causes can be septicaemia, endocarditis or cardiomyopathy
Idiopathic renal haemorrhage	Not uncommon. Unilateral cases may be due to ruptured intrarenal blood vessel
Renal cysts Familial telangiectasia	Seen in Pembroke Welsh Corgi and in cats
Crystalluria	Rare
Radiation injury	Rare
Renal parasites	Not in UK, except in imported animals
Bladder or urethra: Feline lower urinary tract disease	Associated with crystalluria, urolith formation, infection (occasionally) and sebulous plug formation
Punctate cystitis	Cause unknown: possibly due to urinary tract infection
Genital tract: Prostatic disease	Always consider possibility of prostate disease in male dogs – especially prostatitis, hypertrophy or hyperplasia, neoplasia and cysts
Penile and preputial disorders	Particularly trauma, inflammation and neoplasia (transmissible venereal tumour)
Uterine, vaginal and vulval disorders	Particularly normal pro-oestrus discharge, open pyometra, trauma (post-mating, post-spaying, normal parturition, dystocia and foreign bodies)
False positives	Due to interference of bacterial growth with test strip

Table 19.14: Causes of haematuria. (After Bush, 1991.)

Cause	Comments
Causes of haematuria	See Table 19.14
Autoimmune haemolytic anaemia	
Disseminated intravascular coagulation (DIC)	
Splenic torsion	
Toxins	Chlorate, nitrate, paracetamol, benzocaine, propylthiouracil, dimethyl sulphoxide (DMSO), snake venom
Physical causes of lysis	Burns, radiation, intravenous administration of hypotonic solutions
Incompatible blood transfusion	
Haemolytic disease of the newborn	
Feline haemobartonellosis (rare)	

Table 19.15: *Causes of haemoglobinuria. (After Bush, 1991.)*

Finding	Normal	Abnormal	Comments
Red blood cells (RBCs)	None	>5 RBCs per high-power field (hpf)	Dilute urine causes lysis of RBCs Concentrated urine causes crenation of RBCs
White blood cells (WBCs)	None	>5 WBCs per hpf Difficult to differentiate between different types of WBC	Large numbers indicates acute inflammation Dilute urine causes lysis of WBCs Alkaline urine causes lysis of WBCs
Epithelial cells	None	Transitional cells: variable shape and granular cytoplasm	Large numbers suggest inflammation or neoplasia
		Squamous cells: very large and thin cells	Increased numbers during oestrus Can find neoplastic forms
		Renal tubular cells: small, round or comma-shaped cells	Unknown significance
Casts:	Should find only 1-2 hyaline or granular casts per low-power field	Cylindrical shape, of mucoprotein (Tamm–Horsfall) from Loop of Henlé	Take up the shape of the renal tubule in which they form Larger casts originate in larger ducts Large numbers signify severe disease; more in ARF than in CRF
Hyaline			Mucoprotein. Most common form
Cellular			Includes cells (see above)
Granular			Degenerative stage of a cellular cast Most common form seen in renal disease
Waxy			Degenerative stage of a cellular cast. Seen in CRF and ARF
Fatty casts			Degenerative stage of tubular epithelial cells Seen mainly in cats, and are common in nephrotic syndrome
Stained casts: Red			Due to haemoglobinuria
Yellow			Due to bilirubin
Bacteria	None	>3x10⁴/ml before detectable	Contamination of urine samples is common, especially if collected by free flow or catheterization Large numbers suggest a urinary tract infection (but need to culture)
Yeasts/Fungi	None	Hyphae; budding organisms	Usually contaminants of sample
Spermatozoa	Normal finding		Occasionally seen in females
Parasites	None	In UK: eggs of *Capillaria plica*	In imported animals may find eggs of *Dioctophyma renale*, or microfilariae of *Dirofilaria immitis*

Table 19.16: *Findings of examination of urine sediment. (Reference values after Bush, 1991.)*

Crystal/ Urolith	Composition/ Crystal appearance	Urine pH that favours formation	Known predisposing factors	Physical characteristics of uroliths
Struvite	Magnesium ammonium phosphate: 3–6-sided prisms; 'coffin-shaped' (Figure 19.6a)	Alkaline, but occur at any pH	Urinary tract infection by urease-positive bacteria (dogs) In cats, struvite urolithiasis initially occurs in a sterile environment	Radiodense (variable) Smooth, round or faceted
Calcium oxalate	Calcium oxalate dihydrate: envelope-like crystals, octahedral/pyramidal in shape (Figure 19.6c) Calcium oxalate monohydrate: spindles, rings or dumbbell shapes (Figure 19.6d)	Not pH-sensitive Found at any pH	Hypercalciuria: absorptive, renal leak, hypercalcaemia Males > Females Breeds : Miniature Schnauzer, Yorkshire Terrier Ethylene glycol poisoning : monohydrate form usually Low magnesium, acidifying acids	Very radiodense Often rough, with sharp edges, round to oval
Urate	Ammonium biurate: yellow to dark brown aggregations like 'thorn apples' Sodium acid urate Uric acid: diamond -shaped or rhomboid	Acid Acid	Increased urinary urate excretion Breeds: Dalmatian; English Bulldog Liver disease: portosystemic shunts Urinary tract infection with urease-producing bacteria Dalmatians excrete some uric acid in their urine	Radiolucent Smooth, round or oval Green
Calcium phosphate	Calcium phosphate or calcium hydrogen phosphate: amorphous crystals	Alkaline, but occur at any pH	Commonly found as a minor constituent of struvite or calcium oxalate uroliths Metabolic disorders: Primary hyperparathyroidism Renal tubular acidosis	Very radiodense Smooth, round or faceted
Cystine	Cystine: large, flat, hexagonal (Figure 19.6g), colourless	Acid, but occur at any pH	Sex-linked defect in cystine (and lysine) transport by renal tubular cells Breeds: Dachshund, ?English Bulldog	Relatively radiolucent Smooth, usually round or oval
Silica	Silicon dioxide	Less soluble in acid urine	Diet consisting of corn gluten feed or soyabean hulls Ingestion of soil	Relatively radiodense, but often small Characteristic 'Jack stone' shape
Xanthine	Xanthine	Acid	A complication of the use of allopurinol as this drug blocks the conversion of xanthine to uric acid by inhibiting the enzyme xanthine oxidase Breeds: Dalmatian	Radiolucent Small Smooth Green
Bilirubin	Sharp, yellow needles (Figure 19.6h)	Acid	Associated liver disease	
Drug crystals	e.g. Sulphonamides	Acid	Therapeutic doses	Sharp needles: often aggregated

Table 19.17: Common crystals and uroliths found in urine and their significance.

Organism	Antibiotic sensitivity
Staphylococci	Almost 100% respond to penicillin or ampicillin
Streptococci	Almost 100% respond to penicillin or ampicillin
Escherichia coli	80% respond to trimethoprim sulphonamide combination
Proteus mirabilis	80% respond to penicillin or ampicillin
Pseudomonas aeruginosa	80% respond to tetracycline *
Klebsiella pneumoniae	90% respond to cephalexin *

Table 19.18: *Common bacterial causes of UTIs and their antibiotic sensitivities. * Potentially nephrotoxic, so must screen for underlying renal damage prior to administration.*

ible with the presence of an infection and there may be other significant laboratory findings, including the presence of red and white blood cells in the urine. If the infection is acute, with systemic signs, there may be a leucocytosis with a shift to the left on haematological examination. If a UTI does occur, it means that the natural defence mechanisms in place within the tract have been breached.

All animals with clinical signs of lower urinary tract disease (LUTD), including haematuria, increased frequency, polyuria, obstruction due to urolithiasis, and struvite or urate crystalluria, should have their urine cultured to rule in or out the presence of a bacterial infection.

As mentioned above, the nitrite test on commercially available dipsticks is not reliable for cat and dog urine, and cultures are usually best performed in specialist diagnostic centres with experienced staff rather than in a general practice laboratory.

Ideally, urine should be cultured as soon as possible after collection and prior to the administration of any antibiotics. Cystocentesis is the method of collection most authors prefer because it minimizes the likelihood of contamination. The sample should be stored at 4 °C and transported to the diagnostic laboratory within 12 hours. If this is not possible the sample should be mixed with 1% boric acid as preservative.

It is normal practice to culture the sample on blood agar and McConkey or cystine lactose electrolyte-deficient (CLED) agar plates as these between them support the growth of organisms most frequently implicated in UTIs. A growth of at least 100,000 colonies per millilitre is necessary for the result to be highly significant. Counts of 10,000 to 100,000 per millilitre are usually not very significant; however, if the sample has been collected under aseptic conditions by cystocentesis, then counts over 1000 are very significant.

If a significant growth is isolated it is usual to perform sensitivity testing. It is important that the sensitivity discs are set up for concentrations of antibiotic that are likely to be found in urine – not concentrations that are found in blood. Most antibiotics selected for use in UTIs attain a urinary concentration 10 to 100 times greater than their blood concentrations. It is also sensible to include in the sensitivity tests antibiotics with known potency against the common causes of UTI (Table 19.18).

Viral examination

Several viruses may be involved in the development of renal and urinary tract diseases (Table 19.19). Diagnosis is usually confirmed by serology and, rarely, by virus isolation and electron microscopy in specialist referral centres.

Samples need to be collected into suitable transport media for transfer to laboratories (see Chapters 1 and 5).

Virus	Comments
Feline leukaemia virus (FeLV)	May cause: Immunodeficiency leading to pyelonephritis Renal lymphoma (most renal lymphoma cases are FeLV-negative) Uraemia
Feline immunodeficiency virus (FIV)	May cause: Immunodeficiency leading to pyelonephritis Protein-losing nephropathy Uraemia
Feline infectious peritonitis (FIP) virus	May cause: Granulomatous inflammation of kidneys — non-effusive form of FIPV Uraemia
Canine distemper virus	
Cell-associated herpesvirus	Has been implicated as a possible cause of feline urolithiasis by some authors

Table 19.19: *Viruses involved in renal and urinary tract disease.*

RENAL AND OTHER BIOPSY

Biopsy of the kidneys can be an important step in the differential diagnosis of primary renal diseases when clinical signs and other laboratory findings give only non-specific results. An excellent review has recently been published (Macdougall and Lamb, 1996). However, *in vivo* biopsy is not always reliable because of the potential to miss focal lesions unless multiple samples are collected, and furthermore the techniques available are not without the possibilities of serious complications (e.g. intrarenal haemorrhage). Biopsy should therefore only be performed by experienced clinicians with the correct equipment available and with the full consent of the owners.

Indications for renal biopsy are listed in Table 19.20. If biopsy is required then there are some basic principles to follow:

- Avoid taking unnecessary biopsies
- All needle biopsies should be angled so as to avoid penetration of the medulla or hilar region. The easiest way to ensure this is to take biopsies near the poles of the kidney, aiming across the parenchyma rather than aiming towards the renal pelvis
- Following any biopsy of the kidney, manual pressure should be applied for 2–3 minutes to encourage haemostasis after the procedure has been completed. Alternatively, an absorbable haemostatic patch can be applied over the wound during closure. The biopsy site should always be checked for evidence of severe haemorrhage prior to closure of the body cavity
- Always handle biopsy tissues with care, to avoid crushing
- Whenever possible, discuss the case with the diagnostic laboratory in advance of taking a biopsy. They may advise a special fixative for some laboratory examinations
- Always fix tissues as soon as possible after collection
- Prepare smears by squeezing samples obtained by fine-needle aspiration between two microscope slides. Separate and air-dry immediately

- Transfer larger biopsies or longitudinally sectioned kidneys into 10% neutral buffered formalin
- Only use other fixatives such as 10% formol saline, Michel's fixative or 2% buffered gluteraldehyde if advised to do so by your diagnostic laboratory. These are sometimes needed for some forms of examination (see Macdougall and Lamb, 1996).
- Send samples to the diagnostic laboratory of your choice as soon as possible after collection. Try to use laboratories employing personnel experienced at looking at renal biopsies and renal histopathology.

NB Negative results from all forms of biopsy do not rule out the presence of a condition.

Techniques

Nephrectomy
This involves the surgical removal of a whole kidney. It is performed under general anaesthesia, which can be hazardous. The amount of tissue removed is ideal for full histopathological examination.

Nephrectomy is indicated when :

- Only one kidney is diseased
- It is considered that the kidney to be excised has lost all functional reserve
- The kidney has a disease that is localized but which might spread to other organs if not removed (e.g. neoplasia)
- The single kidney has intractable infection. Care is needed not to induce haematological spread or leakage into the peritoneum during surgery.

Nephrectomy should *not* be performed:

- When both kidneys are seriously diseased
- In the presence of neoplasia that is bilateral or which has metastasized
- If the patient is severely azotaemic or exhibits more than two risk factors for the development of ARF in the other kidney.

Indication	Comment
Severe proteinuria, when lower urinary tract causes have been ruled out	Biopsy to confirm the presence of glomerulonephritis or amyloidosis so that specific therapy can be applied
Terminal ARF	Biopsy findings can help in the evaluation of patients that are being considered for peritoneal dialysis. *NB* General anaesthesia should be avoided or carried out only under optimal conditions in these patients, i.e. with intensive care support facilities
Investigation of inherited forms of nephrology	Biopsy may help with prognosis
Uraemia with no specific diagnosis from other diagnostic procedures	Useful when other tests inconclusive or contradictory

Table 19.20: Indications for renal biopsy.

A midline approach is recommended. Nephrectomy should not be attempted using keyhole surgery, as it is easy to damage adjacent major blood vessels. The initial incision needs to extend further cranially for the right kidney than for the left kidney. Loops of small intestine should be packed off with towels moistened with sterile saline and, for the right kidney, the mesentery of the duodenum is reflected across the other loops of intestine to expose the kidney. For the left kidney the mesentery attached to the descending colon is used in a similar fashion.

The thin peritoneum over the kidney is incised and stripped off to expose the area of the renal pelvis. The renal artery, vein, nerves and ureter should be easily identified. The renal artery is a direct tributary of the aorta, and the renal vein goes direct to the caudal vena cava, so care is needed to clamp, section and ligate them properly. A three-forceps technique is preferred for this procedure, with double ligatures being laid over the vessels below the lower crushing clamp.The proximal end of the ureter (which is still attached to the urinary bladder) is ligated and released back into the abdomen.

Incisional (wedge) biopsy

This technique has the advantage that the biopsy can be taken from an area of obvious disease, discoloration, distortion or swelling, as identified by the clinician visibly or on palpation at laparotomy. Incisional biopsy is indicated when: the lesion is not resectable; the affected kidney or mass appears to be normal or non-neoplastic on gross examination; and a diffuse microscopic lesion is suspected from the history and can be identified from a small tissue sample. Ideally, it should not be used if the suspected diagnosis is neoplasia because of the risk of dissemination, but this may be difficult to determine on macroscopic visual examination alone. It should also not be used in cases with chronic infection.

For renal biopsy the surgical technique is initially similar to that for nephrectomy, with a midline approach to expose the kidney. Whenever possible the lesion should be fully exposed so that the biopsy can include apparently unaffected tissue around the margins of the lesion.

A thin wedge of tissue is taken by making two sharp incisions, approximately 2–4 mm apart, into the renal cortex from the greater curvature of the kidney. Care is taken not to make the incision too deep as the medulla should be avoided. The tissue is removed without excessive handling or crushing, and the sample should be put into fixative formalin immediately.

The incised wound is closed using an atraumatic needle with 3-0 to 4-0 absorbable suture material (chromic gut or synthetic). Synthetic sutures rapidly lose strength in the presence of urine.

Fine needle aspiration

Fine needle aspiration (FNA) can be used either at laparotomy or percutaneously. It should only be performed 'blind', by the percutaneous approach, when the kidney or other lesion to be biopsied can be clearly demarcated by palpation; otherwise ultrasonic guidance is necessary. FNA is the preferred choice for obtaining a biopsy at laparotomy when bilateral neoplasia or infection is a suspected diagnosis or when a cyst is present. Under these circumstances care needs to be taken to avoid contamination of the peritoneal cavity or adjacent tissues by packing off properly and by using copious volumes of sterile fluid for flushing out.

A 21 or 23 gauge sterile hypodermic needle of sufficient length for the size of organ, or a spinal needle, with sterile 5 ml syringe is used to aspirate cells. The tissue is sucked up into the lumen of the needle and can then be expelled from the needle by filling the syringe with air and pushing it out on to a microscope slide where a smear is made and air-dried immediately (see Chapter 7). Pressing the tissue between two slides and then separating them is usually an effective way of producing smears, and this can be done by a trained veterinary nurse whilst the veterinary surgeon obtains further samples or closes the wound. As this technique is relatively atraumatic it can be repeated several times.

Samples obtained by FNA are useful for cytology and so it is a very useful procedure for identifying inflammatory or neoplastic cells. FNA samples are less satisfactory for the isolation of collagen and fibroblasts and it is impossible to get undamaged tissue samples suitable for histopathology, so it is a less suitable technique for the identification of lesions with a structural, spatial distribution, such as glomerulonephritis or amyloidosis.

Percutaneous collection of renal tissue

Percutaneous tissue core biopsy samples are obtained by inserting a biopsy needle through a small transabdominal incision under ultrasonic guidance. The technique is claimed to be accurate by its exponents (Hager *et al.*, 1985) and to cause minimal trauma to the patient. A variety of needles is available for this procedure in the UK, including those for use with automatic biopsy guns (see Macdougall and Lamb, 1996). The number of biopsies needed depends upon the diameter of the needle lumen and the following have been recommended :

    14 gauge needle: one biopsy
    18 gauge needle: two biopsies
    20 gauge needle: three biopsies.

For the collection of core samples for full histopathology and other procedures there are a variety of specially designed biopsy needles such as the Vim-Silverman, wide-bore and Menghini needles (see Chapter 1).

Keyhole finger technique

An alternative approach for renal biopsy is the keyhole finger technique, in which the kidney is immobilized against the abdominal wall by a finger inserted through a small incision made just ventral to the kidney. The fine needle or wide-bore biopsy needle is then introduced through a second, adjacent incision.

Hazards of renal biopsy procedures

The kidneys are extremely well supplied with blood vessels originating from the renal artery and it is impossible to avoid cutting arterioles during any of the published biopsy techniques. Post-biopsy haemorrhage is therefore a very serious potential complication and subcapsular haemorrhage is common. For this reason, biopsy should not be performed in patients with clotting defects and a haematological profile for bleeding time (normally bleeding stops in less than 5 minutes in both cats and dogs) and platelet count (reference values: >200 x 10^9/l in dogs, >300 x 10^9/l in cats) should be performed prior to the procedure. If bleeding time is prolonged, further tests should be performed (see Chapter 3 and Bush, 1991).

Fortunately, reports in the literature suggest that the incidence of serious complications is low after renal biopsy (Hager *et al.*, 1985; Leveille *et al.*, 1993; Nash *et al.*, 1993). If the biopsy needle crosses the cortico-medullary junction, more severe damage results – hence this should be avoided.

In inexperienced hands, percutaneous biopsy techniques can result in injury to other tissues, such as the gastrointestinal tract and adjacent major blood vessels, as well as unnecessary trauma to the kidney under investigation. Use of ultrasonography to guide the operator is a great help, but relatively few veterinary clinicians possess the necessary skills to apply this technique at the present time.

Anaesthetic risk for laparotomy

Nephrectomy or incisional biopsy at laparotomy are undoubtedly the best techniques to employ in respect of the quality of the results that can be obtained from the tissue sample obtained. However, these procedures are only valid if the patient is able to withstand a general anaesthetic without a significant risk of developing further complications – notably ARF. Nephrectomy should never be performed lightly, particularly if an alternative procedure is feasible. In almost all cases for which renal or urinary tract biopsy is indicated the patient will have risk factors for the development of ARF. Common risk factors include CRF, impaired renal function, advanced age and prior administration of nephrotoxic drugs.

False-negative results

The sample size from most biopsies is small and so it is possible to miss the critical part of a lesion, even when several biopsies are performed. This is particu-larly likely if the clinical signs are produced by a very localized lesion. However, glomerulonephritis and amyloidosis, which are two of the most common lesions screened for, are usually widespread through-out the kidney and most biopsies will include sufficient evidence of disease to allow a diagnosis to be made (Figure 19.7).

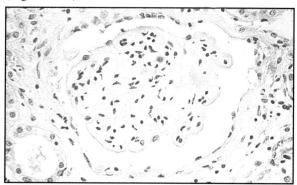

Figure 19.7: *Histological section through a glomerulus, showing changes typical of glomerulonephritis, including sclerosis and mesangial cell proliferation. H&E.*

Examination of biopsy samples

Biopsy samples should be properly preserved and submitted to a diagnostic laboratory with a pathologist experienced in examining renal and urinary tract histopathology (see Chapter 1).

BLOOD CHEMISTRY

The normal reference range values for the blood chemistry parameters recommended to be screened in the dog and cat with a urinary system disorder are summarized in Table 19.21.

Acid–base balance

The kidneys are extremely important in the physiological regulation of the acid–base balance of the body. Inadequate excretion of acid through the kidneys leads to accumulation of acid in the body, 'acidosis'. This occurs in post-renal causes of azotaemia, renal tubular defects, and in ARF and CRF with uraemia, although vomiting can lead to excessive losses of acid and so reduce the degree of acidosis. Acid–base imbalance can be identified by measurement of plasma carbon dioxide concentrations, and also urine pH.

Plasma carbon dioxide

Total carbon dioxide concentration is a stable component in a blood sample, and this is the same as the total bicarbonate content. Increased bicarbonate concentrations may occur following bicarbonate therapy in the treatment of renal failure. The main differential diagnosis considerations are metabolic alkalosis (vomiting, hypovolaemia, diuretics) and respiratory acidosis.

Test	Reference values for dogs	Reference values for cats	Comments
Plasma urea	2.5–7 mmol/l	5–11 mmol/l	High levels due to increased amino acid catabolism or to reduced excretion
Blood urea nitrogen (BUN)	7–25 mg/dl	14–35 mg/dl	Check that laboratory is reporting true BUN and not plasma urea
Plasma creatinine	40–130 µmol/l	40–130 µmol/l	Usually <110 µmol/l
Urea:creatinine ratio in plasma	<0.08 if creatinine in µmol/l and urea in mmol/l	<0.08 if creatinine in µmol/l and urea in mmol/l	
Total plasma protein	57–77 g/l	58–80 g/l	Measurements of serum protein will be about 5% lower because of fibrinogen loss from sample in clotting. Total plasma protein concentrations increase with age. There is an increase in globulin and a decrease in albumin
Plasma albumin	25–40 g/l	25–40 g/l	
Plasma sodium	140–155 mmol/l	145–157 mmol/l	False low concentrations are measured in the presence of hyperproteinaemia or hyperlipidaemia, both of which reduce the aqueous portion of the plasma
Plasma potassium	3.6–5.8 mmol/l	3.6–5.5 mmol/l	False high potassium concentrations may be given in some breeds of dog (e.g. Japanese Akita) or where the blood sample has undergone haemolysis. False low potassium concentrations may be given in cases of hyperproteinaemia or hyperlipidaemia
Plasma chloride	100–120 mmol/l	115–130 mmol/l	
Plasma carbon dioxide (bicarbonate)	17–24 mmol/l	17–24 mmol/l	A delay in analysing samples will lead to a reduction in the carbon dioxide concentration
Plasma calcium (Total)	2–3 mmol/l	1.8–3 mmol/l	Hyperlipidaemia causes false high calcium readings due to increased turbidity. Detergent residues on laboratory equipment may increase or decrease calcium readings. Samples for calcium estimation should NOT be collected into EDTA-, citrate- or oxalate-impregnated bottles as these will bind with calcium and so cause low readings. Heparin is acceptable. Haemolysis also causes false low readings
Plasma phosphate	0.8–1.6 mmol/l	1.3–2.6 mmol/l	These normal values should be doubled for dogs aged under 1 year. Haemolysis will give falsely increased values. Glucocorticoids will give false low phosphate values, as will the use of phosphate binders

Table 19.21: Clinical pathology panel for urinary system disease – reference values. (Values from Bush, 1991.)

Decreased bicarbonate concentrations may occur in metabolic acidosis, early CRF or Fanconi syndrome. The main considerations for differential diagnosis are metabolic acidosis (non-urinary system in origin, e.g. diarrhoea, shock, diabetes mellitus, ethylene glycol poisoning, metaldehyde poisoning, status epilepticus, post-racing in Greyhounds, Addison's disease) and respiratory alkalosis resulting from hyperventilation (fever, hepatic encephalopathy, convulsions, heat stroke).

Azotaemia

Azotaemia is defined as an increase in serum or plasma concentrations of urea nitrogen or creatinine or both (see below). Like most vital organs in the vertebrate body the kidneys have huge functional reserves so that their urine-concentrating ability is only lost when 66% of nephrons have lost their function, and azotaemia does not occur until 75% of nephrons have been lost.

Plasma urea

Whenever endogenous or exogenous (dietary) amino acid breakdown rates increase, there is increased production of urea which has to be excreted through the kidneys. The rate of excretion is dependent upon the glomerular filtration rate (GFR), which is directly proportional to the functional renal mass, but which can be altered by pre-renal factors such as reduced blood flow to the kidneys.

Urea nitrogen concentrations are the same in blood, plasma and serum but the term blood urea nitrogen (BUN) is in common use. Plasma urea concentration, however, is not the same as plasma urea nitrogen because chemically urea only contains 47% of nitrogen. The normal reference ranges for both are given in Table 19.21.

In the presence of renal failure, circulating blood urea levels increase, leading to the typical clinical signs associated with the toxic side effects of uraemia. Animals with anorexia, malnutrition or catabolic diseases will break down their own lean body mass proteins to produce energy. This is particularly important in cats, which are obligate carnivores and unable to downregulate their protein-related catabolic enzymes. They can very rapidly develop very high concentrations of urea in the circulation. Dietary protein intake in excess of daily requirements for replenishing body proteins results in excess amino acids being metabolized for energy, which also increases urea production. Non-renal causes of increased plasma urea are summarized in Table 19.22; non-renal causes of decreased plasma urea are shown in Table 19.23.

A further complication to the interpretation of urea values is that urea is also passively reabsorbed from the renal tubules and even at maximum flow rates up to 40% of filtered urea is thought to be resorbed.

As blood urea concentrations are dependent upon the rate of production as well as rate of excretion and the rate of tubular resorption, blood urea estimation is not by itself a reliable measure of renal function.

It is important to realize that:

- A mild increase in urea concentrations is not necessarily due to renal disease
- Important decisions about patient management should never be made based upon moderately elevated urea concentrations alone
- Plasma urea values over 35 mmol/l are significant
- Plasma urea values over 70 mmol/l indicate a poor prognosis
- A large change in GFR early in the course of renal failure may only cause a small increase in plasma urea concentration (Figure 19.8) whereas a small change in GFR in advanced renal disease may cause large increases in circulating urea concentration.

The rate of production and excretion of urea in the body is not constant; for example, after a high-protein meal maximum urea concentrations are achieved after

Cause	Comments
Haemorrhage into gastrointestinal tract	Endogenous protein breakdown
Catabolic conditions	Cardiac failure Hyperthyroidism Starvation Infection Fever Burns
Catabolic drugs	Glucocorticoids Azathioprine
Drugs that reduce protein synthesis, thus cause amino acids to be broken down	Tetracyclines

Table 19.22: Non-renal causes of increased plasma urea.

Cause	Comments
Low-protein diets	A low urea value under these circumstances is physiologically normal
Liver failure	Lack of production through the urea cycle leads to ammonia build-up and secondary encephalopathy
Portosystemic shunts	As for liver failure

Table 19.23: Non-renal causes of decreased plasma urea.

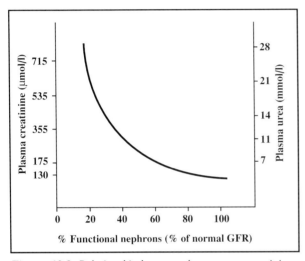

Figure: 19.8: Relationship between plasma urea, creatinine and loss of renal function.

about 8 hours. For this reason samples to be used for urea estimation should be collected after a 12-hour fast. For considerations of the significance of urea estimations see Chapter 4.

Plasma creatinine

Phosphocreatine is an energy source stored in muscle which is broken down to creatinine at a steady rate of about 2% per day, a process that is dependent upon the total lean muscle mass of the individual. The production rate of creatinine is higher in young animals, males and well muscled individuals. Serum creatinine concentrations may increase following trauma (if there is significant muscle necrosis) or strenuous exercise.

Creatinine is excreted unchanged by the kidneys; unlike urea, it is not reabsorbed. In dogs a small amount is actively secreted in the proximal tubules of the kidney. The rate of excretion (clearance rate) of creatinine is not linearly related to the GFR but plasma concentrations are inversely proportional to GFR and therefore plasma creatinine is a much better indicator of GFR and renal function than is plasma urea. On the other hand it provides no information about other types of disorder and so, even when primary renal disease is suspected, both plasma creatinine and plasma urea should be measured to improve the knowledge base for reaching a differential diagnosis and to identify con-

current problems in other organ systems.

One complication in interpretation is that patients with renal failure are often in a catabolic state and, particularly in cats which might also be anorectic, lean body mass is broken down for energy which can lead to an initial rise followed by steady reduction in creatinine production as the muscle mass decreases.

Unfortunately, the alkaline picrate test used in diagnostic laboratories is not specific for creatinine and can also detect chromagens which do not appear in the urine. Up to 50% of the concentration of 'creatinine' detected in serum by this test may in fact be due to chromagens.

Large changes in GFR (see Figure 19.8) early in the course of renal disease may only result in a mild or moderate change in plasma creatinine concentration, whereas small changes in advanced renal disease may cause very large changes in circulating creatinine concentrations. In general terms an elevation in plasma creatinine concentrations will occur when at least 75% of nephrons have ceased to function. Creatinine values of 130–250 µmol/l probably indicate reduced renal perfusion, whilst creatinine values of >250 µmol/l are significant, indicating renal failure or another urinary tract disorder (e.g. ruptured bladder or urethra). Creatinine values over 450 µmol/l indicate a poor prognosis. The degree of elevation of creatinine values cannot be used to determine whether the patient's renal failure is reversible or not, nor whether it is chronic or acute, or non-progressive; nor can it be used to decide if the cause of azotaemia is pre-renal, renal or post-renal in origin. Causes of high creatinine are listed in Table 19.24.

Falsely high creatinine values may be reported if there are high concentrations of ketones present, particularly acetoacetate which is a feature of diabetic ketoacidosis. Some drugs can cause falsely high results. These include cephalosporins (which interfere with the diagnostic test) and salicylates, trimethoprim and cimetidine (which inhibit tubular secretion of creatinine, although this is not very significant).

Electrolyte balance

The kidneys are very important in maintaining electrolyte balance within the body; particularly important are the regulation of sodium and potassium, as imbalance can be life-threatening (see also Chapter 4).

Plasma sodium

Sodium is the main extracellular electrolyte in the body and plasma sodium concentrations are usually homeostatically maintained within a very narrow range. They can be affected by disorders leading to abnormal water loss or water retention, as well as by abnormal sodium intake, sodium loss or sodium retention. High blood sodium concentrations (hypernatraemia) can occur in polyuric disorders, and as a complication of peritoneal dialysis when marked diuresis is induced.

Hyponatraemia can occur:

- In end-stage renal failure, due to urinary sodium losses with decreased intake due to vomiting and diarrhoea
- In ARF, due to excessive drinking during the polyuric phase
- In nephrotic syndrome, when hypoalbuminaemia decreases colloid osmotic pressure, leading to movement of fluid from plasma and causing

Cause	Comments
Non-renal cause: Severe exercise	Only causes a slight increase in plasma creatinine in racing Greyhounds if tested immediately after a race (Snow *et al.*, 1988)

Pre-renal causes:
    Pre-renal ARF
    Reduced renal perfusion due to dehydration, haemorrhage, shock, hypoadrenocorticism, hypo-albuminaemia, cardiac failure
	Plasma creatinine concentrations may reach 250 μmol/l
	Urea:creatinine ratio exceeds 0.08
	Urine SG >1.025 (dog)
	Urine SG >1.035 (cat)

Renal causes:
    Renal ARF
 	
    CRF
	Loss of 75% of functional nephrons results in increased plasma creatinine
	Increased creatinine is evident before there is an increase in urea; can exceed 1000 μmol/l
	Urine SG lower than in pre-renal ARF:
	    66% loss nephrons
	        SG < 1.029 (dog)
	        SG < 1.034 (cat)
	    75% loss of nephrons
	        SG < 1.012 (dog)
	        SG < 1.025 (cat)
	Eventually isosthenuria occurs :
	    SG 1.008 - 1.012
	Urea:creatinine ratio is at or below 0.08
	Other changes to look for: increased plasma phosphate; increased plasma potassium; oliguria then polyuria
	
	Other changes to look for: increased plasma phosphate; low calcium; mild non-regenerative anaemia; low platelet count (thrombocytopenia); lymphopenia; polyuria then oliguria
	By the time plasma creatinine concentrations are elevated the animal is usually in renal failure

Post-renal causes: Post-renal ARF due to urinary obstruction or ruptured lower urinary tract	See text

Falsely high results:
    High ketones
    Drugs	

Table 19.24: Causes of high plasma creatinine concentrations.

decreased blood volume, decreased renal perfusion and stimulation of the renin-angiotensin-aldosterone cascade
- When hypertonic dextrose or mannitol solutions are used in the treatment of renal failure
- When urine leaks into the peritoneal cavity, such as following a ruptured bladder (also causes hypokalaemia).

Plasma potassium

The majority (98%) of the body's potassium is intracellular. Plasma potassium concentrations can change with: potassium intake; potassium loss (renal or gastrointestinal); and movement of potassium from within cells to the extracellular fluid compartment, such as occurs following trauma.

Hyperkalaemia is life-threatening and may occur: in ARF, due to renal or post-renal causes; in metabolic acidosis, due to ARF or CRF; or with excessive potassium supplementation that exceeds the renal capacity to excrete it.

The main differential diagnostic considerations for hyperkalaemia are:

- Hypoadrenocorticism (Addison's disease) – causes potassium retention by decreasing exchange for sodium in renal tubules, and reduced cortisol concentrations allow potassium to move extracellullarly by impairment of the sodium:potassium pump
- Metabolic acidosis due to non-urinary system causes
- Prolonged use of the potassium-sparing diuretic spironolactone
- Low sodium intake
- Massive tissue injury, e.g. crush injuries
- Thrombocytosis
- Drug reactions, e.g. digitalis, succinylcholine, excessive potassium administration.

Hypokalaemia may occur:

- In the polyuric phase of ARF due to excessive water intake. This is especially likely if the patient is anorectic
- In Fanconi syndrome, due to impaired renal tubular resorption
- In other polyuric conditions, e.g. CRF. Hypokalaemia is common in cats with CRF
- Where excessive bicarbonate administration causes alkalosis.

The main differential diagnostic considerations for hypokalaemia are:

- Diarrhoea/vomiting (causes alkalosis)
- Diuretic therapy (urinary potassium losses), especially frusemide, chlorothiazide
- Losses induced by the diuresis following

intravenous fluid therapy
- Mineralocorticoid therapy
- Excessive lactate administration (causes alkalosis)
- Chronic liver disease (causes respiratory and metabolic alkalosis)
- Hyperadrenocorticism (Cushing's syndrome)
- Diabetes mellitus
- Insulin therapy
- Respiratory disease (leading to alkalosis).

Plasma chloride

Plasma chloride concentrations are inversely related to plasma bicarbonate concentrations.

Hyperchloraemia may occur: in metabolic acidosis (e.g. renal failure or Fanconi syndrome); in hypernatraemia; or with overzealous administration of ammonium chloride as a urinary acidifier.

The main differential diagnostic considerations for hyperchloraemia are: metabolic acidosis (non-urinary system causes, e.g. diarrhoea, shock, diabetes mellitus, ethylene glycol poisoning, metaldehyde poisoning, status epilepticus, post-racing in Greyhounds); increased dietary intake or intravenous administration of sodium; and water deprivation.

Hypochloraemia may occur: in metabolic alkalosis; in hyponatraemia (due to overhydration, increased sodium losses); or with overzealous diuresis (frusemide, chlorthiazide or ethacrynic acid).

Mineral balance

The kidneys play a very important role in the maintenance of plasma calcium and phosphate concentrations, and so can influence bone homeostasis (see also Chapter 4).

Plasma calcium

There are three components to the calcium in a blood sample: protein-bound calcium, usually bound to albumin; chelated calcium, e.g. phosphate or citrate; and ionized calcium. Ionized calcium is the biologically active form and accounts for about 50% of the total plasma calcium. Calcium bound to albumin accounts for about 40%, and other calcium salts about 10% of the total calcium. A change in total plasma calcium concentration may not be clinically significant unless the active 'ionized' calcium concentration is significantly outside the normal range. Recently, affordable equipment has become available which is simple to use in a practice environment to measure ionized calcium in whole blood or plasma. Acidosis causes an increase in ionized calcium concentrations, whilst alkalosis causes a decrease in ionized calcium concentrations. Hypoproteinaemia causes a decrease in protein-bound calcium, whilst hyperproteinaemia may increase the protein-bound calcium.

Plasma calcium concentrations are closely regulated by homeostatic mechanisms, involving parathyroid hormone (PTH), calcitonin and vitamin D3.

Hypercalcaemia: This can be a cause of ARF as well as a consequence of ARF and CRF. It may be present:

- In CRF due to:
    decreased renal excretion of calcium
    decreased breakdown of parathyroid hormone by the kidneys
    increased chelated calcium fraction in blood, leading to increased vitamin D activity causing increased calcium absorption from the gastrointestinal tract
- In ARF (renal) in the early diuretic phase. This is usually a temporary observation due to rapid calcium losses. However, hypercalcaemia can also be an important cause of ARF
- After administration of calcium salts such as calcium gluconate in the treatment of renal failure.

The main differential diagnosis considerations for hypercalcaemia are:

- Pseudohyperparathyroidism (paraneoplastic syndrome) due to non-parathyroid malignant neoplasia, especially lymphosarcoma, apocrine gland (anal sac) adenocarcinomas and mammary adenocarcinomas
- Primary hyperparathyroidism(in older animals, due to hyperplasia or neoplasia); (rare)
- Destructive bone tumours
- Osteomyelitis
- Hypervitaminosis D (supplementation, calciferol poisoning)
- Osteoporosis (rare in cats and dogs).

Rare causes are: relative hyperproteinaemia (e.g. in dehydration); dehydration (most cases do *not* develop hypercalcaemia); epilepsy; hypothermia; hypocalcitonism; hypervitaminosis A (e.g. in cats fed liver); hypothyroidism; and hyperthyroidism.

Hypocalcaemia: This may be present in:

- Ethylene glycol poisoning, the calcium being taken up to form oxalate salts which, in turn, cause acute tubular necrosis leading to ARF
- Renal secondary hyperparathyroidism. Reduced GFR, retention of phosphate and reduced calcium absorption from the gastrointestinal tract due to decreased vitamin D conversion to calcitrol in the kidney, causes a mild relative decrease in plasma calcium. This stimulates parathyroid hormone secretion which causes release of calcium from the skeleton and returns plasma concentrations to normal. Many cases therefore present with a normal blood calcium concentration, and occasionally with hypercalcaemia
- Nephrotic syndrome, due to hypoalbuminaemia

and a consequential reduction in protein-bound calcium. In this condition ionized calcium may or may not be affected and so the clinical signs associated with hypocalcaemia may or may not be present
- ARF (postrenal). Urethral obstruction often leads to hypocalcaemia (true for about 50% of cats with lower urinary tract obstruction) . This is secondary to phosphorus retention but can be counteracted by the effects of acidosis, which increases the amount of ionized calcium in circulation.

The main differential diagnostic considerations for hypocalcaemia are:

- Eclampsia (common)
- Ethylene glycol poisoning
- Nutritional secondary hyperparathyroidism
- Glucocorticoids (increase renal excretion of calcium and inhibit vitamin D)
- Phosphate-containing enemas (cats)
- Acute pancreatitis (50% of dogs with this condition)
- Liver disease (reduced albumin production)
- Malabsorption syndrome
- Neoplasia (parathyroid, thyroid, bone, gastrinoma, e.g. Zollinger–Ellison syndrome causing excessive gastrin secretion).

Rare causes are: hypoparathyroidism; thyroid C-cell carcinoma; and tissue trauma.

Plasma phosphate
Phosphate homeostasis is closely regulated by PTH which increases renal excretion and release of phosphate from the skeleton, along with calcium.

Hyperphosphataemia: This often occurs with azotaemia, due to a sudden fall in GFR, e.g. in ARF or urethral obstruction. Hyperphosphataemia is less likely to occur in CRF.
    Causes of hyperphosphataemia include:

- Renal failure, due to decreased excretion in chronic and ARF, and increased activity of parathyroid hormone which causes the release of both calcium and phosphate from the skeleton
- Familial renal disease (e.g. Fanconi syndrome, renal cortical hypoplasia, other inherited nephropathies)
- Rupture of the bladder due to failure to excrete phosphate from the body.

The main differential diagnostic considerations for hyperphosphataemia are:

- Young dogs (under 1 year of age)

- Nutritional secondary hyperparathyroidism (due to high meat or offal ration)
- Hypervitaminosis D (supplementation)
- Primary hypoparathyroidism
- Destructive primary or secondary bone tumours
- Feline hyperthyroidism.

Rare causes are feline hypoadrenocorticism and 'acromegaly' (as a result of progesterone and progestogen imbalances).

Hypophosphataemia: Causes of hypophosphataemia include:

- Diuresis, with associated phosphate loss in the urine
- Fanconi syndrome (rare), due to reduced ability to reabsorb phosphate. In late-stage ARF it develops suddenly with a resulting hyperphosphataemia
- Pituitary dwarfism, with associated reduced renal tubular resorption.

The main differential diagnostic considerations for hypophosphataemia are:

- Cushing's syndrome (33% of dogs have hypophosphataemia due to the effects of cortisol)
- Use of oral phosphate binders
- Glucocorticoid therapy or endogenous production
- Primary hyperparathyroidism.

Rare causes are: rickets/osteomalacia; hypovitaminosis D; diabetes mellitus (dogs); and advanced liver disease.

Parathyroid hormone (PTH) and calcitriol (vitamin D)

Bone homeostasis is severely disturbed in CRF for several reasons:

- Because of phosphorus retention. Increased plasma phosphate complexes with free ionized calcium, causing a relative hypocalcaemia and stimulation of PTH secretion. In some cases, soft tissue calcification will occur and if nephrocalcinosis results this will contribute to advancement of the renal failure
- Because of decreased synthesis of the active form of Vitamin D3 (1,25-dihydroxy-cholecalciferol or 'calcitriol') in the proximal tubules of the kidney. A fall in calcitriol reduces calcium absorption from the gastrointestinal tract, which results in a relative hypocalcaemia, stimulating PTH secretion and releasing calcium from the skeleton by stimulating osteoclast activity. The net effect is that blood calcium concentrations are maintained within the normal range but that calcium is lost

from the skeleton over a period of time, resulting in osteodystrophy ('rubber jaw syndrome').
- Parathyroid abnormalities. PTH secretion occurs even at normal blood levels of ionized calcium. In some cases of CRF in dogs it has been reported that the number of calcitriol receptors in the parathyroid gland falls.

Secondary hyperparathyroidism is a common finding in CRF in cats and dogs, and PTH is usually increased when plasma phosphate concentrations are increased (Barber *et al.*, 1994) but many cats have increased PTH concentrations despite having normal plasma phosphate.

Total plasma protein

The normal reference ranges for total plasma protein in dogs and cats are shown in Table 19.21. These are different to serum concentrations, which are about 5% lower because of the loss of fibrinogen in clotting.

The vast majority of protein in the total plasma protein concentration is made up of albumin and globulin. The albumin:globulin ratio is often used as an indicator of a shift in relative production and loss.

Hypoproteinaemia due to reduced albumin concentrations is a characteristic feature of nephrotic syndrome in which massive urinary losses can be incurred and protein malnutrition is a well recognized cause of hypoproteinaemia in animals with CRF which are anorectic or on protein-deficient rations.

Causes of increased and decreased blood protein are shown in Tables 19.25 and 19.26.

RENAL FUNCTION TESTS

There have been numerous studies performed to identify a simple, cheap and accurate method for measuring renal function, by which one usually means glomerular filtration functionality, but tests can also be performed to determine tubular secretion capabilities, and acidifying capabilities. If a substance is not secreted or resorbed in the renal tubules, measurement of its clearance rate is a measure of GFR because the amount filtered from the blood through the glomerulus equals the amount excreted in the urine. A list of published values for various glomerular function tests (including creatinine clearance) has been compiled by DiBartola (1992); see Table 19.27.

Creatinine clearance

Estimation of the clearance of endogenous creatinine is of particular use when a patient has polydipsia and polyuria but normal plasma urea and normal plasma creatinine. Unfortunately this estimation requires that *all* urine is collected over a reasonable period, usually 24 hours, and this may present practical difficulties in a practice environment.

Cause	Comments
Dehydration	Common cause seen in polyuric disorders including renal failure Confirm dehydration by checking PCV increased, with normal albumin and normal albumin:globulin ratio
Increased globulin concentrations: Primary glomerular diseases	Glomerulonephritis and amyloidosis can increase α, β and γ globulins. Amyloidosis affects α-globulins in particular, e.g. in Abyssinian cats
Non-urinary system causes	Inflammation; liver disease; neoplasia; infections; autoimmune disease
Anabolic steroids	
Increased fibrinogen	
False-positive results	Haemolysis; lipaemia

Table 19.25: Causes of hyperproteinaemia.

Cause	Comments
Overhydration	Associated with fluid administration. PCV is low and albumin:globulin ratio is normal
Protein loss: In urine	Primary glomerular disease (glomerulonephritis and amyloidosis); may lead to nephrotic syndrome Albumin:globulin ratio is reduced as albumin is lost most (due to low molecular weight) Check for increase in cholesterol as well CRF does not usually cause sufficient losses to result in hypoproteinaemia
Gastrointestinal tract	Especially lymphosarcoma, lymphangiectasia; other protein-losing enteropathies
Burns	Preferential loss of serum proteins
Haemorrhage	If severe, albumin:globulin ratio is normal as both are lost Low PCV
Infection	Albumin lost through increased vascular permeability
Decreased protein synthesis: Liver disease	Albumin:globulin ratio decreased as mainly albumin is not being produced
Malabsorption syndrome	Exocrine pancreatic insufficiency or bacterial overgrowth
Protein starvation	Rare
Heart failure	

Table 19.26: Causes of hypoproteinaemia.

Exogenous creatinine clearance (Finco *et al.*, 1981, 1982) involves the administration of massive doses of creatinine subcutaneously or intravenously to minimize the complicating effects of circulating chromagens and this is a potentially useful test.

Urea:creatinine ratio

The ratio of plasma urea to plasma creatinine can be increased in both pre-renal and post-renal causes of azotaemia because at low flow rates tubular resorption of urea may be increased.

The plasma urea:creatinine ratio is normal in ARF of both renal and post-renal types.

The plasma urea:creatinine ratio is high in ARF with pre-renal causes (if there are reduced flow rates there is increased tubular resorption of urea) and in ARF with post-renal causes (if there is urine leakage into the abdomen leading to absorption across the peritoneum).

Test	Dogs	Reference	Cats	Reference
Endogenous creatinine clearance (ml/min/kg)	2.98 ± 0.96 3.7 ± 0.77 2.97 ± 0.42 3.49 ± 0.73 2.10 ± 0.86 2.75 ± 0.57	Finco (1971) Bovee & Joyce (1979) Finco *et al.* (1981) Krawiec *et al.* (1986) Lulich *et al.* (1991) Grauer *et al.* (1985)	2.70 ± 1.2 2.72 ± 0.38	Osbaldiston & Fuhrman (1970) Hoskins *et al.* (1991)
Exogenous creatinine clearance (ml/min/kg)	4.08 ± 0.5	Finco *et al.* (1981)	2.94 ± 0.32 2.56 ± 0.61	Ross & Finco (1981) Rogers *et al.* (1991)
Inulin clearance (ml/min/kg)	3.96 ± 0.58 4.19 ± 1.82 4.72 ± 1.82 3.55 ± 0.14 3.39 ± 0.73	Finco *et al.* (1981) Powers *et al.* (1977) Powers *et al.* (1977) Fettman *et al.* (1985) Krawiec *et al.* (1986)	3.51 ± 0.14 3.83 ± 0.83 3.24 ± 0.14 2.15 ± 0.29 2.31 ± 0.56 3.07 ± 0.77 2.47 ± 0.71	Ross & Finco (1981) Osbaldiston & Fuhrman (1970) Fettman *et al.* (1985) Lulich *et al.* (1991) Lulich *et al.* (1991) Rogers *et al.* (1991) Rogers *et al.* (1991)
Para-aminohippurate clearance (ml/min/kg)	12.23 ± 1.65 10.55 ± 1.5	Powers *et al.* (1977) Powers *et al.* (1977)	10.61 ± 1.71 15.1 ± 3.48	Ross & Finco (1981) Osbaldiston & Fuhrman (1970)
Iothalamate clearance (ml/min/kg)	16.17 ± 2.99	Powers *et al.* (1977)	14.13 ± 5.74	Mercer & Garg (1977)
[^{3}H]-Tetraethyl-ammonium clearance (ml/min/kg)	10.51 ± 0.72	Fettman *et al.* (1985)	8.14 ± 0.53	Fettman *et al.* (1985)
Sodium sulphanilate half-life (min)	58 ± 13 66.1 ± 10.8	Powers *et al.* (1977) Fettman *et al.* (1985)	44.4 ± 5.7	Ross & Finco (1981)
Filtration fraction	0.34 ± 0.02 0.35	Fettman *et al.* (1985) Powers *et al.* (1977)	0.21 0.39 ± 0.02 0.33 0.36	Osbaldiston & Fuhrman (1970) Fettman *et al.* (1985) Ross & Finco (1981) Mercer & Garg (1977)
24 hour urine protein excretion (mg/kg/day)	13.9 ± 7.7 7.9 ± 5.6 7.6 ± 5.5 4.8 ± 3.7 2.4 ± 2.3 2.3 ± 1.2	DiBartola *et al.* (1980) Biewenga (1982) McCaw *et al.* (1985) White *et al.* (1984) Center *et al.* (1985) Grauer *et al.* (1985)	17.4 ± 9.0 12.6 ± 5.4 8.0 ± 3.7 4.9 ± 1.3	Forrester *et al.* (1989) Monroe *et al.* (1989) Hoskins *et al.* (1991) Adams *et al.* (1992)
Urine phosphate: urine creatinine (U_p / U_{cr})	0.17 ± 0.15 0.08 ± 0.04 0.27 ± 0.27 0.29 ± 0.22 0.28 ± 0.24 0.09 ± 0.09	White *et al.* (1984) Grauer *et al.* (1985) McCaw *et al.* (1985) McCaw *et al.* (1985) McCaw *et al.* (1985) Center *et al.* (1985)	0.42 ± 0.23 0.32 ± 0.13 0.22 ± 0.11 0.13 ± 0.04	Forrester *et al.* (1989) Monroe *et al.* (1989) Hoskins *et al.* (1991) Adams *et al.* (1992)

Table 19.27: Glomerular function tests in dogs and cats. (Modified after DiBartola, 1992.)

The plasma urea:creatinine ratio may be decreased following fluid therapy and this is due to decreased tubular reabsorption, not to decreased GFR .

Phenolsulphonphthalein excretion

Phenolsulphonphthalein (PSP) is an organic dye which is excreted through the proximal tubules in normal dogs and cats. About 80% of the administered amount is protein-bound in the plasma so only about 20% is available for excretion by the kidneys and only about 5% is available for glomerular filtration (the rest is secreted by the tubules), so this test is a good measure of tubular secretion. Around 45% of the PSP will be excreted in 20 minutes (the half-life is 18–24 minutes). Excretion of <30% in 20 minutes is abnormal (Finco, 1980).

The technique involves giving 6 mg of PSP in 0.1 ml of solution intravenously; all urine formed in the following 20 minutes is collected and analysed.

Falsely high clearance rates may be caused by reduced cardiac output or dehydration, and falsely low rates by hypoalbuminaemia due to reduced PSP binding.

Sodium sulphanilate excretion

As sodium sulphanilate is excreted solely by glomerular filtration it is a useful indicator of renal function although an accurate GFR is not obtained. An advantage of this test is that urine samples collected over a long period of time are not needed.

The technique involves giving 20 mg/kg (dogs) or 11 mg/kg (cats) intravenously; heparinized blood samples are collected after 30, 60 and 90 minutes. The normal half-life for dogs is reported to be 42–82 minutes, and for cats 37–57 minutes.

Radioisotope excretion

These assays do not require urine collection and are quick to perform. As they use radioactive substances (see Table 19.27) use is limited to licensed referral centres. Nuclear imaging techniques are being used to measure the GFR of individual kidneys in dogs and cats (Krawiec *et al.,* 1986; Krawiec, 1988; Rogers *et al.,* 1991).

Fractional clearance of electrolytes

The electrolyte concentrations in urine depend upon tubular rates of secretion and reabsorption. As creatinine is excreted at a constant rate, a fractional clearance can be calculated from the ratio of electrolyte to creatinine clearance. Normal values are in shown in Table 19.27.

In animals with pre-renal azotaemia and volume depletion, sodium should be retained and the fractional clearance should be very low. In animals with azotaemia due to primary renal disease, the fractional clearance of sodium should be higher than normal.

Water deprivation test

One of the main functions of the kidneys is to concentrate urine to reduce water losses in the presence of reduced fluid intake or excessive fluid losses. If the kidneys fail to do this the animal may become dehydrated and only 15% loss of body fluids can be life-threatening (see also Chapter 17).

The water deprivation test provides very useful information about renal function but it must not be performed in patients that are dehydrated or azotaemic because of the risk of precipitating ARF. Polyuric animals should never be left for any length of time without water because they can very easily dehydrate. The apparently common practice of leaving polyuric

animals overnight without water to see if they can concentrate their urine is to be condemned. This test should only be performed in a supervised hospital ward so that samples can be collected at regular intervals and fluids can be administered rapidly if necessary.

To perform the test properly the urinary bladder should be emptied and the following laboratory tests performed before water deprivation, every 4 hours during the test, and at the end of the test:

- Physical examination:
  moisture on mucous membranes
  skin turgor
  body weight
- Blood sample analysis:
  packed cell volume (PCV) or microhaematocrit
  total protein
  plasma osmolality
- Urinalysis:
  SG
  osmolality.

The osmolality is a measure of the number of particles of solute in a solution and osmolality measurements require the use of an osmometer, which may only be available in a remote diagnostic laboratory. This can delay the results. The SG depends upon the molecular weight of the particles as well as the number of them in a solution. There is no direct relation between urine osmolality and SG.

An increase in total plasma protein concentration is the most reliable test for dehydration (better than PCV or changes in skin turgor or the mucous membranes).

Changes in urine SG are significant observations, as are changes in body weight. A 5% decrease in body weight causes maximum secretion of antidiuretic hormone (ADH). If the patient becomes dehydrated, loses 5% body weight or produces concentrated urine, the test is ended. In normal water-deprived dogs the time to develop dehydration can vary greatly, from 42 to 96 hours; in cats it is around 40 hours. With polyuric disorders the time can be only 3–14 hours. In healthy dogs urine SG changes to 1.050–1.076, and in cats it concentrates to 1.047–10.87. Urine osmolality values of 1787–2791 mOsm/kg (dogs) and 1581–2984 mOsm/kg (cats) have been reported.

Vasopressin is administered subcutaneously at 0.25–0.5 units/kg, to a maximum of 5 units, to animals in which water deprivation results in <5% increase in urine osmolality, <10% increase in SG or 5% loss of body weight. The same parameters are measured after 1 and 2 hours. A positive response to vasopressin administration confirms the diagnosis as central diabetes insipidus. A negative response indicates nephrogenic diabetes insipidus or apparent psychogenic polydipsia.

Modified water deprivation test

The differential diagnosis of polyuria is a common

requirement in small animal clinical practice and a modified water deprivation test can be very helpful:

Step 1: Remove access to water
Step 2: Empty urinary bladder
Step 3: Measure urine SG or osmolality
Step 4: Empty bladder every hour and measure urine SG or osmolality
Step 5: After 24 hours (supervised in hospital) administer 2–3 units of vasopressin
Step 6: Re-sample and test urine after 1 and 2 hours

In normal dogs any further increase in urine osmolality should not exceed 10% after vasopressin is given. In central diabetes mellitus, increases can exceed 250%.

Renal medullary washout is a complication when interpreting water deprivation tests. It occurs when solute concentrations fall in the renal medulla; this affects the ability to concentrate urine because osmotic pressures are abnormal across the tubules. A gradual reduction in water intake has been advocated to try to minimize the effects of washout, but this relies on strict owner compliance in regard to accurate measurement of water intake and food intake, and also means that the test is being performed in a non-controlled environment so the potential for dehydration to occur is a problem.

Hickey–Hare test

The Hickey–Hare test (Lage, 1997) is a useful procedure which can be very helpful in identifying nephrogenic diabetes mellitus. This test is contraindicated in patients with congestive heart failure.

Step 1: Insert an indwelling urinary catheter
Step 2: Administer water by stomach tube, at a rate of 20 ml/kg body weight
Step 3: Calculate urine flow rate (ml/min)
Step 4: Administer hypertonic saline (2.5%) intravenously at 0.25 ml/min per kg for 45 minutes
Step 5: Record urine volume every 15 minutes from start of saline administration until 45 minutes after the administration.

In normal animals there is a decrease in the rate of urine production, due to stimulation of ADH. In nephrogenic diabetes mellitus there is no change or an increase in flow rate. A normal response is found in psychogenic polydipsia and with medullary washout.

Exogenous ADH test

This test is used in patients when water deprivation is too risky. It has the disadvantage that the degree of urine concentration that can be achieved is much less than that achieved with water deprivation, for reasons not fully

understood but probably due to other endogenously produced substances as well as ADH in the presence of water deprivation. Water is made available throughout the test but excessive intake is prevented.

Step 1: Empty bladder
Step 2: Measure urine SG and osmolality
Step 3: Administer 10 milliunits/kg of aqueous vasopressin intravenously over 60 minutes
Step 4: Empty bladder and repeat measurement of urine osmolality and SG at 30-minute intervals over 3 hours.

Urine-acidifying ability (ammonium chloride test)

Ammonium chloride is usually excreted in the urine and creates an acidic pH. This is a test to evaluate the ability of the kidneys to form and excrete an acidic urine.

Step 1: Fast the animal for 12 hours
Step 2: Give 0.1 g/kg ammonium chloride orally
Step 3: Collect urine and check pH at 1-hour intervals, starting 2 hours after dose
Step 4: Stop test when urine pH (based on a meter reading) reaches 6.0. In normal dogs this takes 2–8 hours. In renal tubular acidosis, excessive bicarbonate is lost in urine and so the animal cannot acidify urine properly.

RENAL AND URINARY TRACT DISEASES

Renal and urinary tract diseases may be primary or secondary, and they may also induce serious secondary changes in other organ systems. It is important that other major organs systems should be examined when renal or urinary tract disease is confirmed. Osborne and Finco (1995) recognized nine basic syndromes which together constitute renal or urinary tract disorders.

Acute renal failure

ARF occurs when there is sudden onset (within hours) of oliguria or azotaemia or both together. There are many causes, categorized as follows:

- Pre-renal azotaemia: the kidneys produce a small volume of concentrated urine, which is a physiological response to a pre-renal problem
- Renal azotaemia: due to primary renal disease
- Post-renal azotaemia: due to diseases of the urinary excretory tract.

This system is somewhat simplistic because often animals are presented with more than one form of the disease (particularly older animals), which can make accurate diagnosis and management complicated. For example, old dogs with sudden-onset ARF following obstructive urolithiasis (a post-renal cause) may also have concurrent chronic glomerular disease (a renal cause).

Renal ARF

A typical clinical pathology panel is presented in Table 19.28. There are three definitive causes: acute interstitial nephritis; acute tubular necrosis; and bilateral kidney trauma (rare).

Acute interstitial nephritis: This condition is most often seen in dogs aged between 1 and 5 years and is thought to be associated most frequently with infection with *Leptospira canicola*. However, not all animals that have been in contact with leptospires will develop ARF; in the USA 10–40% of dogs have been exposed to leptospires based upon serology, but they have not developed ARF. Clinical signs include fever, malaise, haematuria, proteinuria, renal pain and uraemia.

Acute tubular necrosis: This condition may be due to:

• Ischaemia. A severe fall in renal perfusion due to hypotension (sometimes due to hypovolaemia) results in irreversible renal damage to the tubular epithelium and basement membrane, leading to necrosis of epithelial cells. This destroys affected nephrons which can no longer produce urine. If urine production is severely reduced, oliguria may result. Secondary tubular obstruction with cell debris and casts further prolongs oliguria
• Nephrotoxins. Risk factors for the development of acute tubular necrosis are well documented (Figure 19.9) and should be screened for during routine pre-anaesthesia examinations. In geriatric patients it is routinely advised to provide intravenous fluids to maintain renal perfusion during general anaesthesia to minimize the risk of developing ARF.

Post-renal ARF

Post-renal ARF develops because of obstruction of urine outflow. The tract can be obstructed anywhere but the urethra is most often the site and calculi are the most common cause. Obstruction can also be due to neoplasia or blood clots. Other causes include anatomical abnormalities, iatrogenic damage at surgery, prostatic enlargement or infection, and trauma. If there is traumatic rupture of the urethra, both ureters or the bladder, there will be post-renal azotaemia but no renal failure. A typical clinical pathology panel for post-renal ARF is shown in Table 19.29.

Pre-renal ARF

Pre-renal ARF may be caused by reduced renal perfusion, severe haemorrhage, dehydration, hypoadrenocorticism, cardiac failure and hypo-

Heavy metals:
  Lead
  Mercury
  Bismuth
  Arsenic

Rodenticides:
  Thallium
  Amphotericin B

Antibiotics:
  Polymyxin/bacitracin
  Aminoglycosides (e.g. streptomycin,
    neomycin, gentamicin)
  Sulphonamides

Organic compounds:
  Carbon tetrachloride
  Chloroform
  Methanol
  Phenol
  Ethylene glycol

General anaesthesia

Analgesics:
  Phenylbutazone
  Phenacetin

Other drugs:
  Cyclophosphamide
  Chlorinated hydrocarbons

Iodide-based contrast media

Figure 19.9: Risk factors for renal ARF.

albuminaemia. A typical clinical pathology panel for pre-renal ARF is shown in Table 19.30.

Chronic renal failure

CRF is present when azotaemia occurs as a result of renal parenchymal disease or injury over a prolonged period of usually months or years. Renal insufficiency only occurs once 66% of nephrons have been lost and clinical signs of polyuria, azotaemia and uraemia are not evident until over 75% of functioning nephrons have been lost.

Early diagnosis is important because it allows for the introduction of measures to delay or prevent further progression of the disease, which tends to be insidious. Diagnosis and prognosis are based upon urinalysis, blood chemistry, haematology and renal biopsy.

In a typical case, the owner usually complains that the animal shows increased thirst or increased frequency of urination, halitosis, and sometimes excessive mobility of the jaw. Clinical signs usually consist of polydipsia, polyuria, a non-regenerative anaemia, renal osteodystrophy, small mis-shapen kidneys, and a stable or progressive azotaemia which develops over many weeks.

Test	Increased value	Decreased value	Comments
BLOOD CHEMISTRY			
Plasma urea	Dogs: >7 mmol/l Cats: >11 mmol/l		Unlike pre-renal causes of ARF urea values may exceed 35 mmol/l
Blood urea nitrogen (BUN)	Dogs: >20 mg/dl Cats: > 32 mg/dl		Unlike pre-renal causes of ARF values may exceed 100 mg/dl
Plasma creatinine	Dogs and cats: >30 μmol/l		Especially significant if value > 250 μmol/l
Urea: creatinine ratio			Usually normal: <0.08 if creatinine in μmol/l and urea in mmol/l
Total plasma protein	Increased if dehydrated	Decreased if proteinuria	
Plasma albumin	Increased if dehydrated	Decreased if proteinuria	
Serum phosphate	Dogs: >1.6 mmol/l Cats: >2.6 mmol/l		In puppies the top end of the normal range can be 3.2 mmol/l
Blood calcium	Occasionally increased	Often low; 2 mmol/l	Hyperphosphataemia causes a fall in calcium level Occasionally calcium concentrations can increase
Plasma potassium	Dogs and cats: >6 mmol/l		Life threatening if exceeds 9 mmol/l
Total carbon dioxide (bicarbonate)		CO_2 falls with acidosis development, and is proportional to the degree of azotaemia	
HAEMATOLOGY			
Packed cell volume (PCV) or microhaematocrit	Increased if dehydrated	Decreased if haemorrhage	
URINALYSIS			
Urinalysis	Presence of : proteinuria; haematuria; casts; oxalate crystals (ethylene glycol poisoning)		
Urine SG		Dogs: <1.029 (early stage) <1.012 (late stage) <1.007 (end stage) Cats: <1.034 (early stage) <1.025 (late stage) < 1.007 - 1.015 (end stage)	Early stage – loss of 66% of functional nephrons Late stage – loss of 75% of functional nephrons End-stage – unable to concentrate urine (isosthenuria)
HISTOPATHOLOGY			
Renal biopsy	Presence of diffuse or focal inflammatory cell infiltration including plasma cells and macrophages		
MICROBIOLOGY			
Microscopy/Culture	*Leptospira canicola; Escherichia coli; Proteus; Klebsiella;* staphyloccci; streptococci; canine adenovirus-1; canine herpesvirus		Leptospirosis is thought to be the main infectious agent causing renal ARF

Table 19.28: *Typical clinical pathology panel in renal ARF.*

Test	Abnormal increase	Abnormal decrease	Comments
BLOOD CHEMISTRY			
Plasma urea	Dogs and cats: >60 mmol/l		
Blood urea nitrogen	Dogs and cats: >170 mg/dl		
Plasma creatinine	Dogs and cats: >400 µmol/l		
Urea:creatinine ratio			Usually normal range (<0.08)
Plasma phosphate	Dogs: > 1.6 mmol/l >2.3 mmol/l		Early stages – normal Loss of 66% of functional nephrons Guarded prognosis
Plasma potassium	Dogs and cats: >6 mmol/l		Life threatening if exceeds 9 mmol/l
URINALYSIS			
Urine SG		Depends upon stage of renal failure	

Table 19.29: Typical clinical pathology panel in post-renal ARF.

The clinician's objectives are to identify the underlying cause and to determine if it is treatable, e.g. infection, partial obstruction or subacute/chronic toxicity, or if progression can be delayed or arrested. Accurate diagnosis requires urinalysis, haematology, blood chemistry and, in some cases, renal biopsy.

Causes of CRF include:

- Chronic interstitial nephritis (infection with adenovirus 1 or *Leptospira*)
- Chronic glomerulonephritis (due to feline leukaemia virus, respiratory viruses, bacteria, systemic lupus erythematosus, pancreatitis, feline infectious peritonitis – dry form)
- Chronic amyloidosis
- Chronic pyelonephritis (*Escherichia coli, Proteus* spp., *Pseudomonas aeruginosa, Staphylococcus aureus*)
- Nephrocalcinosis(secondary to hypercalcaemia)
- Neoplasia (lymphosarcoma, nephroblastomas, carcinomas)
- Familial renal diseases (see Table 19.1).

A typical clinical pathology panel for CRF is presented in Table 19.31. Whilst this information can be very helpful in reaching a definitive diagnosis, histopathological examination of renal biopsy material is necessary to differentiate between the different causes of advanced renal failure.

Nephrotic syndrome

Nephrotic syndrome is characterized by massive protein loss in urine. As the glomeruli usually prevent large amounts of protein from passing across Bowman's capsule into the urine, the primary cause of nephrotic syndrome is glomerular disease of some type: glomerulonephritis (usually secondary to an immune-mediated disorder); or amyloidosis (usually reactive-type (amyloid A) secondary to other chronic diseases).

Nephrotic syndrome should be suspected when an animal has proteinuria, hypoalbuminaemia, hypercholesterolaemia and excessive fluid accumulation in tissues and/or body cavities.

Proteinuria not associated with nephrotic syndrome is usually due to CRF or ARF. Some cases of proteinuria are associated with subclinical urinary abnormalities (see Table 19.11).

A diagnosis of nephrotic syndrome is confirmed by: investigation for evidence of primary renal disease; quantitative and qualitative analysis of proteinuria; characterization of the renal lesion (biopsy); and, as most cases are secondary, investigation of underlying primary disease (e.g. infectious agent, neoplasia, immune-mediated disorders).

Renal tubular defects

Renal tubular defects are caused by:

- Anatomical abnormalities, which result in cystic or polycystic kidneys. These are uncommon and are

Test	Reference range	Abnormal increase	Abnormal decrease
BLOOD CHEMISTRY			
Plasma urea	Dogs: 2.5–7 mmol/l Cats: 5–11 mmol/l	Dogs: 7–35 mmol/l Cats: 11–35 mmol/l Usually in range 14–17 mmol/l for both species	
Blood urea nitrogen	Dogs: 7–25 mg/dl Cats: 14–35 mg/dl	Dogs: 21–100 mg/dl Cats: 36–100 mg/dl	
Plasma creatinine	Dogs and cats: 40-130 µmol/l	Usually high Dogs and cats: 130 – 250 µmol/l Sometimes creatinine is within normal range	
Urea:creatinine ratio		Usually increased in dogs and cats	
Total protein		If dehydrated	If severe haemorrhage
Albumin		If dehydrated	If severe haemorrhage
HAEMATOLOGY			
Packed cell volume		If dehydrated	If severe haemorrhage

Table 19.30: *Typical clinical pathology panel in pre-renal ARF.*

mainly recognized in young animals. The animal usually develops CRF and the anatomical defect is found as an incidental finding

• Functional abnormalities. Disorders resulting in defective secretion or resorption of solutes or water in the renal tubules occur infrequently and may be congenital or acquired. Polyuria leads to reduced vascular volume through dehydration, which causes increased thirst and hence compensatory polydipsia. If the concentration of urinary substances such as glucose (in diabetes mellitus) or bicarbonate (in alkalosis) increases in the absence of a loss of urine-concentrating ability by the kidneys (i.e. in the absence of renal failure) the patient will exhibit only polyuria and not polydipsia.

Other forms of tubular defect can lead to crystalluria and the formation of uroliths.

If the polyuria is severe enough, the blood levels of solutes being lost in the urine can fall sufficiently to cause abnormally low serum concentrations.

Fanconi syndrome

Fanconi syndrome is a familial disease seen mainly in Basenjis but sporadically in other breeds; it results in proteinuria, amino aciduria (including cystine) and hypokalaemia due to reduced renal tubular absorption. Hypophosphataemia can result, due to an inability to resorb phosphate in the renal tubules but usually circulating concentrations are maintained within the normal range. In advanced stages there is ARF and hyperphosphataemia can result. Glycosuria without hyperglycaemia occurs because the renal threshold for glucose is abnormally low and there is poor resorption. Other causes of glycosuria are listed in Table 19.32.

Urinary retention

Urine filtered through the nephrons passes via the collecting ducts to the renal pelvis, then is transported through the ureters to the urinary bladder, and finally through the urethra. Disease of these or adjacent structures can lead to urinary retention, resulting in distension of the tract or leakage into body cavities.

Obstruction may be intraluminal (urolith, blood clot, foreign body); intramural (neoplasia, fibrosis) or extramural (prostatic disease, perineal rupture, reflex dysynergia). Perforation of the excretory pathway may result from trauma, including iatrogenic causes.

Diagnosis is confirmed by plain and contrast radiography, ultrasonography, endoscopy, cytology, biopsy and urodynamic tests.

The consequences of urinary retention are polysystemic clinical and metabolic disturbances resulting in azotaemia and uraemia, and occasionally anatomical changes (hydronephrosis) and functional changes (CRF).

Test	Abnormal increase	Abnormal decrease	Comments
BLOOD CHEMISTRY			
Plasma urea	Dogs usually >7 mmol/l Cats usually >11 mmol/l		
Blood urea nitrogen	Dogs: > 20 mg/dl Cats: > 32 mg/dl		
Plasma creatinine	Dogs and cats: > 130 μmol/l		Especially significant if over 250 μmol/l
Urea:creatinine ratio			Usually within normal range
Plasma phosphorus	>1.6 mmol/l in dogs over 1 year Once 66% of function lost		If exceeds 2.3 mmol/l (in dogs over 1 year age) it is associated with a guarded prognosis
Plasma calcium	May be increased in terminal renal failure	May be decreased in terminal renal failure	Usually within normal range CRF can be caused by hypercalcaemia if >3 mmol/l
Plasma potassium	Can be elevated in advanced renal failure. Also low sodium intake, excessive sodium losses through the gastro-intestinal tract, the use of potassium-losing diuretics (e.g. frusemide) or metabolic acidosis		
Plasma bicarbonate		May fall in decompensated cases	Usually maintained above 19 mmol/l
Plasma sodium	Sudden increases in intake can lead to transient hypernatraemia	Sudden changes in sodium intake or increases in losses (overexuberant use of diuretics) can lead to transient hyponatraemia	Usually within normal limits
SERUM ENZYMES			
Alkaline phosphatase	Increased if renal secondary hyper-parathyroidism		
Amylase	May be elevated		Decreased excretion and/or increased pancreatic secretion with increased gastrin secretion
HAEMATOLOGY			
Red blood cell count		Normocytic, normochromic non-regenerative anaemia	Reduced erythropoietin secretion
White blood cell count		Lymphopenia often due to reduced lymphopoiesis	
Platelets		Thrombocytopenia	Uraemic effects on bone marrow
URINALYSIS			
Proteinuria	Up to 10 g/l		Not always present
Specific gravity		Dogs: < 1.029 Cats: < 1.034	If 66% loss of nephrons

Table: 19.31: Typical clinical pathology panel in CRF.

Urinary tract infection

A urinary tract infection exists whenever bacteria or other organisms successfully colonize an otherwise sterile part of the urinary system. Usually these are aerobic bacteria, such as Enterobacteriaceae, staphylococci and streptococci, but infections with anaerobes, fungi and viruses also occur.

Infectious agents usually gain access by an ascending route from the distal urethra but they can also arrive via the blood. In the case of ascending infections there is a breakdown in natural defence mechanisms prior to the infection occurring, so a urinary tract abnormality precedes the onset of the urinary tract infection.

Inflammation caused by the infectious agent results in increased frequency of urination (pollakiuria), dysuria and renal pain (if pyelonephritis is present).

Inflammatory cells are found in the urine and systemic signs of inflammation are found on haematological examination.

It is important to realize that urinary tract infections can be secondary to other urinary system diseases, and that urinary tract infections can spread to other systems, resulting in septicaemia, prostatitis, discospondylitis, epididymitis or orchitis. Infections may also be associated with the presence of calculi.

Diagnosis is confirmed by the identification of viable organisms in urine or in tissues. Usually urine is examined by direct microscopy or it is cultured, and occasionally tissue samples are cultured and examined histologically. Whenever possible the site of infection should be identified.

Urine pH may be persistently alkaline in the pres-

Condition	Comments
Glycosuria with hyperglycaemia:	
Diabetes mellitus	Glycosuria occurs with all forms, with or without ketoacidosis
Hyperadrenocorticism – especially in cats	Induces development of diabetes mellitus in <10% of dogs but in 75% of cats
'Acromegaly' in bitches	Induces NIDDM; seen in bitches on progestogen treatment or in dioestrus
Hyperthyroidism in cats	Induces NIDDM; glycosuria occurs in >10% of affected cats
Phaeochromocytoma (usually adrenal medulla neoplasm)	Induces NIDDM due to sympathetic stimulation
Drugs (corticosteroids, ACTH, progestogens)	Induce NIDDM
Acute pancreatitis	Usually transient glycosuria
Pancreatic trauma	Road traffic accident; post-pancreatic surgery
Stress (especially in cats)	NIDDM due to the effects of sympathetic stimulation
Parenteral administration of fluids	Especially after dextrose
Convulsions	
Post–xylazine administration (cats)	Inhibits insulin secretion
Insulin overdose	Leads to rebound hyperglycaemia and glycosuria – Somogyi effect (rare)
Chronic liver failure	Rare
Alloxan or streptozotocin therapy	Destroys beta-cells in hyperinsulinaemia cases
Glycosuria without hyperglycaemia:	
Primary renal glycosuria	Inherited defect with low renal threshold for glucose and inability of the tubules to resorb filtered glucose
Fanconi syndrome	Inherited defect with low renal threshold for glucose and inability of tubules to resorb filtered glucose
Familial glycosuria	Inherited defect in Norwegian Elkhound, Cocker Spaniel
ARF	When there is significant renal tubular damage, e.g. nephrotoxins such as gentamicin, post-renal obstruction
Phloridzin therapy	Rare
False-positive results:	
Feline lower urinary tract disease (FLUTD)	Following urethral obstruction in cats an unknown substance in the urine can change the colour reaction for glucose

Table 19.32: *Causes of glycosuria. (After Bush, 1991.) NIDDM = non-insulin dependent diabetes mellitus.*

ence of a urinary tract infection with urease-positive bacteria, but the presence of an acidic urine does not rule out the possibility of the presence of a urinary tract infection.

Treatment should be based upon accurate culture and sensitivity findings and repeat cultures (collected by cystocentesis) are necessary at 5-day intervals to determine when the urine is sterile and treatment can be stopped. It is also useful to monitor for recurrence 10 days after treatment has been stopped. Urinary tract infections frequently recur despite treatment. In some cases of chronic or recurrent urinary tract infection, treatment needs to be continued for 6 months or more to eliminate a deep-seated infection, but this is only valid if regular urine cultures are negative during the treatment. It is not valid to continue with antibiotics if organisms can be cultured during the treatment period. Prostatic infection is a common recurrent problem, in which trimethoprim, erythromycin, chloramphenicol, oleandomycin and doxacycline may be indicated (subject to sensitivity tests) to get the tissue penetration needed to eliminate the infection.

The administration of urinary acidifiers has been advocated as a method of treatment but results have been evaluated on an empirical basis. Modifying urine pH may however influence the efficacy of some antimicrobial drugs.

Leptospirosis

Leptospirosis is a common, important zoonotic disease, although it is not always recognized. Leptospirosis in dogs and cats has recently been reviewed by Greene and Shotts (1990).

The majority of leptospiral infections in dogs and cats are chronic or subclinical, with few noticeable signs. When subacute infection is present the patient exhibits a fever, anorexia, vomiting, dehydration and polydipsia, with hyperaesthesia in some cases. Mucous membranes may be infected and widespread petechial and ecchymotic haemorrhages may develop. Anterior uveitis occurs due to an immunological reaction. Serious sequelae include renal failure, and icterus due to cholestasis, hepatitis or hepatic fibrosis. Intestinal intussusceptions occur in some dogs.

With peracute infections massive leptospiraemia occurs with death. The early signs are pyrexia (39.5–40 °C), shivering and muscle pain. Vomiting, dehydration and vascular collapse follow. Coagulopathies develop, leading to gastrointestinal and respiratory haemorrhages with haematemesis, melaena, haematochezia, epistaxis and petechiae. Hypothermia develops in the terminal stages. The clinicopathological findings in leptospirosis are summarized in Table 19.33. Leptospirosis is a multisystemic disease and this is reflected in the typical laboratory findings.

For laboratory isolation and identification, samples should be taken prior to the administration of antibiotics and, because of the zoonotic risk, strict protective measures should be employed during the collection and examination of samples.

Dark-field microscopic examination of wet-mount preparations is used to identify leptospires. Unfortunately they cannot be stained using simple dye techniques. Also, the characteristic irregular whip-like movements of leptospires can be mimicked by other bacteria and so microscopic identification should be supported by culture and serological testing to confirm the diagnosis. EMJH is a medium that is used for the isolation of leptospires. It contains polysorbate-80 and calf serum or bovine serum albumin; adding antibiotics or 5-fluorouracil facilitates the isolation of some of the many serovars that exist.

Leptospires can be isolated from blood, cerebrospinal fluid (CSF) and urine. They can also be isolated from tissue biopsy samples. Leptospires in CSF and circulating leptospires are most plentiful during the first week of infection; thereafter, urine is the best source for isolation but as leptospires are shed into urine intermittently, repeat testing is often necessary. Cystocentesis is the preferred method of collection for urine, as catheterization introduces natural bacterial contaminants which can overwhelm any leptospires present. Normally voided urine is also usually contaminated.

The following precautions should be taken to ensure viability of the leptospiral organisms during transportation:

- Collect all samples under aseptic conditions into sterile impervious containers, preferably made from glass
- Inject 0.25–0.5 ml of blood, urine or CSF into 10 ml of transport medium
- Place tissues and fluids in buffered saline (dilution of sample by 1:10 v/v), 1% bovine serum albumin or culture medium to negate the effect of any antibodies present in the sample
- Anticoagulate blood with heparin or sodium polyethylene sulphonate. Avoid citrated anticoagulants as these inhibit leptospires
- Alkalinize urine prior to transportation by adding dilute sodium bicarbonate solution
- Use transport media for tissues and fluids, or transport them on ice. DO NOT FREEZE. For research only, leptospiral samples can be frozen and stored at –60 to –70 °C for up to 6 years prior to culture.

Leptospires do not survive for long under postmortem conditions and they are best isolated from sections of macerated kidney, intercellular locations within hepatic cords, pericapillary areas of the central nervous system (when using silver stain) or body fluids saved in a sterile glass container.

The multisystemic nature of leptospirosis is reflected in the typical post-mortem findings (Table 19.34).

Test Comments	
Haematology:	
White cell count	Leucopenia during leptospiraemic phase
	Leucocytosis in typical cases
Thrombocytes	Thrombocytopenia
Erythrocyte sedimentation rate (ESR)	Increased when hyperfibrinogenaemic and hyperglobulinaemic
Blood chemistry:	
Blood urea nitrogen	Increased when renal failure present
Creatinine	Increased when renal failure present
Sodium	Hyponatraemia in most cases
Chloride	Hypochloraemia in most cases
Potassium	Hypokalaemia in most cases
	Hyperkalaemia in terminal stage of renal failure
Phosphate	Hyperphosphataemia in most cases
Glucose	Hypoglycaemia occasionally when liver failure is present
	Hyperglycaemia in terminal stage of renal failure
Calcium	Hypocalcaemia when hypoalbuminaemic
Blood acid–base balance	Metabolic acidosis in severely affected animals, with low serum bicarbonate
Serum bilirubin	High conjugated bilirubin concentrations peaking 6–8 days after onset of disease
Sulphobromophthalein retention	> 5% in acute stage – prior to jaundice and in dogs that develop chronic active hepatitis
CSF examination:	
Protein	Increased when meningitis present (subclinical)
Cells	Increased when meningitis present (subclinical)
Serum enzymes:	
ALT	Increased if liver damage
AST	Increased if liver damage
Lactic dehydrogenase	Increased if liver disease
ALP	increased if liver disease
Amylase	Increases without lipase increase, when from liver or small intestine and decreased renal function
	Very high if intestinal intussusception
Creatine phosphokinase	Increased when skeletal muscle inflamed
Urinalysis:	
Proteinuria	Common
Bilirubinuria	If liver damage; can be high concentrations which precede hyperbilirubinaemia
Casts	Granular often present
Blood cells	Erythrocytes often present
	Leucocytes often present
Serology:	
Microscopic agglutination test	Non-specific test. Titres may be increased with natural exposure and vaccination. A 4-fold increase is needed to confirm a diagnosis, and the test has to be repeated 2–3 times at 2–4 week intervals
ELISA test	IgM ELISA most sensitive 1–2 weeks after infection; vaccinated dogs have low IgM after 1 year
	IgG ELISA most sensitive 2–3 weeks after infection with maximum titre after 4–5 weeks; vaccinated dogs have high IgG after 1 year
Microscopic microcapsular agglutination test	Titres rise for a short period after infection; hence is useful to detect recent infection

Table 19.33: Clinicopathological findings in leptospirosis.

Urolithiasis

Stones that form within the urinary tract are known as uroliths or calculi (Figure 19.10). When crystals are identifiable in urine (see above), oversaturation with the chemical components has occurred, but this can occur *in vitro* due to temperature or pH changes, so the presence of crystalluria alone does not confirm a diagnosis of urolithiasis. Diagnosis can only be confirmed: by finding a urolith in freshly voided urine; on radiography; with ultrasonography; or at surgery. Radiographic contrast studies are sometimes needed to identify the presence of poorly radiodense or radiolucent uroliths.

Accurate and early diagnosis is of paramount importance if successful treatment is to be achieved and if the risk of ARF or CRF is to be avoided. Examination of urine sediment for the presence of crystalluria, as well as urinalysis for pH and for the presence of a urinary tract infection, is important in assisting with the diagnosis, as usually (but not always) large numbers of crystals in a urine sample will be of the same chemical type as the constituents of a urolith.

The only sure way to reach an accurate diagnosis is to perform a quantitative and qualitative analysis of a urolith. Commonly used semi-qualitative analytical kits can produce erroneous results if they fail to detect the presence of calcium; so treatment based on this test alone should be monitored carefully and used with caution. In one study, the test kit failed to detect 62% of calcium-containing uroliths, gave false-positive results for urates in 55% of cystine uroliths, and agreed with less than half of the calcium oxalate, urate and cystine uroliths detected by quantitative methods (Bovee and McGuire, 1984). X-ray diffraction crystallography is more expensive but does give accurate quantitative results. Laboratories performing X-ray diffraction urolith analysis include Birkbeck College, University of London (Dr June Sutor) and University of Minnesota (Dr Carl Osborne).

The aetiopathogenesis of most forms of urolithiasis has yet to be fully elucidated. Predisposing factors include genetics, diet, lifestyle, infectious agents and systemic disease. Uroliths can only form in urine under certain circumstances:

- The chemical components of the urolith have to be present in sufficient quantities to exceed their solubility product. Once crystals precipitate they

Organ system	Findings
Mucous membranes	Injected or icteric; petechiae
Tongue	Ulcerations
Buccal cavity	Ulcerations
Tonsils	Enlarged
Respiratory tract	Oedema
Lungs	Gross: Congestion; diffuse infiltrates; petechiae and ecchymoses on pleural surfaces Histology: Fibrinoid necrosis of blood vessels; perivascular, intra-alveolar and subpleural haemorrhages; mononuclear cell infiltration around pulmonary vessels
Liver	Gross: Enlarged, friable, interlobar markings, yellow-brown discoloration Histology: Focal necrosis which can be widespread and associated with disintegration of nuclei; round hepatocytes with pyknotic nuclei and an eosinophilic, granular cytoplasm; bile stasis and severe hepatocellular injury; fatty change in mild cases; chronic active hepatitis and hepatic fibrosis in chronic cases
Central nervous system	Gross: Petechiae and ecchymoses on leptomeninges Histology: Perivascular haemorrhage; mononuclear cell infiltration; occasionally vascular thrombosis
Gastrointestinal tract	Necrosis and haemorrhage in small intestine with intussusceptions; colonic haemorrhage; acholic faeces in colon
Heart	Histology: focal lymphocytic myocarditis
Spleen	Pale and small
Kidneys	Gross: Enlarged if died during acute phase; pale or yellow on cut surface; renal capsule may adhere to surface of kidney; subcapsular haemorrhages common; focal white spotting may be seen in the cortex Histology: Desquamation of degenerate renal tubular epithelium; swollen glomeruli; necrosis associated with mononuclear infiltrates; diffuse lymphocytic infiltration in chronic cases with macrophages; large numbers of atrophied tubules containing eosinophilic casts; glomeruli sometimes swollen and contain proteinaceous deposits in Bowman's space

Table 19.34: Post-mortem findings in leptospirosis.

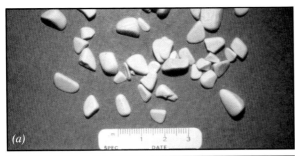

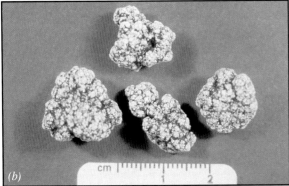

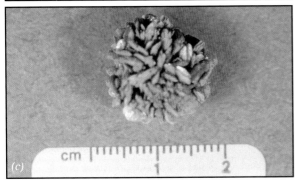

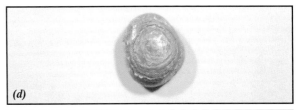

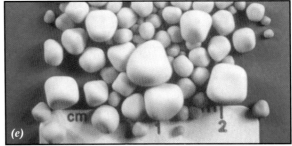

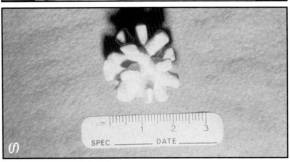

Figure 19.10: (*a*) *Smooth-surfaced faceted struvite uroliths removed from a canine bladder.* (*b*) *100% struvite uroliths with atypical rough surfaces removed from a Dalmatian.* (*c*) *Calcium oxalate urolith from a 3-year-old Lhasa Apso, showing typical sharp-edged surface.* (*d*) *Typical urate urolith: smooth surfaced and green-brown in colour.* (*e*) *Typical smooth surfaced cystine uroliths.* (*f*) *A typical silicate 'Jack Stone'; these can be quite small.*

aggregate and produce micro-uroliths, which gradually grow and often incorporate other substances present in the urine

- Some crystals are affected by urine pH. Struvite crystals rarely form at a pH less than 6.4 and frequently form at pH greater than 7, whereas others (e.g. urates) form best in an acidic urine
- Time is needed for a stone to develop; otherwise the crystals are washed out of the tract during micturition
- In some circumstances there is probably a breakdown in natural inhibitory factors (such as reduced effect of glycosaminoglycans) before crystalluria and urolithiasis can occur
- Uroliths frequently form around a nidus within the urinary tract. Examples include cell debris and foreign bodies such as sutures
- Bacterial infection can predispose to some forms of urolithiasis. Urease-positive bacteria are often associated with struvite uroliths and ammonium urate uroliths.

Urolithiasis should be suspected whenever an animal presents with clinical signs of partial or complete urinary tract obstruction, or haematuria. Staging of the urinary tract signs associated with urolithiasis has been suggested (Davies, 1996) and recommendations for clinical pathology tests at each stage can be made (Table 19.35).

Clinical signs associated with urolithiasis are usually those of lower urinary tract disease but occasionally stones form in the kidney (nephroliths) causing damage, and if uroliths cause partial or complete urinary obstruction ARF can result with serious consequences.

Diagnosis of urolithiasis is usually straightforward but it can be difficult, particularly when the uroliths consist of two apparently paradoxical types. For example, mixed struvite and calcium oxalate stones can form, with one forming an outer shell around the other. It is therefore important that the whole urolith is submitted for laboratory analysis, and that this is done in an organized way so that the composition of different layers can be properly evaluated.

Dalmatians have impaired uricase activity and so excrete uric acid rather than allopurinol in their urine. Prolonged hyperuricosuria may result in uric acid precipitation and the development of calculi. The use of allantoin (a xanthine oxidase inhibitor) to prevent the development of urate uroliths in this breed has resulted in several reports of the development of xan-

Stage	Signs	Recommended laboratory tests
Stage 1: Subclinical	No signs Presence of urolithiasis discovered by chance or crystalluria found on routine urine examination Most often these are struvite or other smooth stones (cystine, urate); less frequently calcium oxalate, as they often have a sharp surface and cause urinary tract inflammation with associated signs	1. Identify crystals by light microscopy 2. If struvite or urate crystals present, culture urine for a urinary tract infection 3. If urate crystals present, perform blood chemistry to rule out liver disease or portosystemic shunt (liver enzymes, blood ammonia, etc.) 4. If calcium oxalate or calcium phosphate crystals present, analyse urine for hypercalciuria and blood for hypercalcaemia 5. If cystine crystals present, consider familial disorder Screen for evidence of early ARF and CRF Start investigative procedures to identify if a urolith is present in the urinary tract (radiography, ultrasonography) If a urolith has been retrieved, send for full qualitative and quantitative analysis
Stage 2: Mild signs	Slight increase in frequency of urination Mild haematuria — blood staining Mild straining at time of urination Slight discomfort at time of urination Increased licking of genital area	Signs consistent with inflammation and/or partial obstruction. Identify crystals as above **AND** 1. Start investigations (radiography, ultrasonography) for the presence of a urolith and its location. Also identify the source of haemorrhage - upper or lower urinary tract. Licking genital area suggests lower tract 2. *Prior to administration of an anaesthetic*, perform a full laboratory screen for evidence of underlying renal disease; otherwise anaesthesia could precipitate acute renal failure
Stage 3: Severe signs	Pollakiuria (continually passing or dribbling urine) Urinary tenesmus Severe haematuria Severe discomfort on urination - vocalization and evidence of pain Bladder often grossly distended on palpation Polydipsia/polyuria if secondary renal failure present General depression, malaise and anorexia	Signs consistent with obstruction and severe damage to urinary tract, possibly with signs of renal failure Urgent need to prevent patient progressing to life-threatening stages 1. If bladder distended, relieve pressure by cystocentesis — take sample for urinalysis and possible culture 2. Establish whether lower urinary outflow tract is patent by urethral catheterization. Note site of partial or complete obstruction 3. Establish intravenous fluid line 4. Then start investigations as for Stages 1 and 2 above **PLUS** a full laboratory blood and urine panel 5. Avoid the administration of any substances that might constitute a risk factor for the development of ARF
Stage 4: Life-threatening signs	Anuria Weakness/collapse Dehydration Bladder either tense and full, or not palpated if ruptured or anuric Uraemic halitosis present Vomiting Seizures Coma	**Life-threatening situation**. Need to act quickly : 1. Establish intravenous fluid line — maximum rate for replacement and maintenance and to induce diuresis. 2. Rush through blood potassium estimation and administer potassium intravenously if hypokalaemia present 3. Check acid–base balance and correct any serious acidosis as soon as possible with bicarbonate 4. Take blood sample for full haematology and appropriate chemistry panel 5. If possible, obtain urine sample for full panel of tests. Insert an indwelling urinary catheter attached to a collection bag. This will help in obtaining urine samples throughout the treatment period and (more importantly) will also allow urine outflow to be monitored 6. Must stabilize patient before contemplate surgery (e.g. for repair of ruptured bladder). Consider peritoneal dialysis

Table 19.35: Staging of signs associated with urolithiasis and clinical pathology panels recommended for each stage.

thine uroliths with urine concentrations exceeding its saturation point.

Feline lower urinary tract disease (FLUTD)

Despite our improved understanding of this syndrome, FLUTD (previously known as feline urological syndrome, FUS), remains a relatively common occurrence in both male and female cats. It manifests a range of clinical signs typical of lower urinary tract inflammation (cystitis and/or urethritis), with or without signs of partial or complete urinary tract obstruction:

- Increased frequency of voiding of urine
- Haematuria
- Urinary tenesmus
- Dysuria
- Licking perineum
- Anuria (if total obstruction)
- Vomiting (if uraemic)
- Coma (if total obstruction) .

Causes can be single or multiple (Table 19.36) but it is generally agreed that FLUTD is a multifactorial disease syndrome.

Many factors have been identified as potential risk factors for the development of FLUTD (Table 19.37) and the severity of the disease can vary from mild signs, such as increased frequency of urination, to life-threatening signs, such as coma associated with complete urinary tract obstruction for 24–72 hours and postrenal ARF (see above). A typical clinical pathology panel is shown in Table 19.38. The syndrome is most often associated with the presence of struvite crystalluria and calculi. Urethral obstruction is most frequent in males and is often caused by urethral plugs of mucoid material which are a mixture of protein and struvite mineral deposits. Mild cases often resolve spontaneously. Recurrence is common unless preventive steps, such as long-term dietary management, are instituted.

It is important to evaluate the patient fully before

Cause	Comments
Metabolic causes	
Uroliths	Mostly struvite, but also calcium oxalate and others

Urethral plugs :
     Struvite crystals only
     Proteinaceous matrix only
     Struvite and matrix
     Matrix and other crystals
	Most common

Infections:
     Bacteria
     Viruses
     Mycoplasma/Ureaplasma ?
     Parasites
	Secondary infections usually
	 Experimental only
	 Not identified yet in cats
	 Not in UK

Immune-mediated	Confirmed ?

Anatomical disorders:
     Urachal anomalies (congenital)
     Ectopic ureters (congenital or acquired)
     Urethral stricture
     Post-urethrostomy	

Neoplasia:
     Benign: mainly in bladder
     Malignant: mainly in bladder
	Older cats

Neurological disorders:
     Primary
     Secondary (e.g. trauma)	

Trauma: Road accident	

Iatrogenic:
     Flushing solution
     Repeat catheterization
     Indwelling catheters
     Post-urethrostomy	

Idiopathic	

Table 19.36: Causes of FLUTD.

Risk factor	Comments
Infections: Bacteria Viruses	The first occurrence of FLUTD is usually not associated with urinary tract infection, but infection may occur following recurrence of FLUTD and/or following catheterization (particularly repeated catheterization) of the urethra to free obstructions. Recurrent infection is more likely after urethrostomy than with dietary management alone Viruses have been implicated by some authors but their precise significance has yet to be elucidated fully
Alkaline urine pH	Struvite crystals form frequently at pH>7 and rarely at pH<6.4
Dietary intake	Rations high in the basic constituents for struvite (magnesium, protein and phosphorus): cats have a relatively high dietary requirement for protein (high in phosphorus) so only the intake of magnesium can be easily controlled Rations that produce an alkaline urine pH
Obesity	May lead to infrequent exercise, hence infrequent urination encouraging the development of crystalluria
Sedentary lifestyle	Infrequent urination, leading to urine stasis encouraging the development of crystalluria
Age	FLUTD usually first occurs at 1–3 years
Breed	Persians have a higher than average incidence Siamese have a lower than average incidence
Anatomic anomalies	Vesicourachal diverticulum is a well recognized congenital anomaly that may be associated with FLUTD. Enlargement of the diverticulum is a result, not a cause, of FLUTD
Vitamin A deficiency?	Theoretical cause: deficiency increases sloughing of epithelial cells into the urinary tract
Nidus	Material in urinary tract lumen acts as a collection site for debris, cells and crystals. Confirmed examples include suture material

Table 19.37: Risk factors for the development of FLUTD.

embarking upon treatment, as administration of incorrect treatment (e.g. acidification of urine) can be detrimental if the diagnosis is not accurate. Acutely obstructed patients should always be treated as medical emergencies, with correction of serious metabolic disorders (e.g. hyperkalaemia, dehydration) and relief of the urinary obstruction being of paramount importance, followed by stabilization. Cystocentesis and retrograde flushing is the author's preferred approach to the completely obstructed male cat.

Abnormal micturition

The inability to store and void urine normally may be primary, or secondary to other disorders such as an increased rate of urine formation (polyuria) or a decreased rate of urine production (oliguria) in animals with renal failure.

Increased frequency of urination without increased urine production (pollakuria) may be seen, as may discomfort on urination (dysuria) or straining to pass the urine (stranguria).

Causes may be anatomical (e.g. ectopic ureters, patent urachus) or functional (e.g. neoplasia, fibrosis, feline idiopathic haemorrhagic cystitis, urethral incompetence, detrusor instability, motor neuron deficits).

Diagnosis is confirmed by the results of radiography – plain and contrast (dynamic studies sometimes needed), ultrasonography, neurological examination, identification of partial obstruction, or cytology.

Subclinical urinary system abnormalities

Routine screening or examination for other reasons may identify subclinical abnormalities when the patient is exhibiting no clinical signs. Common examples of this are: the presence of haematuria, proteinuria or dilute urine on routine examination of urine samples; abnormalities detected on survey radiographs; and abnormalities (e.g. cystic kidneys) discovered during exploratory laparotomy. An exhaustive investigation may not be justified, but the underlying cause should be identified whenever possible because of the potential for many of the common conditions to progress to irreversible renal failure.

REFERENCES AND FURTHER READING

Adams LG, Polzin DJ, Osborne CA *et al.* (1992) Correlation of urine protein–creatinine ratio and 24-hour urinary protein excretion in normal cats and cats with surgically induced chronic renal failure. *Journal of Veterinary Internal Medicine* **6**, 36-40

Risk factor	Comments
URINALYSIS	
Sediment	Red blood cells if inflammation White blood cells if inflammation/infection Crystals: usually struvite, but also calcium oxalate, calcium phosphate, urates Casts: none, unless secondary or concurrent acute renal disease
Bacterial culture	Usually sterile at time of first occurrence Positive culture usually due to secondary infections after recurrent episodes of FLUTD, especially after catheterization or urethrostomy. Urease-positive bacteria most common
Proteinuria	Present due to inflammation
pH	Usually pH 7; rarely below pH 6.4 if associated with struvite crystalluria or urolithiasis
Specific gravity	Usually >1.035 if sterile urine culture; sometimes <1.035 if bacterial infection present
Glycosuria	Up to 33% of obstructed cats have glycosuria of 10–50 mg/100 ml May be secondary to hyperglycaemia (see below)
Hypercalciuria	May be present with/without hypercalcaemia, and in association with calcium salt (phosphate or oxalate) urolithiasis
HAEMATOLOGY	
Blood cell counts	Usually normal
Packed cell volume	Elevated if obstructed and dehydrated
BLOOD CHEMISTRY	
Serum biochemistry	Routine screening tests (including BUN and creatinine) are usually within published reference ranges *unless* • there is ARF due to postrenal causes (see Table 19.29) *or* • there is urate crystalluria or calculi formation secondary to portosystemic shunts or liver disease, in which case liver enzymes may be elevated and postprandial blood ammonia concentrations may also be increased, but BUN may be low
Hyperglycaemia	Blood glucose concentrations may be high due to stress or insulin inhibition in the presence of uraemia
Hypercalcaemia	May be present in association with calcium salt (phosphate or oxalate) urolithiasis
Hyperkalaemia	Rare; moribund obstructed cats

Table 19.38: Typical clinical pathology panel in FLUTD.

Bainbridge J and Elliott J (eds) (1996) *Manual of Canine and Feline Nephrology and Urology.* BSAVA Publications, Cheltenham

Barber PJ (1996) Proteinuria. In: *Manual of Canine and Feline Nephrology and Urology,* ed. J. Bainbridge and J Elliott, pp.75–84. BSAVA Publications, Cheltenham

Barber PJ, Torrance AG and Elliott J (1994) Carboxyl fragmentation interference in assay of feline parathyroid hormone. *Journal of Veterinary Internal Medicine* **8**, 168

Barsanti JA and Finco DR (1979) Protein concentration in urine of normal dogs. *American Journal of Veterinary Research* **40**, 1583–1588

Biertuempfel PH, Ling GV and Ling GA (1981) Urinary tract infection resulting from catheterisation in healthy adult dogs. *Journal of the American Veterinary Medical Association* **178**, 989

Biewenga WJ (1982) Urinary protein loss in the dog: Nephrological study of 29 dogs without signs of renal disease. *Research in Veterinary Science* **33**, 366–374

Biewenga WJ and Van den Brom WE (1981) Assessment of glomerular filtration rate in dogs with renal insufficiency: analysis of the ^{51}Cr-EDTA clearance and its relationship to the plasma concentrations of urea and creatinine. *Research in Veterinary Science* **30**, 158–160

Bovee KC and Joyce T (1979) Clinical evaluation of glomerular function: 24 hour creatinine clearance in dogs. *Journal of the American Veterinary Medical Association* **174**, 488–491

Bovee KC and McGuire T (1984) Qualitative and quantitative analysis of uroliths in dogs: definitive determination of chemical type.

Journal of the American Medical Association **185**, 983.

Bush BM (1991) *Interpretation of Laboratory Results for Small Animal Clinicians.* Blackwell Scientific, Oxford

Center SA, Wilkinson E, Smith CA *et al.* (1985) 24-hour urine protein/creatinine ratio in dogs with protein-losing nephropathies. *Journal of the American Veterinary Medical Association* **187**, 820–824

Chew DJ and DiBartola SP(1986) *Manual of Small Animal Nephrology and Urology* . Churchill Livingstone, New York

Comer KM and Ling GV (1981) Results of urinalysis and bacterial culture of canine urine obtained by antepubic cystocentesis, catheterisation and the midstream voided methods. *Journal of the American Veterinary Medical Association* **179**, 891

Davies M (1996) Management of canine and feline urolithiasis. In: *Manual of Canine and Feline Nephrology and Urology,* ed. J. Bainbridge and J. Elliott, pp.211–212. BSAVA Publications, Cheltenham

DiBartola SP (1992) Clinical evaluation of renal function. In: *Proceedings of 16th Annual Waltham/OSU Symposium,* pp. 7–15. Kal Kan Foods, Vernon, California

DiBartola SP, Chew DJ and Jacobs G (1980) Quantitative urinalysis including 24-hour protein excretion in the dog. *Journal of the American Animal Hospitals Association* **16**, 537–546

Elliott J (1996) Polyuria/polydipsia. In: *Manual of Canine and Feline Nephrology and Urology,* ed. J. Bainbridge and J Elliot, pp. 28–41. BSAVA Publications, Cheltenham

European Society of Veterinary Nephrology and Urology (ESVNU). (1988) *Proceedings of the 3ʳᵈ Annual Symposium*

Fettman MJ, Allen TA, Wilke WL *et al.* (1985) Single injection method for evaluation of renal function with ¹⁴C-inulin and ³H-tetraethylammonium bromide in dogs and cats. *American Journal of Veterinary Research* **46**, 482–485

Finco DR (1971) Simultaneous determination of phenolsulfonphthalein excretion and endogenous creatinine clearance in the normal dog. *Journal of the American Veterinary Medical Association* **159**, 336–340

Finco DR (1980) Kidney function. In: *Clinical Biochemistry of Domestic Animals, 3ʳᵈ edn,* ed. JJ Kaneko, pp. 389–000. Academic Press, New York

Finco DR, Coulter DB and Barsanti JA (1981) Simple, accurate method for the clinical estimation of glomerular filtration rate in the dog. *American Journal of Veterinary Research* **42**, 1874–1877

Finco DR, Coulter DB and Barsanti JA (1982) Procedure for a simple method of measuring glomerular filtration rate in the dog. *Journal of the American Animal Hospital Association* **18**, 804–806

Forrester SD, Lees GE and Russo EA (1989) Urine protein-creatinine ratio determinations in healthy cats. *Journal of Veterinary Internal Medicine* **3**, 130 (abstract)

Grauer GF, Thomas CB and Eicker SW (1985) Estimation of quantitative proteinuria in the dog using the protein:creatinine ratio from a random voided sample. *American Journal of Veterinary Research* **46**, 2116–2119

Greene CE and Shotts EB (1990) Leptospirosis. In: *Infectious Diseases of the Dog and Cat,* ed. CE Greene, pp. 498–507. WB Saunders, Philadelphia

Hager DA, Nyland TG and Fisher PE (1985) Ultrasound-guided biopsy of the canine liver, kidney and prostate. *Veterinary Radiology* **26**, 82

Hill's Pet Products (1989) *Managing Canine and Feline Urolithiasis.* (1989) Veterinary Medicine Publishing Co., Goleta, California

Hoskins JD, Turnwald GH, Kearney MT *et al.* (1991) Quantitative urinalysis in kittens from four to thirty weeks after birth. *American Journal of Veterinary Research* **52**, 1295–1299

Krawiec DR, Badertscher RR, Twardock AR *et al.* (1986) Evaluation of ⁹⁹ᵐTc-diethylenetriaminepentaacetic acid nuclear imaging for quantitative determination of glomerular filtration rate of dogs. *American Journal of Veterinary Research* **47**, 2175–2179

Krawiec DR, Twardock AR, Badertscher RR *et al.* (1988) Use of ⁹⁹ᵐTc diethylenetriaminepentaacetic acid for assessment of renal function in dogs with suspected renal disease. *Journal of the American Veterinary Medical Association* **192**, 1077–1080

Kruger JM, Osborne CA, Goyal SM, Wickstrom SL, Johnston GR, Fletcher TF and Brown PA (1991) Clinical evaluation of cats with lower urinary tract disease. *Journal of the American Veterinary Medical Association* **199**, 211

Lage AL (1977) Nephrogenic diabetes insipidus. In: *Current Veterinary Therapy VI,* ed. RW Kirk, pp. 1102–1106. WB Saunders, Philadelphia

Leveille R, Partington BP, Biller DS and Miyabayashi T (1993) Complications after ultrasound-guided biopsy of abdominal structures in dogs and cats: 246 cases (1984–1991). *Journal of the American Veterinary Medical Association* **203**, 413

Lulich JP, Osborne CA, Polzin DJ *et al.* (1991) Urine metabolite values in fed and nonfed clinically normal Beagles. *American Journal of Veterinary Research* **52**, 1573–1578

Macdougall DF and Curd GJ (1996) Urine collection and complete analysis. In: *Manual of Canine and Feline Nephrology and Urology,* ed. J. Bainbridge and J Elliot, pp. 86–106. BSAVA Publications, Cheltenham

Macdougall DF and Lamb CR (1996) Renal biopsy. In: *Manual of Canine and Feline Nephrology and Urology,* ed. J. Bainbridge and J Elliot, pp. 148–159. BSAVA Publications, Cheltenham

McCaw DL, Knapp SDW and Hewett JE (1985) Effect of collection time and exercise restriction on the prediction of urine protein excretion using urine protein:creatinine ratio in dogs. *American Journal of Veterinary Research* **46**, 1665–1669

Mercer HD and Garg RC (1977) Bioavailability and pharmacokinetics of several dosage forms of ampicillin in the cat. *American Journal of Veterinary Research* **38**, 1353–1359

Monroe WE, Davenport DJ and Saunders GK (1989) 24-hour urinary protein loss in healthy cats and the urinary protein–creatinine ratio as an estimate. *American Journal of Veterinary Research* **50**, 1906–1909

Nash AS, Boyd JS, Minot AW and Wright NG (1983) Renal biopsy in the normal cat: examination of the effects of a single needle biopsy. *Research in Veterinary Science* **34**, 347

Nash AS, Boyd JS, Minot AW and Wright NG (1986) Renal biopsy in the normal cat: examination of the effects of repeated needle biopsy. *Research in Veterinary Science* **40**, 112

Osbaldiston GW, Fuhrman W (1970) The clearance of creatinine, inulin, para-aminohippurate and phenolsulfonphthalein the cat. *Canadian Journal of Comparative Medicine* **34**, 138–141

Osborne CA, Davis LS, Sanna J, Unger LK, O'Brien TD, Clinton CW, Davenport MP (1990) *Urine Crystals in Domestic Animals: A Laboratory Identification Guide.* Veterinary Medicine Publishing Co., Goleta, California

Osborne CA and Finco DR (1995) *Canine and Feline Nephrology and Urology.* Williams and Wilkins, Baltimore

Osborne CA, Polzin DJ, Feeney DA and Caywood DD (1985) The urinary system: pathophysiology, diagnosis, treatment. In: *General Small Animal Surgery,* ed. IM Gourlay and PB Vasseur, pp. 479–658. Lippincott, Philadelphia

Osborne CA and Stevens JB (19??) *Handbook of Canine and Feline Urinalysis.* Ralston Purina, St Louis

Powers TE, Powers JD and Garg RC (1977) Studies of the double isotope single-injection method for estimating renal function in purebred Beagle dogs. *American Journal of Veterinary Research* **38**, 1933–1936

Rogers KS, Komkow A, Brown SA *et al.* (1991) Comparison of four methods of estimating glomerular filtration rate in cats. *American Journal of Veterinary Research* **52**, 961–964

Ross LA and Finco DR (1981) Relationship of selected clinical renal function tests to glomerular filtration rate and renal blood flow in cats. *American Journal of Veterinary Research* **42**, 1704–1710

Scott-Moncrieff CR (1996) Dysuria. In: *Manual of Canine and Feline Nephrology and Urology,* ed. J. Bainbridge and J Elliot, pp. 18–27. BSAVA Publications, Cheltenham

Snow DH, Harris RC and Stuttard E (1988) Changes in haematology and plasma biochemistry during maximal exercise in greyhounds. *Veterinary Record* **123**, 487–489

Waltham/OSU 16ᵗʰ Annual Symposium Proceedings (1992) Nephrology and Urology. Kal Kan Foods, Vernon, California

White JV, Olivier NB, Reimann K *et al.* (1984) Use of protein-to-creatinine ratio in a single urine specimen for quantitative estimation of canine proteinuria. *Journal of the American Veterinary Medical Association* **185**, 882–885

Acknowledgements and sincere thanks for permission to use several of the images in this chapter: Mr D.B.Murdoch; Prof C.A.Osborne; Hill's Pet Nutrition.

Reproductive System

Robert A. Foster

INTRODUCTION

Diagnosis of disease of the mammary glands or the male or female reproductive tract requires an understanding of anatomy, knowing what diseases to expect, and examination of urogenital tract fluids and tissues, using serology, hormonal assays, biochemistry, cytology and histopathology. In many cases ancillary tests are pathognomonic, but many require patience and an understanding that although a positive result is confirmatory a negative result neither proves nor disproves the proposed diagnosis.

Many diseases of the reproductive system are incidental and of no clinical consequence. The challenge for the clinician and pathologist alike is to use the techniques available to determine which conditions are significant. It is fortunate that each part of the tract has a very short list of diseases that are commonly seen and, with few exceptions, have a definitive prognosis.

MAMMARY GLANDS

Many of the diseases of the mammary gland require little in the way of ancillary tests because diagnoses such as agalactia, galactostasis (milk retention) and mastitis are made on clinical grounds. Subclinical mastitis, inappropriate lactation and galactostasis may create a diagnostic dilemma. Results of the cytological examination of milk are infrequently reported and normal reference ranges are not readily available. The presence of neutrophils in milk is normal in bitches that are resorbing milk. Finding degenerative neutrophils containing bacteria, especially in mid-lactation, suggests infectious mastitis (Olson and Olson, 1984).

Mammary masses

Masses in the mammary gland are best examined by excisional biopsy, but fine needle aspiration (FNA) cytology and punch biopsy can be useful in determining the extent of further surgical intervention (Griffiths *et al.*, 1984). Choice of the best therapy, be it removal of one gland, removal of an entire chain of glands plus draining lymph nodes, lumpectomy, euthanasia or no treatment, can be made in the light of the most accurate information available. Masses may first be examined by FNA cytology; based on the findings, the appropriate choice for both the animal and owner can be made.

One of the real tragedies is that many canine mammary diseases are preventable, and the protective effect of early ovarioectomy (Schneider *et al.*, 1969) is well known. Epidemiological data could not establish a similar protective effect in cats.

Not all mammary masses are neoplastic. There are a wide range of changes, including cystic dilation (or ectasia) of ducts, lobular hyperplasia, dysplasia and the peculiar disease of fibroepithelial hyperplasia (mammary hypertrophy) of cats. Mammary hypertrophy is an overgrowth of otherwise normal mammary tissue, in young cats especially (Hayden and Johnson, 1986).

Mammary neoplasia

Mammary neoplasia of bitches has received a large amount of attention because of the potential of using the high rate of spontaneous occurrence as a model for breast cancer in women. Dogs are also one of the species used to test ethical pharmaceuticals for safety and they have thus been studied very closely.

There is still considerable confusion and a lack of uniformity in the way mammary neoplasms are reported and categorized. Studies with long-term follow-ups are inherently difficult to interpret because owners vary in their abilities to detect and act on finding a mass; owners also vary in their willingness to proceed with treatment, and there is a tendency for pets to be euthanased when a diagnosis of carcinoma is made. Some laboratories classify neoplasms based on histological criteria according to the scheme of the World Health Organization (Hampe and Misdorp, 1974). Others have a simplified scheme that includes the anticipated prognosis.

A simple approach is to classify tumours as either benign or malignant, and as epithelial, mesenchymal or mixed mammary tumours.

Epithelial mammary tumours of dogs: Figure 20.1 shows a canine mammary carcinoma. The majority of mammary neoplasms have an epithelial component— be it the majority of the mass, or part of a neoplasm composed of a mixture of both epithelial and mesenchymal elements (Bostock, 1986). The most important prognostic indicator for epithelial tumours is evidence of invasion, regardless of the appearance of the neoplastic cells (Gilbertson *et al.,* 1983; Bostock, 1986). Cytological examination of fine needle aspirates and even punch or core biopsies can rarely provide accurate evidence of invasion, so correlation between cytological evaluation and prognosis of epithelial neoplasms is less than optimal (Allen *et al.,* 1986). The most accurate way to determine an accurate diagnosis and prognosis is to perform an excisional biopsy and have the specimen examined histologically.

The classification of epithelial mammary neoplasms according to the appearance of the neoplastic cells has resulted in dogs being euthanased unnecessarily when a diagnosis of carcinoma was given, because they were assumed to have malignant disease. The published figures of 50% malignant and 50% benign (Bostock, 1975) are probably far too pessimistic (Nerurkar *et al.,* 1989; Hellmen *et al.,* 1993). One simple scheme is to divide epithelial neoplasms into four categories based on presence of invasion and on the appearance of the

Classification	Approximate survival (months)		
	6	**12**	**24**
Benign	100	100	100
Non-invasive carcinoma	100	90	80
Invasive ductular carcinoma	90	60	50
Invasive solid carcinoma	90	30	5
Lymph node metastasis	40	10	0
Sarcoma	50	30	10
Malignant mixed neoplasm	80	80	50

Table 20.1: *Percentage of animals surviving after the diagnosis of mammary neoplasia.*

neoplastic cells: benign mammary tumour; non-invasive carcinoma; invasive carcinoma with evidence of ductular differentiation; and invasive carcinoma without ductular differentiation. Table 20.1 provides a composite of information on prognosis based on some of the published information (Bostock, 1975; Nerurkar *et al.,* 1989; Hellmen *et al.,* 1993).

There is some disagreement about the usefulness of routinely removing the draining lymph node for examination. Metastasis to the lymph node is a powerful prognostic indicator, but the correct node must be sampled, i.e. the inguinal node for the posterior glands and the axillary node for the anterior glands. Crossover can occur. In addition, there may be little benefit in the extra trauma involved with locating the node, especially in an obese patient or if a lumpectomy is chosen as the appropriate approach. An animal with clinical evidence of local invasion would be a good candidate for sampling the draining node to provide additional prognostic information.

Researchers have tried to improve prognosis by using special techniques such as flow cytometry for growth phase analysis and DNA ploidy analysis (Hellman *et al., 1993*), and examination for silver nuclear organizer regions (Bostock *et al.,* 1992) and

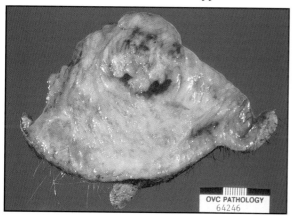

Figure 20.1: *Cross-section of a canine mammary carcinoma. Invasion of neoplasm into surrounding tissues is indicative of a poor prognosis.*

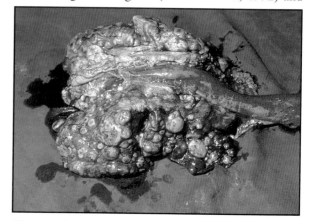

Figure 20.2: *Necropsy specimen of multiple lung metastases from a malignant mammary carcinoma in a 9-year-old Dalmatian bitch.*
Courtesy of Dr R.W. Else

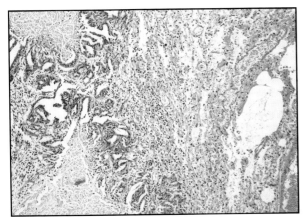

Figure 20.3: *Histopathological section of a lung metastasis from a primary mammary carcinoma; note the tubular carcinoma at top left and necrotic tumour at bottom left. H&E.*
Courtesy of Dr R.W. Else

oestrogen receptors, but these require submission of fresh tissue, or equipment and technologies not currently available to most diagnostic laboratories.

Mixed mammary neoplasms of dogs: Neoplasms that contain both epithelial and mesenchymal components are relatively common and the majority are benign (Hampe and Misdorp, 1974; Bostock, 1975, 1986; Gilbertson *et al.*, 1983; Hellmen *et al.*, 1993). They are a mixture of epithelium and the myoepithelium or fibroblasts of the interstitial tissue. Prognosis is probably best based on the same criteria as that for epithelial neoplasms, or on the 'worst' or most poorly differentiated part of the tumour. Occasionally, both the epithelial and mesenchymal component appear to be neoplastic, and the term carcinosarcoma may be used. Such tumours are very rare and their prognosis, although based on very few cases, is probably the same as the prognosis for the epithelial component (Hampe and Misdorp, 1974).

Epithelial mammary neoplasia in the cat: Feline mammary neoplasia is much more straightforward than the disease in the dog. The majority of neoplasms are carcinomas and the appearance of the neoplastic cells can be used for prognosis (MacEwen *et al.*, 1984; Hayes and Mooney, 1985). Once the diagnosis of carcinoma has been made, and this will be the case in over 90% of cases, it is claimed that survival time can be approximated by measuring the diameter of the mass. Survival times of >3 years, 2 years, and 6 months can be expected with tumours of diameters <2 cm, 2–3 cm and >3 cm, respectively (MacEwen *et al.*, 1984).

Mesenchymal mammary neoplasia: Mesenchymal neoplasms are rare (Hampe and Misdorp, 1974; Nerurkar *et al.*, 1989). In the dog, prognosis is only reported for sarcomas and is poor; 10% may survive 24 months (Hellman *et al.*, 1993). Examples of mesenchymal mammary tumours include fibrosarcoma, chondrosarcoma and osteosarcoma. Benign spindle cell

neoplasms such as haemangiopericytoma occur in the mammary gland and their behaviour is probably as in any other location in the skin; local recurrence may occur due to inadequate excision. FNA and core biopsies should assist in the diagnosis of these neoplasms, but excisional biopsies provide the best material.

THE FEMALE REPRODUCTIVE TRACT

The approaches to the diagnosis of diseases and conditions of the reproductive tract of bitches and queens are very similar and will therefore be discussed together. Some of the conditions that affect the reproductive tract are difficult to diagnose without a knowledge of normal hormonal and physiological processes. These are outlined by Concannon and Lein (1989) and Feldman and Nelson (1996).

The Ovaries

Normal ovulation and cycling

Bitches: There is considerable variation in the length of the various stages of the oestrous cycle in bitches. The lengths of pro-oestrus, oestrus and dioestrus can vary by many days. The most accurate method of determining when each of these stages and ovulation occurs is to measure the concentration of the hormones oestradiol, luteinizing hormone (LH) and progesterone. Samples must be collected sequentially at least every second day.

An important part of clinical practice is determining the time of ovulation. Not only does this provide the best time for insemination, especially if frozen–thawed semen is being used, but it also provides the exact anticipated whelping date. Gestation is around 63 days from the time of ovulation. Ovulation is estimated to occur 48 hours after the LH surge, and fertilization can occur after a further 2–3 days. The LH surge lasts 1–2 days and can be measured directly by sequential sampling every 2 days, or can be deduced to have occurred by observing a rise in plasma progesterone concentration to a level above 6.4 nmol/l. Insemination is best carried out 2–3 days after the day of the LH surge.

The time of ovulation can be estimated by other indirect means. Ovulation occurs the day before identification of the postural reflex of tail flagging and vulval elevation in response to perineal stroking, so insemination on the day after the postural reflex can be stimulated is optimal.

Vaginal cytology is another indirect method of estimating the best time for insemination and is particularly useful if no postural reflex can be elicited. Progressive cornification of the vaginal epithelial cells occurs in pro-oestrus (Figure 20.4). In anoestrus, the dominant cells are the parabasal and intermediate cells. The basal cell is rarely seen on

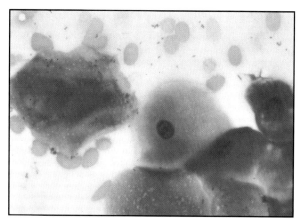

Figure 20.4: Vaginal cytology of a bitch in pro-oestrus. The red blood cells and the dominance of the basal or intermediate cells is characteristic of this stage. (Diff Quik®)

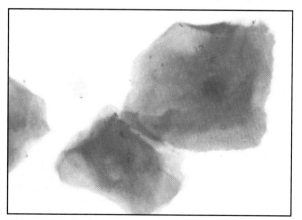

Figure 20.5: Vaginal cytology of a bitch in oestrus. All the cells are superficial squamous epithelium. (Diff Quik®)

smears. In pro-oestrus and with an increasing concentration of oestradiol, the number of intermediate and superficial cells increase, and red blood cells and neutrophils are seen. As oestrus approaches, the number of keratinized cells, which include the superficial cells and some of the superficial intermediate cells, increases to 100% of the epithelial cells (Figure 20.5) and neutrophils are no longer seen. When dioestrus is reached, the percentage of keratinized cells drops by about 20% per day. Insemination is best done when the percentage of cornified cells reaches 90% of the total and then every 3 days until dioestrus occurs (Wright, 1991).

When it is necessary to know the anticipated whelping date or to perform an elective caesarian section, measurement of progesterone and LH concentrations during oestrus will provide the ovulation date; gestation is 63 days. In a pregnant animal, serum progesterone concentration remains at about 16 nmol/l until 24 hours before labour. If the progesterone concentration drops below 6.4 nmol/l, parturition is imminent, or an elective caesarian can be performed.

Queens: Determining the various stages of oestrus in queens is much less commonly practiced than in bitches. Cats are induced ovulators. Ovulation occurs about 24

| Ovarian remnant syndrome |
| Pyometra |
| Trauma |
| Coagulopathy |
| Vaginitis |
| Vaginal/urethral neoplasia |
| Cystitis |

Figure 20.6: Differential diagnosis for bloody vaginal discharge in an ovariectomized bitch.

hours after the mating-induced LH surge. Repeated manual stimulation can also induce a surge in LH. Vaginal cytology can be performed in queens and the changes are identical to those in bitches.

Ovarian remnant syndrome
The ovaries of both bitches and queens are similar in structure and location. In the majority of animals, germ cells and ovarian tissue are located in one distinct structure. Additional accessory ovarian tissue or 'rests' rarely occur. When present they are usually in the ligament of the ovary and their presence is only recognized when a previously ovariohysterectomized animal shows signs of oestrus. 'Ovarian remnant syndrome' may be due to improper or complicated surgery, but proving this is impossible because it occurs after ovariohysterectomy performed by both new graduates and experienced practitioners alike (Miller, 1995). Some cases occur several years after initial surgery. Ovariectomized bitches with a bloody vaginal discharge with or without the signs of oestrus (Figure 20.6) should have vaginal cytologies that show progressive cornification, suggesting the influence of oestrogen.

If the animal is being treated with oestrogens for another problem, oestrogenic therapy should be stopped.

Hormonal assays may provide evidence of ovarian function, and a serum oestrogen of >75 pmol/l is indicative of functional ovarian tissue. Increased oestrogen concentration is present for several days in bitches but may be missed if only one blood sample is taken. A progesterone concentration during dioestrus of >6.4 nmol/l confirms the presence of ovarian tissue in the bitch but not in the queen unless she has been induced to ovulate. Administering gonadotrophin releasing hormone (GnRH) during the follicular phase and then measuring serum progesterone increases the accuracy of the progesterone assay in dogs (Wallace, 1991).

The finding of residual tissue during laparotomy may be difficult and is best attempted while the animal is 'on heat'. Histological examination is necessary to confirm the presence of ovarian tissue.

Ovarian disease

Most ovarian conditions are silent and are only recognized at ovariohysterectomy (see Figure 20.8). Those lesions that induce clinical disease do so because of ascites due to metastasis throughout the abdomen, by induction of signs of excessive hormone secretion, or by forming a space-occupying mass.

Signs of excessive oestrogen response are a manifestation of ovarian disease. Bitches so affected have ventral alopecia, gynaecomastia, enlargement of the vulva and prolonged or persistent oestrous cycles. Causes include functional ovarian neoplasms, follicular cysts or an exaggerated response to normal circulating oestrogens. Diagnosis is usually made on clinical grounds with support from the results of a skin biopsy. Serum oestrogen concentration can be supportive if it is elevated.

Ovarian neoplasia: Primary ovarian neoplasms arise from one or more of the three major tissue types of the ovary: epithelium, germ cells, or the sex cord stromal cells. Germ cell neoplasms include teratoma, usually seen in young animals, and dysgerminoma, usually seen in older animals. Sex cord stromal neoplasms are those that arise from either the granulosa–thecal cells (Figure 20.7) or the Sertoli–Leydig cells. They are the most common type of ovarian neoplasm in the queen (Gelberg and McEntee, 1985) and about half of them are malignant. In bitches, adenocarcinomas are the most common neoplasms seen (Patnaik and Greenlee, 1987; McEntee, 1990).

The signs of persistent oestrus and endometrial hyperplasia that suggest excessive hormone secretion have been seen in most of the types of primary ovarian neoplasia and are not specific for any one type

The uterus

The non-pregnant uterus

Diagnosis of disease of the non-pregnant uterus is usually considered when an abnormality is found on

Hydrosalpynx, hydrometra, mucometra
Serosal inclusion cysts
Endometrial polyps
Endometrial hyperplasia–pyometra complex
Leiomyoma
Lipoma
Minor and major anomalies

Figure 20.8: Uterine diseases detected at ovario-hysterectomy.

routine spaying. The conditions that may be found are listed in Figure 20.8. Less common diseases include mucometra and hydrometra. Confirmation of the diagnosis is best achieved by histological examination of the lesion. The diseases with the most impact on the health of the animal are pyometra and neoplasia.

A rare complication of spaying is the occasional development of colonic obstruction due to the formation of excessive scar tissue from the uterine stump and mesometrium (Remedios and Fowler, 1992).

A common normal finding in bitches is transverse dark bands that are implantation sites. Confirmation of suspicious findings is best done by submitting the lesion for histopathology. For large lesions the uterus is best sampled along the long axis, rather than taking a cross-section. The normal endometrium of the bitch has longitudinal folds and these are occasionally mistaken for abnormalities.

Endometrial hyperplasia and pyometra: There are several types of endometrial hyperplasia. The most important type is the cystic hyperplasia–pyometra complex. This occurs when there are successive oestrous cycles but no pregnancy, or when there is a source of exogenous progesterone. Once cystic endometrial hyperplasia occurs, endometritis and pyometra may develop (Figure 20.9). *Escherichia coli* is

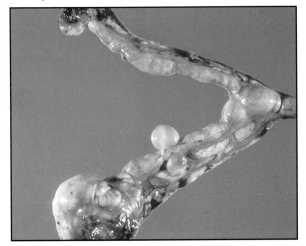

Figure 20.7: Reproductive tract of a bitch with unilateral granulosa cell tumour. The uterine serosal cyst is incidental.

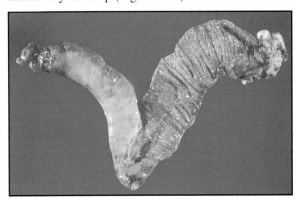

Figure 20.9: Canine cystic endometrial hyperplasia and pyometra. One uterine horn has been opened to show the irregular surface of the endometrium with cystic hyperplasia.

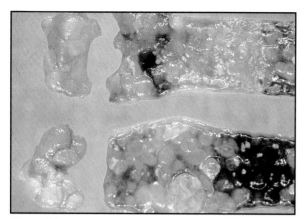

Figure 20.10: *Ovaries and uterine horns from an 8-year-old crossbred bitch with cystic endometrial hyperplasia.*
Courtesy of Dr R.W. Else

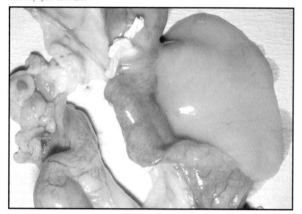

Figure 20.11: *Pyometra in a 14-year-old Labrador bitch with vaginal discharge for 2 weeks.*
Courtesy of Dr R.W. Else

the major pathogen. The size of the uterus in either condition depends on the patency of the cervix.

There is a range of changes, from hyperplasia to acute or chronic ongoing pyometra. Mostly, the disease is seen about 50–90 days after oestrus. The classical signs of pyometra are lethargy, vaginal discharge, polydypsia and polyuria, and an elevated leucocyte count. In practice these may not all be present (Sevelius *et al.*, 1990). In most cases of pyometra there is a leucocytosis, with a shift to the left and toxic change, marrow hyperplasia and toxicity, a mild normocytic normochromic anaemia, extramedullary haematopoiesis of the neutrophilic lineage, renal tubular degeneration, a fatty liver, myeloid metaplasia similar to myeloid leukaemia, adrenal necrosis and haemorrhage, and polyuria and polydipsia with an inability to concentrate urine but with a normal concentration of antidiuretic hormone. A mild proteinuria may be found but there does not appear to be a microscopic lesion of the glomerulus.

In queens, endometrial hyperplasia appears to be age-related and, because cats are induced ovulators, is not related to the presence of a corpus luteum and therefore progesterone. The presence of pyometra or endometritis is associated with a retained corpus luteum and therefore with progesterone (Potter *et al.*, 1991).

Other causes for endometrial hyperplasia are long-term medroxyprogesterone acetate (MPA) administration to shorten or prevent oestrus, oestrogen administration, cystic follicular degeneration, granu-

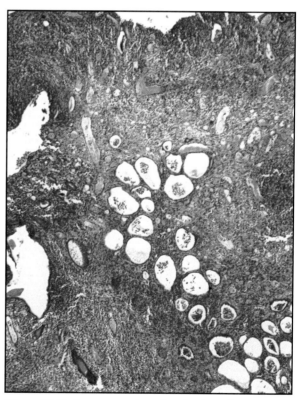

Figure 20.12: *Low-power view of a uterine wall with cystic endometrial hyperplasia. H&E.*
Courtesy of Dr R.W. Else

Figure 20.13: *Low-power view of uterine horn from a bitch with pyometra of acute onset. H&E.*
Courtesy of Dr R.W. Else

losa cell tumours and intersex conditions. Diagnosis of each of these conditions is outlined in the relevant sections of this chapter.

Pseudopregnancy
Pseudopregnancy can occur after oestrus in both young and older bitches. In queens, pseudopregnancy occurs when the queen ovulates but does not conceive, or after repeated manual stimulation. Serum progesterone concentration increases and cannot be differentiated from levels in pregnancy. Oestradiol, LH and prolactin remain at basal levels. Lactation is related to increased prolactin concentrations in blood that can occur when progesterone concentration drops. At ovariohysterectomy focal regions of endometrial enlargement that resemble placental sites are seen. They can be differentiated at biopsy examination by the lack of fetal components.

Uterine neoplasia
Uterine neoplasia is rare. Epithelial neoplasms tend to be malignant. and mesenchymal neoplasms tend to be benign. The diagnosis is usually made after cytological or histological examination at necropsy, or at ovariohysterectomy for another reason. Uterine carcinoma is rarely diagnosed before death (Baldwin *et al.*, 1992).

Hermaphroditism
Hermaphroditism is usually clinically evident and recognizable by such external genital features as an enlarged clitoris, abnormal placement of the vulva and hypospadias. Determining the exact anomaly is not always possible but would involve karyotyping, gross and histological examination of the genitalia, and measurement of serum testosterone to determine chromosomal, gonadal or phenotypic abnormalities (Sommer and Meyers-Wallen, 1991).

The post-partum uterus

Subinvolution of placental sites: Haemorrhage or thrombosis in placental sites is normal. Subinvolution of placental sites is a condition where there is a haemorrhagic discharge or excess lochia for 8–12 weeks after parturition. Normally there is discharge for 2–4 weeks. Anaemia may occur. Treatment can be by ovariohysterectomy or administration of a progestogen. Spontaneous resolution usually occurs (Al-bassam *et al.*, 1981).

Diagnosis of subinvolution of placental sites is confirmed by taking smears of the bloody vaginal discharge and identifying the discharge as blood. The total and differential cell counts of the discharge should resemble those of normal blood. Spontaneous resolution or histological examination of ovariohysterectomy samples that include normal and affected uterus is confirmatory.

Postpartum metritis occurs occasionally in bitches and queens and is especially common after intervention in dystocia. Diagnosis of metritis is made by cytological examination of vulval discharges (see below) or by histological examination after spaying. Systemic signs of neutrophilia are usually not seen but may occur in severe cases.

Abortion
The identification of the cause of abortion in a bitch or queen, or in a kennel or cattery, requires considerable and often extensive and expensive investigation. Most veterinary surgeons concentrate on looking for infectious causes because they are often easier to confirm or reject than some of the other causes.

Investigation of the cause of abortion includes considering the history and physical examination plus the results of ancillary tests as listed in Figure 20.14. Submission of maternal serum and whole fetuses and placentae is preferred. If this is not feasible, a complete set of tissues for histopathology, bacteriology, mycoplasmology and virology should be collected. Samples for identification of infectious agents by cul-

Haematology

Serum biochemistry

Urinalysis

Vaginal cytology

Cranial vaginal culture:

  Bacteria

  Mycoplasma spp.

  Ureaplasma spp.

Serum progesterone concentration

Testing of bitch for:

  Brucella canis

  Toxoplasma spp.

  Neospora spp.

  Canine herpesvirus

Testing of queen for:

  Feline herpesvirus

  Feline calicivirus

  Feline immunodeficiency virus (FIV)

  Feline leukaemia virus (FeLV)

Figure 20.14: Maternal database for the investigation of abortion.

ture, by immunological means such as immunofluorescence or by the polymerase chain reaction (PCR) are best sent as blocks of fresh tissues, chilled (2–4ºC) but not frozen. However, if it will take more than 24 hours for samples to reach the laboratory, they should be frozen and packaged so that they do not thaw.

Maternal serum is often overlooked in submissions but may be very important, especially in cats. Testing serum from bitches for *Brucella canis,* the protozoans *Toxoplasma* and *Neospora,* and for herpesvirus (see Chapter 5) and that from queens for herpesvirus, calicivirus, FIV or FeLV (see Chapter 5) by immunological or molecular methods can provide information that may lead to a diagnosis. It is important to correlate evidence of the presence of a potential pathogen with the clinical syndrome and/or the presence of lesions consistent with the agent. It is only when this correlation is made that the diagnosis is made more certain.

Vaginal discharge from a pregnant animal is a sign that warrants concern. If the discharge is tinged with blood or is green, impending parturition, abortion or pyometra/metritis should be suspected. Diagnostic tests to differentiate the cause of vulvar discharges are described below.

Cervix, Vagina and Vulva

Vulvar discharges
One of the first indications of female reproductive disease is the presence of a vulvar discharge. If it is of a mucous or purulent nature, vaginitis or metritis should be suspected. Bloody discharges have a wide range of causes and may require a thorough investigation involving history and clinical examination, vaginal cytology, vaginoscopy and abdominal imaging (plain and contrast radiography, ultrasonography, computed tomography or magnetic resonance imaging). The conditions that can cause a bloody discharge are listed in Figure 20.15 and are reviewed by Johnson (1989).

Congenital anomalies
Anomalies of the vagina may be of no clinical significance, but some may interfere with breeding, cause infertility or predispose the animal to vaginitis. Diagnosis is made with vaginoscopy or contrast radiography, or at autopsy.

Vaginal prolapse / hyperplasia
Eversion of the vaginal wall can occur in bitches in the oestrogen phase of oestrus, or at parturition. It is caused by excessive oedema, and may involve the ventral floor of the vagina or, in the most extensive cases, the entire circumference of the vagina. It regresses spontaneously and recurs in about 70% of cases. Differentiation from neoplasia is the major reason for submission of material; biopsy and fine needle aspiration are useful for obtaining samples.

Non-pregnant
Oestrus
Cystic ovarian follicles
Ovarian neoplasia
Pyometra
Coagulopathy
Trauma
Neoplasia

Pregnant
Abortion
Parturition
Vaginitis
Metritis
Torsion
Neoplasia
Coagulopathy

Post partum
Lochia
Subinvolution of placental sites
Metritis
Pyometra
Neoplasia
Coagulopathy

Figure 20.15: Causes of bloody vulvar/vaginal discharge in entire animals.

Oestrus
Vaginal hyperplasia/ prolapse
Vaginal polyp
Vaginal neoplasia
Urethral neoplasia
Vulval fold pyoderma
Uterine prolapse
Clitoral hypertrophy
Haematoma

Figure 20.16: Causes of vulvar swellings.

Neoplasia

Most neoplasms of the vagina and vulva can be diagnosed by cytological imprints and examination of fine needle aspirates. Histopathology of biopsy samples can be used for confirmation.

The most common neoplasm of the vagina is the leiomyoma (Figure 20.17) and the cells sampled from such tumours are cytologically benign and stromal in origin. Leiomyoma in the bitch is reported to be responsive to oestrogen, and ovariectomy may be curative.

The transmissible venereal tumour is a notifiable disease in the UK and occurs in many other countries. The transmissible venereal tumour is a type of lymphoid neoplasm that usually regresses spontaneously but is occasionally malignant. Neoplastic cells have 56 chromosomes (normal dogs have 76). Cytological imprints and fine needle aspirates show a characteristic uniform population of round cells with clear vacuoles at the cell membrane. Melanoma can occur in the reproductive tract and tends to be more aggressive than in the skin. Cytological imprints and fine needle aspirates show cells with melanin pigment granules within the cytoplasm.

Epithelial tumours are very rare, especially cervical tumours (compare with women). Papilloma, squamous cell carcinoma, and carcinoma of the canine vestibule have been recorded. The origin of carcinoma of the canine vestibule may be difficult to ascertain. Possibilities include the urinary bladder, vestibular glands and the urethra. Carcinomas of urethral origin usually cause clinical effects because of obstruction rather than metastasis. Metastatic carcinoma of mammary glands may spread up the perineum to involve the vulva. Examination of cytological preparations and biopsy samples are the methods of choice for diagnosis.

Vaginitis

Vulvar discharge of a mucoid or purulent nature is a relatively common finding in young animals. It is uncommon for the discharges to be bloody. Vagino-

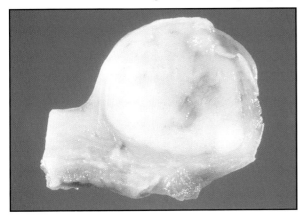

Figure 20.17: *Cross-section of a canine uterine leiomyoma. The well circumscribed appearance and white colour are typical.*

scopy to ensure no underlying (congenital) predisposing condition, and cytological examination exhibiting a blood-free and neutrophil-dominated discharge, are the best methods for confirmation (Johnson, 1989).

Culture of samples from the vagina or uterus of queens or bitches is frequently recommended as an ancillary test. Reports of the bacterial flora of the vagina of healthy bitches and queens list a wide range of bacteria, including potential pathogens such as the aerobic bacteria *Streptococcus* spp., *Staphylococcus* spp., *Escherichia coli*, *Corynebacterium* spp. and *Pasteurella* spp, and the anaerobic Peptococcaceae and *Bacteroides* spp. (Allen and Dagnall, 1982; Clementson and Ward, 1990) Recovery of *Mycoplasma* spp. from bitches is also common. Bacteria are cultured from the uterus of bitches and queens much less frequently than from the vagina. Culture of the vagina would probably also reveal a 'normal' viral population.

Demonstration of a bacterium in high numbers or as the sole agent is not sufficient to ascribe pathogenicity. The total number of bacteria, as determined by counting, increases at oestrus (Baba *et al.*, 1983). One should not ascribe pathogenicity to an agent unless there is supporting evidence of a host response, such as the presence of degenerative neutrophils, inflammation, or the absence of an underlying imbalance or anomaly that allows the normal flora to induce disease.

The finding of prominent lymphoid follicles in the distal vagina and vulva is a common and non-specific indication of antigenic stimulation.

THE MALE REPRODUCTIVE TRACT

Diagnosis of abnormalities in the male genital tract requires an understanding of the normal situation and the judicious use of ancillary diagnostic tests. Diagnostic aides include physical examination, semen evaluation, urinalysis, serological tests for *Brucella canis*, hormonal testing, ultrasonography, microbial testing of semen and prepuce, cytological examination of secreted and sampled tissues and fluids, and incisional and excisional biopsies.

Diseases may be incidental, or they may cause illness or result in infertility. Deciding which are incidental and which are significant can occasionally be a challenge. Infertility and its causes is a major field in itself and semen morphology is adequately covered in reviews by Ellington (1991), Meyers-Wallen (1991), Olson (1991) and Olson *et al.* (1992).

Seminal fluid

Examination of semen, other than for spermatozoal changes, can be useful. Semen may contain microorganisms that are resident in the distal urethra and prepuce. Members of the genera *Staphylococcus, Streptococcus, Escherichia, Proteus, Mycoplasma,*

Ureaplasma, and many others are frequently found in normal healthy dogs, and the total bacterial count can be up to 10,000 per millilitre (Johnston, 1991). Seminal alkaline phosphatase and carnitine are produced in the epididymis and can be used as markers of patency of the epididymal duct and the vas deferens (Olson *et al.,* 1987; Olson, 1991). The pH of normal semen is 6.3–6.7 (Johnston, 1991) and the white blood cell count should be <2000 per microlitre. Cytospin preparations of semen can be examined for the types of inflammatory cells.

Serum hormone concentration
Measurement of the concentration of hormones in serum is not widely available. Reference values are often based on small numbers of animals, and on only a few breeds. Both LH and testosterone concentration vary during the day, so a single sample is not accurate. In normal animals, an injection of gonadotrophin releasing hormone (GnRH) can be used to test the pituitary–gonadal axis. Injection of GnRH should result in an increase in the serum concentrations of follicle stimulating hormone (FSH) and of luteinizing hormone (LH) after 30 minutes, and serum testosterone concentration should peak 60 minutes after injection of GnRH.

Urinalysis
Spermatozoa are frequently found in the bladder and urine of intact dogs; the bladder and urine should be examined in an azoospermic dog to see whether spermatozoa are actually being produced.

Testicular and epididymal disease
Neoplasia is the most common testicular abnormality of dogs that requires submission of diagnostic material. Testicular tissues are the most frequent samples collected. Ultrasonography, and examination of fine needle aspirates and testicular biopsy specimens are used as diagnostic aides, especially in valuable breeding animals. Testicular biopsy has a limited usefulness but may identify the cause or provide a prognosis if the animal is azoospermic. Biopsy is prone to sampling errors because the sample may not adequately represent the affected area. Postoperative haemorrhage can be a complication. Samples for the accurate assessment of spermatogenesis are best fixed in Bouin's fluid, and then transferred to either 10% buffered neutral formalin or 70% alcohol solution after 6 hours.

Orchitis is extremely rare in dogs and cats and most suspected cases are actually epididymitis.

Cryptorchidism
The diagnosis of cryptorchidism is seldom difficult in adult dogs but in puppies the testes may not be fully descended until 35–40 days of age. As well as showing infertility and certain behavioural traits, cryptorchid dogs are more prone to testicular neoplasia and testicu-

lar torsion (Romagnoli, 1991) so confirmation is an important step. The laboratory test of choice is the LH stimulation test or a GnRH challenge test. The presence of testicular tissue is confirmed if there is an increase in serum testosterone after administration of either LH or GnRH.

Cryptorchidism is the major testicular abnormality in cats. A clinical challenge is created when a cat has male characteristics but has no scrotal testes. The demeanour and behaviour of the cat may be such that it is not possible to determine whether the animal is bilaterally cryptorchid, has had one (scrotal) testis removed and still has the other, or has been castrated late in life. The barbs of the penis are testosterone-dependent and are absent in an animal without testicular tissue. Measurement of serum testosterone at and after administration of LH or GnRH is also confirmatory.

Animals with intersex conditions may be phenotypically male. This can be confirmed with karyotyping.

Testicular neoplasia
In most cases, castration is performed and an accurate diagnosis can be made on the gross appearance of the mass. Cytological examination of impression smears or histological examination of formalin-fixed material is adequate for accurate identification. The latter is preferred because mixed or multiple neoplasms may be present and not adequately sampled by cytological methods.

In valuable breeding animals, fine needle aspirates of a mass will assist in differentiation of the neoplastic types. Three main testicular neoplasms of dogs are the Sertoli cell tumour, the interstitial cell tumour and the seminoma. The fourth most common type, but still rare, is a mixed germ cell and stromal cell neoplasm (Patnaik and Mostofi, 1993). Multiple types of neoplasia may be found in one testis (Figure 20.18). Almost all major primary testicular neoplasms in dogs are benign. Exceptions are extremely rare but have been recorded in Sertoli cell tumour and seminoma. Identi-

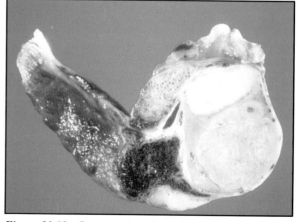

Figure 20.18: *Cross-section of a canine testis with a seminoma, interstitial cell tumour, and testicular atrophy.*

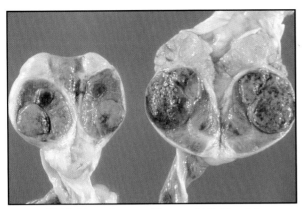

Figure 20.19: *Testes from an 11-year-old Collie with multiple bilateral tumours.*
Courtesy of Dr R.W. Else

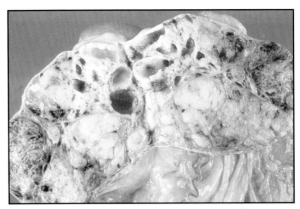

Figure 20.22: *Gross section of a cystic Sertoli cell tumour of the testis of a 12-year-old crossbred dog.*
Courtesy of Dr R.W. Else

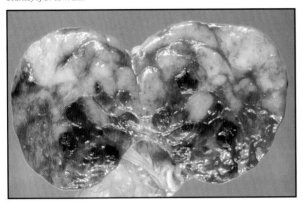

Figure 20.20: *Haemorrhagic seminoma in a testis from an 8-year-old Labrador.*
Courtesy of Dr R.W. Else

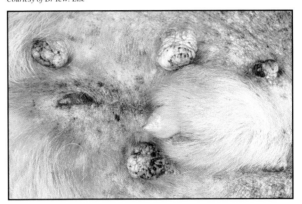

Figure 20.23: *Gynaecomastia in a dog with Sertoli cell tumour (same case as Figure 20.22).*
Courtesy of Dr R.W. Else

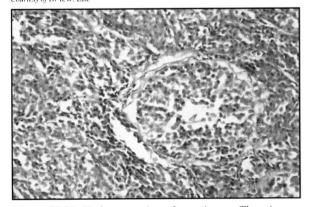

Figure 20.21: *High-power view of a seminoma. There is a remnant of intratubular neoplasia surrounded by diffuse germinal-like cells. H&E.*
Courtesy of Dr R.W. Else

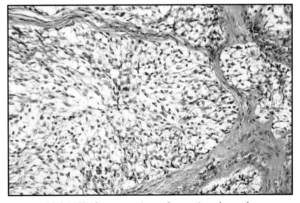

Figure 20.24: *High-power view of a section through a Sertoli cell tumour, showing 'wispy' neoplastic intratubular cells. H&E.*
Courtesy of Dr R.W. Else

fication of metastasis is the only way to determine that the neoplasm is malignant; there are no good cytological or histological markers.

Most neoplasms cause enlargement of the testis. In general, seminomas are white and soft and usually bulge on cut section. Sertoli cell tumours tend to produce a lot of fibrous tissue so they are white and firm. The interstitial cell tumour is yellow, often contains areas of haemorrhage, and is soft. On occasion Sertoli cell tumours, usually when they become very large, may produce a hyperoestrogenism syndrome and feminization (Brodey and Martin, 1958). This is

usually manifested by attractiveness to other male dogs, gynaecomastia and alopecia. Affected animals return to normal after removal of the neoplasm. The signs are not always associated with oestrogen production and not all dogs have raised levels of serum oestrogen. In these instances secretion of inhibin by the neoplastic Sertoli cells inhibits the secretion of FSH and LH by the pituitary, and this in turn inhibits testosterone production (Grootenhuis *et al.,* 1990). Some animals develop bone marrow suppression and a poorly responsive pancytopenia. Feminization is much more common when the neoplasm is larger, and

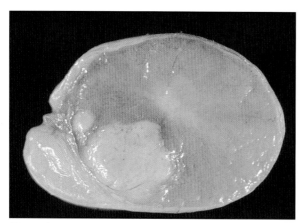

Figure 20.25: *Gross section of a benign interstitial cell tumour of the testis found incidentally on autopsy of a 13-year-old Miniature Poodle.*
Courtesy of Dr R.W. Else

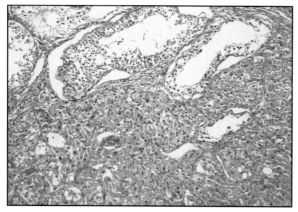

Figure 20.26: *Histopathological section of interstitial cell neoplasia, showing surviving normal seminiferous tubules at the top of the field, with extratubular neoplasia adjacent. H&E.*
Courtesy of Dr R.W. Else

therefore is more common in cryptorchid dogs. It is also in these dogs that an unfortunate sequel of testicular torsion can occur.

Testicular torsion
Torsion of the testis is virtually impossible unless there is incomplete descent. A testicular neoplasm is usually also necessary to provide sufficient weight to maintain the torsion. The usual clinical presentation is acute abdominal pain; the offending mass is blackened due to venous infarction and sometimes not readily identified as testis.

Epididymitis
Epididymitis may present as scrotal pruritus to the extent that a dog will mutilate its scrotum. Epididymitis in dogs is most frequently caused by *Escherichia coli* and other Gram-negative organisms. *Brucella canis* is uncommon but is zoonotic and should therefore always be considered. Epididymitis usually presents initially as a severe clinical disease, but on occasion may then produce a short period of discomfort and lead to a more chronic condition. The chronic condition is usually due to spermatic granulomas.

Animals with epididymitis are frequently infertile. Their semen contains abnormal spermatozoa and inflammatory cells, including lymphocytes and macrophages. Infertility is probably related to the presence of inflammatory cells and exudates in semen, anti-spermatozoal antibody, or an accompanying prostatitis. Fine needle aspirates from affected epididymides are useful to confirm the diagnosis and for culture of the causative agent. Serology for *Brucella canis*, using an enzyme immunoassay or other such test, should be carried out. In affected individuals, removal of the offending epididymis and testis should result in a return to normal fertility if the prostate is not involved.

Inflammatory disease in cats
Severe inflammation of the intrascrotal tissues and organs can occur. Local trauma such as a scratch or a bite wound can cause a suppurative periorchitis. The diagnosis is usually made after castration, and differentiation from feline infectious peritonitis (FIP) is made by examination of the peritesticular fluids (see Chapter 5) and by histopathology. FIP produces a fibrinosuppurative or pyogranulomatous periorchitis or orchitis.

Prostate
The prostate is the only accessory sexual organ of the dog and it is prone to diseases which can be difficult to differentiate. The gland is relatively inaccessible and signs of prostatic disease are not always specific to that organ.

Cats have two accessory sex organs, the bulbourethral gland and the prostate. The diseases that affect the accessory sex glands of the cat are extremely small in number, and very rare, so that the following discussion will be focussed entirely on the disease in dogs.

Clinical signs of prostatic disease in dogs
The major diseases that affect the prostate in dogs are prostatic hyperplasia, prostatic cysts, paraprostatic cysts, bacterial prostatitis and prostatic neoplasia. Enlargement of the prostate due to hyperplasia or some combination of hyperplasia and cyst formation is common in older intact dogs. In its pure form, excessive prostatic enlargement may be either completely incidental and found on rectal palpation, or may cause lethargy, straining to defecate and anorexia. Bacterial prostatitis, in its acute form, causes haematuria, lethargy, and signs of systemic illness. Infertility will occasionally be the only indication. Prostatic neoplasia tends to be insidious and it is only in advanced disease that the signs of tenesmus, stranguria, dysuria, or the cachexia of malignancy are seen. When there is evidence of tenesmus, urethral discharge including haemorrhage, and haematuria, one can focus specifically on the prostate as the origin (Krawiec, 1994).

Diagnosis of prostatic disease in dogs

In addition to the clinical signs, which can be quite vague, rectal palpation is often useful for diagnosis. Hyperplasia tends to produce a prostate that is uniform and smooth-surfaced. Acute prostatitis will usually result in pain on palpation and a 'doughy' feeling to the prostate, with sponginess and a lack of definition due to periprostatic oedema. In prostatic neoplasia, palpable changes will vary from no significant findings to a total inability to palpate the prostate because of extensive periprostatic fibrosis and prostatic infiltrate. Ancillary diagnostic aids that greatly assist in the diagnosis include ultrasonography and cytological examination of urine, prostatic washes, semen, penile discharge, urethral brush biopsy specimens and fine needle aspirates. Punch biopsy, direct incisional prostatic biopsy, or excisional biopsy also yield valuable specimens (Hornbuckle *et al.*, 1978; Barsanti *et al.*, 1980; Wright and Parry, 1989).

Prostatic hyperplasia

The prostate gland has been the focus of much research, especially in the area of prostatic hyperplasia. Dogs and men both develop prostatic hyperplasia as they get older. The hyperplasia in dogs does not usually cause a urinary obstruction as it does in men. The enlargement occurs in an eccentric fashion so that it may act as a ball valve in the pelvic inlet and restrict the passage of faeces along the colon. Enlargement of the prostate with age is progressive and dependent on the presence of testes.

There is little useful information available about the rate of prostatic enlargement for species other than the Beagle (Lowseth *et al.*, 1990). Scottish Terriers are reported to have a normal prostate that is much bigger than in other species (Ladds, 1993).

Castration prior to the onset of signs reduces the number of prostatic diseases to one, i.e. carcinoma (see below).

Prostatitis

Acute prostatitis (Figure 20.28) is a disease that arises from ascending infection and is often caused by *Escherichia coli*. The signs are as described above and are often typical of what one finds in any infectious disease. Chronic prostatitis is frequently a subclinical disease. It may cause a urethral discharge, infertility, recurrent cystitis and haematuria (Cowan and Barsanti, 1989).

The diagnosis of prostatitis is made difficult by the proximity to the bladder and urethra, so that semen can be contaminated with urethral material and urine. A urethral brush and prostatic massage technique (Kay *et al.*, 1989) is probably the most accurate method for sampling prostatic secretion if there is no facility for direct needle biopsy guided by ultrasonography (see Chapter 7).

Paraprostatic cysts

There are a large number of cystic structures that can occur around the prostate. Many of the cysts probably arise as a cystic change in hyperplasia. Cysts that are small and multiple are often clinically silent until they are complicated by infection. Others may become extremely large and have a space-occupying effect. The prognosis for single large cysts is usually very poor because they can seldom be completely removed and marsupialization is fraught with complications.

Prostatic abscess

Prostatic abscesses probably arise from bacterial infection of a prostatic cyst. They may be single or multiple. Signs are usually noticed when the dog becomes clinically ill, and fever, anorexia, pyrexia, and urethral discharge are presenting complaints. Gram-negative bacteria, especially *Escherichia coli*, *Mycoplasma*, *Staphylococcus* and *Streptococcus* spp., may be recovered from semen, prostatic washes or prostatic tissues.

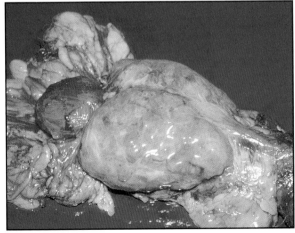

Figure 20.27: *Prostatic hypertrophy due to benign hyperplasia in a 10-year-old German Shepherd Dog with tenesmus.*

Courtesy of Dr R.W. Else

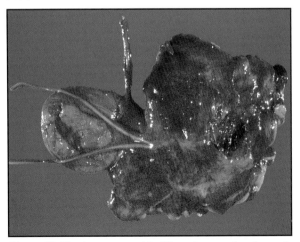

Figure 20.28: *Acute prostatitis. The redness and oedema of the periprostatic tissues give the prostate a 'doughy' feel on palpation per rectum.*

Prostatic neoplasia

There is considerable confusion in the literature regarding the origin of carcinomas. The blanket term 'prostatic carcinoma' is used in some studies but really should be limited to neoplasia that develops from prostatic epithelium. The transitional cell carcinoma is probably the most common and it arises from the prostatic urethra. The neoplasms often have differing clinical syndromes. Transitional cell carcinomas have a tendency to produce widely metastatic disease while maintaining a very small primary tumour. Signs include obstruction to the urethra, erosion of blood vessels and resultant haematuria, or evidence of extensive metastasis. Prostatic adenocarcinoma tends to be a locally infiltrative disease, and results in extensive periprostatic and intrapelvic spread. It tends to be more sclerotic than transitional cell carcinomas. The extensive fibrosis and space-occupying effect can result in stricture of the rectum and colon, resulting in tenesmus and other signs of constipation. Hindleg lameness and weakness, and emaciation are frequently found. Prostatic adenocarcinomas in dogs produce prostate-specific antigen (PSA) inconsistently, so this is not a good marker for the disease in dogs in contrast to the situation in men (McEntee *et al.*, 1987).

Penis and prepuce

Diseases of the penis and prepuce are common. Trauma from car accidents, mating injuries or foreign material within the prepuce present little diagnostic challenge if the area is examined carefully. Where there is extensive trauma to the penis, fracture of the os penis may occur.

Haemorrhagic discharges

Trauma

Foreign body

Prostatic disease

Neoplasia

Urolithiasis

Malformations

Coagulopathy

Purulent discharges

Phaloposthitis

Foreign body

Prostatic disease

Neoplasia

Malformations

Figure 20.29: Causes of preputial discharge.

Preputial discharge is seen frequently and has been reviewed by Hornbuckle and White (1989). Most cases are due to phaloposthitis. Figure 20.29 gives a list of differential diagnoses for preputial discharge.

Phaloposthitis

A non-specific phaloposthitis is probably the most common disease of the penis in the dog. Many dogs develop a mild purulent preputial discharge. As with any external site, the prepuce has a normal flora that contains potential pathogens. Dogs are also prone to develop papilloma virus infection and warts of the penis or prepuce. Transmissible venereal tumour is relatively common in endemic areas, and diagnosis of masses around the prepuce can usually be made from fine needle aspirates, impression smears, or incision or excision biopsy specimens.

In cats, apart from urothlithiasis and obstruction of the penis, diseases that affect the penis are extremely rare.

REFERENCES AND FURTHER READING

Allen WE and Dagnall GJR (1982) Some observations on the aerobic bacterial flora of the genital tract of the dog and bitch. *Journal of Small Animal Practice* **23**, 325-335

Al-bassam MA, Thomson RG and O'Donnell L (1981) Involution abnormalities in the postpartum uterus of the bitch. *Veterinary Pathology* **18**, 208-218

Allen SW, Prasse KW and Mahaffey EA (1986) Cytologic differentiation of benign from malignant canine mammary tumors. *Veterinary Pathology* **23**, 649-655

Baba E, Hata H, Fukata T, Arakawa A (1983) Vaginal and uterine microflora of adult dogs. *American Journal of Veterinary Research* **44**, 606-609

Baldwin CJ, Roszel JF and Clark TP (1992) Uterine adenocarcinoma in dogs. *Compendium on Continuing Education for the Practicing Veterinarian* **14**, 731-737

Barsanti JA and Finco DR (1979) Canine bacterial prostatitis. *Veterinary Clinics of North America: Small Animal Practice* **9**, 679-700

Barsanti JA, Shotts EB, Prose K, Crowell W (1980) Evaluation of diagnostic techniques for canine prostatic diseases. *Journal of the American Veterinary Medical Association* **177**, 160-163

Bostock DE (1975) The prognosis following the surgical excision of canine mammary neoplasms. *European Journal of Cancer* **11**, 389-396

Bostock DE (1986) Canine and feline mammary neoplasms. *British Veterinary Journal* **142**, 506-515

Bostock DE, Moriarty J and Crocker J (1992) Correlation between histologic diagnosis mean nucleolar organizer region count and prognosis in canine mammary tumors. *Veterinary Pathology* **29**, 381-385

Brodey RS and Martin JE (1958) Sertoli cell neoplasms in the dog. *Journal of the American Veterinary Medical Association* **133**, 249-256

Clemetson LL and Ward CS (1990) Bacterial flora of the vagina and uterus of healthy cats. *Journal of the American Veterinary Medical Association* **196**, 902-906

Concannan PW and Lein DH (1989) Hormonal and clinical correlates of ovarian cycles, ovulation, pseudopregnancy and pregnancy in dogs. In: *Current Veterinary Therapy X,* ed. RW Kirk, pp. 1269-1282. WB Saunders, Philadelphia

Cowan CA and Barsanti JA (1989) Chronic bacterial prostatitis in the dog. In: *Current Veterinary Therapy X,* ed. RW Kirk, pp. 1243-1247. WB Saunders, Philadelphia

Ellington JE (1991) Diagnosis, treatment and management of poor fertility in the stud dog. *Seminars in Veterinary Medicine and Surgery (Small Animal)* **9**, 46-53

Feldman EC and Nelson RW (1996) In: *Canine and Feline Endocrinology and Reproduction, 2nd edn,* ed. EC Feldman and RW Nelson, pp.399-480. WB Saunders, London

Gelberg HB and McEntee K (1985) Feline ovarian neoplasms. *Veterinary Pathology* **22**, 572-576

Gilbertson SR, Kurzman ID, Zochrou RE, Hurvitz AI and Black MM (1983) Canine mammary epithelial neoplasms biological implications of morphological characteristics assessed in 232 dogs. *Veterinary Pathology* **20**, 127-142

Griffiths GL, Lumsden JH and Valli VEO (1984) Fine needle aspiration cytology and histologic correlation in canine tumors. *Veterinary Clinical Pathology* **13**, 13-17

Grootenhuis AJ, Sluijs FJ, Klaij IA, Steenberger J, Timmerman MA, Bevers MM, Dieleman SJ and de Jong FH (1990) Inhibin, gonadotrophins and sex steroids in dogs with Sertoli cell tumours. *Journal of Endocrinology* **127**, 235-242

Hampe JF and Misdorp W (1974) Tumors and dysplasias of the mammary gland. *Bulletin of the World Health Organization, International Histological Classification of Tumors of Domestic Animals* **50**, 111-133

Hayden DW and Johnson KH (1986) Feline mammary hypertrophy – fibroadenoma complex. In: *Current Veterinary Therapy X,* ed. RW Kirk, pp. 477-480. WB Saunders, Philadelphia

Hayes AA and Mooney S (1985) Feline mammary tumors. *Veterinary Clinics of North America: Small Animal Practice* **15**, 513-520

Hayes HM and Pendergrass TW (1976) Canine testicular tumors: epidemiologic features of 410 dogs. *International Journal of Cancer* **18**, 482-487

Hellmen E, Bergstrom R, Holmberg L, Spangberg I, Hansson K and Lindgren A (1993) Prognostic factors in canine mammary tumors: a multivariate study of 202 consecutive cases. *Veterinary Pathology* **30**, 20-27

Hellmen E, Lindgren A, Linell F, Matsson P and Nilsson A (1988) Comparison of histology and clinical variables to DNA ploidy in canine mammary tumors. *Veterinary Pathology* **25**, 3, 219-226;

Hornbuckle WE, and White ME (1989) Preputial discharge in the dog. In: *Current Veterinary Therapy X,* ed. RW Kirk, pp. 1259-1261. WB Saunders, Philadelphia

Hornbuckle WE, MaCoy DM, Allen GS and Gunther R (1978) Prostatic disease in the dog. *Cornell Veterinarian* **68**, (Suppl. 7) 284-305

Johnson CA (1989) Vulvar discharges. In: *Current Veterinary Therapy X, ed.* RW Kirk, pp. 1310-1312. WB Saunders, Philadelphia.

Johnston SD (1989) Vaginal prolapse In: *Current Veterinary Therapy X,* ed. RW Kirk, pp. 1302-1305. WB Saunders, Philadelphia

Johnston SD (1991) Performing a complete canine semen evaluation in a small animal hospital. *Veterinary Clinics of North America: Small Animal Practice* **21**, 545-551

Kay ND, Ling GV and Johnson DL (1989) A urethral brush technique for the diagnosis of canine bacterial prostatitis. *Journal of the American Animal Hospital Association* **25**, 527-532

Krawiec DR (1994) Canine prostate disease. *Journal of the American Veterinary Medical Association* **204**, 1561-1564

Ladds PW (1993) The male genital system. In: *Pathology of Domestic Animals, 3rd edn,* ed. KV Jubb *et al.,* vol. 3, pp. 471-529. Academic Press, San Diego

Lowseth LA, Gerlach RF, Gillett NA and Muggenberg BA (1990) Age related changes in the prostate and testes of the beagle dog. *Veterinary Pathology,* **27**, 347-353

MacEwen EG, Hayes AA, Harvey HJ, Patnaik AK, Mooney S and Prasse S (1984) Prognostic factors for feline mammary tumours. *Journal of the American Veterinary Medical Association* **185**, 201-204

McEntee K (1990) *Reproductive Pathology of Domestic Mammals.* Academic Press, London

McEntee M, Isaacs W and Smith C (1987) Adenocarcinoma of the canine prostate: immunohistochemical examination for secretory antigens. *Prostate* **11**, 163-170

Meyers-Wallen VN (1991) Clinical approach to infertile male dogs with sperm in the ejaculate. *Veterinary Clinics of North America: Small Animal Practice* **21**, 609-633

Miller DM (1995) Ovarian remnant syndrome in dogs and cats: 46 cases (1988-1992). *Journal of Veterinary Diagnostic Investigation* **7**, 572-574

Nerurkar VR, Chitale AR, Jalnapurkar BV, Naik SN and Lalitha VS (1989) Comparative pathology of canine mammary tumour. *Journal of Comparative Pathology* **101**, 389-397

Olson PN (1991) Clinical approach for evaluating dogs with azoospermia or aspermia. *Veterinary Clinics of North America: Small Animal Practice* **21**, 591-608

Olson PN, Behrendt MD, Amann RP, Weiss DE, Bowen RA, Neft TM and McGarry JD (1987) Concentrations of carnitine in the seminal fluid of normospermic, vasectomized, and castrated dogs. *American Journal of Veterinary Research* **48**, 1211-1215

Olson PN and Olson AL (1984) Cytologic evaluation of canine milk. *Veterinary Medicine and Small Animal Clinician* **79**, 641-644, 646

Olson PN, Shultheiss P and Seim HB (1992) Clinical and laboratory findings associated with actual or suspected azoospermia in dogs: 18 cases (1979-1990). *Journal of the American Veterinary Medical Association* **201**, 478-482

Olson PN, Wrigley RH, Thrall MA and Husted PW (1989) Disorders of the canine prostate gland: pathogenesis, diagnosis and medical therapy. *Compendium on Continuing Education for the Practicing Veterinarian* **9**, 613-623

Patnaik AK and Greenlee PG (1987) Canine ovarian neoplasms: a clinicopathologic study of 71 cases, including histology of 12 granulosa cell tumours. *Veterinary Pathology* **24**, 509-514

Patnaik AK and Mostofi FK (1993) A clinicopathologic histologic and immunohistochemical study of mixed germ cell–stromal tumors of the testis in 16 dogs. *Veterinary Pathology* **30**, 287-295

Potter K, Hancock DH and Gallina AM (1991) Clinical and pathologic features of endometrial hyperplasia, pyometra, and endometritis in cats: 79 cases (1980-1985). *Journal of the American Veterinary Medical Association* **198**, 1427-1431

Remedios AM and Fowler JD (1992) Colonic stricture after ovariohysterectomy in two cats. *Canadian Veterinary Journal* **33**, 334-336

Romagnoli SE (1991) Canine cryptorchidism. *Veterinary Clinics of North America: Small Animal Practice* **21**, 533-544

Schneider R, Dorn CR and Taylor DON (1969) Factors influencing canine mammary cancer development and postsurgical survival. *Journal of the National Cancer Institute* **43**, 1249-1261

Sevelius E, Tidholm A and Thoren TK (1990) Pyometra in the dog. *Journal of the American Animal Hospital Association* **26**, 33-38

Sommer MM and Meyers-Wallen VN (1991) True hermaphroditism in a dog. *Journal of the American Veterinary Medical Association* **198**, 435-438

Wallace M (1991) The ovarian remnant syndrome in the bitch and queen. *Veterinary Clinics of North America: Small Animal Practice* **21**, 501-507

Wright PJ (1991) Practical aspects of the estimation of the time of ovulation and of insemination in the bitch. *Australian Veterinary Journal* **68**, 10-13

Wright PJ and Parry BW (1989) Cytology of the canine reproductive system. *Veterinary Clinics of North America, Small Animal Practice* **19**, 851-874

Reference Values

The reference values in the following tables have been taken from the BSAVA *Small Animal Formulary, 2nd edition* (1997; edited by Bryn Tennant). These values reflect those commonly used by small animal veterinary surgeons and have largely been used throughout this Manual. Where authors have preferred to use alternative reference values the appropriate sources have been given in the text.

It should always be remembered that any table of reference values of this kind is for guidance only. Whenever a sample is sent to a laboratory for analysis, the laboratory should be asked to provide a reference value for the specific laboratory, the specific test and the specific patient type so that interpretation of the results can be done fairly.

Substance	Dog	Cat
Alanine transaminase (ALT) (IU/l)	<100	<75
Albumin (g/l)	22–35	25–39
Alkaline phosphatase (SAP) (IU/l)	<200	<100
Serum alkaline phosphatase levels may be raised in young dogs.		
Ammonia (µmol/l)	0–60	0–60
Amylase (IU/l)	400–2000	400–2000
Anion gap (mEq/l)	5–20	10–30
Aspartate transaminase (IU/l)	7–50	7–60
Base excess (mEq/l)	+6 to 0	+2 to -5
Bicarbonate (mEq/l)	21–23	15–23
Bile acids (fasting) (µmol/l)	0–15	0–15
Bilirubin (µmol/l)	0–6.8	0–6.8
Bilirubin direct (µmol/l)	0–0.4	0–0.2
Calcium (mmol/l)	2.2–2.9	2.1–2.9
Carbon dioxide total (TCO_2) (mmol/l)	17–27	13–25
Chloride (mmol/l)	105–122	112–129
Cholesterol (mmol/l)	2.7–9.5	1.5–6.0
Cobalamin (B12) ng/ml	225–661	200–1680
Creatinine (µmol/l)	20–110	40–150
Creatine kinase (CK) (IU/l)	0–500	0–600
Folate (mg/ml)	6.7–17.4	13.4–38
Fructosamine (mmol/l)	3.5–5	3–5
Gamma glutamyltranspeptidase (GGT) (IU/l)	0–8	0–8
Globulin (g/l)	22–45	26–50
Glucose (mmol/l)	3.5–5.5	3.5–6.5
Lactate (mmol/l)	0.44–2.22	
Lipase (IU/l)	0–500	0–700
Magnesium (mmol/l)	0.7–1.19	0.82–1.23
Osmolality (mOsmol/kg)	289–313	299–327
pH	7.31–7.53	7.32–7.44
pO_2 (mm Hg) Arterial	85–95	101–112
Venous	35–40	35–40
pCO_2 (mm Hg) Arterial	33–39	28–34
Venous	35–38	32–50
Phosphate (mmol/l)	0.5–2.6	1.1–2.8
Potassium (mmol/l)	3.8–5.8	3.6–5.8
Sodium (mmol/l)	140–158	145–165
Trypsin-like immunoreactivity (ng/ml)	>5	>5
Total protein (g/l)	50–78	60–82
Urea (mmol/l)	3–9	5–10

***Table Appendix 1.1:** Clinical biochemistry.*

HAEMATOLOGY		
Value	**Dog**	**Cat**
PCV (l/l)	0.35–0.55	0.26–0.46
Hb (g/l)	120–180	80–150
RBC (x 10^{12}/l)	5.4–8	5–11
MCV (fl)	65–75	37–49
MCH (pg)	22–25	12–17
MCHC (g/l)	340–370	320–350
Reticulocytes (%)	0–1	0–1
Reticulocytes (x 10^9/l)	20-80	20-60
RBC life (days)	100–120	66–78
ESR (mm/h)	0–2	0–10
M:E ratio	0.75–2.5:1	0.6–3.9:1
Platelets (x 10^9/l)	150–400	150–400
WBC (x 10^9/l)	6–18	5.5–19.5
Neutrophils: bands	0–0.3	0–0.3
Neutrophils: mature	3–12	2.5–12.5
Lymphocytes	0.8–3.8	1.5–7
In young dogs up to 6 months old lymphocyte numbers		
may be increased by as much as 50%.		
Monocytes	0.1–1.8	0–0.85
Eosinophils	0.1–1.9	0.1–1.5
Basophils	0–0.2	0–0.2
MCV (fl) = (PCV x 1000) ÷ RBC.		
MCHC (g/l) = (Hb concentration) ÷ PCV		
HAEMOSTASIS		
Value	**Dog**	**Cat**
One stage prothrombin time (OSPT) (seconds)	7–12	7–12
Activated partial thromboplastin time (APTT) (seconds)	12–15	12–22
Bleeding time (ear) (min)	1–2	1–5
Whole blood coagulation time		
Glass (min)	6–7.5	8
Silicone (min)	2–15	
Capillary tube (min)	3–4	5–5.4
Activated coagulation time (seconds)	60–129	
Fibrinogen (g/l)	2–4.5	1–4
Fibrin degradation products (µg/ml)	<10	<10

Table Appendix 1.2: Haematology and haemostasis.

Value	**Dog**	**Cat**
Specific gravity	1.001–1.070	1.001–1.080
pH	5.5–7.5	5.5–7.5
Volume (ml/kg/day)	24–41	22–30
Osmolality (mOsmol/kg)	500–1200	
	50 min–2500 max	50 min– 3000 max
Sediment: leucocytes (/HPF)	0–5	0–5
erythrocytes (/HPF)	0–5	0–5
casts (/HPF)	0	0
Bilirubin	0-trace	0
Calcium (mmol/l)	1–5	
Chloride (mmol/l)	0–400	
Creatinine (mmol/l)	9–26	10–25
Creatinine clearance (ml/min/kg)	2.8–3.7	2–3
Fractional clearances		
Sodium (%)	0–0.7	0.24–0.96
Chloride (%)	0–0.8	0.41–1.33
Potassium (%)	0–20	6.7–23.9
Calcium (%)	0–0.4	
Phosphorus (%)	3–39	17–73
Glucose/Ketones	0	0
Magnesium (mg/kg/24h)	1.7–3	3
Phosphate (mmol/l)	17–60	
Potassium (mmol/l)	20–120	
Protein (g/l)	0–0.3	0–0.2
Protein semiquantitative	0–trace/1+	0–trace/1+
Protein:creatinine ratio– Normal	<0.2	<0.6
Questionable	0.2–1.0	0.6–1.0
Abnormal	>1.0	>1.0
Sodium (mmol/l)	20–165	
Urea (mmol/l)	23–384	62–312

Table Appendix 1.3: Urinalysis.

Monitoring Laboratory Performance

INTRODUCTION

A laboratory, as with any organization that offers a service or has an end-product, must have in place measures that control, monitor, record and verify its procedures. It must be in a position whereby it can prove to itself and to its customers that the results obtained are accurate, consistent and reliable. Schemes whereby the quality of output can be measured and demonstrated will greatly reduce the probability that the accuracy of the results and their interpretation will be questioned. There are several ways in which this can be achieved.

IN-HOUSE MONITORING

Every laboratory should have in place systems controlling the various aspects of laboratory practice.

Identification of specimens
A unique number should be assigned to every specimen upon receipt. Documentation of specimen details should be thorough and the identification number should follow the sample through every stage of its processing in the laboratory. Several excellent computer software packages are available for this purpose; barcode labels are often useful for sample labeling.

Equipment
Items of equipment need to be maintained regularly to ensure continuing reliability. Accurate maintenance records should be kept and suitably qualified engineers used when appropriate. Easy-to-read temperature monitors should be fitted to incubators, refrigerators and freezers. Freezers should have alarms fitted so that breakdowns can be signalled.

Particular care must be taken with the plethora of kits available nowadays ('near-patient testing'). It is essential that theses are calibrated and monitored by qualified staff and the results obtained thoroughly scrutinized.

Methodologies
All techniques used in the laboratory must be standardized and recorded and available to personnel in the laboratory for 'bench use'. These may be updated in the light of new technology and other modifications. Methodology manuals should be kept and updated.

Reagents
Reagents, chemicals, stocks solutions and test kits must be labelled clearly to indicate the date they were purchased or made up and the expiry date (if appropriate). Hazard warnings should be carried where appropriate.

Staff
Of all the in-house procedures adopted to achieve and maintain quality in the laboratory, the use of properly trained and qualified staff is arguably the most important. The correct mix of skill levels ensures that all the other measures detailed above will be carried out in the most efficient and cost-effective manner. Technical staff training should be pre-planned and documented, and a training log kept by each trainee. The training programmes and log books produced by The Council for Professions Supplementary to Medicine (CPSM) in conjunction with the Institute of Biomedical Sciences (IBMS), although designed for human laboratory medicine, are particularly thorough and are easily adapted for veterinary laboratories. Since the technologies used and the expertise required are virtually identical, it is worth considering that staff employed in veterinary laboratories should be trained and qualified to the same degree as those working in human hospital laboratories.

EXTERNAL QUALITY ASSESSMENT

The procedures and methods of control discussed above are regarded as 'good laboratory practice' and should be adopted for daily working. However, this is only part of the process necessary to ensure the quality of service. External Quality Assessment (EQA) is a means whereby the quality of the output of a laboratory is measured by an external body and can be compared to other laboratories.

Individual schemes work slightly differently but they usually operate by supplying samples to the participating laboratory for analysis and subsequent assessment of the results. Confidentiality is guaranteed by the use of a laboratory identification number known only to the organizer and the participating laboratory. The schemes currently available cover most aspects of laboratory medicine and more are being added. Because these schemes are organized by independent bodies, the credibility given to laboratories who are members of appropriate schemes is high. Indeed, one of the criteria for laboratories being accredited in human medicine is membership of EQA schemes and there is every reason to believe that veterinary laboratories will follow suit. Most schemes have an educational element to them, which is essential if the quality of laboratory output is not only to be maintained but to be improved or if a laboratory is conversely underperforming.

Several schemes are currently available in the UK (addresses at foot of page):

- UK National External Quality Assessment Schemes (UK NEQAS) (designed for human medicine but will accept veterinary laboratories): for serology, drugs assays, general clinical chemistry, haematology, histopathology, hormone assays, microbiology, immunocytochemistry
- MAFF Veterinary QA Schemes: for clinical chemistry, bacteriology, haematology
- Technical External Quality Assessment in Veterinary Pathology (TEQA VP) (designed specifically for veterinary pathology laboratories: for histopathology
- Randox Laboratories (for both medical and veterinary laboratories): for clinical chemistry

TERMINOLOGY

The terms used for describing the quality of function of laboraties are varied and may sometimes be incorrectly; they are not interchangeable. The most commonly used terms are:

- Good laboratory practice (GLP): A managerial concept covering the organizational practices and conditions under which laboratory studies are planned, performed, monitored and reported
- Quality assurance: A formal arrangement for assuring that facilities, equipment, personnel, methods, procedures and documentation conform to agreed standards
- Quality assessment: A system of comparing results from different laboratories by means of an external agency so that performance can be monitored and maintained
- Quality control: A set of procedures within a laboratory which provides for the continual check of the accuracy of tests performed
- Standard operating procedure: Standardized documentation that details a laboratory's activities to ensure accuracy and quality of results; it should cover reagents, equipment and methods

UK NEQAS, Wolfson EQA Laboratory, PO Box 3909, Birmingham B15 3UE
MAFF Veterinary Laboratory QA unit , College Road, Sutton Bonnigton, Loughborough, LE 12 5RB
TEQA VP, c/o Brian Kelly, Department of Veterinary Pathology, University of Edinburgh, Summerhall, Edinburgh, EH9 1QH
Randox Laboratories, Ardmore, Diamond Road, Crumlin, Country Antrim

Necropsy Technique

INTRODUCTION

Postmortem examination should be regarded as an important and beneficial procedure. It is important in the education of new graduates. Where animals die or are euthanased and the diagnosis is in doubt or unresolved, the experienced clinician will wish to check for evidence of disease in various organs. Although private laboratories and government agencies offer necropsy services, many veterinary surgeons perform their own postmortem examinations. It is therefore important that practitioners are knowledgeable on necropsy technique, even if they perform such examinations infrequently, and particularly if there is a legal requirement for such examination.

EQUIPMENT

The following are required:

- Scissors: large, fine, blunt-ended
- Rat-toothed forceps
- Bone forceps: large, fine
- Stainless steel saw (or Desoutter cast cutter)
- Large knife
- Small scalpel
- Sterile swabs
- Sterile containers for bacteriological samples
- Hypodermic needles (20–21 gauge)
- Syringes: 5 ml, 10 ml
- Microscope slides

A cork board and dissection darts are useful for pinning out the carcasses of rodents, cagebirds and neonates.

Protective clothing should include rubber gloves, rubber boots, a protective boiler suit, and a plastic or rubber apron. On some occasions face masks are needed.

PROCEDURE (PROSECTION) FOR CATS AND DOGS

The aim of a postmortem examination is a thorough investigation of all organs and tissues of the different body systems. A standard sequence of examination should be adopted and all organs should be examined, even when clinical history does not indicate disease affecting them. Clinically significant lesions may be missed in hurried and incomplete examinations, while a careful and complete examination frequently reveals unexpected but significant information.

Before starting, all the information available should be considered, including the clinical findings, radiographic evidence and laboratory results. Care should be taken to ensure that the cadaver should is the correct one.

1. Note age, sex, breed and weight

2. External inspection

- Assess the general state of bodily condition
- Examine the anus, genitalia, limbs, skin and mucous membranes of the mouth, nose, eyes and ears

There may be soiling of the skin associated with discharge from the eyes, ears, mouth, nose, anus, vulva or penis. Pale mucous membranes may indicate shock or anaemia. Jaundice may be seen as yellowing of the mucous membranes and sclera. Reddening or haemorrhages of mucous membranes may be present associated with septicaemia or viraemia. Sunken eyes and dehydrated skin may be due to loss of body fluid or may be seen in death from shock. Tumours of the skin, subcutaneous tissue or mammary glands may be visible or palpable. Joints and bones should be checked for normal movement or configuration. Skin wounds or torn claws may be present in cases of road traffic accidents.

Briefly immersing the cadaver in water, particulary for long-coated breeds, will reduce the spread of hair to viscera during the examination which follows.

Abnormalities should be recorded as accurately as possible, as they are found. Decription of lesions should include: number, location, size, colour, and consistency. Samples for histological or microbiological examination, as appropriate, should be taken from each lesion as it is encountered. All samples may not ultimately be submitted for further examination, but lesions will often prove difficult to relocate at the end of a complete examination.

Interpretation of the findings should wait until the post mortem has been completed and, where appropriate, the result of histological and microbiological examinations are known.

3.   Reflect the limbs

- Lay the animal on its back
- Cut the skin and muscle in the axilla and inguinal regions on each side
- Incise and examine the hip joints

The limbs will then lie flat, away from the body which will remain upright and stable.

4.   Midline skin incision

- Incise the skin in the midline from the mandibular symphysis to the pelvis; on a male take the incision to one side of the penis
- Reflect the skin over the ventral and lateral aspects of the carcasse

There may be signs of dehydration, haemorrhage or oedema. The occurrence of subcutaneous oedema may be associated with accumulation of fluid elsewhere in the carcasse.

5.   Reflect the tongue

- Make incisions parallel to the horizontal rami of the mandible on each side
- Cut the lingual attachments
- Reflect the tongue

6.   Examine the superficial lymph nodes

- Examine the following nodes: popliteal (lying caudal to the stifle joint); superficial inguinal (embedded in subcutaneous fat cranial to the pelvis); prescapular (cranial to the scapula); and submandibular (ventral to the angle of the jaw, cranial to the submandibular salivary glands, often bilobed with a branch of the jugular vein between the lobes).
- Incise the lymph nodes
- Examine the cut surfaces for normal differentiation into cortex and medulla, and for lesions

Lesions may be present in a lymph node which is not obviously enlarged.

7.   Expose the trachea

- Remove the muscle from the ventral aspect of the trachea

- Cut the muscles attached to the medial borders of the horizontal rami of the mandibles
- Pull the tongue out ventrally
- Cut through the articulations of the hyoid bones and the soft palate
- Strip the oesophagus and trachea down to the thoracic inlet

8.   Examine the lymph nodes and tonsils

- Examine the retropharyngeal lymph nodes (caudal to the submandibular salivary glands and dorsal to the larynx and tonsils)

Enlarged tonsils protrude from the crypts.

9.   Reflect the skin and open the abdominal cavity

- Make a small incision through the linea alba
- Check for the presence of free fluid in the abdominal cavity
- Collect free fluid present for cytology and/or bacteriology
- Open the abdomen from the xiphisternum to the pubic symphysis
- Reflect the abdominal wall reflected laterally
- Inspect the abdominal viscera *in situ*
- Note the type and volume of any exudate, the appearance of the parietal and visceral peritoneum, the relationship of the major organs, and the presence of any major vascular anomalies

A few millilitres of clear colourless fluid is normally present; normal peritoneal surfaces are smooth and glistening.

10.   Open the thorax by removing the sternum

- Make a small incision in the diaphragm and note the inrush of air (indicating a normal negative pressure in the pleural cavity)
- Note the amount and type of any abnormal pleural fluid
- Separate the diaphragm from the last rib to allow insertion of rib cutters
- Clear a cutting line through the soft tissues of the thoracic wall
- Cut through the ribs with rib cutters from floating ribs to the thoracic inlet, so that about two-thirds of the ventral ribcage is removed
- Cut through the sternal attachments of the mediastinum
- Observe the thoracic viscera *in situ*
- Note the appearance of pleural surfaces, the presence of any thymus or thymic tumour, the lungs, and heart and major blood vessels
- Clear the connective tissue attachments around the trachea and oesophagus at the thoracic inlet

- Apply gentle traction to separate the thoracic viscera from the dorsal aspect of the thorax

11. Structural relationships

- Examine structure and relationship of major structures and organs of the oral cavity, pharynx, thorax and abdomen

12. Examine the thyroid and parathyroid glands

The thyroid gland on each side lies caudal to the larynx on the lateral aspects of the trachea. Usually, in the dog two small pale parathyroid glands can be identified, one close to and one embedded in each thyroid gland. In the cat it is usual to be able to identify one parathyroid gland at the cranial pole of each thyroid.

13. Locate and examine the adrenal gland

The left adrenal gland lies cranial and slightly medial to the left kidney. The right adrenal gland lies nearer the hilus of the right kidney.

- Incise both adrenal glands longitudinally or dissect out carefully

The pale cortex should conform roughly to the shape of the gland. The central medulla is softer and red/brown in colour. The cortex and medulla should be present in about equal proportions.

14. Removal of organs

- Remove the tongue and thoracic organs together, separating them from the oesophagus
- Lift the heart and lungs out of the thorax
- Cut the mesentery close to its dorsal attachments
- Withdraw the oesophagus, stomach, intestines and liver, together with the omentum, spleen and mesentery
- Transect the rectum cranial to the pelvis or, if appropriate, remove the bones of the pelvic floor
- Leave the kidneys and ureters (and ovaries and uterus in entire female animals) *in situ*

15. Examine the alimentary system

Upper alimentary tract

- Inspect the teeth, gums, oropharyngeal mucosa and salivary glands
- Examine the tongue and oesophagus
- Incise the oesophagus along its length and examine the mucosal surface

Gastrointestinal tract

- Examine the structure and relationship of the excised organs

- Cut the omentum and mesentery along their serosal margins and examine the mesenteric lymph nodes
- Incise the stomach along the greater curvature
- Incise the intestines along their length
- Examine serosal and mucosal surfaces
- For bacteriological examination, take swabs or excise a tied-off piece of bowel (8–10 cm long) and place in a sterile container
- Apply gentle pressure to the gall bladder; bile will enter the duodenum from the common bile duct, if the latter is patent
- Remove the oesophagus, stomach and intestines from the other viscera

16. Examine the pancreas

- Examine the pancreas for size, shape, colour and any abnormal features

17. Examine the hepatobiliary system

Bile duct patency can be checked by gentle manual pressure on the gall bladder; this should be done before the liver and duodenum are separated from one another.

- Examine the surface of the liver and the gall bladder
- Make several cuts into all liver lobes
- Incise the gall bladder

Cystic hyperplasia of the gall bladder mucosa is a common incidental senile change in dogs. The gall bladder may be distended in animals which have not eaten recently.

18. Examine the spleen

- Remove the spleen from its omental attachments
- Incise

The spleen may be diffusely or irregularly enlarged.

19. Examine the respiratory tract

- Examine the larynx, trachea and mediastinum
- Palpate and inspect both lungs
- Open the larynx
- Cut down the trachea and major bronchi
- Examine the cut surfaces of the lungs

Multiple transverse gross sections can be helpful.

20. Examine the heart and pericardium

- Examine the pericardial sac
- Cut through the pericardium and collect any excess fluid
- Expose the heart
- Examine the heart for enlargement or abnormality of shape

Enlargement of the right side makes the heart bigger and rounded. An enlargement of the left side makes the heart bigger and longer. The muscle wall of the right ventricle is normally much thinner than that of the left. Enlargement may be a result of dilation of the chamber and/or hypertrophy of the muscle wall. The significance and interpretation of such changes is determined by clinical history and other postmortem findings.

- Dissect the heart by first opening the right side
- Cut down the pulmonary artery, through the pulmonary valve to the apex of the right ventricle
- Cut up the cranial wall of the right ventricle to exit through the tricuspid valve, right atrium and common vena cava, in that order
- Identify the junction of the pulmonary vein with the left atrium
- Observe the mitral valve onfice from this entry point and check for valve or chordal abnormalities (e.g.rupture)
- *Then,* cut open the left ventricle by incising through the mitral valve onfice and lateral ventricular wall
- Finally, expose the aortic valve and aortic root by cutting up the aortic outflow tract to the lateral aspect of the main mitral valve cusp

21. Examine the blood vessels

- Study the position and size of blood vessels
- Examine the luminal surfaces

22. Examine the urinary system

- Examine the kidneys, ureters, bladder (and prostate in the male dog) *in situ*
- Apply gentle pressure to the bladder and check for patency of the urethra

The entire urinary tract may be removed for dissection, or each part excised and examined separately.

- Incise the kidneys longitudinally and strip off the capsule carefully
- Inspect the capsular surface and the cut surface and check that the cortex and medulla are present in a uniform, correct proportion (cortex:medulla 2:1)
- Examine the renal pelvis

The kidneys of the dog and cat differ markedly in shape and colour. The kidney of the cat is pale with prominent surface blood vessels; the capsule strips very readily. The kidney of the dog is bean-shaped and usually dark red; the capsule may be removed easily but occasional fine fibrous strands penetrate the cortical tissue. In neonatal animals the cortex is normally narrow.

- Check for patency and uniformity of ureters
- Check that the ureteral entry points to the bladder are normal
- Examine the serosal and mucosal surfaces of the incised bladder

The ureters may be distended by urine or pus in association with hydronephrosis or pyelonephritis. Anomalous development of the ureters may occur.

23. Examine the genital system

Male
A small amount of discharge from the preputial orifice is normal in dogs. The prostate should be examined at the same time as the bladder and urethra. Differentiation between hyperplasia, infection and neoplasia depends particularly on size, shape and structure. In castrated dogs the prostate is small.

- Incise the scrotum and expose the testes
- Section each testis and epididymis

Normal testicular tissue is fawn coloured, fleshy and bulges on cutting.

Female
- Examine the ovaries and uterus *in situ.*

The ovaries and uterus can be removed by cutting at the cervix, and the vagina may not need to be examined routinely.

24. Examine the musculoskeletal system

Joints
The hip joints are incised at an early stage in postmortem examination. They are the site of specific diseases which are well recognized in different ages and breeds of dog. Other synovial joints are examined when indicated.

- Note the amount and character of synovial fluid, the appearance of synovial membranes and the conformation and appearance of articular surfaces

Examination of the intervertebral disc joints requires opening of the spinal canal. This procedure is best performed after removal of the spinal cord (see below)

Bones
Softness of ribs may be noted when they are cut to expose the bone marrow. In adult animals the marrow is pale pink, fatty and floats in fixative. The hypercellular marrow is more solid, red/pink in colour and sinks in fixative.

Muscle

Atrophy of muscle will occur in any wasting disease and develops locally if nerve supply is damaged.

- Examine the craniomandibular muscles of dogs with a clinical history of dysphagia.

25. Examine the nervous system

The brachial plexus is exposed early on when the axilla is incised. Other nerves may be examined if indicated. Examination of the brain and spinal cord should not be neglected if disease affecting those parts is suspected. In many cases, a grossly evident lesion, e.g. hydrocephalus, a disc protrusion or a tumour mass will be readily seen. In other cases, e.g. encephalitis, no macroscopic lesion may be apparent but marked histological lesions are present.

The brain and spinal cord may be exposed together or the head may be removed by disarticulation of the atlanto-occipital joint.

- Reflect the skin and muscle from the dorsal spinous process of the vertebrae
- Cut through and remove the dorsal parts of the vertebral arches to expose the spinal cord
- Using bone forceps or a saw, cut through the sinus of the frontal bone into the anterior border of the cranial cavity
- Continue the incision on each side along the lateral aspects of the skull to the foramen magnum
- Prise up the roof of the cranium and remove it
- Ensure that the leaf-like projections of the parietal bone between the cerebrum and cerebellum are removed
- Incise the spinal cord caudal to the foramen magnum, so that some brainstem is left attached to the brain

Spinal cord

Ideally the spinal cord, or the portion of it containing a potential lesion, should be fixed *in situ* for 12–14 hours. It may then be removed more easily, without being damaged.

- Remove the spinal cord by grasping the dura at one end and lifting gently to expose the spinal nerves
- Cut the spinal nerves
- Avoid pulling the cord
- Examine the dura and cord for areas of compression, haemorrhage, necrosis, or tumour growth
- Examine the ventral surface of the spinal canal for evidence of protrusion of intervertebral discs
- Cut through and examine one or more discs for evidence of degenerative change.

Brain

The brain may be fixed *in situ* or after removal. Unless samples for microbiology etc. are required, examination of the fixed brain is easier and more rewarding.

- Remove the dura if it remains attached
- Turn the head upside down and cut through cranial nerves and olfactory bulbs
- Allow the brain to fall gently out of the cavity
- Examine the floor of the cranium, the pituitary gland and pituitary fossa

External inspection of the brain (preferably after fixation) will frequently reveal no specific changes. However, tumours or cerebellar hypoplasis, for example, may be visible. Swelling of the brain may cause protrusion of the caudal cerebellum through the foramen magnum. This is evident as a cone-shaped compression.

Examination of the internal structure of the brain is best delayed until it has been fixed for at least 96 hours.

- Section the brain transversely at regular 0.5–1.0 cm intervals
- Examine the ventricles and the white and grey matter

A useful indicator of brain abnormality is the loss of symmetry in the brain, although it is important to ensure the accuracy of gross sectioning in this respect.

26. Examination of ears, eyes and nasal cavity

Ears
- Open the vertical canal
- Examine the external ear canal
- Carefully remove the tympanic bulla with bone forceps to expose the middle ear

Eyes
- Grasp the closed eyelids with forceps
- Incise the lid margins
- Apply gentle traction and cut through the soft tissues surrounding the globe
- Cut the optic nerve

Any soft tissue attached to the eye should be removed before it is fixed. Eyes should be fixed for 24 hours in formalin prior to any gross sectioning.

Nasal cavity
- Divide the skull longitudinally along the middle
- Examine the nasl cavities

The frontal sinuses are also exposed.

Index

Page numbers in italics refer to figures; page numbers in bold refer to tables.

Index **365**

faeces, **100**, 145
Campylobacter jejuni, 106
Candida spp., 107
Canine adenovirus-1, 95
Canine demodicosis, 248, **249**
Canine distemper virus, 94-5
   and renal disease, **307**
Canine enteric viruses, 95
Canine herpesvirus, 95
Canine hypertrophic osteodystrophy, **214**
Canine masticatory myositis, 213
Canine otodectic mange, **249**
Canine parvovirus, *94*
Canine respiratory viruses, 95
Canine sarcoptic mange, **249**
Capillaria aerophila, eggs, *147*
Capillaria plica, **304**
Carbohydrate metabolism, 77-9
   fructosamine, 79
   glucose, 77, *78, 79*
Carbon dioxide, total, **323**
Cardiovascular system *see* Respiratory tract and cardiovascular system
Cat fur mite, **249**
Cerebrospinal fluid, 126
   examination, 236-8
      complications of collection, 236-7
      effects of blood contamination, 238
      indications and contraindications, 236
      interpretation of results, 238
      sample analysis, 237-8
      sample handling, *237*
      sampling procedure, *236*
   leptospirosis, **329**
Cervix, 344-5
Chalazion, 242-3
Chemical profiles, **83**-4
Chemicals, *23, 24-5*
Cheyletiella spp., 247, *251*
Cheyletiella blakei, **249**
Cheyletiella yagsuri, **249**
Cheyletiellosis, **249**, *251*
Chlamydia spp., 107
Chlamydia psittaci, 107
   conjunctivitis, keratitis, 242
   ELISA assay, 9
Chloride, 73
   drugs affecting estimation, **298**
   leptospirosis, **329**
   plasma, **311**, 315
Cholangiohepatitis, 185
Cholesterol, 79, *80*
   liver disease, 167
Chondrodysplasia, **214**
Chronic hepatitis, 184
Cirrhosis, 184
Clinical biochemistry, 61-85
   carbohydrate metabolism, 77-9
      fructosamine, 79
      glucose, 77, *78, 79*
   chemical profiles and test selection, **83**-4
   copper, 82-3
   coughing, 192
   electrolytes, 71-6
      calcium, 74, *75*
      chloride, 73
      inorganic phosphorus, *76*
      magnesium, 73-4
      potassium, *72, 73*
      sodium, *71, 72*

indicators of renal function, 64-5
   creatinine, 64-5
   urea nitrogen, *64*
infective endocarditis, 200
iron, 81, *82*
lead, 82
lipid metabolism, 79-81
   cholesterol, 79, *80*
   triglycerides, 80-1
markers of hepatic disease, 65-9
   alanine aminotransferase, 65, *66*
   alkaline phosphatase, 66
   ammonia, 69
   aspartate aminotransferase, 66
   bile acids, 68-9
   bilirubin, 67, *68*
   gamma-glutamyl transferase, 67, *68*
muscle enzymes, 77
pancreatic disease, 69-71
   amylase, 69-70
   lipase, 70-1
pleural effusions, 197
serum proteins, 62-3
   globulins, *64*
   total protein and albumin, *62-3*
sneezing and nasal discharge, 188
zinc, 82
Clostridium spp., **255**
   faeces, 145
   muscle infection, *207*
Clostridium botulinium, 103-4
Clostridium difficile, 103
   faeces, **100**
Clostridium perfringens, 103
   faeces, **100**, 145-6
Clostridium tetani, 103
Clot retraction, 54
Coagulation time
   coughing, 192
   liver disease, 164, 176-7
   pleural effusions, 195
   sneezing and nasal discharge, 188
Cobalamin, **154**
Coccidioides immitis, 192
Colonoscopy, 160
Combing, *251*
Complement
   concentration, 117
   function testing, 117
Congenital portosystemic shunts, 184-5
Congestive cardiac failure, *198*-9
Conjunctival melanoma, 243, *244*
Conjunctivitis, 241-2
   culture, 241-2
   cytology, 242
   follicular, *244*
   serology, 242
   surgical biopsy, 242
Containers, 20, *21*
Control of Substances Hazardous to Health regulations, *23, 24-5*
Coombs' test, 46, 110-11, *112*
   infective endocarditis, 200
Copper, 82-3
Corticotrophin releasing hormone, **272**
Cortisol, basal levels, 278
Coughing, 189-93
   bronchoalveolar lavage, 191
   clinical biochemistry, 192
   diagnosis, 189
   FeLV and FIV, 192

bilirubin, 67, *68*
gamma-glutamyl transferase, 67
Hepatic necrosis, 184
Hepatitis, 184
  acute, 184
  cholangiohepatitis, 185
  chronic, 184
  copper-associated, 82-3
Hepatobiliary system, *161*-86
  clinicopathological changes, 163-4
      consequences of hepatobiliary dysfunction, *163*
      correlation with clinical signs, *163*, *164*
    diagnostic approach, 164, *165*
    enzyme markers of liver disease, 168-74
      alanine aminotransferase, 169, *170*, *171*
      alkaline phosphatase, *172*, 173-4
      arginase, 172
      aspartate aminotransferase, 171-2
      glutamate dehydrogenase, 172
      lactate dehydrogenase, 172
      ornithine carbamoyltransferase, 172
      sorbitol dehydrogenase, 172
    general screening tests, 165-8
      routine haematology, 165, *166*
      serum biochemistry, 167, **168**
      urinalysis, *166*, *167*
    liver biopsy, 181-3
      cytology, *182*-3
      indications and techniques, *181*, *182*
    liver function tests, 174-81
      ascites, **175**, 176
      bilirubin, **176**, 177-8
      bromosulphthalein retention test, 178
      coagulation times, 176-7
      indocyanine green retention test, 178
      interpretation of, 183, **184**, *185*-6
      P-450 cytochrome oxidase activity, 179
      plasma ammonia and ammonia tolerance test, 178, *179*
      serum bile acids, 179, *180*-1
      serum proteins and albumin, *174*
    normal hepatobiliary function, **162**, *163*
    prognostic indices, *183*
Hepatoencephalopathy, 164
Hepatotoxic drugs, *185*, 186
Hereditary canine myopathy, **205**
Hermaphroditism, 343
Herpesvirus, and renal disease, **307**
Heterodoxus spiniger, **249**
Hickey–Hare test, 321
High-dose dexamethasone suppression test, 280
Histoplasma capsulatum, 192
Howell–Jolly bodies, 40
Humoral hypercalcaemia of malignancy, 217-18
Hydronephrosis, **291**
Hyperadrenocorticism, 67, 213, 215, *279*
Hyperammonaemia, 163
Hyperbilirubinaemia *see* Jaundice
Hypercalcaemia, 75-6, 316
  of malignancy, 217-18
Hyperchloraemia, 73
Hypercholesterolaemia, 67, *80*
Hyperglobulinaemia, *63*, *152*
Hyperglycaemia, 79
Hyperkalaemia, 72, *73*
Hypermagnesaemia, 74
Hypernatraemia, 72, *73*
Hyperphosphataemia, 76, 316-17
Hypersensitivity testing, 115, *116*
Hyperthyroidism, 265, *269*
Hypertriglyceridaemia, *81*

Hypertrophic osteodystrophy, **214**
Hypertrophic pulmonary osteoarthropathy, **214**
Hypervitaminosis A, **214**
Hypoadrenocorticism, 278
Hypoalbuminaemia, *62*-3, *75*
Hypocalcaemia, *75*, 316
Hypochloraemia, 73
Hypocholesterolaemia, *80*
Hypoglobulinaemia, 63
Hypoglycaemia, 78-9
Hypokalaemia, 72
Hypomagnesaemia, 74
Hyponatraemia, *71*
Hypoparathyroidism, 75
Hypophosphataemia, 76, 317
Hypoproteinaemia, *152*, **318**
Hypothalamus, *263*
Hypothyroidism, 114-15, *154*, 264-5, *268*
Hypotriglyceridaemia, 81

Icterus *see* Jaundice
Idiopathic thrombocytopenic purpura, 110
Immune-mediated arthritis, 113, *114*
Immune-mediated arthropathy, *223*
Immune-mediated diseases, 109-20
  arthritis, 113, *114*
  haemolytic anaemia *see* Immune-mediated haemolytic anaemia
  hypothyroidism, 114-15
  laboratory tests for hypersensitivity, 115, *116*
  laboratory tests for immunodeficiency, 116-18
    complement concentration and function testing, 117
    lymphocyte function testing, 118
    lymphocyte phenotyping, 118
    neutrophil and macrophage function testing, 117-18
    serum immunoglobulin concentration, 116, *117*
  laboratory tests for lymphoid neoplasia, 118, *119*
  skin, kidney and joint diseases, *115*
  systemic lupus erythematosus, *113*
  thrombocytopenia, 112
  tissue and blood typing, **119**
Immune-mediated haemolytic anaemia, 45-6, 110-12
  Coombs' test, 110, *111*, *112*
Immune-mediated thrombocytopenia, 112
Immunocytochemistry, 88-9
Immunodeficiency testing, 116-18
  complement concentration and function testing, 117
  lymphocyte function testing, 118
  lymphocyte phenotyping, 118
  neutrophil and macrophage function testing, 117-18
  serum immunoglobulin concentration, 116, *117*
Immunodiagnostic assays, 88-9
  ELISA, 89
  immunofluorescence and immunocytochemistry, *88*-9
  rapid immunomigration tests, 89
Immunofluorescence, 88-9
Immunoglobulins, serum concentration, 116, *117*
Impression smears, 124-5
Incisional biopsy, 11-12, **14**
  kidney, 309
  lymph nodes, 230
Indocyanine green retention test, 178
Infective endocarditis, 199, *200*
Inflammation, interpretation of, 129, *130*, *131*
Inorganic phosphorus, 76
Insulin-like growth factor 1, 275
Insulinoma, *283*
Interface dermatitis, **258**
Interference, 28
Intestinal permeability, 157-9